The Clinical Practice of Pediatric Physical Therapy

From the NICU to Independent Living

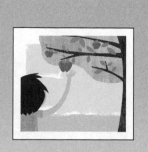

The Clinical Practice of Pediatric Physical Therapy

From the NICU to Independent Living

Mark Drnach, PT, DPT, MBA, PCS

Department of Physical Therapy
Wheeling Jesuit University
Wheeling, West Virginia

Wolters Kluwer Health | Lippincott Williams & Wilkins

Health

Philadelphia · Baltimore · New York · London
Buenos Aires · Hong Kong · Sydney · Tokyo

Acquisitions Editor: Peter Sabatini
Managing Editor: Andrea M. Klingler
Marketing Manager: Allison M. Noplock
Associate Production Manager: Kevin P. Johnson
Designer: Stephen Druding
Compositor: Aptara, Inc.

9 8 7 6 5 4 3 2 1

Library of Congress Cataloging-in-Publication Data

Drnach, Mark.
 The clinical practice of pediatric physical therapy : from the NICU to
independent living / Mark Drnach.
     p. ; cm.
  Includes bibliographical references and index.
  ISBN-13: 978-0-7817-9063-5 (alk. paper)
  ISBN-10: 0-7817-9063-8 (alk. paper)
 1. Physical therapy for children.   2. Children with disabilities—
Rehabilitation.   I. Title.
  [DNLM: 1. Disabled Children—rehabilitation.   2. Adolescent.   3. Child.
4. Continuity of Patient Care.   5. Infant.   6. Long-Term Care.   7. Physical
Therapy Modalities.   WS 368 D782c 2008]
  RJ53.P5D73 2008
  615.8'20832--dc22

                                        2007031803

DISCLAIMER

Care has been taken to confirm the accuracy of the information present and to describe generally accepted practices. However, the authors, editors, and publisher are not responsible for errors or omissions or for any consequences from application of the information in this book and make no warranty, expressed or implied, with respect to the currency, completeness, or accuracy of the contents of the publication. Application of this information in a particular situation remains the professional responsibility of the practitioner; the clinical treatments described and recommended may not be considered absolute and universal recommendations.

The authors, editors, and publisher have exerted every effort to ensure that drug selection and dosage set forth in this text are in accordance with the current recommendations and practice at the time of publication. However, in view of ongoing research, changes in government regulations, and the constant flow of information relating to drug therapy and drug reactions, the reader is urged to check the package insert for each drug for any change in indications and dosage and for added warnings and precautions. This is particularly important when the recommended agent is a new or infrequently employed drug.

Some drugs and medical devices presented in this publication have Food and Drug Administration (FDA) clearance for limited use in restricted research settings. It is the responsibility of the health care provider to ascertain the FDA status of each drug or device planned for use in their clinical practice.

To purchase additional copies of this book, call our customer service department at **(800) 638-3030** or fax orders to **(301) 223-2320**. International customers should call **(301) 223-2300**.

Visit Lippincott Williams & Wilkins on the Internet: http://www.lww.com. Lippincott Williams & Wilkins customer service representatives are available from 8:30 am to 6:00 pm, EST.

This book is dedicated to the child in front of you.
The one you think about when you read through these pages.

Ad Majorem Dei Gloriam

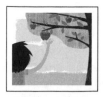

PREFACE

The doctoring profession of physical therapy incorporates the attributes of professionalism, education, evidence-based practice, direct access to services by the consumer, and the concept of the practitioner of choice.[1] It is reflective of the way physical therapists provide services as autonomous clinicians, chosen by families to provide services to their children. The need for a physical therapist to demonstrate these attributes of a doctoring profession is growing ever more necessary as the services to children and people with disabilities in our society evolve. As the clinician of choice, the physical therapist may be called upon to provide effective services to a child to promote healing, wellness, or optimal functioning throughout the child's life and in a variety of practice settings. These settings can range from the hospital to schools and from early intervention to home-based programs.

The United States Congress, in its reauthorization of the Individuals with Disabilities Education Act (IDEA), stated, "disability is a natural part of the human experience and in no way diminishes the right of individuals to participate in or contribute to society. Improving educational results for children with disabilities is an essential element of our national policy of ensuring equality of opportunity, full participation, independent living, and economic self-sufficiency for individuals with disabilities."[2] Physical therapists are in the unique position of being able to influence a child and his family and to promote the health and participation of all children toward attaining independence and self-sufficiency.

The purpose of this book is to provide a comprehensive guideline to the clinical application of the practice of pediatric physical therapy throughout the continuum of care that families of children with disabilities often encounter. The neonatal intensive care unit (NICU), special education programs, and the services and options available after the child reaches the age of 21 years are some of the topics covered within *The Clinical Practice of Pediatric Physical Therapy: From the NICU to Independent Living*. Each of the practice environments presented has a unique structure and purpose that has been established to provide services for a specific need to a child and his or her family. Physical therapy is often identified as a primary or related service to help meet some of those identified needs. This book intends to provide the student of physical therapy or the practicing clinician with a better understanding of his or her role in these practice environments and to identify some of the key influences of patient/client management for children in various settings. A unique aspect of pediatric patient/client management is the influence of the parent or guardian, who has the sole responsibility for making decisions for the child. In many pediatric settings, such as early intervention or hospice, the federal government also influences the purpose and utilization of physical therapy services. The physical therapist must have a working knowledge of the many factors that influence service provision from the perspective of the child, the parent, the program, and the larger practice environment.

As the clinician of choice for the child, the physical therapist may find herself providing services throughout a continuum of care, not solely through one program or agency. She will be the child's physical therapist in whichever setting the child is in and any role he is currently fulfilling. This book presents information intended to reinforce and aid in that vision.

ORGANIZATION

Part I, Foundational Issues, includes three foundational chapters that provide information that will aid in the understanding of the process of the child's development and his role in life, together with the identification of factors that may impair his ability to fulfill that role. This information will aid in the selection and utilization of physical therapy services to optimize a child's abilities within the environment in which he is functioning. Hopefully by doing so we, as practicing clinicians, will broaden our scope of intervention from a narrow treatment approach, with its emphasis on a cure, and embrace a larger view that includes an equally important enablement approach with an emphasis on the acceptance of each child's ability and participation in his family and society.

Chapter 1 presents a history of physical therapy, with an emphasis on the influence that children and individuals with disabilities have had on the early establishment and growth of the profession. It also presents information on disablement and the role of physical therapy in the process of enablement, highlighting the importance of patient/client management and the use of current literature in clinical decision making with an emphasis on function and participation. Chapter 2 presents an overview of child development, highlighting important skills and behaviors seen in the growth and maturation of the child from birth to maturity. The developmental information touches on the classical domains of child development and provides a broad picture of the growing child. Chapter 3 provides a list of pathology-based diagnoses commonly seen in children and the possible impairments and functional limitations that are associated with that particular pathology. Implications for the physical therapist are highlighted as a quick reference.

Part II, Practice Environment, includes Chapters 4 through 10 and provides information on the provision of physical therapy services through various settings and programs. The information presented in these chapters follow a similar sequence to allow the reader to see the similarities and differences in the patient/client management process across settings. The chapters are presented in a developmental order to provide the reader with the understanding of the variety of services through which a child may transition on his way to adulthood. This is done to emphasize the importance of the role of the physical therapist in enabling the child to develop into an adult who will have equality of opportunity, live as independently as possible, and achieve an optimal level of economic self-sufficiency. Understanding these programs and the laws that fostered their creation and influence their structure allows the physical therapist to better understand and to participate more fully in them.

Part III, Selected Topics, contains Chapters 11 through 14, which discuss selected topics relevant to the practice of physical therapy with children that a new clinician may find helpful. Back care and exercise, the basics of pharmacology, common legal issues that pertain to children, and common financial concepts in health care are topics that aid in the delivery of services to children and their families and are relevant to all the practice settings.

FEATURES

Each chapter begins with *Learning Objectives,* which are intended to assist the reader with the study of this information. *Points to Remember* are included throughout the chapters to aid in learning the information and to emphasize the key issues that are addressed. *Parent Perspectives* provide real-world scenarios from a parent's point of view, providing the reader with another aspect of the factors that influence the environment and clinical decisions made in the care of a child. *Case Studies* are included to show the clinical application of the information. Each chapter ends with a *Summary* of the information and questions that allow the reader to self-evaluate his or her command of the information. The chapter *Appendices* provide examples of data collection tools or methods of data collection, evaluations, or key documents that are utilized in clinical decision making. These provide one example of how the information presented in the chapter can be applied to clinical practice.

Standardized tests and the interventions mentioned are not all-inclusive; they are intended to provide general examples of the kinds of data and common interventions used. These are incorporated into the chapters to provide general information and options for the reader. The interventions in the book are referenced according to the *Guide to Physical Therapist Practice,* with some degree of evidence-based information provided. The focus of the chapters is on the structure of the practice environment and the identification of general interventions that may be appropriate. The reader is encouraged to reference the current literature for information on the efficacy of specific interventions used in her clinical practice. This information is appropriately obtained through a review of the current peer-reviewed literature.

The chapters alternate between the use of the pronouns he or she when referring to the physical therapist and the child, with consistent use of the pronouns throughout the chapter. This is to make the text both fluid and inclusive.

I hope this book will both teach and serve as a reference for students and clinicians on the provision of physical therapy services to children. It is intended to clarify the major delivery systems in order to make the reader better understand the influences, expectations, and outcomes of the various settings in which children and families are served. By understanding the continuum of practice environments, hopefully we, as clinicians, will improve our contributions to children as they grow older, ensuring equal opportunity and full participation in society as individuals … who happen to have a disability.

Mark Drnach

REFERENCES

1. *American Physical Therapy Association Vision Statement for Physical Therapy 2020.* Alexandria, VA: American Physical Therapy Association; 2000.
2. Individuals with Disabilities Education Improvement Act of 2004. 20 USC 1400. Title I. Sec. 601(c)(1).

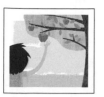

ACKNOWLEDGMENTS

Writing a book is not a solitary activity. I could not have completed this project without the love and support of my wife Joann. She gave me something that eludes many parents: more time. I am very grateful for the many opportunities she made available and the encouragement she provided. She is the great love of my life and enriches it in so many ways. In addition, the patience and understanding of our four children—Alek, Grace, Luke, and Rachel—helped make it possible to write at home.

I would also like to acknowledge the influence of my parents Joseph and Margaret Drnach. They inspire me to take chances and to understand that success is in the act of doing. Their unfailing support for any endeavor I undertake is a constant source of energy that has made my life an adventure. That adventure has led to many encounters with interesting and influential people, one of whom is Ellen Kitts, MD. I would like to thank her for her unknowing affect on my clinical life and for her insight with the overall direction of this book, along with several of the chapters it contains. She is a good friend and an excellent mentor.

I would also like to thank Lippincott Williams & Wilkins for approaching me to write this book and for providing the support and guidance in its production, and I acknowledge the support of Wheeling Jesuit University, which provided me with additional time at work to write and to edit. Their involvement helped me to maintain some balance between my professional and personal life during this process.

Thanks to Wendy Kelly for her critique and feedback on several chapters of this book, to Angela Bryant for her help with the glossary, to all those individuals who agreed to be photographed for this book, and to the authors and publishers who granted permission to reproduce figures, tables, pictures, or charts that helped me to clarify a point or to summarize information.

Thanks also to you, the reader, for purchasing this book. I am glad to share with you my perspective and understanding of providing services to children. I hope this book adds to your understanding of the variety of practice environments encountered by families and children and, in some small way, improves the physical therapy services you provide.

Finally, I would like to acknowledge the many children and families who have motivated me to be a better clinician. As many physical therapists who work in pediatrics will attest, the interactions with this patient population make it difficult at times to call it work. For their many influences, challenges, and moments of joy, I am grateful.

MD

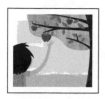

REVIEWERS

DENISE ABRAMS, PT, MA
Chairperson
Physical Therapist Assistant Program
Broome Community College
Binghamton, NY

ROY LEE ALDRIDGE JR., PT, EDS
Associate Professor of Physical
    Therapy
Arkansas State University
State University, AR

LARRY CHINNOCK, PT, EDD, MBA
SPT Program Director
Loma Linda University
Loma Linda, CA

BETH ENNIS, PT, EDD, PCS
Assistant Professor
Bellarmine University
Louisville, KY

SUSAN L. ESKRIDGE, MS, PT
Doctoral Student
Joint Doctoral Program, Epidemiology
San Diego State University and
    University of California, San Diego
San Diego, CA

SHANEY FAINI, PT
Independent Practitioner
Wheeling, WV

ELLEN M. GODWIN, PT, PHD, PCS
Associate Professor/Associate Director
Long Island University
Brooklyn, NY

BARBARA A. JOHNSON, PT
Movement Analysis Laboratory
    Clinician/Adjunct Faculty
Shriners Hospitals for Children/
    University of Utah Division of
    Physical Therapy
Salt Lake City, UT

KRISTEN KLYCZEK
Adjunct Faculty
Member, Clinician
SUNY University at Buffalo
Buffalo, NY

CELESTE RUGGIERI JONES, BA, MS, PT
Clinical Assistant Professor
Physical Therapy Program
University of Rhode Island
Kingston, RI

JOHN J. SCANDURA, MS, PT, CSCS
Physical Therapist
National Training Center at South
    Lake Hospital
Clermont, FL

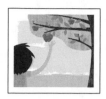

CONTRIBUTORS

**CATERINA ABRAHAM,
PT, MPH, OCS**
Academic Coordinator of Clinical
 Education
Wheeling Jesuit University
 Department of Physical Therapy
Wheeling, WV

CAROL ANTONELLI-GRECO, DO
Clinical Associate Professor of Family
 Medicine
West Virginia School of Osteopathic
 Medicine
Lewisburg, WV
Greco Osteopathic Medical Associates
Family Medicine
Wheeling, WV

TASIA BOBISH, PT, PHD
Physical Therapist
Children's Hospital of Pittsburgh
Pittsburgh, PA

**MELISSA S. BOZOVICH,
PT, DPT, ATC**
Physical Therapist/Athletic Trainer
NovaCare Outpatient Rehabilitation
 and Sports Medicine
Bentleyville, PA

THERESA M. CHAMBERS, PT, DPT
Physical Therapist
Independent Practitioner
Barnesville, OH

JOEL E. CLARK, PT, DPT, CSCS
Physical Therapist
Fayette County Public Schools
Lexington, KY

CHRISTINE L. CONSTANTINE, RN
Hospice Administrator
Albert Gallatin Home Care and
 Hospice Services, LLC
Uniontown, PA

MICHAEL J. DRNACH, MBA
Director, Ambulatory Services
Children's Hospital of Pittsburgh
Pittsburgh, PA

NIKKI KIGER, PT, MPT
Physical Therapist/Clinical
 Coordinator
Easter Seals Rehabilitation Center
Wheeling, WV

**MAUREEN MCKENNA,
PT, PHD, LPC**
Assistant Professor of Physical
 Therapy
Wheeling Jesuit University
Wheeling, WV

MEG STANGER, PT, MS, PCS
Director of Physical Therapy and
 Occupational Therapy
Children's Hospital of Pittsburgh
Pittsburgh, PA

**BRYAN J. WARREN,
JD, MS, MSPT, PT**
Corporate Counsel and Senior Director
The Human Motion Institute
Musculoskeletal Management
 Systems, LLC
Pittsburgh, PA

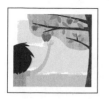

CONTENTS

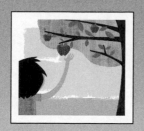

PART I

FOUNDATIONAL ISSUES

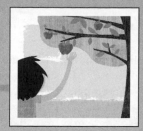

C H A P T E R **1**

Physical Therapy and Children

Mark Drnach

LEARNING OBJECTIVES

1. Describe some of the key influences on the development of the profession of physical therapy.
2. Summarize key pieces of federal legislation and their influence on the models of service delivery for physical therapy.
3. Understand the patient/client management model as outlined in the Guide to Physical Therapist Practice.
4. Plan a sequence for the delivery of physical therapy interventions.
5. Identify factors that influence the frequency and duration of services in a plan of care.
6. Identify and define standard terminology used in the clinical setting to describe a level of assistance, balance, or coordination.
7. Evaluate the use of evidence-based practice (EBP) in the clinical setting.

This chapter will present information on some of the key issues that have influenced the development of the profession of physical therapy and on how the practice of physical therapy has grown beyond the walls of the traditional hospital setting where it began treating patients and has spread into the community and homes of clients where physical therapists enable people to fulfill their intended roles in life. Several key factors in this process have included epidemics, wars, and many times federal legislation. Federal laws have significantly impacted not only the market for physical therapists but also have established a framework for the delivery of physical therapy services in federally funded programs.

The health care community and society have been influential as well, with the emergence and expectation of EBP. This chapter presents this concept from a clinical point of view and highlights how information could be used in the decision-making process. Gathering information in an objective and consistent manner aids in the validation of the tests, measurements, and interventions that physical therapists use with specific patient populations.

HISTORICAL PERSPECTIVE: DEVELOPMENT OF THE PROFESSION AND PRACTICE OF PHYSICAL THERAPY

The treatment of children has been an influential aspect in the development of the profession of physical therapy. The epidemic of **infantile paralysis** or **poliomyelitis** (polio) in the late 1800s and early 1900s, affecting children in the New England States for the first time in 1894,[1] was one of the early factors that led to the development of the profession of physical therapy in the United States of America. The application of physical modalities and therapeutic procedures were incorporated into the medical management, which then consisted mainly of bed rest and immobilization, of children affected by this disease.[1] The earliest providers of these interventions were teachers of physical education, gymnastics, or corrective exercise, who, in collaboration with the physician, provided interventions that included massage, muscle training, and corrective exercise.[2] Mary McMillan, considered to be the first physical therapist in America, was born in the United States and educated in Liverpool, England. There she received a bachelor's degree from the Liverpool Gymnasium College in physical culture and corrective exercise (physical education) and worked in Liverpool's Children's Hospital with patients who had polio, spasticity, and scoliosis.[2] Moving to Connecticut in the United States in 1915, she continued her work as the Director of Massage at the Crippled Children's Hospital in Portland, Maine. The therapeutic and restorative interventions provided by these early physical reconstruction aides were further required to address the impairments and functional limitations of soldiers injured or disabled in World War I. Interventions were required to enable these men returning from war to function in the growing industrialized society. Along with this growing need for personnel came the need for standardization in training and education. In 1917, the establishment of the Division of Special Hospitals and Physical Reconstruction in the Office of the Surgeon General of the U.S. Army Medical Corps provided a standard education for preparation of clinicians who were given the title **reconstruction aide**.[2] Marguerite Sanderson was hired as the director of the Reconstruction Aide Program. Mary McMillan joined here to head the program established at the Walter Reed General Hospital[3] but soon moved to Portland, Oregon, to train at Reed College. Here efforts to train an increasing number of women to aid in the rehabilitation of men wounded in the war helped to meet the demand of the newly created and growing profession of physiotherapy.[4] By 1919, 45 hospitals in the country employed >700 reconstruction aides.[5]

Poliomyelitis

The epidemic of poliomyelitis in the late 1800s and early 1900s was one of the early factors that led to the development of the profession of physical therapy. Treatment of this disease included massage, muscle training, and corrective exercise provided by reconstruction aides.

In 1921, the American Women's Physical Therapeutic Association was founded with Mary McMillan as its president. The purpose of the organization was to establish a professional and scientific standard for those engaged in the profession of physical therapeutics.[6] In 1922, the name was changed to the American Physiotherapy Association (APA) in recognition of the men who also practiced physiotherapy.

In the 1930s, in order to more closely align with the medical profession and make a clear distinction between the profession of physiotherapy and other professions such as nursing, occupational therapy, or chiropractics, the APA agreed to allow the American Medical Association's (AMA) Council on Medical Education to accredit physiotherapy schools. In the agreement, the APA also consented to the title of "physiotherapist technician" and the requirement to work only under the direct supervision of the physician.[4] In hindsight this may seem like an inappropriate move for professional autonomy, but in the context of an emerging profession during the Great Depression of the 1930s this was a move toward professional legitimacy and survival.

The continuing polio epidemic and the outbreak of World War II in the 1940s placed further demands on the limited number of qualified physiotherapy technicians and facilitated a period of major growth in the profession. This era also saw a change in the medical specialty that focused on physical therapeutics and rehabilitation. A physician who specialized in this area used the title of physical therapy physician. In 1945, this medical specialty officially became known as physical medicine, with the physician adopting the title of physiatrist. This made the title of physiotherapy technician unnecessary, and clinicians adopted the title of physical therapist. In 1946, the APA changed its name to the American Physical Therapy Association (APTA).

Not only epidemics and wars influenced the development of the physical therapy profession during this era: Social movements resulting in federal legislation and advances in medicine and rehabilitation impacted the scope of the profession as well. Ironically, it was a polio survivor, President Franklin D. Roosevelt, who in 1935 signed the **Social Security Act** into law. This legislation is one of the most significant pieces of social legislation in the United States establishing federal aid for public health and welfare assistance, maternal and child health, and children with disabilities services.[7] It would give rise in subsequent years to the programs of Medicare and Medicaid. Another significant piece of federal legislation came about in 1946 with the passage of the **Hill–Burton Hospital Construction Act.** This legislation had a major influence on the expansion of the hospital industry and the physical therapy departments that they housed. It required hospitals with >100 beds to also have a physical therapy department (the primary setting for physical therapy practice during this era), which had a major influence on how services were provided to patients.

The polio epidemic reached its peak in the United States in 1952 with >21,000 paralytic cases being reported that year.[8] The polio virus enters the body via the nose or mouth (via fecal–oral or oral–oral transmission) and travels to the intestines, then to the bloodstream. Replication of the virus in motor neurons of the anterior horn cell and brain stem result in cell destruction and the general manifestation of paralysis associated with this disease. Early efforts to develop a vaccine failed, due to the fact that the researchers were unaware that, instead of one strain of virus, there were three. In 1953, Dr. Jonas Salk discovered a vaccination that would prevent poliomyelitis. His discovery, known as the Salk vaccine, went on to virtually eradicate the disease in the United States. Physical therapists continued to provide interventions to those individuals who were paralyzed by the disease, and also addressed other disabling conditions such as cerebral palsy. During this time, the practice of physical therapy took on an additional perspective in the treatment of patients with neuromuscular diseases. Margaret Rood, a physical therapist and an occupational therapist, had a major influence on the treatment approach to patients with central nervous system (CNS) disorders. Her rehabilitation approach focused more on the neurophysiologic bases than the more traditional orthopedic approach.[9] The work of Margaret Knott and Dorothy Voss also emerged in the 1950s. Their developmentally based intervention for movement, Proprioceptive Neuromuscular Facilitation (PNF), became another intervention provided by the physical therapist[10] along with the works of Signe Brunnstrom in the treatment of hemiplegia[11] and Dr. Karl and Berta Bobath with their specialized handling techniques for children with cerebral palsy.[12] In the 1950s and 1960s, the traditional interventions provided by physical therapists were broadened to include a more neurophysiologic and developmental approach to the treatment of movement disorders, based on the understanding of the CNS at that time. This understanding included a direct relationship between the neurologic maturation of the CNS and motor behavior as seen through a developmental sequence, where sensory input preceded motor output, and the presence of a hierarchical relationship of the CNS structures, where the cortex ultimately controlled complex movements.[13] These contributions provided the foundation of how physical therapy would be provided to people with movement disorders for decades to come. The profession of physical therapy was expanding its repertoire of interventions to address the changing needs of the patient population.

The 1950s saw additional legislative influences with the passage of physical therapy licensure laws in many states. By 1959, 45 states had a **Physical Therapy Practice Act**;[6] today, all 50 states have such an Act, which is intended to protect the public from imposters or fraudulent billing practices when the services are not rendered by a physical therapist or physical therapist assistant. It is important to note that these laws do not prohibit competent personnel from using interventions associated with physical therapy, such as passive range of motion (PROM), positioning, or therapeutic exercise, as long as the person providing them does not represent himself or herself as a physical therapist or as an individual providing physical therapy. Many state practice acts provide information regarding the practice of physical therapy under the supervision of a physician.

Direct access is the ability to access physical therapy services without a physician's referral. It is a growing trend in the United States, with the majority of states currently allowing for some form of direct access of physical therapy services by the consumers in that state. Today, many states, but not all, allow for some form of direct access to physical

therapy services. Some states put limits on the amount of time a physical therapist can provide services before a physician's prescription to continue to treat is needed. It is important for the practicing physical therapist to abide by the laws of the state as well as the laws of the federal government.

POINT TO REMEMBER

State Physical Therapy Practice Act

All states have a practice act for physical therapists. It is the physical therapist's professional and legal obligation to understand and abide by the state practice act in the state where the services are provided (see Additional Online Resources).

In the 1960s, the U. S. Congress passed the landmark Civil Rights Act of 1964 and saw the enactment of Title XVIII (Medicare) and Title XIX (Medicaid) of the Social Security Act of 1965. **Medicare** is the largest source of federal funding for medical services for people older than 65 years.[7] **Medicaid** is the largest source of funding for basic medical services for the poor. The Medicaid program is a joint federal and state program, administered by the state, which can determine eligibility requirements, covered benefits, and fee schedules. Unlike Medicare, which reimburses providers through an intermediary (such as Blue Cross Blue Shield), Medicaid reimburses providers directly. In addition to Medicare and Medicaid, the Social Security Act also includes Supplemental Security Income (SSI), which provides a fixed monthly payment to eligible children and individuals older than 65 years who are disabled, blind, or have limited resources.[14]

With the creation of Medicare and Medicaid adding to the increasing demand for physical therapists, the APTA moved forward in the process of creating the physical therapist assistant, a process that began in the late 1940s. At that time, many physical therapists were utilizing aides in their departments but desired someone with more education specific to physical therapy. The title of **physical therapist assistant** was adopted by the APTA in 1973. The physical therapist assistant helps the physical therapist in the provision of physical therapy interventions. The role is defined by the APTA as

"a technically educated health care provider who assists the physical therapist in the provision of selected physical therapy interventions. The physical therapist assistant is the only individual who provides selected physical therapy interventions under the direction and supervision of the physical therapist. The physical therapist assistant is a graduate of a physical therapist assistant associate degree program accredited by the Commission on Accreditation in Physical Therapy Education (CAPTE)."[15]

In the 1970s and 1980s, physical therapists and physical therapist assistants were using a combination of neurophysiologic techniques to solve motor problems and to address the impairments of the children they were treating.[13] The basis of the interventions continued to rest on the understanding of the CNS and its influence on motor behavior. During the 1960s through the 1990s (and continuing today), research advanced the understanding of human movement providing insight into the heterarchical (instead of hierarchical) relationship of cortical and subcortical structures of the CNS. The dynamic systems theory of motor development, along with the theories of motor control and motor learning, expanded the understanding of movement and influenced how physical therapists addressed movement deficits in the clinic. The acquisition of a motor behavior and skill was seen not so much as a linear process that was closely associated with neural maturation but as a dynamic process in which new behaviors emerge as old behaviors lose their stability or primary influence as a result of a change in one of the many systems that impact movement (e.g., cognitive, musculoskeletal, sensory, neuromuscular).[16] These newer theories view the child not as a passive recipient of therapeutic interventions but as an active problem solver whose motor behavior is goal directed and whose knowledge of performance and results aid in his motor learning. To integrate this understanding into practice, the physical therapist would have to modify her interventions, structuring meaningful activities with active child participation into the treatment session. This approach would be beneficial in the various settings in which the physical therapist will find herself, with the passage of several significant pieces of federal legislation that expanded the market for physical therapists.

The Influence of Federal Legislation on the Practice Environment

The practice environment of physical therapy is engulfed in a larger health care system that evolved with the development of the United States of America, the roots of which can be found in the "can do" spirit of the early American settlers, and the philosophy that the body is a machine that can be fixed.[7] This culture fostered the growth and development of the world's most sophisticated and technologically advanced health care system, which celebrates the often heroic and costly medical procedures to save or extend life, but has generally downplayed the less heroic preventative procedures that can improve the quality of life for many.

Today the recipient of this health care is more informed and involved in the decision-making process than ever before. It is important to understand the patient's point of view about what health care can do for him, or for a parent, or for his child. Interestingly, in the 1950s, Parson[17] suggested that people in Western developed countries demonstrated predictable behaviors when they were ill. His theories are still recognized as contributing to understanding behaviors around illness today. Parson noted that a society makes certain

assumptions about people who are ill. People who are ill or sick are not solely responsible for their condition, and it is not within their power to get better. Being ill exempts the individual from normal personal and social obligations in proportion to the severity of the illness. Being sick is undesirable, and people who are ill should take the appropriate actions and enlist the help of competent people to aid in recovery. They are also obligated to comply with the treatment and advice given to them. It is in this environment that the medical model of service delivery has evolved (Box 1-1A). The patient is by definition the person who is ill (or the child with polio or cerebral palsy) and seeks out the consult of a physician, who writes a prescription for physical therapy to address the patient's problem, to fix it. This model of service is practiced today in several states that require a referral by a physician in order for a patient to access a physical therapist. It is practiced in many hospital settings and outpatient clinics and reinforced by third party payment systems that require a referral from a physician as a requirement for receiving payment for treatment.

POINT TO REMEMBER

Parson's Assumptions on Being Ill

People who are ill:

1. are not solely responsible for their condition, and it is not within their power to get better;
2. are exempt from normal personal and social obligations in proportion to the severity of their illness;
3. should take appropriate actions and enlist the help of competent people to aid in their recovery; and
4. are obligated to comply with the treatment and advice given to them.

Then something happened in 1975. At the federal level, the practice of physical therapy in the public educational environment was more clearly defined with the passage of Public Law (PL) 94-142: The **Education for All Handicapped Children Act** (see Chapter 8). This law provides for a "free and appropriate public education" for all children with disabilities, beginning whenever the individual state provides public education to children who are not disabled (age 5 or 6 years, depending on the state). Contained in PL 94-142 are several provisions commonly encountered in the special education classroom today, including the Individualized Education Program (IEP), which is the contract between the parents and the school district that directs the delivery of services to the eligible student. The IEP facilitated the development of another model of service delivery: The educational model (Box 1-1B), which includes not a patient, but a student, and an

BOX 1-1
Models of Service Delivery

A. The Medical Model (1920s)
Physician (via prescription)
↓
Physical Therapist (a health care service)
↓
Patient

B. The Educational Model (1970s)
Educational Team (IEP)
↓
Physical Therapist (a related service)
↓
Student

C. The Early Intervention Model (1980s)
Early Intervention Team (IFSP)
↓
Family
↓
Early Intervention Provider (Physical Therapist)
↓
Child

Key Pieces of Federal Legislation

1935—The Social Security Act
1946—The Hill–Burton Hospital Construction Act
1965—The Social Security Act, Title XVIII (Medicare) and Title XIX (Medicaid)
1975—The Education for All Handicapped Children Act (currently the Individuals with Disabilities Education Act)

educational team, which includes the parent of the student, the teacher, and the physical therapist. A physician can also be part of this team, but it is not mandatory. Several states require a physical therapist to obtain a physician's referral in order to provide services (via the Practice Act), making the need for physician involvement necessary when physical therapy services are utilized.

As with many other federal laws, periodic reauthorization is required to assure continued appropriations and to provide an opportunity to re-evaluate the components of the law for necessary updates, clarifications, or deletions. PL 94-142 was reauthorized with amendments in 1986 as the **Education of the Handicapped Act Amendments** or PL 99-457, which contained a significant update extending educational services to children aged 3 to 5 years. Part H of this law (currently Part C of the Individuals with Disabilities Education Improvement Act; PL 108-446) included the provision of early intervention services to eligible families or children, from birth to 3 years of age. (Some states provide these services until the child is eligible for kindergarten.) This law mandates a model of service delivery different from the medical and educational models, with an emphasis on family-centered services in the natural setting (see Chapter 6). The program of early intervention is governed by the Individualized Family Service Plan (IFSP) (Box 1-1C).

These models of service delivery require the physical therapist to fulfill certain roles and responsibilities depending on the setting and the applicable laws that influence the behavior of people working in that system. Understanding the practice environment and the external influences that shape it will allow the physical therapist to clearly understand her role in various settings and enable her to educate others to the appropriate utilization of physical therapy services. In some models, the focus is not on the child as a patient who is to be treated, but on the child as a student who is to learn or the child who is a member of a family. In many early intervention programs, the physical therapist works with the members of a family to assist them in the care and development of their child in the typical environments in which the child lives or plays. In the educational system, the physical therapist works with the classroom staff and the student to optimize the ability of the student to function and learn in the school environment. In the hospital or outpatient setting, the physical therapist works with the medical staff and child to assist him in the recovery of his health and in the acquisition of functional or developmental activities. These various settings and utilization of physical therapy require the physical therapist to broaden her view of the child in front of her into the larger context of the child as a member of a family or a student in a classroom. This shift fits well with the evolution from an impairment-based approach to treatment, which focuses primarily on the physical impairments to movement, to a function-based approach, which focuses on enabling the child to function in his environment despite any inherent physical impairments.

THE PRACTICE OF PHYSICAL THERAPY

Team Practice Models

Understanding how the physical therapist practices in these settings and the expectations of the team members is vital to efficient and effective team functioning. The physical therapist can assume various responsibilities depending on the type of team. Historically the physical therapist has worked on **multidisciplinary** teams with physicians who prescribe the physical therapy for an identified patient. As a member of a multidisciplinary team, the physical therapist works with other disciplines, especially with the examination and ongoing assessment, but generally provides interventions solely within the physical therapist's traditional role. Educational programs may utilize a broader multidisciplinary team including, in addition to the physical therapist, the student, his parents, educators, a speech language pathologist, and psychologist as members of the team. In some educational settings as well as with early intervention programs, the members of the team incorporate a **transdisciplinary** team approach. Collaboration among team members, which may include sharing of traditional intervention roles among members of the team and cross-training, is a key characteristic of this type of teaming. Typically one professional is the primary service provider who is trained and supervised by the other member(s) of the team and incorporates the delegated interventions into a treatment session. In rural areas, or in areas that lack health care providers, states with direct access may find the physical therapist working independently of other disciplines. This team of one professional discipline is a **unidisciplinary** team, which may be seen in private practice settings today.

When working on a team, the members can improve their efficiency by delineating the responsibility of certain aspects of the plan of care (or IEP or IFSP) to specific qualified team members. In an educational setting, the physical therapist may be primarily responsible for the positioning and mobility aspects of a student's IEP as well as his participation in community field trips and in the adaptations to his physical education class. The speech language pathologist may be responsible for the same student's communication program as well as his oral motor program during lunch, or the use of assistive technology in the classroom and community. Each responsibility should be dictated by the skills of the provider, with role release (other team members assuming the role traditionally assigned to one specific discipline) being assumed by capable and willing members to the benefit of the child.

These are fluid characteristics of practice that the physical therapist adopts given the individual child and situation. Certain practice models are expected in specific environments, such as a family-centered, transdisciplinary approach in some states' early intervention programs, but the child's needs and the capability of the physical therapist can influence the way in which services are provided. There is no one best way to provide services. It is the responsibility of the physical therapist to promote the proper utilization of physical therapy services in any given practice environment given the unique attributes of each child and situation. Understanding

how to function on a team begins with understanding how to practice as a physical therapist.

A Guide to Physical Therapist Practice

In 1997, the APTA published the first edition of the **Guide to Physical Therapist Practice** (the Guide),[18] which provides an outline of the profession of physical therapy's body of knowledge (Part One) and describes the boundaries within which physical therapists design and implement appropriate plans of care for specific patient–client diagnostic groups (Part Two). Although unidisciplinary in its approach to patient management, the Guide provides clarification on who physical therapists are and what they do, the types of tests and measures they perform, and the types of interventions they provide. The framework that the Guide uses to describe the practice of physical therapy is based on the Nagi model of disablement (the process of becoming disabled) (Fig. 1-1A).

The process of disablement from a medical model, which is the dominant approach in the history of health care in the United States, has an emphasis on pathology-based causes of impairments that can lead to a disability. This model reflects a treatment approach to the disability with the aim of ameliorating the pathology or impairment in order to cure or lessen the disability. This construct emphasizes the factors that impact a person more from an individual perspective than from the environmental or societal aspects of disability.[19] Disability, as defined by the Guide, is the inability or restricted ability to perform actions, tasks, and activities related to self-care, home management, work (job, school, play), community, and leisure roles in the individual's sociocultural context and physical environment.[15] In addition, the Guide defines impairment as a loss or abnormality of anatomic, physiologic, mental, or psychological structure or function. A model of disablement, adapted by the APTA[15] from Guccione, identifies other factors that affect the disablement process and recognizes the importance of such factors as personal motivation, social support, architectural barriers, education, and income on the process (Fig. 1-1B).

Medical models of disablement emphasize disability as a result of a pathology for which interventions are aimed to treat the underlying disorder or impairment. Medical care is viewed as the main issue related to disability, and at a political level emphasizes the need for health care policy reform.[20] A social model of disability views disability not only as an attribute of an individual but as a collection of conditions, many of which are created by society and act as barriers to the individual's participation in society. Social reform is viewed as the main issue related to disability, and at a political level there is a need for social action and human rights legislation to promote full participation of people with disabilities in all areas of social life.[20]

Nagi Model of Disablement

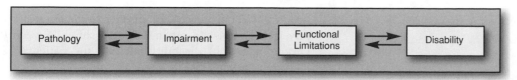

A

Expanded Disablement Model

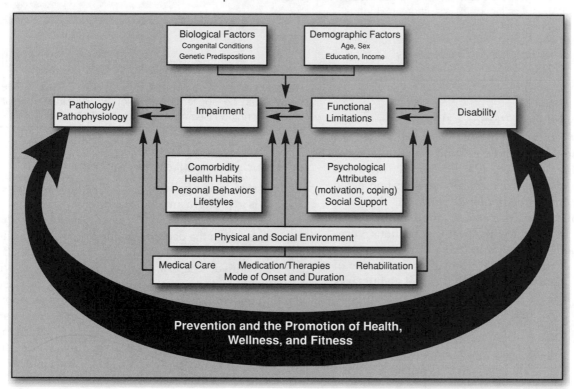

B

Adapted from Guide to Physical Therapist Practice. 2nd ed. 2003:24 with permission of the American Physical Therapy Association. This material is copyrighted, and further reproduction or distribution is prohibited.

International Classification of Functioning, Disability and Health (The ICF Model)

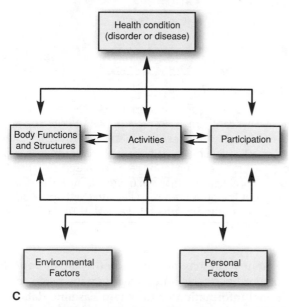

C

World Health Organization. ICF Introduction. Geneva. Switzerland: World Health Organization, 2002:18. With permission.

Figure 1-1 ■ Models of disablement and enablement. **A:** Nagi Model of Disablement (from Nagi S. Some conceptual issues in disability and rehabilitation. In: Sussman M, ed. *Sociology and Rehabilitation.* Washington, DC: American Sociological Association; 1965;100–113). **B:** Expanded Disablement Model from the *Guide to Physical Therapist Practice, Second Edition,* 2003; 24 (adapted from Guccione A. *Arthritis and the process of disablement. Phys Ther.* 1994;74:410). **C:** Interactions between the components of the International Classification of Functioning, Disability, and Health. A biopsychosocial model integrating medical and social aspects of disablement.

Disablement

The medical model of disablement emphasizes pathology that leads to disability. Health care reform is necessary to address this disabling process. A more social model of disablement emphasizes a collection of conditions that influence a person's ability to function in society with an emphasis on societal factors that handicap a person. Civil rights legislation is necessary to address this disabling process.

The World Health Organization's (WHO) *International Classification of Functioning, Disability and Health* (ICF)[20] is an integration of the medical and social models of disablement (Fig. 1-1C). The ICF has moved away from being a "consequences of disease" classification (1980 version) to become a "components of health" classification.[20] As a clinical tool, this classification matrix can be used to match treatment with specific conditions, vocational assessment, rehabilitation, and outcome evaluation. The ICF is structured around the components of body functions and structure, activities (related to tasks and actions by an individual), and participation (involvement in a life situation). According to the WHO:

> Functioning and disability are viewed as a complex interaction between the health condition of the individual and the contextual factors of the environment as well as personal factors. The picture produced by this combination of factors and dimensions is of "the person in his or her world." The classification treats these dimensions as interactive and dynamic rather than linear or static. It allows for an assessment of the degree of disability, although it is not a measurement instrument. It is applicable to all people, whatever their health condition. The language of the ICF is neutral as to etiology, placing the emphasis on function rather than condition or disease. It also is carefully designed to be relevant across cultures as well as age groups and genders, making it highly appropriate for heterogeneous populations.[20]

The ICF model describes how people live with their health condition. It is another reflection of the trend to focus on the individual and the factors that enable that person to live life to its fullest, taking into consideration not only his abilities but also the environmental and social constraints that may impair those abilities. As a clinical tool the ICF has applications in the development of a more detailed description of a person with a disability and the factors that contribute to that disability.[21] The model also has applications in childhood disability,[22,23] physical therapy, and rehabilitation medicine.[24,25] The ICF framework, as well as the other models of disablement, provides the rehabilitation disciplines with a universal language to discuss disability.[26] Understanding the multifaceted aspects of disablement can assist the physical therapist in making relationships between the various factors of disability and aid the patient/client management process.

ICF

The WHO's ICF model is a universal classification of disability and health with applications for intervention studies, research, policy development, and economic analysis. The model can be applied to all people regardless of their health condition (see Additional Online Resources).

THE PATIENT/CLIENT MANAGEMENT PROCESS

The first step in the patient/client management process (Fig. 1-2) is to perform an examination. An examination is the collection of data that will be used to make an evaluation and assists in the decision-making process regarding the necessity and type of physical therapy services that may be required. The examination process begins with the collection of demographic information and the reason why the child and/or his family is seeking the services of a physical therapist. This can include identification and prioritization of the goals that the family has, which may be their reason for seeking physical therapy services. It is also important to identify motivators for the child. What is he interested in at present? What and how does he like to play? The examination process may also include observation of the child as he moves and interacts with his environment. How does he move? Are his movements typical of a child his age? What is he doing that is atypical? What systems or barriers are associated with this lack of movement?

Why the Guide?

The Guide provides a framework for clinical decision making in physical therapy. To provide high-quality pediatric physical therapy services, therapists should consider the Guide; other documents, such as federal and state legislation; the practice setting; and research-based evidence to aid in clinical decision making. (From: Using APTA's Guide to Physical Therapist Practice in Pediatric Settings. Practice Committee of the Section of Pediatrics, APTA, 2003.)

The examination may also include the use of appropriate standardized tests and measurements taken to gain additional information or to obtain baseline data to be used in the decision-making process. Which tests and

Diagnosis
Both the process and the end result of evaluating examination data, which the physical therapist organizes into defined clusters, syndromes, or categories to help determine the prognosis (including the plan of care) and the most appropriate intervention strategies.

Evaluation
A dynamic process in which the physical therapist makes clinical judgments based on data gathered during the examination. This process also may identify possible problems that require consultation with or referral to another provider.

Prognosis
(Including Plan of Care)
Determination of the level of optimal improvement that may be attained through intervention and the amount of time required to reach that level. The plan of care specifies the interventions to be used and their timing and frequency.

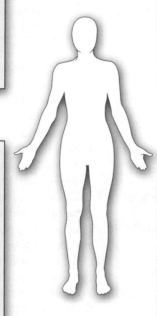

Examination
The process of obtaining a history, performing a systems review, and selecting and administering tests and measures to gather data about the patient/client. The initial examination is a comprehensive screening and specific testing process that leads to a diagnostic classification. The examination process also may identify possible problems that require consultation with or referral to another provider.

Intervention
Purposeful and skilled interaction of the physical therapist with the patient/client and, if appropriate, with other individuals involved in care of the patient/client, using various physical therapy procedures and techniques to produce changes in the condition that are consistent with the diagnosis and prognosis. The physical therapist re-examines to determine changes in patient/client status and to modify or redirect intervention. The decision to re-examine may be based on new clinical findings or lack of patient/client progress. The process of re-examination also may identify the need for consultation with or referral to another provider.

Outcomes
Results of patient/client management, which include the impact of physical therapy interventions in the following domains: pathology/pathophysiology (disease, disorder, or condition); impairments, functional limitations, and disabilities; risk reduction/prevention; health, wellness, and fitness; societal resources; and patient/client satisfaction.

Figure 1-2 ■ Patient/client management model (Adapted from Guide to Physical Therapist Practice. 2nd ed. 2003:35 with permission of the American Physical Therapy Association. This material is copyrighted, and further reproduction or distribution is prohibited).

measurements are chosen will depend in part on the availability of these examination instruments and the therapist's competency in administering the test. In the selection and administration of a test or measurement the physical therapist should be aware of the **psycho-metric properties** of the test or measurement. Psychometric properties are the quantifiable attributes, such as validity and reliability, that relate to the item's statistical strength or weakness (Box 1-2). The user of the test should know how the test is constructed and if the test is

BOX 1-2
Psychometric Terminology

Validity–Meaningful
Construct validity–How was the test made?
Content validity–Are the parts of the test meaningful?
Criterion-related validity–Is the test result justified by comparison to another measurement? Predictive and concurrent validity are forms of criterion-related validity.
   Predictive validity–What do the results of this test say about the future?
   Concurrent validity–Is the test result justified by comparison to another measurement done at the same time?
Reliability–Repeatability
Intra-rater–When one person takes repeated measurements (between me and myself)
Inter-rater–When different people take repeated measurements (between me and you)
Test-retest–Repeatability of the test to provide a consistent result over time (stability of the test to provide a consistent answer)
Equivalence reliability–Test produces the same result when an equivalent test or instrument is used
Sensitivity–How well a diagnostic test can identify a specific condition when the specific condition is present
Specificity–How well a diagnostic test can identify the absence of a specific condition when the specific condition is not present

appropriate for the intended purpose. Tests and measurements may be performed to identify delays in the acquisition of developmental skills, to identify atypical behaviors, to assess progress made during the course of intervention, or to predict an outcome. There are a variety of standardized tests applicable to children, each fulfilling a different purpose: to be discriminative, predictive, or evaluative.[27] A discriminative test allows the user to identify whether a particular problem causes the child to differ from a typical population. The Peabody Developmental Motor Scales (PMDS-2)[28] is one test that discriminates between the motor skills of the child tested and the skills of a group of same aged children. A predictive test is used to determine what the child's future status may be based on the items tested. The Movement Assessment of Infants (MAI) when done at 4 months of age is used to predict cerebral palsy in children 3 to 8 years old.[29] Finally, an evaluative test is performed to assess a child's change over time, particularly with intervention. The Gross Motor Function Measure (GMFM) is an example of a test that evaluates the motor function of a child with cerebral palsy, over time.[30]

POINT TO REMEMBER

To Examine, to Evaluate, or to Assess

Examination—Typically the collection of data and information from various sources, including the medical record, the patient's history, a systems review, tests, and measurements.

Evaluation—A professional judgment based on the examination findings providing a snapshot of the patient at one moment in time.

Assessment—Typically, an ongoing process of measurement providing information on the progress of the patient.

Tests that are **norm-referenced** are standardized to groups of children with similar characteristics. Therefore, the test result for a particular child who is being tested is compared to those for the group of children for whom the test was designed. The fact that the test is norm-referenced means that the results of the test for one child could be compared to a normal distribution of scores of the group (a bell-shaped curve). When compared to a group of typically developing children, the test result can provide a developmental age for the child and help with the identification of appropriate developmental activities. Norm-referenced tests are diagnostic. They take a snapshot of a child at a particular moment in time and compare his performance with that of a reference group. Examples of norm-referenced tests for children include the Bayley Scales of Infant Development[31] for children 1 to 42 months, the Denver II[32] for children 1 week to 6 years, the Pediatric Evaluation of Disability Inventory (PEDI)[33] for children 6 months to 7 years, and the Bruininks–Oseretsky Test of Motor Proficiency[34] for children 4 to 14 years old.

Criterion-referenced tests measure mastery of a skill in a child. The reference points used may or may not be dependent on a reference group. Therefore, the test result for a particular child who is being tested is compared only to his other test results, over time. These tests look at individual performance and are sensitive to the effects of intervention. Examples of criterion-referenced tests for children include the MAI,[29] The Carolina Curriculum for Infants and Toddlers with Special Needs,[35] the GMFM,[30] and the School Function Assessment.[36]

POINT TO REMEMBER

Types of Tests

Discriminative—Identifies whether a particular problem causes the child to differ from the typical population.
Evaluative—Identifies if a child has changed over time.
Predictive—Identifies what the future status of a child may be based on the results of the items tested.

The results of the physical therapist's tests and measurements are then evaluated for their importance and relevance to the current impairments to movement or learning and the limitations to a child's expected function. This is the professional process of evaluation.

The Guide separates the process of examination, which includes the collection of data, and the **evaluation,** which includes the clinical judgments made from the information gained from the examination data. Understanding these discrete components highlights the importance of information from a variety of sources, possibly collected by several other competent individuals, which is used by the physical therapist in the evaluation of the child. The term 'evaluation' is sometimes interchanged with the term 'assessment.' For clarification throughout this book, evaluation is used to emphasize a judgment made based on the examination data. Assessment is an ongoing measurement that provides information on the progress of the child.

The next step in the patient/client management process is making a **diagnosis.** This allows the physical therapist to categorize a child into a specific group, aiding in the selection of interventions and possible outcomes. The physical therapist makes a diagnosis by evaluating the results of the examination, which include a history, a systems review, and the results of tests and measurements that she performed on the child. She then groups the collection of impairments and functional limitations and identifies which impairment is the most limiting to the child. What impairs the child the most leads to the primary diagnosis or practice pattern that best describes the current categorization of the child. Using the knowledge she has and the ability to administer specific tests and measurements, she can diagnose a child with impaired neuromotor development; impaired joint mobility, muscle performance, and ROM associated with connective tissue dysfunction; or impaired respiration associated with airway clearance dysfunction (to name a few). By classifying a child into a practice pattern or diagnostic group, the physical therapist can better identify the appropriate interventions, which will hopefully provide more appropriate, efficient, and cost effective care.

When the evaluation is completed, the physical therapist can then make a prognosis through a re-evaluation of the parent's reasons for seeking physical therapy and the identification of any additional goals developed as a result of the evaluation. The prognosis made is for a particular **episode of care** (a sequence of care provided to address a given condition) at this particular time, and is based on clearly identified goals and the interventions that can be used to achieve them.

POINT TO REMEMBER

Making a Diagnosis

Making a diagnosis aids the physical therapist in the selection of interventions and the identification of possible outcomes. The physical therapist categorizes a child into one (or more) of the four practice patterns:

Musculoskeletal

Neuromuscular

Cardiovascular pulmonary

Integumentary

The **interventions** for the child's plan of care come from the skill level and knowledge of the physical therapist. Interventions are the tools that a physical therapist uses to produce a change in the patient or client. Interventions range from education to the application of modalities or manual techniques. A listing of interventions used by physical therapists can be found in the Guide (Box 1-3). Ultimately the effectiveness of the intervention is measured by the effect it had on achieving the parent's and/or child's goals. The interventions used by the physical therapist to facilitate or aid in this process could be the same interventions used in a variety of settings such as

BOX 1-3
Interventions

Coordination, Communication, Documentation
Patient/Client-Related Instruction
Procedural Interventions
   Therapeutic exercise
   Functional training in self-care and home management, including ADLs and IADLs
   Functional training in work (job, school, play), community, and leisure integration or reintegration, including IADLs, work hardening, and work conditioning
   Manual therapy techniques, including mobilization and/or manipulation
   Prescription, application, and, as appropriate, fabrication of devices and equipment (assistive, adaptive, orthotic, protective, supportive, or prosthetic)
   Airway clearance techniques
   Integumentary repair and protective techniques
   Electrotherapeutic modalities
   Physical agents and mechanical modalities

From the American Physical Therapy Association. *Guide to Physical Therapist Practice,* 2nd ed. Rev. American Physical Therapy Association; 2003:98.

outpatient clinic, early intervention program, or the hospital setting. It is the primary purpose of physical therapy that varies from one setting to another. There is no distinction between what type of interventions are used in various settings, such as educational versus medical.[37]

In the direct application of interventions to a child, a physical therapist can follow a logical sequence of steps that can make the process more understandable, especially to a new graduate or clinician working with children. The delivery of the hands-on interventions can be broken down into the following steps: neurologic issues (neuro) → ROM (range) → strength → function. This neuro–range–strength–function approach can be used not only to clarify a sequence of interventions but also to assure that impairments are addressed and that the interventions provided are ultimately associated with some functional activity or outcome. This may help the new clinician in structuring a hands-on treatment session.

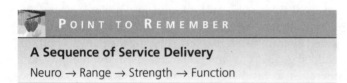

POINT TO REMEMBER

A Sequence of Service Delivery
Neuro → Range → Strength → Function

The first consideration is to address any neurologic issues that are evident at the time. Neurologic issues can include factors such as pain, hypertonia, hypotonia, visual or hearing impairment, or motivation. Interventions may include managing pain, structuring the immediate environment or activity to motivate the child to move, providing external support or positioning to allow for or promote certain movements, or applying inhibitory or facilitatory techniques that address abnormal muscle tone. Using interventions to decrease pain or to momentarily alter a child's muscle tone can allow for more passive or active ROM. ROM activities such as stretching, applying a brace or orthotic, or just positioning a child to stretch certain soft tissues is a logical next step after the neurologic issues have been addressed, allowing for additional or more comfortable movement. One example of this sequence can be seen in donning an ankle foot orthotic (AFO) on a child with hypertonia in the gastrosoleus muscle complex. This process may be made easier if the child's hypertonic lower extremity is positioned in hip and knee flexion and if stretching is done prior to the application of the orthotic.

The logical time in the treatment sequence to strengthen the muscle throughout the available ROM is after stretching the muscles and soft tissues. Strengthening of muscles could be encouraged in both open- and closed-chain movements. Progressing a sequence of a child lifting blocks with his right upper extremity and

placing them on a table (an open-chain activity for the right upper extremity), to placing his right upper extremity on the floor and encouraging a weight shift over the extremity, transitions the activity to a closed-chain exercise. Strengthening is done through repeated movements by the child, who is motivated to move by his desire to please an important adult in his life, to receive positive reinforcement, or through his own internal motivation to achieve the end result. Structuring the activity or providing manual guidance to encourage the child to move through the available ROM assists in strengthening the muscle. If upper extremity strengthening is a goal of the intervention, then encouraging a child to weight shift and weight bear through his upper extremities, as well as to repeatedly reach and manipulate objects may aid in that process. Prior to strengthening, the alleviation or decrease of any neurologic issues or limitations in ROM may make the strengthening activities more productive. Increasing muscle strength should be linked to an age-appropriate functional skill. The ability to reach and manipulate an object or toy can be associated with the ability to don and doff a shirt or manipulate a spoon to eat. It may improve the efficiency of creeping across the floor or negotiating stairs in the house. Linking the strengthening activities to a functional outcome will help the parent or caregiver understand the association and reason for the intervention. Mobility and manipulation also promote motor learning, which requires daily practice and repeated trials.[38] Multiple attempts at a motor activity in a variety of situations, prompted by the parent or caregiver, will allow the child to learn from the errors he makes and ultimately to succeed in the most efficient manner. Daily opportunities to work on these skills are paramount in improving the child's expression and efficient utilization of a specific skill. These opportunities require caregiver understanding, acceptance, and education, not only in one strategy, but in multiple strategies that will provide the child with the opportunity to learn the skill.

This sequence is an attempt to clarify how a treatment session can be organized, but it is not a linear model. The physical therapist may begin with a functional activity that the child is presently interested in and enjoys, such as playing with building blocks. She may place them and the child on the floor, a place where the child typically plays with them, which will provide an opportunity for him to weight bear and weight shift through his upper extremities. This activity may have an affect on his muscle tone, ROM, and strength. Prompting the child to reach to his limit of balance and assume or maintain certain postures that provide a means to accomplishing a task may also promote increases in ROM and postural control. Repeatedly stacking blocks, or encouraging movements to obtain more blocks to stack (such as rising to stance or climbing up a step to retrieve a block) can be a strengthening activity. Having the child solve the problem of obtaining more blocks (by hiding them under a container, or putting them in a clear container with a lid) can be used to promote learning. Educating the caregiver or parent on the environmental setup, handling, and goals of the activity while participating in this type of play may encourage repeated application of this type of exercise. Having the child help you to put the blocks away after you are finished playing will incorporate another functional activity into your treatment sequence. The ongoing process of examination and evaluation with regard to the barriers or facilitators of a functional task aids in the evaluation of the effectiveness of the intervention and treatment session. The information obtained can also assist in the evaluation of the frequency and duration of the services provided.

MAKING DECISIONS ON FREQUENCY AND DURATION OF SERVICES

Physical therapists, as well as pediatricians,[39] are frequently presented with the question of how much therapy is needed for a child and how long it will be provided. The ability of the physical therapist to make a reasonable recommendation on the frequency and duration of treatment depends on several variables that influence the decision on how frequently and for what duration physical therapy services are recommended. This may include such factors as the severity of the child's impairments and functional limitations, the potential for improvement in motor function, the availability of a willing and capable caregiver, the availability and use of assistive technology, as well as the effectiveness of physical therapy on the identified goals.[40–43]

Another factor to consider in this process is the significant attribute that differentiates a pediatric patient from an adult patient. In pediatrics, it is the parent that is the decision maker. Unlike an adult, a child is dependent on his parents for all of his needs. The parents have an invested emotional interest and ultimate responsibility for the care and growth of their child. The concerns, goals, resources, schedule, and availability of the parent play a larger role in affecting the frequency and duration of treatment for a pediatric patient. The parent makes the decisions regarding when and how the child will get to the therapy session, incorporating the physical therapy recommendations into the family's daily schedule, and carrying out the home exercise program, as well as paying for the services. On the other hand the acquisition and expression of motor skills is a significant aspect in the child's role as a son or daughter, and a significant reinforcer for the parents as well.

These physical, social, and emotional factors influence the frequency and duration of physical therapy services more than they do in the adult patient population. In the current environment of EBP and cost control, justification of frequency and duration based solely on the available published evidence would be very limited. With multiple factors being considered by various decision makers (the child, therapists, parents, administrators, third party payers, etc.), it is understandable that there is wide variation in this aspect of clinical decision making. Are the appropriate factors in this process being considered? Are they being weighted correctly? Is the most effective intervention being provided? Clarity and communication regarding the factors relating to frequency and duration decisions should aid in the process of developing an appropriate level of services for a child and his parents.

Frequency

In the process of determining the frequency of services the physical therapist should first identify what the family expects from physical therapy. It is imperative that the family is aware of physical therapy's benefits and limitations. The frequency and duration of treatment will be based on the clear and understandable goals and expectations set up at the initial meeting for this specific episode of care. Agreement with the parents concerning the established goals is necessary for a manageable plan of care that can be timely, and in the end, evaluated for its effectiveness.

Interventions should encourage a functional and active lifestyle of the child outside the clinical setting. The family's participation and understanding of their role, and how it affects the outcome of physical therapy interventions, is an important factor in the decision of how frequently and for what duration services are provided. Determining the frequency and duration of care is a dynamic process with several variables that can alter the course of treatment. These variables can include the availability of a willing and capable caregiver, the effectiveness of the available interventions on the identified impairments, financial constraints, or the availability and use of assistive technology. Identification of variables and their influence on the outcomes is important to keep in mind during the treatment process.

If frequent intervention is needed in order to effect a change, the ability and compliance of the caregiver is vital to the establishment of the frequency of physical therapy visits. If strengthening is the key to goal achievement and there is no willing and able caregiver, then the frequency of physical therapy may be 3 to 5 days a week. If a caregiver is willing and able, then 1 time a week may be all that is necessary to monitor and progress the program. If the caregiver is competent in the management of the child's condition and current program, then 1 time a month may be all that is needed to evaluate the effectiveness of the plan of care. The ability to work as a team is an important factor in determining the frequency as well as the duration of intervention.

POINT TO REMEMBER

Factors that Influence Frequency

Factors that influence frequency can include:

- severity of impairments
- functional limitations
- potential for improvement
- availability of a willing and able caregiver
- use of assistive technology
- effectiveness of interventions
- parent's values and priorities

Duration

The duration of the episode of care is determined by the goals established in the initial evaluation. If a child is not yet sitting independently and his goal is to walk independently, his duration of treatment can be expected to be longer than if the child is cruising along furniture. A well-established plan of care that outlines the expected sequence of events that would move the child to his established goals, using reasonable timelines for improvements in range, strength, motor skills, and function, would help to create a logical timeframe and assist in the identification of limitations or barriers to the attainment of the established goal.

It is also helpful to include the child's height and weight in the initial evaluation. During the episode of care, the factor of growth can be objectively measured. How it affects ROM, muscle strength, and function can also be more objectively discussed. Another factor that may not be given its appropriate level of importance is the cognitive ability of the child. Although this is a sensitive issue, and a controversial one for young children, it nonetheless is an important component in learning motor skills. The possibility that a cognitive limitation is impairing the acquisition of motor skills should not be ignored. This should be discussed with the parent, physician, and the child's teacher, if appropriate.

Changes in the family's situation, concerns, schedules, and priorities are also important when planning for the duration of treatment and in the evaluation of the outcome of therapy. Physical therapy interventions should be chosen to facilitate function in the child, which should be lifelong in its duration. Also, factors that may influence the frequency or duration of services should be identified and monitored throughout the episode of care. Factors such as an illness in the child, the consistent availability of a caregiver, or compliance with the home program may significantly impact the intended outcome of services. Management of the duration of the episode of care should be monitored through appropriate and

objective documentation, which can be used to educate the parents or other team members, monitor progress toward the intended goals, and aid in determining the effectiveness of the interventions provided throughout the episode of care.

POINT TO REMEMBER

Factors that Influence Duration

Factors that influence duration can include:

- established goals
- efficiency in the delivery and assessment of the effectiveness of the intervention
- compliance with recommendation
- changes in the family's situation
- change in the child's health
- family's financial resources

DOCUMENTATION

Showing evidence that physical therapy interventions make a significant difference in a child's acquisition of developmental or motor skills is a challenge for the profession of physical therapy today. The first step in this process begins with the ability of the physical therapist to accurately observe the child and then objectively document what was observed.

Documentation is an essential component of practice in physical therapy and is a key factor in the child (patient) management process. By definition, documentation is any entry into a child's record that identifies that care or a service has been provided.[44] Documentation occurs at every visit or encounter and is used to record a child's performance during a particular treatment session and his response to interventions during the episode of care. This documentation should contain information regarding the effectiveness of the physical therapy services during the session and justification for the services rendered. Also reflected in this information should be the rate of goal or skill acquisition. Many of the services provided by the physical therapist are aimed at making quantitative and qualitative changes in a child's ability to move and interact within his environment. Capturing and communicating this information is essential to the success of physical therapy programs, outcome research, and efficacy studies in clinical practice.

In order to promote this success, written information should be clear, concise, and organized, and it should reflect current practice. Documentation, when used to justify an intervention or as evidence toward outcomes, requires a high standard of reliability and validity.

Additionally, it has to be understood by all members of the health care team associated with the management of the child's care. Today, it is not uncommon for physical therapy services, in some settings, to be delivered by more than one physical therapist or physical therapist assistant. In addition, other caregivers will implement specific strategies or activities in daily routines at home or at school. In order to promote consistency this should involve the use of understandable terminology, clear communication, and collaboration among all the members of the team, including the family. The Guide defines terms commonly used in physical therapy to assist in this process (Box 1-4). The APTA also has published guidelines on the use of documentation[44]. (Additional terms and information can be accessed in the Guide or through the APTA web site.)

Today, physical therapists and administrators are working in an environment of regulations and the need to justify the costs of services, trying to balance cost and quality effectively. The participation of the physical therapist is crucial in this process to provide meaningful information on the child's current status, the projection for future visits, and the rate of progress that the child is making in the plan of care.

Clear documentation of efficacy related to the variable parameters of therapy continues to be elusive.[39] Although objective tests and measurements are available, one area in need of clarification and uniformity in documentation is with terminology. The following is an example.

> Jennifer is a 4-year-old girl who requires a moderate amount of assistance to transfer from her bed (supine) to standing. She also demonstrates poor balance in stance, is unable to ascend stairs without using a handrail, and has poor coordination in her upper extremity movements, during her self-feeding tasks.

What does it mean when it takes a moderate level of assistance to complete this task? It may depend on the caregiver's definition of moderate assistance. According to the University of Iowa Level of Assistance Scale with Associated Ordinal Grades this would mean that two points of contact are needed for the safe performance of the activity[45] (Box 1-5). Another scale, the Functional

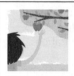

BOX 1-4
The Guide Terminology

Episode of care–All physical therapy services that are (i) provided by a physical therapist, (ii) provided in an unbroken sequence, and (iii) related to the physical therapy interventions for a given condition or problem or related to a request from the patient and/or client, family, or other health care provider.

Episode of maintenance–A series of occasional clinical, educational, and administrative services related to maintenance of current function.

Episode of prevention–A series of occasional clinical, educational, and administrative services related to prevention; the promotion of health, wellness, and fitness; and the preservation of optimal function.

Discharge–The process of ending physical therapy services that have been provided during a single episode of care, when the anticipated goals and expected outcomes have been achieved.

Discontinue–The process of ending physical therapy services that have been provided during a single episode of care, when (i) The patient/client, caregiver, or legal guardian declines to continue intervention; (ii) the patient/client is unable to continue to progress toward the anticipated goals and expected outcomes because of medical or psychosocial complications or because financial and/or insurance resources have been expended; or (iii) the physical therapist determines that the patient/client will no longer benefit from physical therapy.

Adapted from American Physical Therapy Association. *Guide to Physical Therapist Practice*, 2nd ed. Rev. American Physical Therapy Association; 2003:678–679.

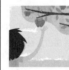

BOX 1-5
Levels of Assistance

Independent:	No assistance or supervision is necessary to safely perform the activity with or without assistive devices or modifications.
Minimal:	One point of contact is necessary for the safe performance of the activity, including helping with the application of the assistive device, orthotic, or prosthetic and/or the stabilization of the assistive device, or 25% effort on the caregiver's part is needed to complete the task.
Moderate:	Two points of contact are necessary (by one or more people) for the safe performance of the activity, or 50% effort on the caregiver's part is needed to complete the task.
Maximal:	Three points of contact are necessary (by one or more people) for the safe performance of the activity, or 75% effort on the caregiver's part is needed to complete the task.
Dependent:	The patient is totally dependent and does not assist.

Adapted from: Shields R, et al. An acute care physical therapy clinical practice database for outcome research. *Phys Ther*. 1994;74:463–470.

Independence Measure (FIM)[46] interprets moderate assistance as requiring the child to assist in 50% to 74% of the effort to complete the task. Gauging the effort provided by the child is more subjective than using points of contact and could lead to various reports from different providers or caregivers on the amount of assistance provided or required to complete a task.

In the measurement of balance, a physical therapist may determine whether various systems are impaired, but there are no standard definitions used to quantify the degree of impairment. Although many tools have been developed to accurately assess balance in children, results from a survey of the Section on Pediatrics of the APTA[47] suggest that these tools are not commonly used. The survey's purpose was to explore preferences of pediatric physical therapists for evaluation and treatment of balance dysfunction in children. It appears that a majority of physical therapists prefer to rely on nonstandardized testing of balance, based on results of the survey.[47] Researchers propose that physical therapists do not or cannot take the time necessary for longer standardized tests. Standardized tests for balance may not be appropriate for every evaluation. A similar survey-based study regarding balance evaluation methods concluded that the most commonly used method to assess balance in the clinic was a good/fair/poor rating scale.[48] Grading a child's balance by using nonstandardized functional balance grades based on subjective definitions can lead to entirely different interpretations from one physical therapist to another.[49] The above reasons emphasize the need to use an objective, clinically applicable terminology that can effectively communicate impairments in balance in lieu of a standardized test. Box 1-6 provides one example of functional definitions for a level of impairment in a child's balance.

Historically, the physical therapy examination of coordination occurs through direct observation of the child with an evaluation of the quality of movement performed during a task. In the upper extremity, this can include coordination tests such as the finger-to-nose test, finger opposition, or alternately flexing and extending the wrist. In the lower extremity, the heel-to-shin test, alternate dorsiflexion, plantarflexion of the ankle, or marching in place can be used to examine coordination. From these observations the physical therapist is able to determine if the child's coordination is impaired. Does the impairment in coordination affect the child's ability to function? Box 1-7 provides one example of functional definitions for a level of impairment in a child's coordination.

These functional definitions of impairments in balance and coordination are one way of clarifying the terminology used in clinical practice. Clarity is the first step in the process of evaluating the effectiveness of the interventions provided. What is done with the data and information collected and how they are managed are also

BOX 1-6
Definitions of Impairment in Balance

The following definitions can be separated into static and dynamic balance. If the child's balance is evaluated using an assistive device, it should be noted in the documentation. The degree of impairment is based on the reported frequency of loss of balance.

Normal: Able to maintain static and dynamic positions against maximal resistance. Displays age-appropriate balance reactions. Independent in balance activities without limiting functional ability. Able to weight shift in all directions without limitations.

Mild: Able to maintain static positions against moderate resistance. Independent in dynamic balance activities but experiences an occasional loss of balance, without consequence. Loss of balance does not occur daily. May limit some functional ability. No support needed for routine activities. Occasionally uses an assistive device for some activities. Weight shift limitations are evident.

Moderate: Requires supervision or contact guarding during static and dynamic activities secondary to daily loss of balance. Balance deficit limits functional ability. Needs an assistive device to perform activities safely.

Severe: Requires physical assistance to maintain static and/or dynamic balance. Unable to move trunk from midline without some level of assistance secondary to loss of balance.

Absent: No evidence of any balance reactions and/or responses in either static or dynamic positions.

vital to this process. Utilizing what was documented is just as important as capturing information clearly and objectively.

Utilization of Daily Documentation

At each visit, documentation is required that should be organized in some consistent format. Organizing information into subjective, objective, assessment, and plan (SOAP notes) is one way of structuring that information. The SOAP note format separates the documented information into subjective information, objective information, the overall assessment of the current interventions, and a plan for the future.

Subjective information should be limited to that which is relevant to the plan of care, or which could have a significant impact on the treatment plan. Two key

BOX 1-7
Measurement in Impairment in Coordination

For the extremity tested: Based on the patient's age and the degree to which the impairment limits performance of the extremity in ADLs.

Normal: Able to demonstrate age-appropriate recip-rocal movement patterns at the expected speed and rhythm. Does not limit functional activities.

Mild: Able to demonstrate age-appropriate recip-rocal movement patterns at a decreased speed and/or rhythm. Does not significantly limit daily functional activities, but may alter the quality of movement.

Moderate: Able to demonstrate age-appropriate recip-rocal movement patterns at a decreased speed and/or rhythm. Limits daily functional activities.

Severe: Attempts to perform but cannot complete age-appropriate reciprocal movement pat-terns. Significantly limits functional activities.

Absent: No evidence of any ability to demonstrate reciprocal movement patterns.

points in the subjective area are the parent's report on the current health status of the child since the last visit and the effectiveness of any interventions from the last visit. Also included are the current behavior of the child and any information that may influence the child's perfor-mance in the treatment session today.

Objective information is the core of the clinical note. Objective information should clearly demon-strate the changes in the child's status as it relates to the established plan of care. When using a narrative format, the objective measures are listed as they relate to the goals stated in the initial evaluation. This may require repeated reference to the initial evaluation. A more efficient format may be to compile the goals and objective measures onto one form or flow chart. This would organize the objective information so that the therapist "at a glance" could determine the patient's progress toward the stated goals. It eliminates redun-dancy and can be used to estimate the rate of progress toward the goals. Flow charts, without additional explanation, do not meet the requirements of docu-mentation according to the APTA, but they are an effective means of organizing objective information in the child's record.

Assessment of the patient's response to treatment should also include an assessment of his progress in the overall plan of care. Interpretations of the objective measures and the rate at which the patient is progress-

ing should be noted. Referring back to the previous example:

Jennifer has improved in her transition skills, requiring minimal assistance to negotiate the stairs with the use of the handrail. Her moderate impairment in upper extremity coordination remains unchanged since her initial evalua-tion. She has met 66% (2 of 3) of the goals stated in her plan of care.

Noting that the level of impairment in coordination has not improved in the last 2 weeks should trigger an assessment of the effectiveness of the current interven-tions for this condition. It also brings up the following questions: (a) How long should a physical therapist allow a child not to make progress before assessing the effectiveness of the intervention? and (b) How often should the intervention be changed before it is deter-mined that the child will no longer benefit from it? These are pertinent questions that are facilitated through clear documentation.

After the assessment, a plan should be developed to include what is expected at the next treatment session. This plan provides the child and physical therapist with expec-tations for the next session, and may save time at the beginning of the treatment session. By reviewing the previ-ous session's documentation, the physical therapist can see what was planned for this visit. This review aids in plan-ning by making sure that the recommendations or trials of new interventions take place as discussed, which promotes an efficient delivery of services. The timely delivery of ser-vices will affect the duration of the episode of care.

The **outcome** or result of the provision of physical therapy services should be viewed in the context of the established episode of care. Were the goals identified at the initial evaluation met? If they were, is the child now functioning at the expected level for his age or ability? Are there current medical or health issues that would limit the child from progressing further at this point? Are there activities in place to foster continued progress as the child matures? If goals were not met, why not? What rea-son can be given for not meeting a goal set at the initial evaluation? Was the goal inappropriate? Was the inter-vention ineffective? Was there cooperation and compli-ance with daily exercise programs and activities? After the initiation of therapy, was the identified goal no longer a priority for the family? It is also important to note the difference between the terms "discharge" and "discontin-uation of services" (Box 1-4). Discharge occurs when the expected outcomes have been met. Discontinuation occurs when the parent or guardian declines further ser-vices, the physical therapist determines that the child can no longer benefit from services, or the child is unable to continue with services because of health or other reasons. These definitions can provide more clarity to the outcome of the physical therapy services, identifying all of the fac-tors that influence the episode of care.

Episode of Maintenance

The discontinuation of physical therapy services can be frightening for some families. Remember Parson's assumptions: The family seeks out competent help to make the child well, and now this episode of care is over. For a child with an acute injury, such as a broken leg, or one who has undergone a posterior spinal fusion to correct scoliosis, the completion of physical therapy is indicative of progress and a return to relatively typical family functioning. For a child with a chronic condition, such as cerebral palsy, or one who has had a spinal cord injury, the completion of therapy may be viewed as acceptance of a level of functioning that is not optimal or anticipated. Families may resist, or seek additional therapy elsewhere. This situation highlights the importance of education and where an episode of maintenance may be applicable. A child with a lifelong disability may require physical therapy throughout his life to optimize his level of functioning as he develops and changes with time. Providing the family with a list of signs or symptoms that should prompt them to call the physical therapist for services is helpful in this process. This list could include topics such as the maintenance of the child's current level of functioning, utilization of assistive technology, or proper fit of orthotics. Providing a family with this information, and how to initiate therapy services in the future, can provide a better understanding of the utilization of physical therapy services, not only during the episode of care, but also in the maintenance of a child's current level of functioning and in the promotion of a child's general health (Box 1-8).

Evidence-Based Practice

Are the physical therapy interventions effective? Is the physical therapist providing the most beneficial interven-

---

BOX 1-8
An Example of Parent Information Regarding an Episode of Maintenance

1. Lauren will maintain her current level of fitness evident by her ability to walk and stay with her group or family on community outings.
2. Lauren will adhere to her home exercise program and progress as advised.
3. Lauren will maintain her ability to negotiate the stairs at her school allowing her to move in a timely manner between classes.
4. Lauren will continue to use her AFO daily without any irritation to her skin.

If Lauren has any questions or difficulty with the above recommendations, please contact me at the number provided.
Professionally,
Pam Evans, PT

---

tion for the identified impairment? Is the optimal amount of services being provided to produce a positive outcome? These questions can be challenging, yet are necessary with the ever increasing scrutiny and questioning by payers and policy makers on the efficacy of the interventions provided by health care providers, not only physical therapists. It has become increasingly necessary for the physical therapist to be knowledgeable on the effectiveness of current interventions, to be objective and clear in her documentation, and to self-evaluate the delivery of interventions provided to children and their families.

The application of **evidence-based medicine** (EBM) according to Straus[50] is composed of four factors: (i) clinical expertise, (ii) evidence from the literature, (iii) the patient's values, and (iv) the patient's unique circumstances. It is a combination of the utilization of published research evidence and clinical expertise. Evidence from the literature has taken the forefront on EBM recently and for valid reasons. The use of valid and reliable tests and measurements in the evaluation process and in subsequent reports aids in the evaluation of the effectiveness of the interventions. Are the interventions that are being applied having a positive effect on the identified impairment? Are there valid studies that show the intervention's effectiveness? How does the physical therapist know if the intervention is effective with her patient? Objective and clear documentation of the individual child's response to a particular intervention is a starting point for self-evaluation on the effectiveness of a particular intervention for that child.

The physical therapist also has the option of accessing published literature that addresses the use of the specific intervention with the particular patient population that is being treated (Box 1-9 selected databases). According to a study done by Jette and colleagues,[51] who surveyed a random sample of physical therapists who were members of the APA, a large majority agreed that the use of EBP was necessary and helpful in their clinical practice, and that the quality of patient care was better when evidence was used. The biggest barrier to implementing EBP was the lack of time. Making the reading of at least one or two research articles each month a priority can do much to add to a physical therapist's professional knowledge and EBP. When reviewing the literature, the physical therapist should also be aware of the inference made when applying results from the literature to clinical practice. The physical therapist should examine the study done and evaluate its appropriateness for her particular needs. Questions such as: Are the tests and measurements used appropriate? Are they reliable and valid? Does the application of the interventions make sense to me? Are the interventions available to me? How similar is the population studied to my patient? Having evidence in the literature is only one part of EBP. Does the intervention coincide with the values of the family, child (patient), and their individual circumstance? Therapeutic

BOX 1-9
Some Databases for Evidence-Based Practice

Hooked on Evidence
http://www.hookedonevidence.com/
The APTA's database containing current research on the effectiveness of physical therapy interventions.

PEDro
http://www.pedro.fhs.usyd.edu.au/index.html
PEDro is the Physiotherapy Evidence Database. It provides access to bibliographic details and abstracts of randomized controlled trials, systematic reviews, and evidence-based clinical practice guidelines in physical therapy.

Medline
www.ncbi.nlm.nih.gov/PubMed
A service of the National Library of Medicine and the National Institutes of Health.

Netting the Evidence
http://www.sheffield.ac.uk/~scharr/ir/netting/
A site designed to facilitate evidence-based health care by providing support and access to helpful organizations and useful learning resources.

Agency for Healthcare and Research Quality (AHRQ)
http://www.ahrq.gov/
United States Department of Health and Human Services. AHRQ site that contains links to clinical information and government findings on EBP, outcomes, effectiveness, effective health care, and more.

Center for Evidence-Based Medicine
http://www.cebm.utoronto.ca/
The goal of this web site is to help develop, disseminate, and evaluate resources that can be used to practice and teach EBM in undergraduate, postgraduate, and continuing education for health care professionals from a variety of clinical disciplines.

horseback riding, aquatic therapy, and certain positioning devices can be time consuming and unique in their application. A family may not value these interventions in lieu of established family routines or activities. In the case of hospice, a family may have come to terms with the palliative care approach for a child; therefore, the application of strengthening exercises may not be appropriate or of value, even if the literature shows that exercises can improve function.

Clinical expertise is another factor to consider. Certain manual therapy techniques, fabrication of orthotics, aquatic therapy techniques, and sensory integration intervention, for example, require specialized training beyond entry-level education. Acquiring these skills adds to the physical therapist's clinical expertise and repertoire of readily available interventions. Clinical

expertise also includes the knowledge of the role of the physical therapist in the particular setting. Understanding the laws that influence the delivery of services, the reason why physical therapy is utilized in the particular setting and the role and abilities of other people in this setting, maximizes the appropriate utilization of physical therapy services. It is the blend of all of these factors that promotes EBP.

POINT TO REMEMBER

Components of Evidence-Based Medicine and Practice

Clinical expertise
The patient's values
The patient's circumstances
Evidence from the literature

The following is an example from the literature of the use of evidence in clinical practice:

> In the initial examination of a child with cerebral palsy, ROM, functional motor skills, and the extent of the disability may be examined. The tests and measurements chosen for the examination were the following: goniometric measurements (a measurement of impairment), the GMFM (a measurement of functional limitation), and the FIM for Children (WeeFIM; a measurement of disability). The psychometric properties of these tests were reviewed for their appropriateness for this child. The information was gathered from a variety of sources that were available to the physical therapist. For the literature search, the user manual for the standardized tests, published articles (obtained through Medline and the *Physical Therapy Journal*), and The Guide to Physical Therapists Practice (CD version. Pub Med.) were used.

Much of the literature on the psychometric properties of goniometric measurement using a universal goniometer (UG) is with adult patients. Content validity is based more on the examiner's knowledge of anatomy and the anatomic markers used when aligning the goniometer.[52] Criterion-related validity using radiographs shows a high correlation in the extremities and cervical spine, but variable correlation when measuring the lumbar spine.[52] Additional studies found the criterion validity of a UG with a parallelogram goniometer to be $r = 0.975$–0.987, depending on what movement is being measured.[53] Studies looking at the construct validity of ROM have been done and show a correlation between ROM impairments and functional limitations.[52] An additional study by MacDermid and colleagues[54] looked at the construct validity of pediatric passive range of motion and pain variables. The authors found a correlation coefficient of

$r = 0.79$–0.94 between a movement diagram for shoulder rotation and goniometric measurement. Studies that look at the reliability of goniometric measurements vary in their results, depending on the patient population and the joint being studied. Intra-rater reliability has been found to be higher than inter-rater reliability. The standard deviation when using a UG on adult patients has been documented as 5 degrees.[52] Few studies that look at the reliability of goniometric measurements in children with disabilities come to a different conclusion. In a study by Stuberg[55] variations of 10 to 15 degrees were found in inter-rater measurements of children with cerebral palsy. Intra-rater reliability was found to be acceptable for specific motions of the lower extremity. This review of the literature on ROM measurements taken with a UG concludes that it should be done in a consistent manner by the same examiner. Changes of ± 10 to 15 degrees over time in a child with cerebral palsy may not signify a meaningful change.

The GMFM is a standardized observational criterion-referenced test that evaluates (on a 4-point Likert scale) the movement of a child with cerebral palsy. It was designed to assess how much of an item a child can accomplish and to measure the change in gross motor function over time. A 5-year-old child with typical motor abilities would be expected to be able to complete all of the items contained in the test.[30] Thirteen physical therapists from two pediatric rehabilitation centers in Canada were included in this process to establish content validity.[30] Construct validity of the GMFM was studied by Bjornson and colleagues,[56] who found a strong correlation between the measurements of change by the GMFM and the external criterion of video-based evaluations. The authors of this study go on to present various studies that have demonstrated (i) a correlation with the GMFM and muscle power in the lower extremities, and (ii) the relationship of GMFM scores to cognitive levels, intensity of therapy, and gait velocity. Russell and colleagues[57] studied the concurrent validity (a form of criterion-based validity) by correlating the total GMFM score with video-based evaluations ($r = 0.82$), the therapist's judgment ($r = 0.65$), and the parent's judgment ($r = 0.54$). This study also concluded that the GMFM would be responsive to both positive and negative changes in a child. Reliability studies concluded that repeated testing can be done consistently with the inter-rater reliability of intraclass correlation coefficient (ICC) $= 0.99$ and the intra-rater reliability of ICC $= 0.99$.[30] In another study by Bjornson and colleagues,[58] the authors described the test-retest reliability of the GMFM within a 1-week time period. The results, in addition to supporting the GMFM's reliability, found that children with cerebral palsy exhibit stable gross motor skills during repeated measurement. This understanding is necessary in order to differentiate between true clinical changes and normal variability in a child's performance. This review of the literature on the GMFM concludes that the use of this tool to evaluate the functional motor abilities, and to quantify the change in motor function in a child with cerebral palsy, would be appropriate.

The WeeFIM is a criterion-referenced test that systematically measures a child's disability and the level of assistance required in daily activities. The test was developed for children with developmental delays and disabilities. The test can be administered to children without disabilities from 6 months of age to 7 years, and children up to 18 years old who have a cognitive impairment, with a mental age <7 years.[59] The ICC value for total content validity, including areas of help needed and time, was determined to be $r = 0.95$, $r = 0.88$, respectively.[60] Several studies have compared the WeeFIM to other standardized tests for children to assess concurrent validity. The results ranged from moderate to excellent correlation, with the Amount of Assistance Questionnaire (AAQ) demonstrating an $r = 0.91$ in all subscales and total score.[61] The WeeFIM and the PEDI are the most commonly used measures of functional performance in children. The PEDI, as noted in the section on the GMFM, is one of the two tests commonly used in pediatrics that have demonstrated reliability and validity in response to change in children. In a study by Ziviani and colleagues,[62] the concurrent validity of the WeeFIM to the PEDI was studied when used with children with developmental disabilities and acquired brain injury. Spearman correlation coefficients between the two tests were >0.88 for self-care, transportation (locomotion), and communication (social function). The reliability of the WeeFIM was examined by Ottenbacher and colleagues[63] who found that ICCs for individual test items ranged from 0.90 to 0.99. The ICC for the six subscales ranged from 0.94 for social cognition to 0.99 for transfers and locomotion. The results of equivalence reliability testing showed an ICC for WeeFIM totals of 0.98, which suggest that the WeeFIM can be administered in alternate ways (face to face or by telephone) with high confidence that the results will still be trustworthy.[63] Statistical responsiveness was high up to 8 years of age, with greatest values from 2 to 5 years old (ICC > 0.80).[64] Test-retest reliability ranged from ICC $= 0.97$ to ICC $= 0.99$ for total scores.[65] Inter-rater reliability had an ICC of 0.98,[65] with $r = 0.80$–0.96. This review of the literature on the WeeFIM shows that the use of this tool to evaluate the level of a child's disability and to track the changes in his level of care (assistance) needed over time would be appropriate.

From this activity the physical therapist can conclude that the analysis of changes in the GMFM and WeeFIM would be appropriate to evaluate the child's changes in motor function and level of disability during this episode of care. Changes in ROM measurements may or may not be as meaningful.

C A S E   S T U D Y

Patient/Client Management Using the Guide Format

Patient/client's name: Tricia
Medical diagnosis: Closed head injury
Physical therapy setting: Outpatient

EXAMINATION

History

Tricia is a 17-year-old Caucasian girl who sustained a closed head injury 4 months ago as a result of an accident while riding an all terrain vehicle (ATV) that resulted in damage to her cerebral cortex. Prior to her accident she attended the local high school where she was on the honor roll and participated in the school's volleyball and track programs. She is also a member of her church youth group. Tricia lives with her parents and two younger siblings in a split entry style home here in town.

Her mother reports that her development has been typical. Tricia has no significant past medical history and has been a very healthy and active adolescent. Currently she is taking oral Baclofen and a multivitamin.

Tricia plans on going to college after she completes her high school education. At present, she reports that she is independent with her activities of daily living (ADL), requiring additional time to complete. She requires the assistance of another person to perform the necessary mobility functions to utilize the community and school environment.

Current Condition (Chief Complaint): Tricia reports her main problems at this time are the following: inability to transfer from her wheelchair independently, decreased wheelchair mobility for long distances or when she needs to go fast, decreased ability to step up a step in school, decreased walking speed and distance making it difficult to move around the classroom.

Systems Review

Cardiovascular and/or Pulmonary:

Heart rate (HR)	82 bpm
Blood pressure (BP)	124/74
Respiratory (RR)	12 bpm
Edema	Absent

Integumentary: Unremarkable

Musculoskeletal: Tricia is hemiplegic on the right. Gross ROM is within functional limits (WFL). Gross strength is WFL on the left, decreased on the right. She is 5' 8" tall and weighs 134 lbs.

Neuromuscular: Tricia requires a roller walker to ambulate. Gait is slow and unsteady. She requires verbal cues to coordinate the movement of the walker and advancement of lower extremities. She demonstrates a step-to gait pattern with her left lower extremity; the hip joint is internally rotated. Impairments in her balance and coordination are noted. Transfers require a moderate level of assistance upon observation.

Communication, Affect, Cognition, Learning Style: Tricia's affect is impaired. She tends to laugh at inappropriate times and situations. Her language is impaired in speed. She is oriented × 3. Tricia reports that she learns best through demonstration and written information.

Tests and Measures

Aerobic Capacity and Endurance: Tricia is able to propel her wheelchair 100 feet in 90 seconds, with several verbal cues to go in a straight line. She is able to ambulate 100 feet in 3 minutes with a standard walker and minimum assistance to keep the walker moving forward in a straight path. She is able to stand with one hand assist for up to 10 minutes before she reports fatigue.

Anthropometrics: Body mass index (BMI) = 20.4 lbs/in^2 (normal)

Assistive and Adaptive Devices: Tricia uses an AFO on the left, which has an articulating ankle joint. She uses a roller walker to assist with ambulation and a folding manual wheelchair with a planar seat system for long distances. These devices fit appropriately at this time. Tricia uses a shower chair when bathing.

Circulation: Capillary refill time in her toes is <3 seconds (normal).

Cognition: By report of her teacher, Tricia is functioning at the fifth grade level in reading, math, English, and sciences. She demonstrates an impairment in her ability to identify numbers with three units, and reads very slowly. She also speaks more slowly than expected. She is enrolled in a special education program at the local high school. She is scheduled for a visual perceptual test next month.

Cranial and Nerve Integrity: Not impaired.

Environmental, Home, and Work Barriers: Tricia lives in a split entry house with seven steps to enter with a hand railing on the left. There are five steps to negotiate after you are in the front door, which also has a hand railing on the left. There is access to the house from a back door, which is attached to a deck with two steps to enter. There is a hand railing on both sides of the steps. A 12-foot ramp has been added to allow Tricia to enter by being pushed up the ramp in her wheelchair. In the house, her bathroom and bedroom are on the first floor. Her bathroom has a walk-in shower with a small threshold, by parent report. The first floor of the house is carpeted with hard wood floors in the kitchen and dining area. The home environment is accessible by parent report.

The high school she is attending is a two-story building with an elevator. Class schedule requires a change of classes within 2 minutes. This will require her to travel a distance of up to 400 feet, at times, depending on her schedule.

Ergonomics and Body Mechanics: Tricia has difficulty in transferring from supine to sitting. She requires minimum assistance to transfer from side lying to sitting. Mom reports that at home Tricia will roll out of bed, onto her knees, and then transfer into stance using the bed for support. In sit-to-stand transfers, Tricia does not weight shift forward sufficiently without assistance of another person.

Gait, Locomotion, and Balance: Tricia ambulates with a roller walker. Her gait pattern on the left shows a decrease in pelvic trunk dissociation, a decrease in step length, a decrease in stance phase, and an increase in internal rotation of the hip joint during swing-through. Her left foot demonstrates a toe–heel pattern with the foot in supination. During the examination, Tricia walked 100 feet requiring physical assist to maintain her balance three times.

Joint Integrity and Mobility: Active ROM of her right hemibody is within functional limits. Her left hemibody was WFL with the following exceptions:

	PROM	AROM
Shoulder flexion	180	150
Shoulder abduction	180	130
Shoulder internal rotation	70	55
Shoulder external rotation	90	70
Forearm supination	70	30
Elbow extension	−10	−10
Wrist extension	50	50
Hip flexion	120	30
Hip extension	30	0
Hip internal rotation	45	10
Hip external rotation	45	10
Knee extension	0	−15
Knee flexion	125	100
Ankle dorsiflexion	10	−5
Ankle plantarflexion	50	30
Inversion	15	0
Eversion	15	0

Motor Function: Tricia demonstrates impairments in motor control in her left hemibody, especially noted in her inability to move through her available ROM, stabilize, and demonstrate controlled mobility in the developmental transition from side lying to stance, and in the decreased efficiency with ambulation. This impairs her from functioning with adequate speed and efficiency.

Muscle Performance: Muscle strength in her right hemibody is 5/5 for all gross muscle groups of her upper and lower extremities. Manual Muscle Testing (MMT) of the left is deferred secondary to the presence of muscle spasticity. Functional strength in the left upper extremity is noted by the following:

Able to touch the back of your head	Able
Able to touch your low back	Unable
Able to fully supinate your forearm	Unable
Able to oppose your thumb to fingers	Able
Able to independently stand from sitting	Unable
Able to step up a 6-inch step	Unable

Reflex Integrity: Deep tendon reflexes (DTRs) on the right for biceps, triceps, knee, and ankle jerks were +2. DTRs on the

left for biceps and triceps jerks were +2, and for knee and ankle jerks were +3.

Self Care and Home Management: Tricia is able to isolate tip-to-tip opposition with each hand. She has limited supination on the left, which does require her to compensate with increased shoulder external rotation. She is able to meet her own hygiene needs, bathe, and dress, which she completes in 45 minutes, by report. She is independent in self-feeding with appropriate utensils.

Sensory integrity to light touch and sharp–dull discrimination is intact with the exception of her left foot, which shows a decrease in light touch and sharp–dull discrimination in the entire foot. The pattern of impairment does not follow any peripheral nerve or dermatome pattern.

EVALUATION

Impairments: Tricia presents with impairments in her cognitive function, language fluency, active ROM with spasticity (Ashworth +2), decreased trunk strength with impairment in trunk co-contraction and rotation, impairments in transitional skills, and a decreased endurance in ambulation. She is impaired in the sensory integrity in her left foot. Moderate impairments in balance and coordination were observed.

Functional Limitations: Her clinical presentation shows functional limitations in bed mobility, transitional skills from sit to stand, ambulation, stair negotiation, and wheelchair propulsion. These limit her participation in school, sport, and community activities.

DIAGNOSIS

Diagnostic Pattern: Impaired motor function and sensory integrity associated with a nonprogressive disorder of the CNS acquired in adolescence
Rationale: Tricia is most limited by her lack of motor control and motor function secondary to an injury to the CNS, which was acquired when she was an adolescent.

PROGNOSIS

Plan of care.

1. Tricia will demonstrate the ability to transition from supine to sitting independently in order to improve in her bed mobility and prepare to transfer out of bed each morning.
2. Tricia will be able to transition from sit to stand independently in order to transfer to other surfaces and to access her home and school environments more efficiently.
3. Tricia will increase in her ability to propel her wheelchair over level surfaces to 200 feet in 90 seconds maintaining a straight path of travel in order to efficiently move from one classroom to the adjoining classroom during school, and to keep up with her peer and family members when on community outings.
4. Tricia will demonstrate the ability to step up seven 6-inch steps with the assist of the handrail in order to be able to negotiate steps at home, at school, and in the community.

Expected range of visits for this episode of care given this Guide Practice Pattern is 10 to 60 visits. (Note: The course of treatment and range of visits is anticipated for 80% of the patients/clients who are classified into this pattern, during a single episode of care.)[15]

INTERVENTIONS

Coordination, Communication, and Documentation: Contact the school's special education program to coordinate with any physical education or related services being offered.

Contact physician who prescribed Baclofen to coordinate Tricia's physical performance with any changes in her medication regimen. Also consult regarding impairment in sensation in her left foot.

Patient/Client–Related Instruction: Instruct mother and other relevant family members in proper lifting and body mechanics to assist with transfers. Instruct in proper foot care with left foot secondary to impairment in sensory integrity. Demonstrate and provide Tricia written information regarding the exercises and motor activities that she is to practice.

Procedural Interventions

Therapeutic Exercise:

1. Left hip extension exercises in side lying with no resistance added. Tricia shows a 30° lag in hip extension. Hip extension strength is key in promoting one-legged stance in gait and to transfer from sit to stand.
2. Left hip flexion exercise in side lying with no resistance added.
3. Reversed chaining, moving from left side prop on extended upper extremity to side-lying. This exercise is done to promote ROM and strength of the upper extremity and trunk to aid with bed mobility.
4. Left terminal knee extension exercises without resistance. Tricia shows a lag of 15°. Incorporate eccentric exercises and Active Assistive Range of Motion exercises (AAROM) into this program to promote terminal knee extension to aid in transfers and gait.

Functional Training: Self Care (Home)

5. Perform sit-to-stand transfers cueing for proper weight shift and movement into stance. From stance return to sit, slowly utilizing eccentric control. Work daily on transfers from bed to stand, couch to stand, bath chair to stand.
6. Once in stance, perform step-up exercises beginning with 1-inch step; progress as tolerated.

Functional Training: Community and Work

7. When visual perceptual issues are clarified, work on propelling wheelchair in a straight path. Decreasing the need to correct for deviations will decrease time to go from one point to another. Work on shoulder extension and flexion muscle strength and bilateral symmetric use of upper extremities. Family may encourage Tricia to propel her wheelchair up the ramp at home. This will add resistance to wheelchair propulsion and work on improving this skill. Distance and time can begin with those

related to her classroom locations. If Tricia has math class in a room 30 feet away from her homeroom, work on improving her efficiency over 30 feet.

8. Stand in walker and work on gait pattern. Incorporate manual techniques and cues to increase rotation of pelvis and trunk. Have Tricia step forward to a target on the floor to help in increasing step length and hip external rotation during swing-through. Work on weight shift to improve stance phase on left. Then work on walking faster, using audio feedback to maintain a rhythm in her gait.

Determining Frequency and Duration The educational interventions (patient/client-related instructions) would be reasonably expected to take two or three visits: one to instruct, one to follow-up, and an additional follow-up visit, if necessary (three visits). In the procedural interventions, seven incorporate strengthening exercises, which should be done at minimum three times per week for at least 6 weeks (24 visits). The last intervention incorporates motor learning and motor control. Motor learning activities require daily practice, which is ideally incorporated into a home exercise program. Teaching these activities may take a week (five visits), then periodic follow-up to make sure that they are being executed appropriately, one time a week for 4 weeks (four visits).

The longest duration is 6 weeks. Frequency could be five times per week for 1 week then three times per week for 5 weeks, for a total of 20 visits. With an able and willing caregiver, the frequency could be three times per week for 1 week, then two times per week for 3 weeks, then one time per week for 2 weeks (for a total of 11 visits). Both of these visit numbers fall within the reasonably expected range of visits that 80% of the patients classified into this Practice Pattern would need to achieve the goals created for this episode of care. The availability of partners in this process and the continued health and cooperation of the patient are important aspects of this prescription.

OUTCOMES

After this episode of care, it is anticipated that Tricia will be able to more fully participate in her family life by transferring independently from her bed into her wheelchair, and by negotiating the steps to get into her home. Tricia will also increase in her mobility speed using her wheelchair in school and in the community, allowing her to efficiently move from one classroom or place to another, in a reasonable amount of time.

Reflection Questions

1. What are some of the typical activities associated with college life? Identify the impact of the impairments and functional limitations identified in the examination with Tricia's ability to participate in college life.
2. Prior to her injury, Tricia was involved in the high school sports of track and volleyball. Considering her impairments, how could she continue to participate in organized sports? As a physical therapist, what do you see as your role in this process?

3. For this episode of care, 20 physical therapy visits are anticipated. The health insurance that covers Tricia allows for only 10 physical therapy visits. The family has no other source of funding. How would this affect the established treatment plan?

SUMMARY

The science and art of physical therapy, as well as its professional roots, are connected to the polio epidemic and the two World Wars at the beginning of the 20th century. These events greatly influenced the development of the profession known today as physical therapy. Historically provided in collaboration with the physician, the practice of physical therapy had a strong orthopedic emphasis. Through scientific discoveries and expanded therapeutic applications, the emphasis of the interventions provided by the physical therapist has broadened to encompass neuromuscular, cardiovascular, pulmonary, and integumentary systems as well. In addition to the growth of scientific knowledge, the practice of physical therapy also expanded into a variety of practice settings made available through major federal legislation such as Medicare, Medicaid, and the Individuals with Disabilities Education Act. Federal programs provided to the elderly, poor, and children with disabilities have influenced not only who is entitled to physical therapy services but also how those services will be provided, whether through home-based programs in early intervention or school-based programs at the local high school. State legislation has also influenced the practice of physical therapy, with many states permitting access to physical therapy services without the prescription of a physician. These factors require the physical therapist to practice with more autonomy, knowledge of the practice setting and the applicable laws, and competence in providing effective evidence-based interventions that can enable a child to function and fulfill his role in the family, classroom, or society.

REVIEW QUESTIONS

1. Today a physician who specializes in physical medicine and rehabilitation is referred to as a
   a. doctor of osteopathic medicine
   b. physiatrist
   c. pathologist
   d. psychiatrist
2. As a physical therapist, you are considering taking a job with the local school district. The Education for All Handicapped Children Act mandated a "free and appropriate public education" for all children, including children with disabilities. Which of the following would be the most appropriate document to identify the amount of physical therapy services that was recommended for a student in a special education program?
   a. IEP
   b. physician's prescription
   c. IFSP
   d. plan of care
3. You are a physical therapist working in the public schools. A student, John, is to receive physical therapy as part of his special education services. You inform John's teacher that physical therapy cannot start until you get a referral from the physician. Which of the following statements is true?
   a. Requiring a physician's referral to provide physical therapy services is a condition of the State's Practice Act. The therapist is responsible for obtaining a prescription before providing services as defined in the Practice Act.
   b. Requiring a physician's referral to provide physical therapy services in the school setting is not necessary because a federal law mandates physical therapy services to eligible students.
   c. Requiring a physician's referral to provide physical therapy services is not necessary in any state.
   d. Requiring a physician's referral to provide physical therapy services is only necessary if you are utilizing a physical therapist assistant.
4. You are a physical therapist working in an early intervention program with an occupational therapist and a speech language pathologist. All of the therapists perform a developmental evaluation in their specific disciplines and write goals for the infant collaboratively. Each then provides an individual intervention with some support for areas beyond their traditional scope of practice. This would be most reflective of which type of teaming?
   a. Unidisciplinary
   b. Multidisciplinary
   c. Transdisciplinary
5. Which of the following most reflects the Nagi model of disablement for a 3-year-old child with cerebral palsy?
   a. cell death of white matter in cortex of brain–impaired movement on the right side of the body–inability to roll–inability to participate in day care or preschool programs
   b. impaired movement on the right side of the body–inability to roll (due to cell death of white matter in cortex of brain)–inability to participate in day care or preschool programs
   c. cell death of white matter in cortex of brain–inability to roll–impaired movement on the right side of the body–inability to participate in day care or preschool programs
   d. inability to participate in day care or preschool programs–inability to roll–impaired movement on the right side of the body–cell death of white matter in cortex of brain

6. Which of the following would be the most appropriate diagnosis, made by a physical therapist?
   a. medial meniscus tear
   b. osteogenesis imperfecta
   c. impaired joint mobility associated with local inflammation
   d. demyelinating disease of the CNS

7. In the examination process of a 14-year-old adolescent's status post spinal fusion secondary to idiopathic scoliosis, the physical therapist may utilize information for the examination from which of the following sources?
   a. results of MMT
   b. radiology reports
   c. laboratory values
   d. all of the above

8. You are working in a clinic with your colleague Joe. As part of your examination of a 5-year-old boy, you perform the GMFM. This standardized test has high intra-rater reliability. Because of this psychometric property
   a. you know that the results will be reliable if you are the one to perform the examination at a future date.
   b. you know that the results will be reliable if Joe performs the examination at a future date.
   c. you know that the results will be reliable regardless of who performs the examination at a future date.
   d. you know that the results of this standardized test will be reliable when compared to another standardized test, such as the Bruininks-Oseretsky Test of Motor Proficiency.

9. Sally is a 7-year-old girl who sustained a hairline fracture of her right humerus, secondary to a motor vehicle accident (MVA). She has been hospitalized secondary to complications. Presently her treatment plan includes the following goal: Sally will demonstrate 90° of active right shoulder flexion to assist with her ADLs. A summary of objective documentation is as follows:

   April 5: Initial evaluation. Patient demonstrates 50° of active and passive ROM of the right shoulder, with pain at end range.

   April 6: Patient demonstrates 60° of active and passive ROM of the right shoulder, with pain at end range. She reports fatigue with ambulation beyond 50 feet.

   April 7: Patient demonstrates 70° of passive and active ROM in her right shoulder.

   April 8: Call from her case manager requesting update.

   Using the information above, choose the best answer to the question below.

   How many more visits would you expect it would take until she reaches her goal of 90° of active shoulder flexion?
   a. 1
   b. 2
   c. 3
   d. 4

10. Jack is a 5-year-old boy who is status post dorsal rhizotomy. He requires the assistance of one person moving him forward at both shoulders to transition from sit to stance. Using the University of Iowa's Level of Assistance Scale, you would document that Jack requires which of the following levels of assistance?
    a. Minimum
    b. Moderate
    c. Maximum

A Guide to the Patient–Client Management Process

PATIENT/CLIENT MANAGEMENT OUTLINE

Examination

HISTORY

- General Demographics
- Current Condition (Chief Complaint)
- Past Medical and Surgical History
- Health Status (can be by family report)
- Family History
- Growth and Development
- Occupation, Employment, School, and/or Play
- Social History (culture, resources) and Social Habits (risks, physical activity)
- Medications
- Other Clinical and Laboratory Tests
- Living Environment
- Functional Status and Activity Level

SYSTEMS REVIEW

- Cardiovascular and Pulmonary
  HR
  BP
  RR
  edema
- Integumentary
  integrity
  color
  scar
- Musculoskeletal
  symmetry
  gross ROM
  gross strength
  height
  weight
- Neuromuscular
  gait
  balance
  gross coordination
  transfers and transitions
- Communication, Affect, Cognition, Learning Style
  affect
  language
  learning preferences
  oriented ×3

TESTS AND MEASURES (IN ALPHABETICAL ORDER)

- Aerobic Capacity and Endurance
- Anthropometrics (body composition and dimensions)
- Arousal, Attention, and Cognition
- Assistive and Adaptive Devices
- Circulation
- Cranial and Peripheral Nerve Integrity
- Environmental, Home, Work, School, and/or Play Barriers
- Ergonomics and Body Mechanics
- Gait, Locomotion, and Balance
- Integumentary Integrity
- Joint Integrity and Mobility
- Motor Function (motor control and motor learning)
- Muscle Performance (strength, power, and endurance)
- Neuromotor Development and Sensory Integration
- Orthotic, Protective, and Supportive Devices
- Pain
- Posture
- Prosthetic Requirements
- ROM
- Reflex Integrity
- Self-Care and Home Management
- Sensory Integrity
- Ventilation and Respiration (gas exchange)
- Work, Community, and Leisure Integration or Reintegration (including instrumental ADLs [IADL])

Evaluation

- Impairments
- Functional Limitations

Diagnosis

- Practice Pattern

Prognosis

- Plan of Care

Intervention

- Coordination, Communication, and Documentation
- Patient/Client-Related Instruction
- Procedural Interventions (listed according to the frequency of use)
  - Therapeutic Exercise
  - Functional Training: Self Care and Home
  - Functional Training: Community and Work
  - Manual Therapy

- Prescription, Application, and Fabrication of Equipment and Devices
- Airway Clearance Techniques
- Integumentary Repair and Protection
- Electrotherapeutic Modalities
- Physical Agents (mechanical modalities)

Outcomes

- Results

From the American Physical Therapy Association. *Guide to Physical Therapist Practice*, 2nd ed. Rev. American Physical Therapy Association, 2003.

REFERENCES

1. Scott R. *Foundations of Physical Therapy. A 21st Century-Focused View of the Profession.* New York: McGraw-Hill; 2002:1.
2. Pinkston D. Evolution of the practice of physical therapy in the United States. In: Scully RM, Barnes MR. *Physical Therapy.* Baltimore: Lippincott Williams and Wilkins; 1989.
3. Moffat M. The history of physical therapy practice in the United States. *Journal of Physical Therapy Education.* 2003;17:15–25.
4. Linker B. Strength and science. Gender, physiotherapy, and medicine in early-twentieth-century America. *J Women's History.* 2005;17:105–132.
5. United States Army Medical Services. *Medical Department of the United States Army in the World War.* The Surgeon General's Office. Washington, DC: Government Printing Office; 1923.
6. Murphy W. *Healing the Generations: A History of Physical Therapy and the American Physical Therapy Association.* Lyme, CT: Greenwich Publishing Group Inc.; 1995.
7. Sultz H, Young K. *Health Care USA. Understanding Its Organization and Delivery.* 4th ed. Boston: Jones and Bartlett; 2004.
8. Centers for Disease Control and Prevention. *Health Topic: Polio.* Department of Health and Human Services. 2005:89–100. Available at http://www.cdc.gov/nip/publications/pink/polio.pdf. Accessed January 9, 2006.
9. Rood MS. Neurophysiological reactions as a basis for physical therapy. *Phys Ther Rev.* 1954;34:444–449.
10. Knott M, Voss DE. *Proprioceptive Neuromuscular Facilitation.* Philadelphia, PA: Harper and Row; 1956.
11. Brunnstrom S. Associated reactions of the upper extremity in adult patients with hemiplegia. *Phys Ther Rev.* 1956;36:225–236.
12. Bobath B. Treatment principles and planning in cerebral palsy. *Physiotherapy.* 1963;49:122–124.
13. Stuberg W, Harbourne R. Theoretical practice in pediatric physical therapy: past, present, and future considerations. *Pediatr Phys Ther.* 1994;6:119–125.
14. United States Social Security Administration. Social Security Online. Supplemental Security Income Homepage. Available at http://www.ssa.gov/notices/supplemental-security-income. Accessed January 3, 2006.
15. American Physical Therapy Association. *Guide to Physical Therapist Practice.* 2nd ed. Rev. Alexandria, VA : American Physical Therapy Association; 2003:24.
16. Kamm K, Thelen E, Jensen J. A dynamical systems approach to motor development. *Phys Ther.* 1990;70:763–774.
17. Parson T. *The Social System.* New York: Free Press. 1951:436.
18. American Physical Therapy Association. *Guide to Physical Therapist Practice.* 2nd ed. *Phys Ther J.* 2001;81:1.
19. Clifton D. Disablement models. In: *Physical Rehabilitation's Role in Disability Management: Unique Perspectives for Success.* St. Louis, MO: Elsevier Saunders Publishers; 2005.
20. World Health Organization. The International Classification of Functioning, Disability and Health—Introduction. 2002;1–25. Retrieved May 31, 2006, from http://www.who.int/classification/icf/intros/ICF-Eng-Intro.pdf.
21. Ustun TB, Chatterji S, Bickenbach J, et al. The International Classification of Functioning, Disability and Health: a new tool for understanding disability and health. *Disabil Rehabil.* 2003;25:565–571.
22. Simeonsson R, Leonardi M, Lollar D, et al. Applying the International Classification of Functioning, Disability and Health (ICF) to measure childhood disability. *Disabil Rehabil.* 2003;25:602–610.
23. Battaglia M, Russo E, Bolla A, et al. International Classification of Functioning, Disability and Health in a cohort of children with cognitive, motor, and complex disabilities. *Dev Med Child Neurol.* 2004;46:98–106.
24. Stucki G, Ewert T, Cieza A. Value and application of the ICF in rehabilitation medicine. *Disabil Rehabil.* 2003;25:628–634.
25. Steiner W, Ryser L, Huber E, et al. Use of the ICF model as a clinical problem-solving tool in physical therapy and rehabilitation medicine. *Phys Ther J.* 2002;82:1098–1107.
26. Jette A. Toward a common language for function, disability, and health. *Phys Ther J.* 2006;86:726–734.
27. Wescott SL, Lowes LP, Richardson PK. Evaluation of postural stability in children: current theories and assessment tools. *Phys Ther J.* 1997;77:629–645.
28. Folio MR, Fewell RR. *Peabody Developmental Motor Scales. Examiner's Manual.* 2nd ed. Austin, TX: Pro-Ed; 2000.
29. Chandler L, Andrews M, Swanson M. *The Movement Assessment of Infants: A Manual.* Rolling Bay, WA: Infant Movement Research; 1980.
30. Russell D, Rosenbaum P, Gowland C, et al. *Gross Motor Function Measure Manual.* 2nd ed. Hamilton, Ontario, Canada: Gross Motor Measures Group, McMaster University; 1993.
31. Bayley N. *Bayley Scales of Infant Development.* 2nd ed. San Antonio, TX: The Psychological Corporation; 1993.
32. Frankenburg WK, Dodd J, Archer P, et al. *Denver II Technical Manual.* Denver, CO: Denver Developmental Materials; 1990.
33. Haley SM, Coster WJ, Ludlow LH, Haltiwanger JT, Anrellos PJ. *Pediatric Evaluation of Disability Inventory.* Boston, MA: New England Medical Center Hospitals; 1992.
34. Bruininks RH. *Bruininks-Oseretsky Test of Motor Proficiency. Examiner's Manual.* Circle Pines, MN: American Guidance Service; 1978.
35. Johnson-Martin N, Jens K, Attermeier S, Hacker B. *The Carolina Curriculum for Infants and Toddlers with Special Needs.* 2nd ed. Baltimore, MD: P H. Brooks Publishing Company; 1986.
36. Coster W, Deeney T, Haltiwanger J, Haley S. *School Function Assessment.* San Antonio, TX: The Psychological Corporation; 1998.
37. McEwen IR, Shelden ML. Pediatric therapy in the 1990s: the demise of the educational versus medical dichotomy. *Occup Phys Ther Pediatr.* 1995;15:33–45.
38. Shumway-Cook A, Woollacott M. *Motor Control: Theory and Practical Application.* Baltimore MD: Lippincott Williams & Wilkins; 2001.

39. Michaud L; Committee on Children with Disabilities. Clinical Report. Prescribing Therapy Services for Children with Motor Disabilities. *Pediatrics*. 2004;113:1836–1838.
40. Kaminker MK, Chiarello LA, O'Neil ME, Dichter C. Decision making for physical therapy service delivery in schools: a nationwide survey of pediatric physical therapists. *Phys Ther J*. 2004; 84:919–933.
41. O'Neil ME, Palisano R. Attitudes towards family-centered care and clinical decision making in early intervention among physical therapists. *Pediatr Phys Ther*. 2000;12: 173–182.
42. Effgen S. Factors affecting the termination of physical therapy services for children in school settings. *Pediatr Phys Ther*. 2000;12:121–126.
43. Montgomery P. Frequency and Duration of Pediatric PT. *Physical Therapy Magazine*. 1994;2:42–47.
44. American Physical Therapy Association. Position on Authority for Physical Therapy Documentation. HOD 06-98-11-11 (Program 32) [Initial HOD 06-97-15-23]. Alexandria, VA: American Physical Therapy Association; 1997.
45. Shields RK, Leo K, Miller B, Dostal W, Bar R. An acute care physical therapy clinical practice database for outcome research. *Phys Ther J*. 1994;74:463–470.
46. Guide for the Uniform Data Set for Medical Rehabilitation (Adult FIM™). Version 4.0. Buffalo, NY: State University of New York; 1993.
47. Wescott SL, Murray KH, Pence K. Survey of the preference of pediatric physical therapists for assessment and treatment of balance dysfunction in children. *Pediatr Phys Ther*. 1998;10:48–61.
48. Nellis J, Mutilva M, McGinnis PQ. Assessment of balance evaluation methods utilized by physical therapists in the state of New Jersey. *Phys Ther J*. 1999;79:S15.
49. Farrel T. Where do you stand on balance? *Phys Ther J*. 2000;80:S4.
50. Straus S, Richardson WS, Glasziou P, Haynes RB. *Evidence-Based Practice. How to Practice and Teach EBM*. 3rd ed. Edinburgh: Elsevier Churchill Livingstone; 2005.
51. Jette D, Bacon K, Batty C, et al. Evidence-based practice: beliefs, attitudes, knowledge, and behaviors of physical therapists. *Phys Ther J*. 2003;83:786–805.
52. Norkin C, White DJ. *Measurement of Joint Motion. A Guide to Goniometry*. 3rd ed. Philadelphia: F. A. Davis Company; 2003.
53. Brousseau L, Balmer S, Tousignant M, et al. Intra- and intertester reliability and criterion validity of the parallelogram and universal goniometer for measuring maximum active knee flexion and extension of patients with knee restrictions. *Arch Phys Med Rehabil*. 2001;82:396–402.
54. MacDermid JC, Chesworth BM, Patterson S, Roth JH. Validity of pain motion indicators recorded on a movement diagram of shoulder lateral rotation. *Aust J Physiother*. 1999;45:269–277.
55. Stuberg WA, Fuchs RH, Miedaner JA. Reliability of goniometric measurements of children with cerebral palsy. *Dev Med Child Neurol*. 1988;30:657–666.
56. Bjornson KF, Graubert CS, Burford VL. Validity of the Gross Motor Function Measure. *Pediatr Phys Ther*. 1998;10: 43–47.
57. Russell D, Rosenbaum P, Cadman D. The Gross Motor Function Measure: a means to evaluate the effects of physical therapy. *Dev Med Child Neurol*. 1989;31:341–352.
58. Bjornson KF, Graubert CS, McLaughlin J. Test-retest reliability of the Gross Motor Function Measure in children with cerebral palsy. *Phys Occup Ther Pediatr*. 1998;18:51–61.
59. Guide for the Uniform Data Set for Medical Rehabilitation (Wee FIM^sm). Version 1.5. Buffalo, NY: Research Foundation–State University of New York; 1991.
60. McAuliffe CA, Wenger RE, Schneider JW, Gaebler-Spira DJ. Usefulness of the Wee-functional independence measure to detect functional change in children with cerebral palsy. *Pediatr Phys Ther*. 1998;10:23–28.
61. Ottenbacher KJ, Msall ME, Lyon N, et al. Functional assessment and care of children with neurodevelopmental disabilities. *Am J Phys Med Rehabil*. 2000;79:114–123.
62. Ziviani J, Ottenbacher KJ, Shephard K, Foreman S, Astbury W, Ireland P. Concurrent validity of the Functional Independence Measure for Children (WeeFIM) and the Pediatric Evaluation of Disabilities Inventory in children with developmental disabilities and acquired brain injuries. *Phys Occup Ther Pediatr*. 2001;21:91–101.
63. Ottenbacher KJ, Taylor ET, Msall ME, et al. The stability and equivalence reliability of the functional independence measure for children (WeeFIM). *Dev Med Child Neurol*. 1996;38:907–916.
64. Msall ME, DiGaudia K, Duffy LC, et al. Normative sample of an instrument for tracking functional independence in children. *Clin Pediatr*. 1994;33:431–438.
65. Ottenbacher KJ, Msall ME, Lyon N, et al. Interrater agreement and stability of the functional independence measure for children (WeeFIM): use in children with developmental disabilities. *Arch Phys Med Rehabil*. 1997;78:1309–1315.

Additional Online Resources

Access your state's Practice Act via your state's Board of Physical Therapy, which can be found at http://fsbpt.org/licensing/index.asp.
Information on the ICF model can be found at http://www3.who.int/icf/ (accessed October 19, 2006).

CHAPTER 2

The Child

Mark Drnach and Theresa Chambers

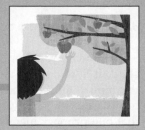

LEARNING OBJECTIVES

1. Understand the definition and concept of family.
2. Define what a ritual is and what a routine is in a family.
3. Understand the basic processes of human gestation and birth.
4. Identify key elements of child development in all domains, from infancy to adulthood.
5. Understand the importance of good nutrition throughout childhood.
6. Be aware of the current issues of inactivity and obesity in children.
7. Understand the importance of fitness in children.

In the practice of pediatric physical therapy it is necessary for the physical therapist to have a framework of developmental expectations, skills, and behaviors that provides a structure for the examination, evaluation, and the development of a plan of care. This chapter presents the general development of a child from conception to physical maturity, noting the key aspects of development toward adulthood. The developmental skills are grouped according to the different stages of a child's life; as an infant, a toddler, a child, and as an adolescent. It should be emphasized that development is not a strict linear process, nor does the expression of certain developmental skills always proceed in a strict sequential order. Development is a dynamic process that ebbs and flows as the child moves along the stream of skill development. The information in this chapter is organized to provide a broad picture of the child as she develops skills that enable her to participate in the world around her. The emphasis is on the acquisition of general developmental skills that play an integral role in learning and functioning within the family, on the playground, in the classroom, or in the workplace. When she is playing, she has the opportunity to learn, to move, to manipulate, to communicate, and to interact with her environment and others. The learning that takes place during these encounters will aid in the development of the many roles she will assume in her life—as a daughter, sibling, or friend—and as an individual person functioning in a family, a classroom, and ultimately in society. This chapter begins with a fundamental and key concept for any child: the family.

CHILDREN AND FAMILIES

Children are not just born into the world, they are born into families; the family is an integral part of the child's life. A young child experiences her first social interactions and develops her first relationships with the members of her immediate family and develops an understanding of the world based on her family's unique set of standards, perspectives, and beliefs. Parents play an integral role in the family, acting as the primary educators, disciplinarians, and advocates for their child. Parents also make major decisions on behalf of the family. The parent or parents often have the single greatest influence on the child's development and functioning as an adult.

When providing physical therapy services to a child, it is important to remember that each member of the family may be individually involved in the child's health care in a variety of ways. Some families may prefer that one primary member be solely in charge of the care and decision making, whereas other families may want every family member to be involved. Remember that many of the interventions provided to a child are difficult to isolate from the family context. What impacts the child impacts every other member of the family as well.

Defining the Family

The concept of what constitutes a family has changed over time. An ideal family was once viewed as a two-parent household consisting of a mother, a father, and one or more children. The father played the role of disciplinarian and provided the primary means of economic support. The mother played the role of educator and nurturer, caring for the children and managing the household while the father was at work. The children fulfilled the roles of sons or daughters by participating in family activities, as students by attending and learning in school, and as friends and siblings by developing meaningful relationships. Today, the concept of what makes a family is much broader and encompasses other individuals who significantly add to the functioning of the family unit. A family can consist of one or more parents; same-sex parents; a blended family; foster care family; adoptive family; an aunt, uncle, grandparent, or other family member raising a child; or even an older sibling caring for and rearing a younger one.[1] Since the 1940s, single-parent families have become more socially acceptable.[2] A parent in this situation, typically the mother, must provide contributions to the family that encompass all aspects of family management and child care. The single parent must fill the role of disciplinarian, breadwinner, decision maker, educator, nurturer, and manager of the household, often providing for the family with fewer resources than those available to two-parent families.

Families also can change depending on their current situation. Medalie and Cole-Kelly[3] recognized the importance of defining families with certain medical issues in order to aid in health care delivery by physicians in family practice. Their approach highlights the dynamic nature of families and provides some insight for the health care provider about the clinical significance of family functioning (Box 2-1). Their definition of a **primary family** in the context of routine health care includes those members living in the same house, who have a biological relationship to the patient or who are involved in the care of that person. **Secondary family** definitions emerge when major health issues arise. These are more evident in situations of illness, death, when difficult decisions regarding health care need to be made, or when violence or abuse is suspected. These definitions are important because they

BOX 2-1
Family Definitions

Family Definition	Clinical Application
Primary	
Biological	Identification of biological relationships and issues that may factor into the medical diagnosis. Identification of genetic tendencies in the family.
Functional	Identification of an able and willing caregiver. Is the home environment accessible and safe? Who is the party responsible for care and payment for services?
Secondary	
Crisis	Identification of other family members to assist with crisis situation.
Bereaved	Preparation of patient and family for death and identification of who is appropriate to provide follow-up services.
Cultural	Determines beliefs and possible reasons for behaviors. Understanding of priorities and expectations of the family.

Modified from Medalie J, Cole-Kelly K. The Clinical Importance of Defining Family. Editorial. *Am Fam Phys.* 2002;65:1277–1279.

touch upon the many environments and situations that are encountered in the provision of health care services to children.

Today biological or residential relationships are not the sole determining factor of who is considered part of the family. The family is dynamic and can be viewed as a separate entity from each of the contributing members. The primary caregiver is very influential in a child's life, as are other people with whom she interacts, especially as she ages and develops through adolescence. A family as a whole can be greater than all of the individual members combined. The **Family Systems Theory** originated by Murray Bowen acknowledges this concept. This theory assumes that all members of the family are involved in each other's lives, so what happens to one member will affect the entire family. Family members function as a group, deciding who is included in the family and establishing rules of family behavior.[1,4] With this in mind, the physical therapist should consider not only the child's behavior, but also the behavior of relevant family members and the significance of a behavior in the context of the family (Box 2-2). Each member of a family functions as part of a team: Each member has a specific role to play. Just as the parents are usually (but not always) in a leadership role within the family, each child also has uniquely

BOX 2-2
Components of the Family Systems Theory

- All families have rules that must be followed to maintain order.
- The family's individual characteristics are based on its belief system, moral values, and strategies for dealing with problems.
- The family decides who is included in the family group.
- Realize that over time, the family structure will change as new members come and old members leave.
- Family members function as a group to provide education, health care, social interactions, financial assistance, love, and play time for each of its members.
- Each family contains subsystems around which it is formed. These subsystems include interactions between individuals associated with the family, such as the marital relationship between partners, interactions between the child and her parents, sibling interactions, and interactions with extended family, friends, and other outside individuals.

defined roles depending on the structure of her family. The role that the child plays defines that child's "occupation" and is defined by the family's unique structure. A child is often expected to fill many different roles based on the complex relationships within the family. These **family activities of daily living** (FADL) can be seen as an extension of ADL, which apply to an individual's ability to perform personal care and hygiene activities, and instrumental ADL (IADL), which apply to those skills necessary to function with some level of independent living, such as shopping for food or managing a bank account. **FADL** can be defined as those activities that are the work of the family unit. They are done in collaboration with, or for the benefit of, other members of the family. Examples are seen in the activities associated with getting ready for school in the morning, the preparation of meals, household chores, and house maintenance. Who is responsible for each activity and how these are accomplished contribute to the overall functioning of the family.

POINT TO REMEMBER

Defining a Family

A family can be defined in many different ways and may include people not traditionally associated with being members of a family. Who is included can vary depending on the current situation and the needs of the parent. It is important to remember that what impacts the child impacts every other member of the family.

These family activities can also be viewed in the context of family routines and rituals. Family **routines** are defined as those interactions within the family that occur frequently, are episodic, have a clear beginning and end, and reflect the broader concept of family organization.[5] According to Fiese et al.,[6] routines function to organize and coordinate the behaviors and actions of individuals and to bring about order in the family unit. There is some literature that suggests establishing routines can have a positive influence on the functioning of individual family members.[7] Serpell et al.[8] found that families who read to their young children had a positive effect on their basic reading skills as third grade students. It is generally believed that order, established boundaries of behavior, and consistency in a child's life are positive attributes of child rearing. **Rituals** are defined as family routines that convey a message about who the family is as a group.[6] Family rituals have a social–emotional component that conveys feelings of belonging and continuity across generations. Routines give life order, whereas rituals give it meaning.[7] Common family rituals are associated with holidays such as Thanksgiving Day in the United States, Cinco de Mayo in Mexico, or religious holidays such as Hanukkah and Christmas. They are seen in family traditions and celebrations that typically reflect the culture of the family. It is important to recognize that what may seem to be a routine to a nonfamily member may hold more value as a ritual to the family, imparting a sense of family identity.[9] In some families, the act of the oldest child working in the family business is more of a ritual than the routine of employment (Fig. 2-1). It is what is important to the family. The physical therapist should be aware that, at times, imposing a seemingly simple change in a perceived routine may in fact require the family to adapt in the way it views itself.[7]

Inevitably, all families change over time. New family members are born, children mature and assume the

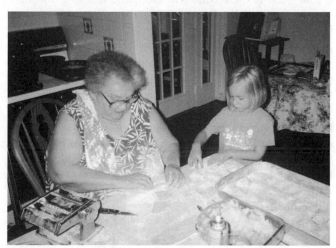
Figure 2-1 ■ A grandmother and granddaughter participating in a family activity of making perogies. The importance of the activity to the family can make what appears to be a routine more of a ritual.

role of adults, and older members of the family become ill or die. The role that the child holds within the family may change as the family changes. **Adaptability** refers to how well a family responds to change. In all cultures, rituals such as weddings, baby showers, bar mitzvahs, and funerals serve the purpose of helping the family members to adapt to change and to understand that their roles will be changed after the ceremony has occurred. These rituals also draw on the entire family to lend emotional support to the members undergoing this change.

POINT TO REMEMBER

Routines and Rituals

Routines give family life order whereas rituals give family life meaning. As families change, routines and rituals can aid in the transition.

PRENATAL DEVELOPMENT

A significant change in the family occurs when a woman realizes she is pregnant, especially if it is for the first time. Not only will an additional family member affect her family, but also the woman, who now assumes the role of a mother.

The most dramatic time in the course of human development has to be the gestational period. **Gestation** is the period of time during which an embryo develops within the mother's womb. This is the most radical change in human existence. During this period, a single cell grows into a complex and functional human being all within 37 to 42 weeks time (average gestational age is 40 weeks). This period of phenomenal change is divided into three periods for the expectant mother: Weeks 1 through 12 of pregnancy are the **first trimester**, weeks 13 through 26 are the **second trimester,** and weeks 27 through 40 are the **third trimester.** The developing human is known as an **embryo** for the first 8 weeks and afterwards is referred to as a **fetus** until birth. This is a time of great change, not only for the fetus, but also for the expectant mother. Although the uterus nurtures and offers protection to the developing fetus, fetal development is also influenced by social, psychological, and environmental factors to which the mother is exposed. She too will undergo physical, psychological, and social changes as her pregnancy ensues. The intricate relationship among these factors and the physical transformations happening within the mother, influences the development of the fetus into an infant.

The First Trimester (First 12 Weeks)

The **germinal period** (2 weeks in duration) of development begins at conception when a mature ovum (egg),

with its 23 chromosomes, is fertilized by the sperm, with its 23 chromosomes. This usually occurs in the fallopian tube. The **embryonic period** (6 weeks in duration) begins after the first 2 weeks as the zygote is implanted into the uterine wall, commonly on the upper one third of the posterior wall of the uterus. (The most common variation is when an implantation occurs in the inferior portion of the uterus. This is commonly referred to as placenta previa, a low-lying placenta that covers part or all of the opening of the uterus. This condition can give rise to excessive bleeding and separation of the placenta from the uterus that can result in a premature or problematic delivery. Implantation outside the uterus is termed an **ectopic pregnancy** and ultimately ends in the death of the fetus.) The embryo at this point has two discrete layers, the **endoderm** (an inner layer that gives rise to the digestive and respiratory systems) and the **ectoderm** (an outer layer that gives rise to the skin and nervous system). Appearing in the 3rd week is the **mesoderm** layer (a middle layer that gives rise to the skeletal, muscular, and circulatory systems). Every part of the human body is formed from these three layers. Between the 4th and 8th weeks, many changes take place as the embryo transforms into a human-like shape with arm and leg buds appearing. Facial structures, including the jaw, mouth, palate, nose, eyelids, and external ear begin to form. Rapid growth of the brain also takes place; its three main divisions are obvious: forebrain, midbrain, and hindbrain. Blood is being pumped by the heart, which can be seen beating on an ultrasound image. The embryonic period comes to an end by the 8th week when the fundamental organs of all major body systems, as well as the gross organization of the nervous system, have been established. The embryo is 5 cm long and weighs 9 g.[1,10–13]

During the **fetal period** (32 weeks in duration), beginning the 9th week of the first trimester, the fetus increases in cell number and size and several of the newly formed organ systems remodel. By the 10th week, facial features and external genitalia are distinct. The lungs, which are present, are not functional until approximately weeks 20 to 24, when the alveoli form and production of surfactant begins.[1,10,12] Exposure to teratogens at this point will not necessarily result in death, as it would with earlier exposure (Table 2-1). For the fetus, sexual differentiation becomes visible through ultrasound imaging by week 12, and the kidney and digestive systems begin to function.

The mother undergoes changes during this time period as well. During the 3rd week of pregnancy, she may notice a missed menstrual period, possibly her first indication that she is pregnant. Throughout the first trimester, she may experience more fatigue than usual, "morning sickness" (which can occur at any time of the day), and cravings for particular foods. The size and coloration of her breast may change due to the increased

TABLE 2-1 Fetal Development and Teratogens

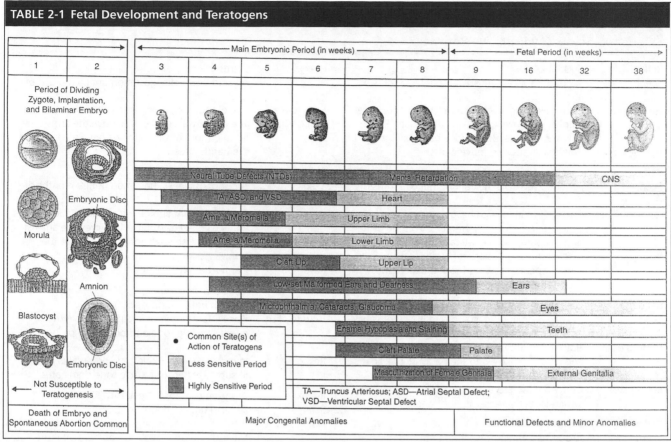

Gray denotes highly sensitive periods when major birth defects may be produced.

Summary of Critical Periods in Prenatal Development. Reprinted from Moore KL, Persaud TVN. *The Developing Human: Clinically Oriented Embryology*, 6th ed. Critical Periods, 548, © 1998, with permission pending from Elsevier.

amounts of estrogen and progesterone in her system. The increased levels of progesterone also slow the movement of the intestines that may cause periods of constipation. She may also experience more frequent episodes of urination throughout the day due to an increase in the size of her uterus, which may press on her bladder, and an increased blood flow to the kidneys. These symptoms of pregnancy could also be attributed to other factors such as stress, a stomach virus, or a urinary tract infection, especially if the woman is not planning on becoming pregnant or is afraid of the possibility. Ambivalent feelings are common at this stage.

The Second Trimester (13 to 26 Weeks)

Fetal growth is rapid during the first part of this trimester. By week 20, the fetus's body structure will be approximately in proportion to its newborn appearance. Spontaneous movements of the fetus are sufficient to be noticed by the mother. Bones and muscles continue to develop. Now that the major organs and systems have been formed, the following months will be spent on growing and preparing for birth. The fetus can hear the mother's voice. Reflexes such as the suck and swallow

reflex develop, and the brain undergoes significant growth (Box 2-3).

The mother is now visibly pregnant. At approximately 20 weeks gestation (the midpoint of the gestation period) she can feel the fetus move. This action reinforces the understanding of the presence of the fetus and may heighten the feelings associated with the pregnancy. At this time the mother and father may have concerns regarding the health of the fetus and what they would do if the baby is not healthy.[10] Morning sickness may subside, and the feeling of fatigue may lessen. This is sometimes referred to as the "good trimester" as the mother feels better than she did in the first trimester and she begins to feel the baby inside her. However, some other symptoms (such as constipation and swelling in the legs) continue, and she may experience back pain or sciatic pain as her body and posture change.

The Third Trimester (27 to 40 Weeks)

During this time, the fetus is beginning to prepare for birth; the weight triples and length doubles as body stores of protein, fat, iron, and calcium increase. There is

BOX 2-3
Some Key Primitive Reflexes

Reflex:	Suck-Swallow	**Reflex:**	Startle
Seen:	Around 28 weeks' gestation until 5 months of age.	**Seen:**	Around 28 weeks' gestation until 5 months of age.
How to elicit:	Place child supine with head in the midline. Place a finger or nipple into the infant's mouth. Press down on tongue. Best if done before infant is fed.	**How to elicit:**	Make a sudden, loud noise or tap the sternum.
Response:	Rhythmical sucking movements.	**Response:**	The infant will startle. Will move the arms similar to a Moro but the elbows remain flexed and the hands closed.
Reflex:	Rooting	**Reflex:**	Plantar Grasp
Seen:	Around 28 weeks' gestation until 6 months of age.	**Seen:**	Around 28 weeks' gestation until 9 months of age.
How to elicit:	Place child supine with head in the midline. Using your finger, stroke the peri-oral skin at the corner of the mouth, moving laterally toward the cheek.	**How to elicit:**	Place the infant supine with head in midline and legs relaxed. Apply a firm pressure against the metatarsal heads, or directly below the toes.
Response:	After stimulation, there is head turning and mouth opening toward the stimulated side. Best if done before infant is fed.	**Response:**	Plantar flexion of all toes.
		Reflex:	Tonic Labyrinthine
Reflex:	Galant	**Seen:**	At birth until 6 months of age.
Seen:	Around 32 weeks' gestation until 2 months of age.	**How to elicit:**	Place infant prone or supine. Observe the infant's muscle tone and posture in prone and supine.
How to elicit:	Hold the infant in prone position with one hand and gently stroke along the paravertebral line from the thoracic to lumbar region.	**Response:**	In prone, flexor muscle tone dominates. In supine, extensor muscle tone dominates.
Response:	Concavity toward the stimulated side. Look for symmetrical response on right and left.	**Reflex:**	Asymmetrical Tonic Neck (ANTR)
		Seen:	At birth until 6 months of age.
Reflex:	Positive Support	**How to elicit:**	Place the infant supine with head in midline. Have the infant follow an object from one side to the other, or turn her head slowly to one side, and hold in this position
Seen:	Around 35 weeks' gestation until 1 to 2 months of age.		
How to elicit:	Support infant in the vertical position with examiner's hands under the arms and around the chest. Allow the infant's feet to make contact with the tabletop or other flat surface.	**Response:**	The infant's arm and leg on the jaw side extend while the arm and leg on skull side flex.
Response:	Simultaneous contraction of flexor and extensor muscles in the legs so as to bear weight through the lower extremities. The child supports only a minimal amount of body weight.	**Reflex:**	Palmar Grasp
		Seen:	At birth until 6 months of age.
		How to elicit:	Place the index finger of the examiner into the hands of the infant and gently press against the palmar surface.
Reflex:	Spontaneous Stepping	**Response:**	The infant's fingers will flex around the examiner's index finger.
Seen:	Around 27 weeks' gestation until 2 months of age.		
How to elicit:	Support the infant in the vertical position with examiner's hands under the arms and around the chest. With the infant's feet touching the table surface, incline the infant forward and gently move the infant forward.	**Reflex:**	Landau
		Seen:	Around 4 to 5 months until 1 to 2 years.
		How to elicit:	Examiner supports the infant prone, horizontally in the air.
Response:	The infant will make alternating, rhythmic, and coordinated stepping movements.	**Response:**	The infant's head and hips extend in sequence.
Reflex:	Moro	**Reflex:**	STNR
Seen:	Around 28 weeks' gestation until 4 months of age.	**Seen:**	Around 6 months of age until 12 months of age.
How to elicit:	Place the infant supine, with head in the midline, arms on chest. The head is gently lifted but not the infant's body. Allow the infant's head to drop backward, quickly supporting the head so it does not bang against the surface.	**How to elicit:**	Place the infant in a prone position supported by the trunk, over the examiner's knee, or in quadruped, if appropriate. The examiner passively flexes and extends the infant's head.
Response:	Abduction of the arms with extension of the elbows, wrists and fingers, followed by subsequent adduction of the arms at the shoulders and flexion at the elbows.	**Response:**	Flexion of the head produces flexion of the arms and extension of the legs. Extension of the head produces extension of the arms and flexion of the legs.

acceleration in the functional development of the respiratory system, preparing the fetus to breathe air. The development of the lungs begins to accelerate at 31 weeks gestation and is not entirely complete until 39 to 40 weeks. Although the mother may be anxious to have her baby by now, it is important to remember that every week in utero increases the baby's chance of survival after birth because the lungs continually develop throughout the third trimester.

Accumulation of body fat will also help with temperature regulation when the baby is exposed to the external environment. By week 34, the fetus should weigh approximately 2500 g (5.5 lb) and have established the ability to regulate her body temperature.[1] After week 35, the fetus should be ready to switch from fetal circulation to self-circulation with spontaneous closure of the ductus arteriosus (the fetal opening between the pulmonary trunk and the aorta that normally closes within the first hours of birth). By 36 weeks, respiratory difficulties are uncommon. By the end of this trimester, the baby is positioned head down in preparation for birth. Any presentation other than head down is referred to as a **breech** presentation, which may make vaginal delivery more problematic.

During the third trimester, the mother may experience more frequent urination, back pain, edema in the lower extremities, fatigue, and shortness of breath.[12] She may experience false labor pains or **Braxton Hicks** contractions. By the end of the third trimester, the mother is more aware of the activity of the fetus and may assign certain personality traits to the infant. The mother becomes increasingly uncomfortable, finding it difficult to take deep breaths and/or get comfortable sleeping at night. She may have increased frequency of urination, constipation, heartburn, hemorrhoids, and/or noticeable swelling (edema) in the ankles, hands, and face. Colostrum (a precursor to breast milk) may leak from her breasts. She may be heard verbalizing that she is ready to have the baby!

 POINT TO REMEMBER

Gestation

Human gestation lasts approximately 40 weeks and is divided into trimesters.

First trimester (First 12 weeks). All major body systems are established.

Second trimester (13 to 26 weeks). Body proportions grow to newborn proportions.

Third trimester (27 to 40 weeks). Body weight triples and length doubles. Body fat accumulates which aides with body temperature regulation. At 36 weeks, lungs are developed.

PRENATAL AND BIRTH INFLUENCES

During an examination of an infant or toddler, the history of the gestational period and birth aid in understanding the current examination findings. This information can be gained by a review of a medical record, but is more commonly acquired by maternal report.

External Influences

Throughout the gestational period, many environmental factors influence the development of the fetus. This influence can have a negative or negligible effect, depending on the timing of the exposure and the degree to which the fetus is exposed (e.g., infections, cigarette smoke, alcohol, caffeine). A group of detrimental environmental factors, known as **teratogens**, may hinder growth and/or lead to malformation and neurological problems (Table 2-1). This group of common agents are recalled by the acronym **TORCHHS** (**T**oxoplasmosis, **O**ther Infections, **R**ubella, **C**ytomegalovirus [CMV] Infection, **H**uman Immunodeficiency Virus [HIV], **H**erpes Simplex Virus, and **S**yphilis).

Toxoplasmosis is an infection caused by the *Toxoplasma gondii* organism and is most commonly transmitted by inadequate hand washing after handling cat feces or by eating undercooked pork, lamb, or eggs. Approximately 25% of women who become infected during pregnancy pass the infection to the developing fetus. The risk of congenital abnormalities is low after 20 weeks gestation and may include damage to the heart, brain, and lungs; it may also cause an eye infection (chorioretinitis) that may produce blindness. Only 10% of people with toxoplasmosis are symptomatic; if suspected, treatment should begin immediately.[1,11,14,15]

Other infections include **Varicella** (chicken pox). There is a 25% chance that a mother who is exposed to chicken pox during pregnancy will pass it to the fetus, but there is only a 2% risk of birth defects, which may include skin scarring, limb reduction defects, muscle atrophy, and neurological abnormalities.[1,14,15]

Rubella is a mild, febrile, highly infectious viral disease most commonly seen in childhood. A mother who acquires the infection while pregnant could pass it to the fetus. The fetus is most susceptible during the first trimester, at moderate risk during the second trimester, and at very low risk during the third trimester. Effects of exposure to this teratogen include congenital heart defects in the fetus, vision and hearing loss, microcephaly, mental retardation, cerebral palsy, and thrombocytopenia with "blueberry-muffin" skin lesions. Newborn infants also may be contagious.[14,15]

CMV is one of a group of herpes viruses that are the most common causes of congenital infection. It is asymptomatic in the majority of cases. The disease may be transmitted from the mother to the fetus through the placenta or during passage through the birth canal. The extent of damage is related to the timing of the infection; earlier infections warrant more defects that can lead to varying degrees of neurologic and sensory impairments, below-average intelligence, behavioral problems, and microcephaly. The infant may also acquire CMV by ingesting CMV-positive breast milk. Infected newborn infants are often contagious.[14,15]

HIV is a viral infection that suppresses the function of the immune system and is characterized by the onset of opportunistic infections. It is transmitted from person to person through body fluids, specifically blood and semen. More than 85% of children born to mothers infected with either HIV or acquired immunodeficiency syndrome (AIDS) contract the disease during gestation, birth, or the postnatal period through ingestion of infected breast milk. Breastfeeding is not recommended if the mother is suspected of having HIV or AIDS. HIV has a shorter incubation period in infants and children, and manifests itself in the presence of opportunistic infections, failure to thrive, lymphoma, or neurodevelopmental deficits.[14,15] A common opportunistic infection is pneumocystis carinii pneumonia (PCP), caused by the fungus *Pneumocystis jiroveci*. PCP can infect the lymph nodes, lungs, liver, spleen, and bone marrow. If left untreated, PCP can lead to respiratory failure and death.[16]

Herpes Simplex Virus is a viral infection that causes lesions in the genital areas and can be passed to the fetus in utero, but infections are more common during the birthing process. The mother may be asymptomatic at the time of delivery. Transmission of the virus can be prevented when a **cesarean section** (C-section) is performed. Infected infants may show growth retardation, skin lesions, retinal abnormalities, conjunctivitis and microcephaly. If left untreated, encephalitis may occur. The infected mother and infant should be kept in contact isolation.[14,15]

Syphilis is both an acute and chronic infectious disease caused by the bacterium *Treponema pallidum* and is transmitted by direct contact, usually through intercourse. Maternal syphilis has a high probability of crossing the placenta and can lead to treatable syphilis in the infant. Treatment of the mother before week 16 of pregnancy can prevent transplacental fetal infection. Manifestations of syphilis include jaundice, recurring rashes, anemia, hepatosplenomegaly, rhinitis, and meningitis. If the infant is suspected of acquiring syphilis from the mother, antibiotics must be promptly administered.[14,15]

Environmental factors also influence the fetus. Cigarette smoking doubles a woman's risk of developing placental problems, which include placenta previa and abruption of the placenta (in which the placenta peels away, partially or almost completely, from the uterine wall before delivery). Both problems can result in heavy bleeding during delivery that can endanger the mother and baby. Chemicals in cigarette smoke can cross the placenta and restrict a baby's normal growth. Smoking increases the incidence of spontaneous abortion and stillbirths. Babies who are exposed to smoke during gestation are shorter, have lower birth weights, suffer from more lower-respiratory illnesses and ear infections, and are three times more likely to die from **sudden infant death syndrome** (SIDS; sudden infant death from an unknown cause) than are other babies. A child exposed to smoking at home during the first few years of life also is at increased risk of developing asthma.[17,18]

The role of the father, as well as other family members, in prenatal development should not be overlooked. Secondhand smoke from the father's cigarette may affect the developing fetus. Also, his use of alcohol and drugs in the home environment may influence the mother's behavior and participation in these activities.[18]

When a pregnant woman drinks alcohol, the alcohol passes swiftly through the placenta to the baby. In the fetus's undeveloped body, alcohol is broken down much more slowly than in an adult's body. As a result, the alcohol level of the baby's blood can be even higher and can remain elevated longer than it can in the mother's blood. Each year, approximately 1 in 750 infants are born with **fetal alcohol syndrome** (FAS), a combination of physical and mental birth defects resulting from the mother consuming alcohol during pregnancy.[12] These women either drink excessively throughout pregnancy or have repeated episodes of binge drinking. FAS is one of the most common known causes of mental retardation and the only cause that is entirely preventable. Infants with classic FAS are abnormally small at birth and usually remain undersized throughout life. They may have petite, narrow eyes, a short or upturned nose and small, flat cheeks. Their organs, especially the heart, may not form properly. Many infants with FAS also have a brain that is small and abnormally formed, and most have some degree of mental disability. Many have poor coordination and a short attention span, and exhibit behavioral problems. The effects of FAS last a lifetime. Even if not cognitively impaired, adolescents and adults with FAS have varying degrees of psychological and behavioral problems and often find it difficult to hold down a job and live independently.[12]

There are 10 times as many infants born with **fetal alcohol effects** (FAE) than with FAS. These infants may have some of the physical or mental birth defects associated with FAS, but to a lesser degree. In general, alcohol-related birth defects are more likely to result from drinking during the first trimester due to the significant growth and development of fetal organs during the early weeks of pregnancy; however, drinking at any stage of pregnancy can affect brain development.[14]

Caffeine, when used in excess, can cause fetal growth retardation and fetal loss. Caffeine may be transported across the placenta and membranes to the fetus and amniotic fluid, where concentrations may be greater than the concentration within the mother's body. Risks for miscarriage and fetal growth retardation increase only with daily doses of caffeine >150 mg.[11]

POINT TO REMEMBER

Environmental Influences

Common detrimental environmental influences that may affect the developing fetus include TORCHHS, tobacco smoke, alcohol, and caffeine.

POINT TO REMEMBER

The Birthing Process

The birthing process can be broken down into three stages: labor, delivery of the infant, and delivery of the placenta. A full-term infant is born after 40 weeks' gestation, is an average of 20 inches long, and weighs 7 pounds.

Environmental factors are one thing to consider during the examination of the infant's history. The birthing process itself is also important. It can be exciting as well as traumatic. Information about the birthing process and any complications in that process are an important component of the examination of an infant.

The Birthing Process

The process of giving birth can be divided into three stages: labor, delivery of the baby, and expulsion of the placenta. It is believed that the timed release of **corticotrophin-releasing hormone** (CRH) from the hypothalamus causes a release of **oxytocin** from the posterior pituitary. A rise in oxytocin facilitates contractions of the uterus to help with the expulsion of the fetus and, subsequently, the placenta. This release and buildup of oxytocin initiates the process of labor. **Relaxin**, a hormone produced by the corpus luteum that plays a roll in the relaxation of connective tissue throughout pregnancy, results in the ability of the pelvic outlet to expand to allow for the passage of the fetus. (The elevated levels of this hormone may also lead to other musculoskeletal malalignment and pain often seen with pregnancy.)

Occasionally, a mother may experience false contractions or Braxton Hicks contractions, which may be felt as early as the second trimester. These "warm up" contractions are usually alleviated with rest. True contractions of labor are not. Labor contractions gradually intensify and increase in frequency. Contractions help with **effacement** (thinning of the cervix) and dilation of the cervix (from the size of a finger tip to 10 cm). This process typically takes several hours to complete. When the cervix has dilated 8 to 10 cm, the women's body is ready to deliver the baby.

Delivery begins with **engagement**, when the baby's head passes through the pelvic outlet, and descends through the birth canal. Passage of the baby's head and/or shoulders requires the most dilation of the birthing canal. The obstetrician may perform an **episiotomy** (surgical opening of the area from the vagina to the rectum) to prevent uncontrolled tearing of the pelvic floor structures. Delivery of the placenta is the final, and shortest stage of the birthing process. Complete delivery of the placenta is necessary to avoid excessive bleeding. At times, a procedure known as a **D and C (dilate and curettage)** is performed to remove any part of the placenta that was not delivered naturally.

A full-term infant may weigh anywhere from 5.5 to 10 pounds (average 7 pounds) and be anywhere from 18 to 22 inches long (average 20 inches).

Precipitous labor and delivery occur in approximately 10% of all deliveries. Precipitous labor is a rapid cervical dilation accompanied by severe, violent contractions that results in the birth of the baby usually within 1 hour. The baby is sometimes injured during this rapid, uncontrolled labor.[11,19]

In some cases, the mother is unable to give birth vaginally, so a C-section must be performed. **C-section** refers to the delivery of a fetus by abdominal surgery requiring an incision through the uterine wall. Indications for a C-section include failure of the birthing process to progress, pelvic disproportion, fetal distress, pregnancy-induced hypertension, mothers with placenta previa or abruption of the placenta, prolapse of the umbilical cord, diabetes mellitus, herpes simplex virus, severe Rh-factor incompatibility, failed forceps delivery, failed induction of labor, and sometimes a repeat C-section. The risk of maternal mortality associated with C-section delivery is three to four times greater than that of vaginal delivery.[11]

Malpresentation of the fetus when the head has not descended first is known as a **breech** presentation and may also require a C-section. The major causes of infant deaths in breech births are cord prolapse, other cord complications, and cerebral hemorrhage. Sudden stresses that may be highly damaging are placed on the infant's cranium. Other injuries include damage to the spinal cord, liver, adrenal glands, or spleen. The risks to the mother and child during vaginal delivery with breech presentation are much higher than with a head first presentation. The extent of the risk depends on the type of breech presentation. Breech births are defined by the lower extremity posture of the infant. **Frank breech** is when the hips are flexed and legs are extended so that feet approximate the jaw. **Complete breech** occurs when the legs are fully crossed at level of buttock as though the fetus is preparing to perform a "cannon ball" (dive). **Footling breech** is where one or both legs are extended through the birth canal. Low birth weight, prematurity, and intrauterine growth retardation put the malpositioned fetus at a higher risk for head entrapment and complications of a traumatic delivery.

Many injuries can occur to the infant during the birthing process. The most common birth injury is due to stretching the head away from the shoulder; this can cause damage to the nerves in the brachial plexus.

Injuries, congenital pathologies, and common pediatric conditions are presented in Chapter 3.

MOTOR DEVELOPMENT

After the fetus has left the relatively weightless environment of the womb, she is confronted with gravity and a variety of sensations that she must begin to process in order to make sense of her new environment. The development of movement and the acquisition of developmental skills is a fascinating and multifactorial process that may be influenced by a variety of factors such as genetics, environmental and learning opportunities, experiences, and health. The process of how a child develops functional skills on the journey toward independence is the keystone in the practice of pediatric physical therapy. The reader is referred to various sources that address this topic in more detail. This chapter will touch only briefly on some of the more influential theories of **motor development**.

Theories of Motor Development

The maturation of the nervous system,[20–25] the environmental experiences of the infant,[26] the infant's cognitive skills,[27] and the complex interaction of the human organism with external stimuli[28–35] have all been identified as having an influence on the development and expression of motor skills. The theories on how humans develop motor skills have themselves developed and changed over time as new knowledge on how and why movements are learned and executed is discovered. Several key theories have had an influence on physical therapy, especially as it is applied to children with disabilities. The **neuromaturation theories** of motor development (Gesell et al.)[20–24] correlated changes in motor development with observable changes in the central nervous system (CNS). According to this theory, every movement occurs as a direct result of CNS activity. Because of this, the level of maturity of the CNS is key to motor development. Motion begins with simple reflexes that are seen in the newborn and progresses in a linear manner until it eventually develops into organized voluntary movements.

The presence and subsequent integration of primitive reflexes as well as the **myelinization** of the lateral corticospinal tracts, which may take up to 24 months, give support to this theory. Myelinization is the process by which some of the nerve fibers throughout the body are coated with a layer of protein and lipids that acts to increase the rate of signal transmission along the nerve fiber.

Cognitive theories of development (Skinner[26] and Piaget[27]) introduced and emphasized the influence of the environment and the cognitive ability of the child in motor development. A child's ability to understand what is asked of her and her motivation to succeed in a movement task that is provided give support to this theory. Practicing physical therapists will recall a child who had the range of motion (ROM) and strength to perform a motor task, but was impaired cognitively and lacked the understanding or motivation to complete the task or make it a skilled behavior. It appears logical that a child has to have the opportunity to experience and react to a motor task in order to develop a motor skill. If a child never had the opportunity to ride a bike, how would she learn to ride a bike? If an infant does not have the opportunity to climb stairs in the home, how does she learn to perform this skill?

A current and increasingly acceptable theory is the **Dynamic Systems Theory** (Thelen et al.,[28–35] Bernstein[36]), according to which movement acquisition is dependent on multiple systems including the external environment as well as the internal biological environment of the child. Having an adequate musculoskeletal system, neuromuscular system, visual perceptual skills, cognitive ability, and the appropriate environmental stimuli are all factors in the development of the most efficient way to move to achieve some action or goal. This theory is more heterarchical than the hierarchical theory of neuromaturation, giving equal weight to each of the systems involved.

The theories that a physical therapist accepts or understands can influence the interventions that he selects and the goals of therapy that are established. Understanding the systems approach to motor development emphasizes the need to examine and evaluate a variety of factors that can have an influence on a child, such as physical maturity or cognitive ability.

Developmental Domains

Development is not a linear or isolated process, but rather a collection of acquired skills that are developed then refined in the process of maturation. Each of the components of this collection of skills is referred to as a different domain of development. A child's environment may influence, positively or negatively, the rate at which these skills are acquired or mastered. Learning requires preparation on the part of the child to perceive and accept new information. Practice requires using the new information in a variety of ways, allowing for trial and error on the part of the child. Feedback and reinforcement of the proper use of information and the proper response of the child is required for appropriate and effective acquisition and application of a skill. Finally, broad application is required for the transfer of a newly acquired skill to other settings or situations that will build upon the knowledge base and lead to the acquisition of new information and additional skills.

Children develop skills in the areas of motor, language, cognitive, social–emotional, and self-help skills as they mature. This categorization of developmental attributes is known as the five **domains of development**.[37,38]

During the first 12 to 15 months, a child's development of skills rapidly proceeds, making significant gains almost monthly, which allows for the identification and listing of expected developmental skills at certain times.

Although this chapter presents these skills within certain time periods, the reader should be sensitive to the individual development of the infant, and see the acquisition and expression of skills as a march toward mastery, which will wax and wane as the child internalizes and develops efficiency in the expression of a skill. Child development is not a rigid set of linear steps, but rather a symphony of movements, expressions, words, and activities, which move the child from a totally dependent being to an independent person.

POINT TO REMEMBER

Developmental Domains

Developmental domains include: motor (both gross and fine), language, cognition, social–emotional development, and self-help skills.

CHILD DEVELOPMENT

Child development occurs in several distinct but interrelated stages throughout the child's life. The first stage is that of the newborn infant, and this is the stage when the child develops basic control over her own body. As the child grows and develops, she also learns to manipulate objects in her environment in increasingly complex ways. These abilities are gained through interactions between the child and her environment and are influenced by many different factors.

The Newborn and Infant

The major developmental tasks from birth to 6 months of age are focused on basic control and regulation of the body; the diurnal/nocturnal cycle; autonomic and motor skills; and state of alertness or arousal.[39] Over the first 3 months, the infant increases her periods of alertness, allowing for relationship building with her primary caregiver. On average she is sleeping approximately 16 hours per day. The primary task of the infant at this stage is to secure a relationship with her caregiver to assure feeding, shelter, and protection. This relationship also helps her to develop a sense of trust in her environment. This bonding process will be the foundation from which she will launch a variety of motor skills and venture out to explore and learn about her environment.

At birth, a full-term infant (referred to as a neonate for the first 2 weeks) will present with a flexed body posture, especially noted in the extremities. This is termed **physiological flexion**, a by-product of intrauterine positioning. A neonate will demonstrate the ability to briefly lift her head when in the prone position. This act of cervical extension is necessary to aid in opening the airway and orienting the mouth to the food source. The act of repeated cervical extension helps to develop the extensor

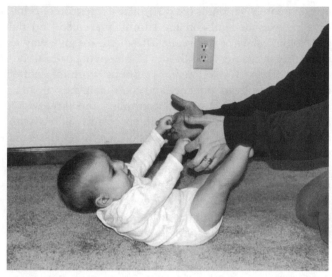

Figure 2-2 ■ Pull to sit of a 6-month-old infant. Notice the ability to control the head at the beginning of the movement.

muscles of the head, neck, and posterior trunk and elongate the flexor muscles of the neck and upper anterior trunk. Voluntary cervical flexion, most noted when the infant is pulled into a sitting position (pull to sit [PTS]), develops. As a newborn, she will show complete head lag during PTS, and progressively develop better head control until approximately 5 months of age, when there will be no head lag noted when she is PTS (Fig. 2-2). Throughout the first 6 months, the infant will work on extension, then flexion, which leads to the ability to co-contract these proximal muscle groups. Development of co-contraction of the flexor and extensor muscles of the cervical regions allows for better head control. When it develops in the trunk, it allows for stability of the trunk, which is necessary for the infant to sit on the floor independently (a hallmark around 6 months). When done in the pelvic region, it allows for kneeling or the maintenance of quadruped.

Around 4 months of age, side-lying provides asymmetrical proprioceptive and tactile input, and encourages midline orientation of the hands. It also stimulates lateral head righting. Lateral head movements are only possible when there is a balance of neck flexor and neck extensor muscles.[40]

During the first 6 months, reflexes are evident as part of the infant's early movements (Fig. 2-3). Although the purpose of these reflexes are unclear, they are believed to be protective in nature (e.g., moro), a mechanism to find and take in food (e.g., rooting and sucking), and may be the foundation for more advanced motor skills that develop later on in life (e.g., spontaneous stepping). They do provide some information on the maturity of the CNS and follow a pattern of obliged expression (obligatory) and integration. The majority of these primitive reflexes are integrated by 6 months, with the noted exception of the symmetrical tonic neck (STNR) reflex, which is integrated at approximately 9 months (Box 2-3). The expression of primitive reflexes depends on the stimuli presented and the physiologic state of the infant. These reflexes give way to voluntary movement and the development of postural control in various developmental positions. Postural control leads to an ability to sequence and coordinate movement to allow for more efficient and controlled mobility, which allows the child to move through space and interact with her environment. Later expressions of primitive reflexes are seen with injury to the CNS. When they are present after the time when they are expected to be integrated, they are referred to as **pathological reflexes**.

Righting reactions also develop during the first 6 months. These midbrain reflexes orient the head to the horizontal, or a body part that is rotated or displaced from the symmetrical posture back into proper alignment. They allow the infant to make her body posture up-"right" (perpendicular to the horizontal) and help to maintain her center of mass over the base of support (Fig. 2-4). They are elicited by several stimuli including visual, vestibular, and somatosensory stimuli (Box 2-4).

Righting reactions are typically seen between 4 and 6 months with their maximum influence seen around 10 to 12 months of age. They persist until approximately 5 years of age when a child can transition supine to stance without trunk rotation.[40]

As the CNS continues to develop and insulate its network of neurons with myelin (the neural insulation that allows for more rapid and efficient delivery of neural

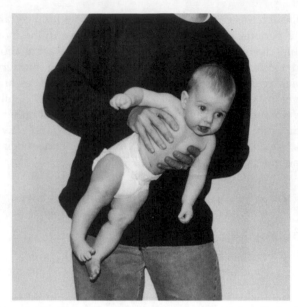

Figure 2-4 ■ The righting reactions of a 6-month-old infant. Notice the attempt to bring the head perpendicular to the horizontal.

impulses), the infant learns to move in more controlled patterns of flexion and extension. The development of this movement from head to toe leads to trunk flexion, which tilts the pelvis posteriorly, bringing the lower extremities into the visual field of the infant, and she "finds her feet" at approximately 4 months of age. This visual stimuli and movement is repeated, stretching the low back and hip extensor muscles, leading to further activation of these muscle groups and the development and expression of a **Landau posture.** (The infant is prone, and her shoulders and hips extend above the horizontal.) This mass movement of the trunk and pelvis can eventually lead to an unexpected roll to the side. The infant may cry at this sudden and unexpected shift in her body alignment, and the parent will notice that the infant has rolled. Rolling prone to supine and supine to prone typically occurs between 5 and 6 months of age. At 4 months of age, an infant will demonstrate the ability to prop up on her elbows when prone. She will progress in this skill until she can raise her chest off the floor and shift her body weight, allowing her upper extremities the freedom to explore objects in front of her. This activity shifts the body weight onto her belly and thighs, a posture essential for the future development of independent sitting.[41]

Not only is the infant developing control of her trunk muscles, she is also developing the use of her upper extremities. She will learn to **reach**, then **grip**, and finally to **manipulate** the objects within her environment. This is done sequentially, and then refined into a synchronistic fashion as seen in adults (Box 2-5). Reaching and grasping objects initially is a reflexive activity, which resembles a swiping type of movement. Vision, especially binocular vision, which develops around 4 months of age, is key to guide the hand toward an object. Vision guides reaching

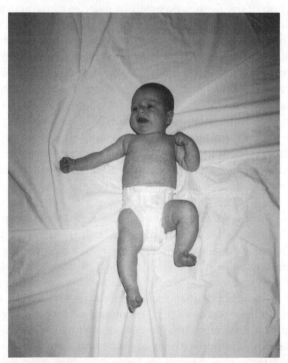

Figure 2-3 ■ The appearance of an ATNR in a 1-month-old infant. The trunk can also be influenced with lateral flexion toward the flexed upper and lower extremities or skull side.

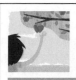

BOX 2-4
Righting Reactions

Reactions of the body to an external stimuli that orient the head to the horizontal or rotation of a part into a symmetrical alignment with the rest of the body. Age of onset and integration may vary slightly.

Reaction:	Body on Head Righting
Seen:	Around 2 months until 5 years of age.
How to elicit:	Place the infant prone or supine.
Response:	The infant's head will orient to the vertical.
Reaction:	Optical Righting
Seen:	Around 2 months until 5 years.
How to elicit:	Suspend the infant vertically, then tip 45° in any direction.
Response:	The head will orient to the vertical.
Reaction:	Labyrinthine Righting
Seen:	Around 2 months of age. Reaction may persist throughout life.
How to elicit:	With the infant's vision occluded, suspend the infant vertically, then tip 45° in any direction.
Response:	The head will orient to the vertical.
Reaction:	Neck on Body Righting
Seen:	Around 4 months until 5 years.
How to elicit:	Place the infant supine and passively turn her head to one side.
Response:	Her body will turn to align with her head and neck.
Reaction:	Body on Body Righting
Seen:	Around 4 months until 5 years.
How to elicit:	Place the infant supine and rotate her upper or lower body.
Response:	Her body rotates to align with rotated body part.

Modified from O'Sullivan S, Schmitz T. *Physical Rehabilitation Assessment and Treatment,* 4th ed. Philadelphia: FA Davis Co.; 2001:187.

BOX 2-5
The Development of Reaching

Age	Hand Movement
0 to 3 months	Hands primarily closed. Grasp is reflexive. Demonstrates swiping.
4 months	Can grasp rattle with gross grasp. Reaching under visual control. Development of binocular coordination for depth perception.
5 months	Raking and squeeze grasp noted. Will orient hand toward object during reaching. Ulnar-palmer grasp evident.
6 months	Radial palmar grasp developing. Beginning opposition which will provide for 70% of normal hand function. Thumb and finger dissociation allows for opposition and poking.
7 to 8 months	Lateral pincher grasp. Picks up tiny objects with fingers. Voluntary release noted. Will be well established by 15 months of age.
10 months	Pokes with index finger. Has inferior pincer grasp: Thumb opposes to volar surface of index finger.
12 months	Controlled release evident. Pad to pad, then tip to tip opposition (superior pincer grasp).

and the orientation of the hand for grasping, whereas proprioception guides the manipulation of the object. By 6 months, the infant is developing the fundamental movement of humans—the ability to place the thumb opposite of the finger (opposition). This skill should allow her to pick up an object such as a toy. By 6 months, she may have developed the skill of holding her bottle with both hands while feeding. This, along with sitting independently, is another major milestone in development, reflecting the beginning of independence.[42]

In addition to the trunk and extremities, the infant is also developing movements of the eyes and mouth that will aid in the infant's ability to provide eye contact with her caregivers, take in visual information from her environment, and to talk, eat, and communicate through facial expressions. Deviations in the ability to move the eyes in harmony can lead to impairments in the ability to see accurately and may impair the motivation to move about the environment. A newborn infant will demonstrate common eye deviations, such as crossed eyes, as she learns to use the small muscles of the eye, much the same way she learns to use her extremities. By 2 to 3 months of age, an infant, while supine, would be expected to follow an object in her visual field 180 degrees. This is a common developmental skill known as tracking. By the end of 4 months, she may have noticed her hand and will watch it as she moves it in front of her face. She will show a preference for looking at people instead of objects and will be able to recognize her mother. By 6 months of age, the infant's vision may be 20/20.

Not only is she developing eye muscle control, she is developing control of the most versatile muscles of her body: her tongue and the muscles of her face. By 2 months, she will smile and make cooing sounds; at times she will make vowel sounds and may squeal. By 5 months, she will laugh. These motor skills carry a lot of social connotation and are reinforcing to the parents. Her tongue movements will mature over the next several years to allow for the development of language, but at this stage the tongue moves mainly in an in/out pattern, to allow sucking and swallowing. For the first 6 months the tongue and jaw move as one unit.

By 5 months of age, the infant should have doubled her birth weight. By her first birthday, she will have tripled her birth weight and measure around 30 inches in length.

POINTS TO REMEMBER

The First 6 Months

Major focus on basic control and regulation of body functions
Evidence of primitive reflexes
Jaw and tongue move as one unit
Binocular vision develops
Rolls
Doubles birth weight by 5 months
Laughs
Holds bottle with both hands
Sits on the floor independently

The Infant

Throughout the first 6 months of development, the infant learns to self-regulate and to gain control of the axial muscles with some degree of efficiency to allow for the development of postural symmetry. Her upper extremity skills at this point allow her to engage in two-handed activities, such as holding a bottle. From 6 to 12 months, the infant continues to advance in skill acquisition, demonstrating some unique characteristics typical of this stage of development. Having developed some trunk control, the infant learns to rotate her trunk in sitting, protect herself from falling, raise her center of mass up off the ground, and move about her immediate environment. Further development of the use of her upper extremities allows for separate hand functions and improved object manipulation.

Rotational movements are key at this point in allowing the infant to transition from one developmental position to another. She will learn to maintain a developmental position before she learns to assume the position. At 6 months of age, an infant will sit on the floor independently, but it may take another month or two to learn how to get into the sitting position from the prone or supine position. Rotational movements require more control and incorporate an asymmetrical use of muscle groups. These movements are more difficult to master than co-contraction of muscle groups, which is done to maintain a developmental position. During this 6-month period, the infant will learn to move into sitting, into

quadruped, pull up into stance, and cruise (walk sideways) along furniture. She will even demonstrate the ability to stand alone briefly, and may take a few steps on her own. Her center of mass is "protected" from moving off her base of support by protective reactions that keep her from falling to the floor. **Protective reactions** are generally single-plane movements incorporating little or no rotation and are elicited when a child is suddenly, and quickly, pushed off of her base of support. Protective extension in sitting develops in the anterior direction (6 to 7 months), then laterally (7 to 8 months), then posteriorly (8 to 9 months). Movement of the extremities is in the same direction of the displacing force, unlike **equilibrium reactions** in which the movement is in the opposite direction. Equilibrium reactions incorporate rotational movements of the trunk and proximal muscles. These reactions emerge after the infant has learned to assume the developmental position independently. Assumption of developmental positions requires rotational movements as well. The purpose of equilibrium reactions is to restore the center of mass over the base of support. These reactions occur in a developmental position approximately 1 to 2 months after the infant learns to assume the position. In prone, they are evident at 6 months of age, supine at 7 months, sitting by 8 months. Equilibrium in standing, an exception to the general rule, is seen at approximately 21 months of age.

The emergence and use of these reactions is accompanied by an increase in mobility skills. Following the ability to sit is the ability to maintain a hands and knees position, or quadruped. In this position an infant learns to move her elevated center of mass forward and backward (rocking in quadruped) and side-to-side, which allows her to free up her weight-bearing upper and lower extremity and creep forward. Creeping (moving forward on her belly; think commando crawl) and crawling (moving forward on hands and knees) require a coordinated movement of the upper extremities, trunk, pelvis, and lower extremities. This complex movement demonstrates dissociation of the right and left sides of the body. In some infants, consistent symmetrical movement of the lower extremities is noted during creeping. This moving of the knees forward at the same time while in quadruped has been termed "bunny hopping" and has been associated with disorders of the nervous system, such as cerebral palsy (see Chapter 3). Creeping stretches the gluteal and low back muscles—two key areas needed for the next developmental skill of kneeling. Full kneeling (both knees on the ground with hips extended) places the center of mass anteriorly over the base of support, making it easier to fall forward than backward. Rising to stance at this stage will require the assistance of the upper extremities and is accomplished by pelvic and hip dissociation and the assumption of a half kneel (the weight-bearing knee determines if the child is in right or left half kneel), or by taking weight off the lower extremities and pulling up with the upper extremities, using both legs to push into stance through a squatting position. This maneuver requires the lower extremities to perform the same motion of flexion into extension, at the same time. Now in stance, holding on with both hands, the infant may bounce up and down, working the muscles that got her into this position, and may shift her weight from left to right. When she takes the weight off of one leg, she may move it to the side then shift weight onto that leg, allowing her body to move sideways while holding onto a surface. This is called "cruising," which is typically done with the lower extremities externally rotated and the knees kept in extension.

In addition to the dramatic gross motor skills she is learning and demonstrating, she is also learning to use her hands for manipulation of the objects she encounters. She can now transfer objects from one hand to the other. The skill of thumb and finger opposition, which requires thumb and finger dissociation, also progresses. By 7 to 8 months, she is using a lateral pincer grasp, and is able to pick up tiny objects with her fingers (Fig. 2-5). She is also demonstrating more of a voluntary release of objects, noted when she is asked to give her caregiver an object she is holding. By 9 months of age, the child may be able to "wave good-bye," but indiscriminately. She should also be able to hold a spoon, but will not be able to successfully feed herself. By 10 months of age, she will use an isolated index finger to poke and explore objects. She further develops fine motor skills, demonstrating thumb opposition to the volar surface of the index finger, referred to as an inferior pincer grasp. By 12 months of age, she will demonstrate a controlled release of the objects in her grasp and will be able to oppose her thumb pad-to-pad, then tip-to-tip prehension, demonstrating a superior pincer grasp. This improved manipulation of objects allows her to grasp certain food items and finger feed.

Between 9 and 12 months of age, the concept of object permanence, the ability to understand that objects not seen are still in existence, develops. This awareness, which is accompanied developmentally by the ability of the infant to move away from her caregiver, by crawling into another room, often leads to anxiety when the primary caregiver is absent (separation anxiety) or when new people are present in the infant's environment (stranger anxiety). These processes are typical and should be expected. They pass within a few months.

The infant will also develop improved oral motor skills enabling her to maneuver food in her mouth to chew and swallow solid foods. Her tongue movements will develop allowing for lateralization of foods in the mouth, which is necessary for chewing, and the formation of a bolus for swallowing. By 12 months, she will have developed improved lip closure allowing her to drink from a cup. For the first 6 months, the tongue and jaw moved as one unit, but now move separately, allowing for the development of further language skills. At this stage, the infant is making vowel sounds and producing the words "da da" or "ma ma" (generally at 10 months and by 12 months to her mother or father appropriately).

By 8 months, an infant should understand the meaning of the word "no," although her actions may not always abide by the command. Her ability to internalize the meaning and consequences of her actions is still developing. Receptive language precedes expressive language. An infant will understand her first words around 6 to 9 months and will be able to understand "wave bye-bye" when asked at 9 to 12 months of age.

At 2 months of age, an infant will turn her head in response to a sound. By her first birthday she should demonstrate, with adult accuracy, the localization of sounds made in her immediate environment.

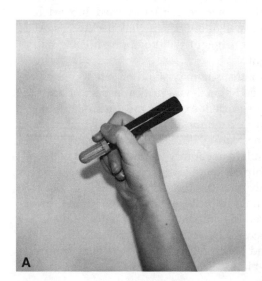
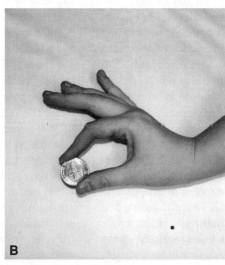

Figure 2-5 ■ **A:** Lateral pincer grasp is used to hold a marker. **B:** Superior pincer grasp is used to hold a coin.

The Toddler

Different parts of the body grow at different rates. The trunk grows the fastest during the first year of life. After the first year, the legs are the fastest growing part of the body.[40]

During the period from 12 to 36 months, the infant will develop the skills of walking, climbing, running, talking, dressing, feeding, and a variety of cognitive and self-help skills that will further propel her toward independence.[42] The rapid acquisition of skills continues with a noticeable change in her ability to move about her environment and to talk. Typically at 12 months of age, an infant will take her first steps, becoming a toddler. These steps are significantly different than the ones she will use as an adult. She walks forward with her elbows flexed, shoulders abducted and externally rotated and shoulder girdles retracted (a guarded position). She will demonstrate decreased rotation during ambulation. (Remember that rotation develops later, allowing for the child to assume stance from the floor, without upper extremity assistance. That occurs around 15 months of age.) She will have a wide base of support and advance her lower extremities with increased hip and knee flexion, shortening the stride length, and demonstrating foot flat contact instead of heel strike with the unweighted limb. Her cadence at 12 months is approximately 175 steps per minute, compared to 153 steps per minute at 36 months. (A 7-year-old will demonstrate approximately 144 steps per minute, and an adult cadence is approximately 114 steps per minute.)[43]

The acquisition of independent ambulation is unique in its social emphasis as the infant demonstrates the skills necessary to overcome the forces of gravity and to sufficiently control her posture in space to move forward in stance. This is another hallmark of independence. The age at which an infant takes her first steps, whether at 9 months or 18 months, depends on a variety of internal and external factors. An infant's general health, body weight,[44] cultural practices,[45] environmental influences, and the development of postural control are a few of the necessary components needed for the development of independent walking. Other factors such as genetics, maturation of the nervous system, and cognitive development also play a role in the development of this skill. The process of acquiring and mastering the skill of efficient ambulation takes 6 years to become adult-like (7-year-old child); at this time, a mature gait pattern is evident in the way the child walks.[44,45] As she continues to grow, the velocity of ambulation, her stride length, and step length will all increase as the cadence of her gait decreases. During the process of physical maturation, she will grow in height while her legs become longer, and her center of mass will move more superior from her base of support making her more unstable and dependent on postural control, muscle strength, and equilibrium reactions to maintain an upright position.

Learning to take her first steps is only the beginning of the development of higher level skills that will include postural control at the end ranges of movement, allowing her to squat while she is playing and to use her arms and legs to creep up steps or climb onto low furniture (15 months of age). By 18 to 24 months, she will begin to walk faster and to run with a noted decrease in rotation of her trunk and pelvis. At this time, she is also developing the skill to jump with both feet, an activity which is a progression of strength, seen in her ability to squat and climb, to an activity demonstrating power (a product of force and velocity). Power gives her the ability to throw her center of mass higher, leaving the surface and security of the ground.

At 24 months of age, this increased strength will allow her to ascend and descend stairs marking time (one step at a time), and to demonstrate another activity incorporating power, this time in her upper extremity, throwing a ball overhand. (It may take another 12 months for her to consistently hold out her arms in anticipation of catching a ball thrown to her.) Increased hip extensor muscle strength will allow her to walk backwards. At 24 months of age, her height will be approximately half of her adult height.

By 30 months, she may stand on one foot momentarily. One-legged stance is a critical aspect of ambulation, requiring sufficient extensor muscle strength to stabilize the lower extremity allowing for advancement of the non-weight-bearing limb.[46] Increasing strength and power will result in her ability to jump forward with both feet (broad jump). If there are steps in the home, the parents may notice that the toddler jumps off the last step when descending. Improvements in strength and power are incorporated into improved coordination of the lower extremities seen in the ability of a 3-year-old to pedal a tricycle, ascend stairs reciprocally (step over step) and walk a straight line.

Not only is she improving in the use of her lower extremities during this time period, she is also learning to use her upper extremities to drink from a cup, scoop with a spoon, and to remove her shoes (18 to 24 months). By now, she will be able to turn the pages of the book that is being read to her. At 2 years of age, a toddler may manipulate a doorknob to open a door and remove a lid by unscrewing it from the container. Added dexterity of the upper extremities and the emerging cognitive skills in identifying major body parts will allow the 30-month-old to put on shoes and pants and to assist with posturing in anticipation for donning clothes during dressing. She will be able to hold a crayon with her thumb and index finger. By 3 years of age, she will be able to use a fork for self-feeding, copy a circle while drawing, and use scissors to cut paper. Hand preference is typically noted by the third year.

The period between 18 and 24 months will show an explosion in expressive language. Language reflects both cognitive and social–emotional development and lays the foundation for literacy and future academic skills.[10] After the realization of what words represent, a toddler will expand her vocabulary from approximately 15 words at 18 months to 100 words at 24 months.[10]

The emergence of verbal language is the transition in the child's life from learning primarily through sensory and motor experience to learning through more cognitive activities. The need for direct sensory or motor experiences to understand and learn is shifting toward the use of symbols and relationships to understand the world around her. By 18 months, object permanence is well understood by the child, as is "cause and effect" relationships. These skills further her ability to solve problems and encourage further and more extensive exploration and manipulation of her environment. This heightened activity and inquisitiveness is often mislabeled "the terrible twos."

As she acquires an understanding of the meaning of words, she will connect them to make a more complete thought or request. As a general rule, between the ages of 2 and 5 years, the number of words in a child's sentence is her age in years.[10] For example, a child who is 2 years old will speak using two-word sentences, a child who is 3 years old will use three-word sentences, and so on. A delay in expressive language by the age of 24 months is significant.

Another major development in her independence during this period is her ability to control her bowel and bladder. Voluntary control of the bowel and bladder sphincter muscles emerges around 18 months of age. (This occurs about the same time she learns to pucker her lips to give a kiss.) Parents will notice extended periods of dryness and predictable times of bowel movements. On average, she will have control of her bowel and bladder by 30 months of age, but there is a wide variation in the acquisition of this skill. Daytime control precedes nighttime control. Some signs that she is ready for toilet/potty training include: being dry for 2 hours at a time during the day, waking up dry after a nap, predictable bowel movements, her ability to indicate that she has to go to the bathroom, and her ability to follow simple one-step directions. By 4 years of age, she should be able to use a toilet by herself. Episodes of bedwetting may continue.[47]

Social interactions also progress during this period. A child will begin to pretend (around 12 to 17 months) to give a baby doll a bottle, or will play with toy cars. Not only is she using her refined motor skills, she is also demonstrating the use of symbolic thought and creativity. A toddler will demonstrate the ability to play alone, termed solitary play. By 3 years of age, she may also demonstrate parallel play, playing with the same toys as the child next to her, and possibly doing the same activity, but not interacting. The child learns social–emotional skills through her play interactions. A 2-year-old child may begin to demonstrate behaviors that would be considered empathetic to adults, but her ability to see another child's point of view still remains limited. She is a very concrete thinker with rules being absolute. Sharing, which is often encouraged by adults and carries a higher level of cognitive thought and reasoning, is seen as equal treatment by a child at this stage.

POINTS TO REMEMBER

The Toddler at 1 to 3 Years

First steps may occur between 9 and 18 months.
Strength and power develop to climb steps, throw objects, and run.
Manipulation improves allowing for the use of feeding utensils and other household objects.
Cognitive skills emerge, reflected in identification of body parts, cause and effect relationships, and the use of language.
There is rapid growth in language skills between 18 and 24 months.
The number of words used in a sentence is roughly the child's age.
Bowel and bladder management develops between 18 and 30 months with wide variation.
A 2-year-old is approximately half her adult height.
The child demonstrates solitary play (2-year-old) and parallel play (3-year-old).

The Young Child

The major developmental skills acquired during this stage include an increased mastery of language, increased socialization and self-control, and the continued progression toward mature movement patterns. The activity level of a 3-year-old is higher than at any other time in her entire life. The toddler, now considered a preschooler, is no longer limited in her learning by sensory motor experiences, but is developing a dependence on perception and preoperational (prelogical, symbolic) skills as well.[27] She will understand that the word "bed" is a symbol for her bed, and she will string words together to convey thoughts and needs.

Although her immediate family and parents remain the main influence in her social–emotional development, her involvement in preschool activities during this stage brings her into contact with peers and situations where she must learn to adapt and conform to new rules and relationships. "I'll do it myself" is a common saying for a preschooler as she attempts to have an influence on her environment. Attempting skills that are unrealistic at this age can lead to frustration and outbursts of temper tantrums.[39] Learning from these situations helps the child develop self-control and prepares her for functioning outside of the family. Oppositional behavior is common in children 2 to 3 years of age, but should gradually subside as the child learns more about rules, boundaries, consequences, and self-regulation.

During this phase, she will begin to rely more on somatosensory input to move, particularly between the ages of 3 and 6 years.[48] The movement skills that she will work on and acquire include the ability to get onto and off of a tricycle (3½ years. Remember rotation). Her improved ability to stabilize one side of her body will allow her to stand on one foot longer than 3 seconds (by 6 years, she will be able to do this for 10 seconds) and hop on one foot. As her strength increases, so does her power, enabling her to broad jump and hop on one foot by the age of 4 years. She will also run with noted upper extremity reciprocal movements and will be coordinated enough to perform a somersault. The equilibrium reactions that emerged during infancy are now mature.

At 4 years of age, a child will have the fine motor skills to brush her teeth, use scissors, and throw a ball overhand with more trunk rotation. She will be able to dress herself, managing zippers and complete the process with few errors.[42] At 4½ years, she will begin to print letters.

By the age of 5 years, she will improve in her lower extremity coordination, demonstrating the ability to skip, ride a two-wheeled bike, and roller skate. She will be able to throw a ball to a friend or at a target 10 feet away and catch it upon return. She will demonstrate eye–foot coordination by being able to drop kick a ball. She will also be able to run and kick a ball without loss of balance, demonstrating an improvement in dynamic postural stability.[42]

By the age of 6 years, the child will be able to hop in patterns (play hopscotch) and gallop. These motor achievements can be related to brain development and myelination of neurons in the area associated with balance and coordination. There is a transitional period between 4 and 6 years of age when responses may be slower and more disorganized, resulting in noticeable balance changes.[49] During these years, the child is learning to coordinate somatosensory input with visual input which may result in transient periods of minor "clumsiness" and incoordination. This is also accompanied by growth spurts that occur around this age.[48]

The foundation for literacy is also established in the preschool years. Letter formation and reading words in a book from left to right and top to bottom are activities that the preschooler is exposed to repeatedly when read to by an adult. A 4-year-old will begin to use the past tense when she speaks. She will be able to state her age, know the primary colors, and understand spatial relationships such as: on, under, in front of, and behind. By 5 years, she will incorporate future tense into her conversations, have a vocabulary of approximately 2000 words, know her home address, identify her left from her right, and count to 20. Children who master language early may elicit wordy and complex explanations from adults who incorrectly assume that their language skills are directly related to their cognitive level. Adults should take note that a 5-year-old is still a very concrete thinker and lacks the ability for abstract or logical thought.

During this phase, play becomes more complex and structured. A child (age 3 to 4) will demonstrate associative play, which serves to increase social–emotional skills through interactions with other children; however, there is little organization to this type of play. In this type of play, the child is more focused on her playmates than on the activity itself. Imaginative play scenarios will reflect activities of daily living, allowing the child to prepare for taking on those roles herself one day. By 4 to 5 years of age, she will participate in cooperative play, which includes organized games with a sense of a team and the aim of winning. Her imaginative play will incorporate activities she has not experienced, such as being a racecar driver or traveling to the moon. This aids social–emotional development by allowing the child the opportunity to put herself in someone else's place through play scenarios and to develop more advanced social skills. She will begin to interact more with other children than she has in the past. She may also prefer certain playmates to others as she begins to actively involve other children in her play.

Her entrance into preschool at this time significantly exposes her to other children and their illnesses and behaviors. Although some children attend daycare at an early age, preschool is often the first structured exposure the child has to others outside the family. Through the activities of attending school, performing with others, and making friends, the child continues to develop her role as an individual.

As the child prepares to enter the system of formal education, around 6 years of age, she will also experience the loss of her first tooth and eruption of her first molars. She will experience, on average, a loss of approximately four baby teeth per year. She will also demonstrate more modesty around 4 to 6 years of age.[10]

Vision dominates the influence of postural control in the child until the age of 3 years, when the somatosensory system has matured sufficiently to utilize proprioceptive input in this process. From age 4 to 6 years, there is an increase in the use of somatosensory and vestibular information to maintain postural control. Adult-like balance responses and gait characteristics are seen between 7 and 10 years.[40,49] At 6 years of age, she will weigh, on average, 46 pounds and be 46 inches tall.[12]

POINTS TO REMEMBER

The Young Child, 3 to 6 Years

There is a high activity level at 3 years.
Symbolic, prelogic thought develops.
Contact with peers increases.
Mastery in developmental domains, in self-control, and in socialization increases.
The foundation for literacy skills is established.
Equilibrium reactions mature.
The 4½-year-old prints.
The child demonstrates associative play (4-year-old) and cooperative play (5-year-old).
An average 6-year-old is 46 inches tall and weighs 46 pounds.

The Child

Primary developmental tasks during the elementary school years include the acquisition of symbol-associative learning (reading, writing, mathematics, and spelling), rule-governing play, increased awareness of social expectations, and mastery of more complex cognitive and academic tasks with school being an important and influential environment.[39]

School Readiness is a concept that a child should demonstrate certain developmental skills determined to be necessary in order to succeed in the school environment. Some examples may be the ability to follow simple directions, communicate wants and needs, or the ability to manipulate the tools of education (opening a book, holding a crayon, etc.). There is no standard set of skills for all children. Variations in school readiness criteria can vary from state to state or from school district to school district. School readiness also includes factors of the family, community, and school. All of these factors are influential in promoting success in the educational environment.

One universal aspect of school readiness is physical maturation. Physical growth of the child during this stage occurs in spurts approximately 3 to 6 times per year.[10] Head growth is slower, reflective of slower brain growth during this stage. Myelinization of the nervous system is generally complete around 7 years of age.[10] Along with the growth in size, increases in muscular strength, coordi-

nation, and endurance also occur, allowing the child to perform a jumping jack (7 years), stand on one foot with her eyes closed (7 years), play basketball, or learn to play a musical instrument with some degree of efficiency. Between 6 and 10 years of age, the child will master the adult forms of running, throwing, and catching. Refinement of these skills will depend on the amount of practice and instruction provided to improve and refine these specific skills. By 9 years of age, she will be able to vertically jump 8 to 10 inches, and by 11 years, she will be able to broad jump 5 feet. By age 11, girls will be taller than boys; this is the only time in their lives, on average, when they will be taller than boys given their growth spurt around the age of 10 years.

By 6 to 7 years of age, the child's fine motor skills will also improve, allowing her to use a knife to put peanut butter on bread, or to cut food. By the age of 7, she will begin cursive writing. By the age of 10 to 12 years, she will demonstrate basic manipulative skills similar to an adult. By the age of 12, she may have acquired the basic ADLs needed to be independent.[1] Performing regular chores in the home will provide an opportunity for the child to participate in the family, which can support her development of self-esteem as well as foster the development of IADLs. These are ADLs that involve more cognitive functioning and management. Examples include planning, shopping for and preparing meals, managing a checkbook, following a schedule, or using public transportation.

During this phase, the child is moving from preoperational thinking to more concrete operational thinking (logical thinking). She becomes less dependent on what she sees and will begin to understand basic concepts. She will be able to understand conservation problems (an understanding that a mass or group of objects will remain constant, or be conserved, regardless of its shape or size of the container) and place things and events in serial order.[39] This shift in thinking is gradual, and the elementary student may frequently be heard using the reasoning "just because" to explain her answers.[12] She is still unable to understand abstract or hypothetical questions.

By first and second grades (6 and 7 years), she will start reading; by third grade (8 years), she will read more fluently, out loud, but without much meaning. The child enjoys playing board games and develops expert knowledge in an area such as sports or cars. By the fourth grade (9 years), she will start to use reading as a means of learning. Some of her cognitive skills have become automatic, allowing her to read a paragraph and, not only understand each word, but comprehend the paragraph's meaning. Some children at this age become avid readers. Printing evolves into the composition of sentences. The acquisition of knowledge also builds her developing sense of self-esteem.

As her use of language progresses, her vocabulary increases, but she will still have a problem with subtle changes of intonation in a sentence.[12] She may not fully understand sarcasm. Throughout this phase, the child will show a preference for spending time with same-sex friends, seek their acceptance, and increase her separation from her parents. As the child reaches the end of this stage (10 to 12 years), she will value her privacy. She may be preparing for the second most drastic change in her life since her gestation: puberty.

POINTS TO REMEMBER

The Child, 6 to 12 Years

Growth spurts are noted three to six times per year.
There are increases in muscle strength, power, coordination, and endurance.
The child performs ADLs.
A 6-year-old can read. By 9 years, she is using reading as a means to learn.
A 7-year-old begins cursive writing.
Concrete operational (logical) thinking develops.
Between 7 to 10 years, an adult gait and balance pattern develops as well as mature forms of running, throwing, and catching.
A 12-year-old has the manipulation skills of an adult.

The Adolescent

The word adolescence is derived from the Latin word *adolscere*, which means, "to grow in maturity." Puberty is the process of developing the capability to reproduce. The onset of this process is not fully understood; however, several factors are known. An increased sensitivity of the pituitary gland to gonadotropin-releasing hormone (GnRH); a release of GnRH, leutinizing hormone (LH), and follicle-stimulating hormone (FSH) during sleep; along with an increased rise in levels of gonadal androgens and estrogens appear to be the precipitating factors that trigger the rapid physical changes seen in puberty.

During this phase, the adolescent will grow to near maturity. Girls will reach their adult size around age 17 to 18 years. Boys will reach their adult size between 18 and 21 years.[50] Changes in muscle distribution, fat, and circulatory and respiratory systems lead to increased stamina and endurance in the adolescent.[39] Sexual maturity ratings (SMR) were developed by Tanner to provide some indication of the state of physical maturation of the adolescent (see Table 2-2). Mastery over increased strength and coordination enable the adolescent to calibrate and coordinate her movements, allowing her to perform several activities at once, such as those required to drive a car. The accomplishment of motor skills is refined into performance skills, taking into consideration efficiency and effectiveness of the movement on the desired outcome.

Of all the changes associated with adolescence and puberty, the physical changes associated with reproductive maturity are some of the most dramatic. These outward

TABLE 2-2 Sexual Maturity Ratings

SMR Stage	Distribution of Pubic Hair
1	Preadolescent
2	Sparse, lightly pigmented, straight
3	Darker, begins to curl
4	Coarse, curly and abundant but less than adult
5	Adult distribution, spread to medial surface of thighs

Modified from Tanner J. *Growth at Adolescence*, 2nd ed. Oxford, England: Blackwell Scientific Publications; 1962.

changes are referred to as primary and secondary sex characteristics. Primary sex characteristics associated with puberty in girls may begin between the ages of 7 and 13 years (average is age 10) with the initiation of breast development. Menarche usually occurs 2 years later.[39] Puberty in boys begins between the ages of 9 and 13.5 years, with the onset of pubic hair and growth of the penis and testicles.[39] Spermarche occurs around the age of 13 years.[12]

Secondary sex characteristics are the visible signs of maturation that distinguish the sexes but do not involve the sex organs directly. These include for boys the presence of chest and facial hair, broader shoulders, increased muscle mass, and a prominent Adam's apple. For girls, these include enlarged breasts, pubic hair, and wider hips.

The period of adolescence can be viewed in three distinct periods: early, middle, and late adolescence[10] (Table 2-3). In early adolescence, the adolescent is focused on her physical appearance and is spending more time with her peers. Conformity with her peer group may be noticed in the way she dresses and the activities in which she participates. Parents notice her desire for greater autonomy from the family by her attitude, mood swings, disagreements, and anger expressed verbally with occasional outbursts. Girls develop friendships based more on sharing confidences, whereas boys tend to make friends based on shared activities and competition. At this time the adolescent is developing formal operational learning, abstract thought, and hypothetical deductive reasoning. She is able to think about what is possible and devise several strategies to solve problems as she learns concepts like algebra. She is developing the ability to think logically and rationally. Physical growth in middle adolescence is most remarkable, with an average growth in height of 3 inches per year. This period is associated with SMR 3. Girls will enter this growth period first, followed by boys, typically 2 to 3 years later, and will continue for the boys 2 to 3 years after the girls have stopped growing.[35] Growth of the hands and feet precedes that of the trunk, giving the teenager an awkward appearance. As boys go through puberty, their percentage of body fat tends to decrease, whereas in girls it tends to increase. By 16 years of age, the adolescent can perform IADLs like household chores, making meals, taking care of pets,

TABLE 2-3 Central Issues in Early, Middle, and Late Adolescence

Variable	Early Adolescence	Middle Adolescence	Late Adolescence
Age (yr)	10–13	14–16	17–20 and beyond
SMR*	1–2	3–5	5
Somatic	Secondary sex characteristics; beginning of rapid growth; awkward	Height growth peaks; body shape and composition change; acne and odor; menarche; spermarche	Slower growth
Sexual	Sexual interest usually exceeds sexual activity	Sexual drive surges; experimentation; questions of sexual orientation	Consolidation of sexual identity
Cognitive and moral	Concrete operations; conventional morality	Emergence of abstract thought; questioning mores; self-centered	Idealism; absolutism
Self-concept	Preoccupation with changing body; self-consciousness	Concern with attractiveness, increasing introspection	Relatively stable body image
Family	Bids for increased independence; ambivalence	Continued struggle for acceptance of greater autonomy	Practical independence; family remains secure base
Peers	Same-sex groups; conformity; cliques	Dating; peer groups less important	Intimacy; possibly commitment
Relationship to society	Middle-school adjustment	Gauging skills and opportunities	Career decisions (e.g., drop out, college, work)

*See text and Figures 14.1 and 14.2.
SMR, sexual maturity rating.
Behrman R, Kliegman R, Jenson H. *Nelson Textbook of Pediatrics*, 16th ed. W.B. Saunders Company; 2000:53, with permission from Elsevier.

babysitting, shopping, or taking her own medication. She will begin to think more seriously about what she wants to be when she becomes an adult. In late adolescence, she may spend more time with the opposite sex, developing the interpersonal skills for intimacy more so than peer acceptance. Mastery over movement and proficiency with communication drives expansion of the social skills needed for independent living and the activities of an adult in our society. Some traditional roles and rituals of adulthood include economic and emotional independence from parents, living apart from the family, participating in society by voting, and getting married[51,52] (Chapter 10). Career decisions become more pressing as the adolescent contemplates her role in society, as a student, worker, or parent. To get to this point requires developmental progression of the child and the parent.

The Adolescent, 12 to 18 Years

Menarche (average age 10 years): Girls physically mature around 17 to 18 years.
Spermarche (average age 13 years): Boys physically mature around 18 to 21 years.
Formal operational (logical, abstract) thought develops.
The adolescent performs IADLs.
The role as an adult is pondered.

The Development of the Parent

Parenting (the act of teaching and raising a young child) is not taught. It is based on experiences of childhood, cul-

tural habits, and individual family parenting behaviors. It is "on the job training" that changes and grows as the child and family change and grow. Parenting requires understanding, patience, discipline, and adaptation. As the child continues on her journey toward independence, the parent journeys also, from care and nurturing toward letting her be independent. Parents develop along with their children, responding to different challenges that children at various ages encounter and changing their style of parenting as their family changes and matures.[53] Often parents strive for perfection, but there is no perfect child, perfect parent, or perfect family. Successful parenting begins with self-appreciation of the role of parenting and its important role in nurturing a child toward individuality and independence. Establishing routines may have a positive effect on child development. Parents who stick to routines, even through difficult situations, may be more successful at dealing with those stressful situations.[6] Parent involvement in reading activities with a child has found to be related to the child's reading skills in the third grade.[8] Established routines can also increase satisfaction in the role of parenting in young mothers.[54]

Setting rules and applying consistent discipline may help a child understand her boundaries and the consequences to her actions. Honest and direct answers to her simple questions can help her understand her role and capabilities in her early years. Providing a nurturing and stable environment with established routines, an understanding of her development, and why she behaves the way she does, along with the provision of proper nutrition and rest, and honest praise for her developing sense of self and independence are a few of the basic needs of the developing child provided by the parent.

POINTS TO REMEMBER

Parenting

Skills in parenting develop as the child and family develop. Establishing routines may have a positive effect on child and parent development.

PARENT PERSPECTIVE

REFLECTIONS ON RAISING A CHILD

A baby in the home needs constant attention. Everyday you must feed, bathe, change diapers, and spend time bonding, as well as completing all your other work. It is a family effort, especially when your baby is sick. Not too long ago, when your baby got sick you would call the doctor and if it were an emergency you would even go to the doctor's house instead of the hospital. The doctor would give the baby a shot and some medicine and whatever the doctor told you to do you would do it without question. Of course you would stay up all night and hold your baby and worry. It seems as a parent you always worry about your baby, especially when he is sick. But holding your baby, and the look and feel of utter dependence on you is worth all the effort and work.

When your child is old enough to go to school, you notice the amount of dependence on you has diminished. You have to let go a little. He will start to interact with other children and hopefully learn to share. Teaching him good manners and discipline are important and hopefully make an impression on him, especially as he grows into a teenager. The teenage years can be the most trying for the parent as well as the most rebellious for the child. A parent must be more patient, understanding, and trusting. Drugs, friends, and your child's attitude towards his elders are a greater worry at this time. Your teenager is going to try to "be an adult" and may do things he should not do. As the parent you have to be very diligent for any signs of problems.

College years and young adulthood are also different and difficult times for the parent. The parent must learn to let go and allow her child to learn from his own mistakes. Sometimes it is hard to stand by and watch. Hopefully your child's early training will help him cope with the new problems and challenges he faces. When your child is married and has children of his own, hopefully he will treat them with love, tolerance, and patience.

If you try and give your child the basics of love, social graces, and how to appropriately interact with people, your child will be better equipped to cope with growing up and being on his own. If your child works hard to achieve his goals in the workforce or college, you can take pride in knowing that your years of hard work as a parent have paid off.

—*Margaret B. (77 years old), a great-grandmother.*

NUTRITION

Proper nutrition is essential for growth and development and the maintenance of a healthy lifestyle throughout all stages of life. Proper nutrition is necessary from the time a child is conceived, and continues to play a major role in a person's health throughout the rest of her life. Parents play an important role in the introduction of dietary choices to their child. Making sure that a child gets an adequate amount of rest and eats the appropriate variety and quantities of food is a major aspect of parenting. A physical therapist can screen for any nutritional concerns during the examination of the child. Gathering information on body height and weight, eating habits, and developmental level of the child, as well as the financial resources available to the family to purchase food items, can be part of the initial evaluation process. Comparing the age of the child and the amount and type of foods she consumes can provide a general understanding of her nutritional intake. If any questions or concerns arise during this process, referral to the proper professional (a physician or dietician) may be warranted.

During the first 4 months of life, breast milk or formula is the only source of nutrition that the infant needs. At first, the newborn may eat only 2 to 3 ounces spaced out every 2 to 3 hours throughout the day. Most infants will wake several times during the night to eat because a newborn infant's stomach is not large enough to hold enough food to satisfy her for long periods of time. A healthy infant should ingest a total of 16 to 20 ounces of formula in a 24-hour period.[55] Older infants will begin to eat more food less often as their stomach begins to grow. Most 4-month-old infants will eat 4 to 6 ounces of formula at each feeding and eat 4 to 5 meals per day.

At 5 months of age, the infant can begin to eat a greater variety of foods. The variety and quality of food intake can be monitored by tracking the number of servings eaten in each of five food groups: protein, vegetables and fruits, carbohydrates, dairy products, and fats and oils. The U.S. Department of Agriculture Food and Nutrition Center suggests starting infants on cereal between 4 and 7 months of age.[56] (It is important to remember that breast milk or formula remains the most important source of nutrition throughout the entire first year.) At 5 months of age, the mother can begin to introduce fruit juice and strained fruits and vegetables into the infant's diet. According to the American Academy of Pediatrics, infants can start to eat solid foods around 6 months of age, but they are not needed until 9 to 12 months. An infant at this age will require something more solid in her stomach at each meal in addition to her formula. Plain, strained vegetables should be started first, then strained fruits.

Infants at this age have different tastes than adults. They do not need added sugar or salt on their food. Only one new food should be introduced at a time in case the infant has an allergic reaction to the food. (This way, the parents are able to distinguish which food the infant was not able to tolerate.) Fruit juice can also be introduced at this time and should be limited to 2 to 4 ounces of juice per day, watered down at first until the infant gets used to it. It is best to wait until the infant is 8 to 10 months old before starting the infant on orange juice because of the high acidity of the juice. By 5 months, the infant should be breastfeeding six to eight times per day or drinking four to six, 6- to 8-ounce bottles of formula per day. She may eat 2 to 4 tablespoons of infant cereal, fed with a spoon, twice daily, 2 to 4 tablespoons of strained vegetables, and 2 to 4 ounces of fruit juice each day in addition to her formula. By 6 months of age, she should be breastfeeding for four to six feedings or drinking three to five, 6- to 8-ounce servings of formula, eating 2 to 4 tablespoons of infant cereal twice daily, 2 to 4 tablespoons of strained vegetables, 2 to 4 tablespoons of strained fruit, and 2 to 4 ounces of fruit juice daily. Also, at this age, the infant may start to hold her own bottle. A cup should be introduced by 6 months of age.[57]

At around 7 or 8 months, the infant can start to eat strained meats and egg yolk. Egg whites should not be given until 1 year of age. A normal diet at this age includes three to four, 8-ounce bottles of formula or four to six breast feedings throughout the day, 3 to 5 tablespoons of infant cereal, fed with a spoon, twice per day, 4 to 8 tablespoons of strained vegetables, 4 tablespoons of strained fruit, 2 to 4 ounces of fruit juice, and 1 to 3 tablespoons of strained meat or egg yolk each day.[58]

Infants who are 9 to 12 months old begin to eat with their fingers. This is a good age to begin to introduce table foods. Early table foods should be soft and easy for the infant to chew. During this period of time, the infant should be gradually weaned off strained foods so that by 1 year of age, she is eating entirely table foods. The infant should be given a cup throughout the day and should have progressively fewer bottles so that by 1 year of age she is weaned off the bottle altogether and drinks exclusively from a cup. During this time period, the infant should be taking a total of 24 to 32 ounces of formula throughout the day. She should eat 4 to 8 tablespoons of infant cereal, two to three servings of bread or cereal, 4 ounces of fruit juice, two servings of fruit, two servings of vegetables (4 tablespoons = 1 serving of fruits or vegetables), and 2 to 8 tablespoons of pureed or chopped soft meat, fish, egg yolk, cheese, yogurt, or mashed beans every day.[59] The following is a guide to the number of servings recommended for a 1-year-old infant.[60]

Dairy	4 servings	A serving for a toddler this age consists of ½ cup of milk or ¾ oz of cheese
Vegetables	1 to 2 servings	¼ cup cooked, ½ cup raw
Protein	1 to 2 servings	1 tablespoon of meat, 1 egg, ½ cup cooked beans
Fruit	3 servings	¼ cup cooked, ½ cup raw
Carbohydrates	6 servings	½ slice bread, ¼ cup pasta, rice, or cereal
Fats and Oils	Use sparingly	

POINTS TO REMEMBER

Intake for Infants

0 to 4 months	16 to 20 oz in 24 hours
5 to 6 months	18 to 32 oz in 24 hours + cereal, fruit, and vegetable baby foods
12 months	eats table foods and drinks from cup

As growth starts to slow down, most 18-month-olds will begin to eat less and may refuse to eat at mealtime. Because the toddler is eating less, her parents should monitor what food she does eat to ensure that it is healthy. At 18 months of age, the recommended servings for a toddler are the following:[61]

Dairy	4 servings	A serving for an infant this age consists of ½ cup of milk or ¾ oz of cheese
Vegetables	2 servings	¼ cup cooked, ½ cup raw
Protein	2 servings	1 tablespoon of meat, 1 egg, ½ cup cooked beans
Fruit	3 servings	¼ cup cooked, ½ cup raw
Carbohydrates	6 servings	½ slice bread, ¼ cup pasta, rice, or cereal
Fats and Oils	Use sparingly	

At 2 years of age, a child may not eat a lot of food at one time and may start to develop a taste for sweets. At this age, a child can drink low fat or skim milk. Remember that eating habits started now will last throughout the child's lifetime. Parents should continue to offer healthy foods to their 3- and 4-year-old child and offer water to drink when the child is thirsty. Recommendations for a 4-year-old child include the following servings of food:[62]

Dairy	5 servings	A serving for an infant this age consists of ½ cup of milk or ¾ oz of cheese
Vegetables	3 servings	¼ cup cooked, ½ cup raw
Protein	2 servings	1 tablespoon of meat, 1 egg, ½ cup cooked beans
Fruit	3 servings	¼ cup cooked, ½ cup raw
Carbohydrates	7 servings	½ slice bread, ¼ cup pasta, rice, or cereal
Fats and Oils	Use sparingly	

Children between the ages of 5 and 11 years need increasingly larger portion sizes as they age. Parents can help their children stay healthy by offering healthy foods at mealtimes and ensuring that snacks are limited to one or two per day, which also consist of healthy foods. Children should also be encouraged to exercise regularly and spend a limited amount of time watching television or a computer screen. Children who are overweight should not be placed on a formal diet unless recommended by their physician. They should simply be offered healthy food choices with limited between-meal snacking.

As the child grows, her caloric intake also increases. Active adolescent girls may require up to 2,400 calories per day, and active adolescent boys may require up to 3,000 calories per day. Adolescents and adults need a balanced diet including the following number of servings:[56]

Dairy	*3 servings*
Vegetables	*2½ servings*
Protein	*2 servings*
Fruit	*2 servings*
Carbohydrates	*6 servings*
Fats and Oils	*Use sparingly*

It is important to note that, although water is void of vitamins and minerals, it is the most important nutrient; without it the human body would die within 3 days. Water is used to support the chemical reactions in our bodies, it transports nutrients and eliminates waste, it helps maintain body temperature, and it is necessary for proper bodily functions. The absence of water will result in death quicker than the absence of any other nutrient. For an adult, six to eight 8-oz glasses of water are recommended per day.[63]

Helping a family understand the importance of basic nutrition and exercise for their child is one step in addressing the current national issue of childhood inactivity and obesity.

INACTIVITY AND OBESITY

In infants and children who are of normal weight for their age, an increase in weight is usually due to an increase in

adipose cell size and number. The main increase is seen between 6 months and 2 years of age, and again between 8 and 10 years of age. **Obesity** can be defined as having an excess of body fat >35%, a body weight >20% of the ideal body weight, adjusted for age and height, or a body mass index (BMI) ≥30 (Box 2-6).[64] Obesity in children can be attributed to a host of topics ranging from time spent watching television to decreased participation in physical education.[64,65]

In the younger age groups, inactivity or decreased physical activity due to time spent on computers, video games, and other fewer calorie-burning activities predominates as the environmental cause of obesity. The increasing prevalence of inactivity in school-aged children has reached alarming rates over the past several decades. As a result of inactivity, children are experiencing higher levels of obesity than ever before.[66] On average, a child or adolescent will spend 6.5 hours per day or 45.5 hours per week watching television or playing video games.[67] In addition, there has been a decrease in daily physical education within the school setting over the past decade. In 1991, 42% of students attended daily physical education. Since then, it has declined to only 32% of students attending in 2001.[68] According to the Federal Interagency Forum on Child and Family Statistics, 16% of school-aged children (6 to 18 years of age) were considered overweight from 1999 through 2002. This is a significant increase from 1988 through 1994, when only 11% of

BOX 2-6
Body Mass Index

Body mass index (BMI) is a measure of physical health provided by the National Institutes of Health.[73] BMI is calculated as a person's weight in pounds divided by their height in inches squared. This number is then multiplied by a value of 703 to obtain the final score. Numerous online calculators can be found to determine one's BMI. The values obtained from calculating a BMI fall within a range of scores from <18.5 (underweight) to >30 (obese). The ideal range for a person is 18.5 to 24.9. Opponents of the BMI point to the idea of body type (ectomorph, mesomorph, and endomorph) as one of the factors limiting the value of BMI scores. Although there may be some validity to the arguments for and against the use of the BMI, the practicing clinician should recognize its value as a screening tool within the framework of the patient examination.[74]

Tools and tables to calculate BMI values for selected heights and weights for children 2 to 20 years of age can be found at the U.S. Centers for Disease Control and Prevention. Calculated BMI Values for Selected Heights and Weights. Available at: http://www.cdc.gov/nccdphp/dnpa/growthcharts/bmi_tools.htm (accessed October 31, 2006).

school-aged children were considered overweight.[69] Both of these figures are in stark contrast to the approximately 4% of children and adolescents considered overweight from 1963 through 1970.[66] These statistics are based on a cutoff point at the 95th percentile of BMI from the National Health Examination Survey, which was recently developed by the Centers for Disease Control and Prevention (CDC).[65] Additional data collected by the National Health and Nutrition Examination Survey showed that 20.6% of children aged 2 to 5 years and 30.4% of adolescents aged 12 to 19 years in the United States are obese.[64] Childhood and adolescent obesity have been directly linked to adulthood obesity.[65] The CDC directly correlates adulthood obesity with increased risk for hypertension, dyslipidemia, type II diabetes mellitus, coronary heart disease, stroke, gallbladder disease, osteoarthritis, respiratory problems, and some cancers. These statistics do not arise from one single source. A myriad of problems have attributed to this drastic increase in child and adolescent obesity over the past several decades. The implications for the parent and the physical therapist are evident. There is a need for not only interventions that would address the issue of inactivity, but the prevention of obesity at the earliest age possible. Introducing a child to proper nutrition and physical activity as a way of living, instead of in the form of dieting and exercise, should be the goal of any parent or any pediatric wellness and fitness program. Physical therapists are in a unique position to promote fitness in children, through family and community education, as well as with interventions provided through the various practice settings, such as community fitness centers, outpatient clinics, the child's home, and school.

Fitness in Children

The American College of Sports Medicine (ACSM) and the National Strength and Conditioning Association (NSCA) have position statements regarding the role of physical fitness in prepubertal children and adolescents. Both organizations identify the need for properly designed and supervised exercise programs. The benefits of these programs are numerous: increases in strength, motor skills, sports performance, injury prevention, psychosocial well-being, and most importantly, the establishment of a pattern of physical activity that can be carried over into adulthood.[70,71] The goal of physical activity in prepubertal children should not be one of obtaining a high level of sport performance. Exercise or physical activity should promote a wide range of physically stimulating activities that will encourage the child to be active for the rest of her life.

The frequency and duration of exercise for children in elementary school varies greatly from that of adolescents in high school. The common prescription of 30 minutes of exercise three times per week no longer holds true for everyone. The National Association for Sport and Physical Education (NASPE) is a part of the greater coverage of the American Alliance for Health Physical Education Recreation and Dance (AAHPERD). Both AAHPERD and NASPE provide guidelines for school-aged children with regard to physical activity and recreation.[72] Recently NASPE has revised its current recommendation for exercise duration to reflect the impact of the growing epidemic of childhood obesity. The current guidelines recommend that children participate in at least 60 minutes, up to several hours, of age-appropriate physical activity on all, or most, days of the week. The duration should be in smaller increments of 15 minutes or more at a time.[72] Allowing the child a variety of activities as well as spreading them out over the course of a day, will encourage the child to view activity as fun, not work. The ACSM recommends physical activity for adolescents to be at least 30 minutes a day, most days of the week.

POINTS TO REMEMBER

Fitness for Children

Physical activity should be promoted to encourage a child to adopt an active lifestyle that can be carried over into adulthood.

Physical activity for school-aged children is done in 15-minute increments for a cumulative total of at least 60 minutes of activity per day, every day.

CASE STUDY

Child Development

Client's Name: David
Physical Therapy Setting: David's home

EXAMINATION

History

David is a 10-month-old boy who was born at 32 weeks' gestation. He is the first child of Carole and Gareth. Currently neither David nor his father has any contact with his biological mother Carole. David's father has legal custody of his son. By the father's report, the gestational period and birth were unremarkable with the exception of time. At 32 weeks' gestation, Carole's water broke and an uncomplicated delivery followed. David received oxygen at birth and remained in the hospital for 1 week for observation. No further complications developed. David's birth weight was 5 pounds 9 ounces. David's chronological age is 10 months; corrected chronological age is 8 months. David does have a history of ear infections (×1) and respiratory infections (×2). He does not have a medical diagnosis. He is currently not on any medications. David's father has no concerns regarding David's hearing, and reports that he passed the hearing screen at birth. Immunizations are up-to-date by parental report.

David is enrolled in the Kiddie Corner Daycare Center that he attends 5 days a week, for 8 to 10 hours per day while his father is at work. In addition, Gareth's mother provides childcare periodically in David's home. David lives with his father in a one-floor apartment. There are no steps in the house.

Current Condition/Chief Complaint: The father has concerns regarding David's developmental skills. He wants to make sure he is "developing OK."

Systems Review

Cardiovascular/Pulmonary: David does not show any signs of cardiovascular insufficiency or pulmonary impairment upon visual examination.

Integumentary: There are no visible scars or abnormal findings upon examination. At present David does not have a diaper rash.

Musculoskeletal: Gross ROM is within functional limits. Gross strength appears to be age appropriate.

Neuromuscular: Upon observation, David's movements appear coordinated and appropriate for his age.

Communication, Affect, Cognition: David was awake and in his playpen upon my arrival. He looked at me when I entered the room and smiled appropriately. David appears to be attentive to the objects and people in his immediate environment, looks when spoken to, smiles and laughs to appropriate stimuli. He is able to make his needs known to his father.

Tests and Measures

Anthropometrics: Current weight is 14 pounds 14 ounces. Cognition: David responded to his name when his father called him. He was observed shaking a toy and laughing appropriately. He does react to the command "No!" but generally continues the task. David maintained eye contact with me and followed my movements in the room. His father reports that he does have periods when he is more anxious around new people.

Muscle Performance: David's muscle tone is normal with no resistance to passive stretching noted in either his upper or lower extremities. He was negative for ankle clonus.

Joint Integrity and Mobility: Ligamentous laxity/joint play is equal bilaterally, examined in the elbow and knee joints. David's spine appears straight upon visual examination. His hip joints appear located with symmetrical hip abduction noted. His lower extremity alignment shows slight varus at the knees, bilaterally. Leg lengths appear equal.

Locomotion and Balance: David's primary means of mobility is by crawling, moving his upper and lower extremities reciprocally. He will transition into sitting on the floor and displays protective extension forward and sideways. Protective extension backwards is inconsistent. David is able to sit on the floor and play with his toys, incorporating trunk rotation and weight shifting onto an upper extremity without loss of balance. Righting and equilibrium reactions are age appropriate.

Neuromotor Development: David can roll and crawl and will attempt to move into a hands and knees position, for which he was successful twice during the examination. When David is supine he attempts to bring his feet to his mouth.

David will hold and bite finger food. He is able to hold his bottle with two hands. During the examination David held two objects, one in each hand, and brought them together (banging). He did bring his pacifier to his mouth and sucked on it appropriately. David will attempt to pick up small objects from the floor using a lateral pincer grasp. He attempted to find a covered toy, but did not do so consistently.

David does produce vowel and consonant sounds. He does call his father "da da" by report. In addition he was heard saying "ba," "ma," and several throaty vocalizations.

Reflex Integrity: Primitive reflexes appear integrated with the exception of the STNR, which is non-obligatory, and plantar grasp. The STNR does not appear to affect David's ability to crawl.

Self-Care: David can hold his own bottle. He will remove his socks independently. He is cooperative with dressing and bathing. He will hold a spoon and bring it to his mouth.

EVALUATION

Impairments: None were identified.

Functional Limitations: None were identified.

DIAGNOSIS

David displays age-appropriate developmental skills for an infant who is 8 to 9 months of age.

PROGNOSIS

I instructed the father to (a) allow David to sit on the floor, with a pillow behind him, to play; (b) when putting him in his playpen, place David in a sitting position and allow him to play in that position; and (c) encourage David to retrieve toys in his immediate environment. I reviewed age-appropriate developmental skills and the skills that should be expected over the next 3 months. The father was instructed to contact me if he had any questions in the future regarding David's development or what was discussed today.

PLAN OF CARE
Interventions

Instruction: I provided David's father with information on typical development.

Physical therapy services are not recommended at this time. Dad was in agreement with this recommendation and was encouraged to contact me if he had any further questions about David's acquisition of developmental skills in the future. A phone number was provided. A follow-up phone call will be made within 3 months to make sure that David is progressing.

Reflection Questions

1. What daily activities can the father and son engage in to promote the development of David's gross motor skills in the next 3 months?
2. How would the absence of one parent affect the daily routines of the home?
3. What influence do you think the daycare center would have on David's health and development?

SUMMARY

The growth and development of a child is a complex yet coordinated symphony of factors that promote the development of skilled movements, promoting learning and functioning toward independence as an adult. Many factors are involved, but one that stands out is the influence of the family. The family is a dynamic group that can change depending on the current situation, and may consist of a combination of responsible related and unrelated persons who care for the child or support a member of the family. The physical therapist, in the evaluation process, should be aware of this important aspect of the child in front of him. Information about the family as well as the prenatal period and birth of the child are helpful in understanding the current parental concerns and the examination findings. In addition, the physical therapist should also have a basic understanding of child development from conception to adulthood, and appreciate the many factors that can influence motor development such as the musculoskeletal system, neuromuscular system, visual perceptual abilities, cognitive ability, and the appropriate environmental stimuli. This understanding will aid the physical therapist in the prognosis and selection of interventions used in this episode of care.

A general outcome of physical therapy services for all children would be to function at the best of their ability and to be healthy. This outcome would include adherence to a balanced diet containing the proper proportions of each of the five food groups along with daily physical activity. Physical therapists are in a unique position to promote fitness and health in children through their close associations with families and the services they provide to all children.

REVIEW QUESTIONS

1. A family is best defined by which of the following definitions?
   a. any individual who significantly adds to the functioning of the family.
   b. any individual who is related to the mother or father.
   c. a mother, father, siblings, and any individual residing in the same house.
   d. a mother, father, and siblings.

2. In taking a history of a child, the mother informs you that she just found out that she is pregnant and in her first trimester. Which of the following, if she is exposed to it, can be passed to the fetus, possibly causing heart defects, vision, and hearing loss?
   a. rubella
   b. toxoplasmosis
   c. cytomegalovirus
   d. herpes simplex

3. A family routine is best identified by which of the following?
   a. the sense of organization the activity brings to the functioning of the family.
   b. the family's religious traditions and celebrations.
   c. the emotional aspect of the activity that reflects the family's sense of belonging.
   d. the activities continuity across generations of the family.

4. Of the following, which would most likely be defined as a family ritual?
   a. a father painting a new nursery.
   b. the eldest daughter in the family preparing a family meal.
   c. a mother reading a bedtime story to her 3-year-old daughter.
   d. the family gathering and eating Thanksgiving Day dinner each year.

5. Your new patient is a 27-year-old female. Upon review of the patient's medical record, you note that she has a history of two ectopic pregnancies. This means that
   a. these pregnancies were terminated due to an exposure to teratogens.
   b. these pregnancies lasted <30 weeks.
   c. implantation of the fertilized egg occurred in the inferior aspect of the uterus.
   d. implantation of the zygote occurred outside the uterus.

6. Joseph is a healthy 6-month-old child who was born full term. During your examination, which of the following would you expect to find?
   a. When pulled to sitting from supine, Joseph will demonstrate complete head control without evidence of a head lag.
   b. When placed supine on the floor, Joseph would be able to assume sitting on the floor independently.
   c. When placed in supported stance, Joseph will demonstrate a high guarded position.
   d. Joseph will demonstrate the ability to creep forward.

7. You are performing an examination on Luke, who is 1 month old. When he is placed in supported stance and slightly tilted forward, he moves his legs as though he is stepping forward. This would be an example of
   a. positive suppport.
   b. spontaneous stepping.
   c. creeping.
   d. cruising.

8. The most remarkable physical growth in adolescents is seen in which period of adolescence?
   a. early adolescence.
   b. middle adolescence.
   c. late adolescence.
   d. throughout all periods of adolescence, equally.

9. Which of the following would be the most appropriate exercise prescription for a 4-year-old child who is overweight?

   a. go bike riding on her two-wheeled bike for 30 minutes a day, 3 days a week.

   b. go for a hike with her father every Saturday for a minimum of 60 minutes.

   c. perform 15 minutes of walking in the morning before she gets onto the school bus, and then 30 minutes of active play time when she gets home from school. Promote 15 minutes of activity in the evening after dinner.

   d. participate in the local soccer program, which meets 2 days a week for 90 minutes for practice or games.

10. You are developing a treatment plan for Cathy, who is 15 years old. The family is considering purchasing a wheelchair to help with family outings. The ability of the assistive device to allow for growth is a factor in the purchase of this equipment. Which of the following statements is correct?

    a. Females generally reach their adult size at 10 to 13 years.

    b. Females generally reach their adult size at 13 to 14 years.

    c. Females generally reach their adult size at 17 to 18 years.

    d. Females generally reach their adult size at 18 to 21 years.

Key Developmental Milestones*

Age	Key Developmental Skills
Birth	Can respond to environmental stimuli such as sound, touch, and light
3 Months	Smiles, laughs, coos; grasps objects
6 Months	Says single syllables such as "Ba," "Ma," or "Da"; sits unsupported; reaches for objects; shows anticipation of the outcome of an event; can hold bottle with two hands
9 Months	Begins to understand words; imitates adult speech by attempting to say parts of words; stands while stabilized by holding onto furniture; pinches objects between thumb and finger; attempts to elicit a positive response from caregiver by smiling (cooing, etc.); shows many emotions such as happiness, anger, fear, and surprise
1 Year	Begins to recognize which name corresponds to each person in her life; stands unsupported; imitates adult speech; may walk alone; may deliberately perform actions to gain a desired result; becomes very attached to primary caregiver; may develop a fear of strangers
18 Months	Vocabulary quickly expands, may use two-word sentences; stacks two blocks; may walk up stairs (step-to-step fashion); explores environment with the security of a caregiver; may begin potty training
2 Years	Uses many two-word phrases; firm attachment has formed to primary caregiver; able to jump in place, runs
3 Years	Speech is mostly intelligible, may use three-word sentences; has difficulty stopping suddenly to change direction; can jump short distances of only 15 to 24 inches; can climb stairs (alternating feet); can hop on two feet
4 Years	Can draw a circle; may begin printing letters; has better control of stopping and turning; can jump 24 to 33 inches; can descend stairs (alternating feet); can hop on one foot; many children attend preschool
5 Years	Can stop and change direction quickly; can jump 28 to 36 inches; shame and pride develop as key emotions of this stage; most children attend kindergarten; most gross motor skills are perfected; fine motor skills are still being developed; basic preliminary concepts of reading are learned; writing is unskilled and needs much practice
6 Years	Can skip; can throw an object while shifting weight onto the other foot; most children are in kindergarten or first grade; may learn to ride a two wheeled bike
7 Years	Balancing on one foot with the eyes closed; can walk with a 2-inch-wide base of support; can do coordinated jumping jacks; can hop and jump within a small defined area; most children are in first or second grade
8 Years	Can hop from one foot to another and can hop in a given pattern (3 times on one foot and 2 times on the other, for example); can throw a baseball up to 40 feet; most children are in second or third grade; children may begin puberty; most fine motor skills are usually perfected by this age
9 Years	Boys can throw a ball up to 70 feet; most children are in third or fourth grade; children may begin puberty
10 Years	Can catch a ball; most children are in fourth or fifth grade; children may begin puberty
11 Years	Standing long jump can be done; most children are in fifth or sixth grade; children may begin puberty
12 Years	3-foot standing high jump can be done; most children are in sixth or seventh grade; majority of children go through puberty by this age; interest in the opposite sex increases; strong peer relationships are developed; fear of peer rejection and desire for acceptance is common
13 Years	Most children are in seventh or eighth grade; child begins to spend more time with friends than with family
14 Years	Most children are in eighth or ninth grade; more time is spent with friends than with family; begins to question who they are and what purpose they serve
15 Years	Most children are in ninth or tenth grade; more time is spent with friends than with family
16 Years	Most children are in tenth or eleventh grade; desire to learn to drive is common as children struggle for independence; more time is spent with friends than with family; children may desire to hold a job after school due to a desire for additional independence; can perform IADLs
17 Years	Most children are in eleventh or twelfth grade; more time is spent with friends than with family; may contemplate their role as an adult; girls typically reach adult size from 17 to 18
18 Years	Some children may turn 18 in twelfth grade; more time is spent with friends than with family; boys typically reach adult size from 18 to 21

*The expression of the key developmental skills may vary between children.

REFERENCES

1. Koontz-Lowman D. Family and disability issues through infancy. In: Cronin A, Mandich MB. *Human Development and Performance Throughout the Lifespan.* New York: Thomson Delmar Learning; 2005.
2. The Centers for Disease Control and Prevention. National Vital Statistics Reports. March 1995;43(9). In: Gender Issues Research Center. Available at: http://www.gendercenter.org/mdr.htm. Accessed July 15, 2005.
3. Medalie J, Cole-Kelly K. The clinical importance of defining family. *Am Acad Fam Phys.* 2002;65:1277–1279. Available at: http://www.aafp.org/afp/20020401/editorials.html. Accessed July 18, 2005.
4. Kaplan H, Sadock B. *Synopsis of Psychiatry.* 8th ed. Baltimore, Maryland: Williams & Wilkins; 1998.
5. Howe GW, Reiss D, Yuh J. Can prevention trials test theories of etiology? *Dev Psychopathol.* 2002;14:673–694.
6. Fiese BH, Tomcho TJ, Douglas M, Josephs K, Poltrock S, Baker T. A review of 50 years of research on naturally occurring family routines and rituals: cause for celebration? *J Fam Psychol.* 2002;16:381–390.
7. Denham S. Family routines: a structural perspective for viewing family health. *Adv Nurs Sci.* 2002;24:60–75.
8. Serpell R, Sonnenschein S, Baker L, Ganapathy H. The intimate culture of families in the early socialization of literacy. *J Fam Psychol.* 2002;16:391–405.
9. Segal R. Family routines and rituals: a context for occupational therapy interventions. *Am J Occup Ther.* 2004;58:499–508.
10. Behrman RE, Kliegman RM, Jenson HB. *Nelson Textbook of Pediatrics,* 16th ed. Philadelphia: W. B. Saunders Company; 2000.
11. Stephenson RG, O'Connor LJ. *Obstetric and Gynecologic Care in Physical Therapy,* 2nd ed. Thorofare, NJ: SLACK, Inc.; 2000.
12. Feldman RS. *Development Across the Lifespan,* 3rd ed. Upper Saddle River, NJ: Pearson Education, Inc.; 2003.
13. Health-Cares.net. First trimester of pregnancy. Available at: http://womens-health.health-cares.net/pregnancy-first-trimester.php. Accessed September 14, 2005.
14. *Stedman's Concise Medical Dictionary for the Health Professions.* Illustrated 4th ed. Philadelphia: Lippincott Williams & Wilkins; 2001.
15. Long T, Toscano K. *Handbook of Pediatric Physical Therapy,* 2nd ed. Lippincott Williams & Wilkins; 2002.
16. Project Inform. PCP Prevention. Available at: http://www.projinf.org/fs/pcpproph.html. Accessed October 4, 2005.
17. Shah T, Sullivan K, Carter J. Sudden infant death syndrome and reported maternal smoking during pregnancy. *Am J Public Health.* 2006;96:1757–1759.
18. Melvin CL, Gaffney CA. Treating nicotine use and dependence of pregnant and parenting smokers: an update. *Nicotine Tob Res.* 2004;6:S107–S124.
19. Kisner C, Colby LA. *Therapeutic Exercise Foundations and Techniques.* Philadelphia: F. A. Davis Company; 2002.
20. Gessel A. *Infancy and Human Growth.* New York: Macmillan; 1928.
21. Gessel A, Thompson H, Amatruda CS. *Infant Behavior: Its Genesis and Growth.* New York: McGraw-Hill; 1934.
22. Gessel A. *The Mental Growth of a Pre-school Child: A Psychological Outline of Normal Development from Birth to the Sixth Year, Including a System of Developmental Diagnosis.* New York: Macmillan; 1928.
23. Gessel A. *The Embryology of Behavior.* New York: Harper & Row; 1945.
24. Gessel A, Amatruda CS, Castner BM, Thompson H. *Biographies of Child Development: The Mental Growth Careers of Eighty-four Infants and Children.* New York: Arno Press; 1975.
25. Gessel A, Halverson HM, Thompson H, et al. *The First Five Years of Life.* New York: Harper & Row; 1940.
26. Skinner BF. *The Technology of Teaching. The Century Psychology Series.* New York: Appleton-Century-Crofts; 1968.
27. Piaget J. *The Origins of Intelligence in Children.* New York: International Universities Press; 1952.
28. Thelen E. Coupling perception and action in the development of skill: a dynamic approach. In: Bloch H, Bertenthal BI, eds. *Sensory-Motor Organization and Development in Infancy and Early Childhood.* Dordrecht, The Netherlands: Kluwer Academic; 1990.
29. Thelen E. Motor development: a new synthesis. *Am Psychol.* 1995;50:79–95.
30. Thelen E, Adolph KE, Arnold L. Gesell: The paradox of nature and nurture. *Dev Psychol.* 1992;28:358–380.
31. Thelen E, Corbetta D. Exploration and selection in the early acquisition of skill. *Int Rev Neurobiol.* 1994;37:75–102.
32. Thelen E, Corbetta D, Kamm K, Spencer JP, Schneider K, Zernicke R. The transition to reaching: mapping intention and intrinsic dynamics. *Child Dev.* 1993;64:1058–1098.
33. Thelen E, Kelso JA, Fogel A. Self-organizing systems and infant motor development. *Dev Rev.* 1987;7:39–65.
34. Thelen E, Ulrich BD. Hidden skills: a dynamic systems analysis of treadmill stepping during the first year. *Monogr Soc Res Child Dev.* Serial Number 223. Vol. 56;1. Chicago, IL: University of Chicago Press; 1991.
35. Thelen E, Ulrich BD, Jensen JL. The developmental origins of locomotion. In: Woollacott MH, Shumway-Cook A, eds. Columbia, SC: University of South Carolina Press; 1989.
36. Berstein N. *The Coordination and Regulation of Movements.* Oxford, UK: Pergamon Press; 1967.
37. Gagne RM. *The Conditions of Learning.* New York: Holt, Rinehart, and Winston; 1977.
38. Gagne RM. Domains of learning. *Interchange.* 1972;3:1–8.
39. Culbertson JL, Newman JE, Willis DJ. Childhood and adolescent psychologic development. *Pediatr Clin North Am.* 2003;59:741–764.
40. Martin T. Normal development of movement and function: neonate, infant, and toddler. In: Scully RM, Barnes MR. *Physical Therapy.* Philadelphia, PA: Lippincott Company; 1989.
41. Green EM, Mulcahy CM, Pountney TE. An investigation into the development of early postural control. *Dev Med Child Neurol.* 1995;37:437–448.
42. The U.S. National Library of Medicine and the National Institutes of Health. Developmental milestones. Available at: http://www.nlm.nih.gov/medlineplus/ency/article/002348.htm. Accessed on September 14, 2005.
43. Campbell SK, Vander Linden DW, Palisano RJ. *Physical Therapy for Children,* 2nd ed. Saunders Company; 2000.
44. Adolph, K. Learning in the development of infant locomotion. *Monogr Soc Res Child Dev.* Serial number 251. Vol. 62:3. Chicago: University of Chicago Press; 1997.
45. Cintas HM. Cross-cultural variation in infant motor development. *Phys Occup Ther Pediatr.* 1988;8:1–20.
46. Thelen E, Ulrich B, Jensen J. The developmental origins of locomotion. In: Woollacott M, Shumway-Cook A, eds. *Development of Posture and Gait Across the Lifespan.* Columbia, SC: University of South Carolina Press; 1989.
47. American Academy of Pediatrics. Causes of Bed-wetting. Available at: http://www.aap.org/pubed/ZZZ30FMNH4C.htm?&sub_cat=1. Accessed January 3, 2006.
48. Wescott SL, Lowes LP, Richardson PK. Evaluation of postural stability in children: current theories and assessment tools. *Phys Ther.* 1997;77:629–645.

49. Woollacott MH, Shumway-Cook A. Changes in posture across the life span: a systems approach. *Phys Ther.* 1990;70:799–808.
50. Porter RE. Normal development of movement and function: child and adolescent. In: Scully RM, Barnes MR, eds. *Physical Therapy.* Philadelphia, PA: JB Lippincott Co; 1989.
51. Steinberg L. *Adolescence,* 4th ed. New York: McGraw-Hill; 1996.
52. Dunlap JB. Construction of adulthood and disability. *Ment Retard.* 2001;39:286–296.
53. Schor EL, ed. *Caring for Your School-Aged Child: Ages 5 to 12. The Complete and Authoritative Guide.* Elk Grove Village, IL: The American Academy of Pediatrics; 1995.
54. Leon K, Jacobvitz DB. Relationships between adult attachment representations and family ritual quality: a prospective, longitudinal study. *Fam Process.* 2002;42:419–432.
55. Ohio Department of Health. Feeding Your Baby: 0–4 Months. Form number FB2; October 2002. Obtained from the WIC office in Belmont County, Ohio.
56. United States Department of Agriculture (USDA) Center for Nutrition Policy and Promotion. Steps to a Healthier You. Available at: www.mypyramid.gov. Accessed July 15, 2005.
57. Ohio Department of Health. Feeding Your Baby: 5–6 Months. Form number FB4; January 2003. Obtained from the WIC office in Belmont County, Ohio.
58. Ohio Department of Health. Feeding Your Baby: 7–8 Months. Form number FB6; April 2002. Obtained from the WIC office in Belmont County, Ohio.
59. Ohio Department of Health. Feeding Your Baby: 9–12 Months. Form number FB7; January 2003. Obtained from the WIC office in Belmont County, Ohio.
60. Ohio Department of Health. Feeding Your One Year Old. Form number C-1; April 2002. Obtained from the WIC office in Belmont County, Ohio.
61. Ohio Department of Health. Feeding Your 18 Month Old. Form number C-2; April 2002. Obtained from the WIC office in Belmont County, Ohio.
62. Ohio Department of Health. Feeding Your 4 Year Old. Form number C-5; April 2002. Obtained from the WIC office in Belmont County, Ohio.
63. Marcus B. *Human Nutrition.* Lincoln, NE: Cliffs Notes; 1997.
64. Crespo CJ, Arbesman J. Obesity in the United States. *Phys Sportsmed.* 2003;31:23–28.
65. U.S. Department of Health and Human Services: Centers for Disease Control and Prevention. Overweight and Obesity: Health Consequences. Available at: http://www.cdc.gov/nccdphp/dnpa/obesity/consequences.htm. Accessed June 15, 2005.
66. U.S. Department of Health and Human Services: Centers for Disease Control and Prevention, and The National Center for Health Statistics. *Health, United States.* 2004:245.
67. University of North Carolina School of Public Health. Get Kids In Action. Kids and screen time. Available at: http://www.getkidsinaction.org/2_activity/screentime.php?n=6. Accessed June 3, 2005.
68. U.S. Department of Health and Human Services, Maternal and Child Health Resource Center. *Child Health U.S.A.* 2003;44.
69. Federal Interagency Forum on Child and Family Statistics. America's Children in Brief: Key National Indicators of Well-Being, 2006. Available at: www.childstats.gov/americaschildren/hea.asp. Accessed October 31, 2006.
70. National Strength and Conditioning Association. Youth Resistance Training Position Statement. Available at: www.nsca-lift.org/Publications/posstatements.shtml#Youth. Accessed June 17, 2005.
71. American College of Sports Medicine. *ACSM's Guidelines for Exercise Testing and Prescription,* 6th ed. Baltimore, MD: Lippincott Williams & Wilkins; 2000.
72. Corbin CB, Pangrazi RP, Beighle A, Le Masurier G, Morgan C. *Physical Activity for Children: A Statement of Guidelines for Children Ages 5-12.* Available at: http://www.aahperd.org/naspe/template.cfm?template=ns_children.html.
73. U.S. Department of Health and Human Services and The National Institutes of Health. Calculate Your Body Mass Index. Available at: http://www.nhlbisupport.com/bmi/bmicalc.htm.
74. Dietitians of Canada, Canadian Paediatric Society, The College of Family Physicians of Canada, Community Health Nurses Association of Canada Nutrition Committee, and Canadian Paediatric Society (CPS). The use of growth charts for assessing and monitoring growth in Canadian infants and children. *Paediatr Child Health.* 2004;9:171–180.

Additional Reference

United States Centers for Disease Control and Prevention: National Center for Health Statistics. Growth Charts. Available at: http://www.cdc.gov/growthcharts/

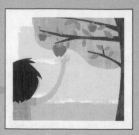

CHAPTER 3

Practice Patterns and Pediatrics

Carol Antonelli-Greco, Melissa S. Bozovich, and Mark Drnach

LEARNING OBJECTIVES

1. Define and understand the process of making a diagnosis.
2. Understand the diagnoses made by physicians and physical therapists for common conditions found in the pediatric population.
3. Understand how the combination of the medical and physical therapy diagnosis aids in clarifying the clinical presentation of a child.
4. Be aware of the general medical management of common pediatric conditions.
5. Understand the implications for physical therapy in the identified pathology-based diagnosis, including assignment of a practice pattern, general safety issues, common impairments, functional limitations, typical interventions, and general outcomes for each diagnosis.

The most common use of the term "diagnosis" is in the profession of medicine when a physician identifies a specific pathology or disease. It is what a physician does when describing a collection of symptoms to a known or accepted label. The process of deciding and making a diagnosis can aid in understanding the current health of the child in terms of what is happening in his body, which is out of the ordinary or expected. Unfortunately, a pathology-based diagnosis does not provide much information about the physical impairments or functional limitations that the child may be experiencing. Is the child who has cerebral palsy (CP) lying in bed or out running in the backyard? Is the child with diabetes able to participate in the family's hiking activities? Is the adolescent with cystic fibrosis (CF) able to climb the stairs at school? A diagnosis based on pathology is very important but does have some obvious limitations.

A physical therapist makes a diagnosis based on the results of an examination. She groups the impairments and functional limitations into one or more defined categories or practice patterns that best describes the clinical presentation of the child. Making a diagnosis aids the physical therapist in making a reasonable prediction of the outcome of specific interventions for a specific individual (e.g., impaired motor function and sensory integrity associated with a nonprogressive disorder of the central nervous system [CNS] vs. CP). It is not the process per se, but what is being observed and how it is measured and categorized.[1] Making a diagnosis aids in clinical decision making by the physical therapist as well as the physician, especially when deciding on the appropriate selection of interventions. The physical therapist and the physician make a diagnosis using the same process of decision making, but differ in the type of label or diagnosis given based on their professional scope of practice. Both the physician and physical therapist categorize a child's condition in a way that will direct their intervention; the physician more along the traditional lines of cellular or systems level, and the physical therapist more along the lines of impairments and functional limitations of the child.

Working together, the diagnoses made by the physician and the physical therapist can provide a more descriptive and clinically relevant picture of the child. A child with a diagnosis of CP and impaired neuromotor development is different than a child with a diagnosis of CP and impaired motor function without impairment in neuromotor development. Working collaboratively, the physician and the physical therapist can identify the pathology and subsequent limitations of the child due to the pathology. This collaboration would provide a broader picture of the child, not only in terms of what is wrong with his body or body system, but what is impairing his ability to move or function throughout the day. A more descriptive diagnosis that categorizes not only the "what" (pathology) but the "how" (functional limitation) of the disease would lead to the development of a plan of care that would optimize the child's capability and ability to function in whatever role he has in society.[2]

This chapter presents common pediatric pathologies and the medical management associated with that pathology, providing the reader with a general understanding of this aspect of the child's health and care. In addition to the medical management, the chapter will identify a reasonable practice pattern that could apply to a child with a specific pathology. Although the process of diagnosing and placing a child in a particular practice pattern can vary, according to the individual presentation of the child, the practice pattern identified was chosen by the author to provide a more comprehensive picture of the child. Other children with similar pathologies may be placed in other practice patterns. The pediatric conditions are grouped according to the practice pattern most likely associated with the condition or disease and then listed in alphabetical order for easy reference.

PARENT PERSPECTIVE

My odyssey into the world of developmental apraxia of speech began in July. My son was 2½ years old and was diagnosed as functioning at the level of a 4 month old. I received this devastating news via fax. As one may understand, my world came to a screeching halt. I didn't understand the medical terminology in the fax, I wasn't familiar with the "scales" the letter was referring to. I only knew that something was wrong. I just kept reading the sentence that said, "(he) performed below average in all areas..." over and over again.

I didn't know what to do or where to turn. I immediately drove to the local Easter Seals office, gave the fax to the receptionist and sat on their couch and cried. I have since learned that developmental apraxia of speech (DAS) is a neurologically based speech disorder. I have learned that DAS is caused by a subtle brain impairment. My son did not have any birth or prenatal injury that would suggest a possible cause for DAS.

The most frustrating part of our experience with DAS has been the diagnostic side. Many pediatricians were not familiar with the symptoms and were slow to diagnose. When we were finally given a concrete diagnosis, finding additional information was difficult, at best. It has been imperative to our family to research DAS. What are the best treatments? Who are the specialists in our area? What other areas of development are affected? These were a few of the subjects we researched as a family to help our son.

—J. Harris, mother

■ Physical Therapy Practice Pattern: Musculoskeletal

ARTHRITIS: JUVENILE RHEUMATOID ARTHRITIS

Juvenile Rheumatoid Arthritis (JRA) is a disease associated with chronic inflammatory changes of the synovium. It also presents with extra-articular manifestations. JRA is a childhood disease with two distinct peaks, initially in the 1- to 3-year-old age group and again in the early teenage years. Diagnosis should be made when arthritis is present for at least 6 weeks in children 16 years old or younger.[3]

There are three types of JRA that are grouped according to clinical presentation during the first 6 months of the illness. The first group is a *pauciarticular disease* and is the most common type. It is characterized by arthritis that is limited to four or fewer joints. Large joints are mainly affected, and the distribution of the arthritis is asymmetrical. Two subgroups of pauciarticular JRA exist. The first is primarily in young girls who often have chronic *uveitis* (inflammation of the iris), and the second is in older boys who are at high risk for developing spondyloarthropathies. Pauciarticular JRA is an autoimmune disease.[3] In younger children, in whom the peak onset is age two, the larger joints are most commonly affected. The knees are the most frequently involved joints, followed by ankles and elbows. Hips are rarely involved. Pain is uncommon and the diagnosis may be made after months of asymptomatic swelling, which leads to contractures. Localized growth disturbance may occur as the result of asymmetric joint disease. This joint disturbance is particularly noticeable in the knees because of the overgrowth in the length of the affected leg. In older children, pauciarticular arthritis usually occurs after 8 years of age. It involves the joints of the legs in an asymmetric pattern. *Enthesopathy* (disease process that occurs at the site of the tendon insertion) of the Achilles tendon, patellar tendon, or plantar fascia often occurs. The knee is the most commonly involved joint with the first metatarsal phalangeal joint and ankle being next. The hips are also commonly involved. The patient usually displays a decreased exercise capacity, low-grade aches and pains, and malaise. Early on in the illness, most children have pain at the points of insertion of tendons and ligaments. Joint swelling develops later in the course of the disease.

The next most common group is the *polyarticular disease*, which predominately affects girls. It is characterized by arthritis that involves five or more joints, including typically the small joints of the hands and feet. Large joints are commonly affected. The cervical spine, temporomandibular joint (TMJ), and sternoclavicular joint may also be affected. Onset of the arthritic symptoms may be slow and insidious with gradual joint stiffness, swelling, and loss of motion. It may also present as a sudden onset of warm, swollen joints, which are not usually *erythematous* (marked by redness). Joint swelling results from periarticular edema, joint effusion, and synovial thickening. Some joint tenderness may be present to touch and painful with motion, but usually severe pain is not present. Young children are usually irritable and can present as typically posturing to guard painful joints from movement. Early in the disease, the joints become limited in range of motion due to muscle spasm, joint effusion, and synovial proliferation. As the disease progresses, limited range of motion results from actual joint destruction, ankylosis, and contractures of soft tissue.

The least common form of JRA is *systemic* onset JRA. It is the only form of JRA that affects boys as frequently as girls. The age of onset is 16 years or younger. These children appear sick and have high temperatures of 103°F for many weeks. Systemic symptoms of red rash, splenomegaly, hepatomegaly, and lymph node swelling are present. Joint and muscle pain are common. Arthritis is usually absent during the first weeks up to 6 to 8 months after the illness. Later in the course of the disease, chronic polyarticular arthritis appears. JRA, therefore, becomes a diagnosis of exclusion in this form of the disease, with the need to rule out other diseases with similar presentations.

Medical Treatment

The outcome of JRA is usually favorable for most children. Medical treatment includes NSAIDs (nonsteroidal anti-inflammatory drugs) to lessen the arthritis pain, inflammation, and fever. Systemic corticosteroids are used for serious sequelae such as pericarditis and obstruction of airways. Intra-articular corticosteroids may also be used to control arthritic symptoms of individual joints. In addition to drug therapy, physical therapy, splinting, and psychological support of the patient and family are imperative for overall treatment of this often intense and prolonged disease.

Physical Therapy

Practice Pattern: *Impaired Joint Mobility, Motor Function, Muscle Performance, and Range of Motion Associated with Connective Tissue Dysfunction*

Safety Issues: *The physical therapist should be aware that a child with JRA may have severe pain, fatigue, and stiffness, and therefore, should be conservative in treatment options.*

Common Impairments: *The most common impairment is decreased joint range of motion, usually involving the lower extremity more often than upper extremity. The child may also experience swelling or effusion, muscle weakness, and decreased endurance. Postural deviations may also occur due to body positioning.[4,5]*

Functional Limitations: *The child may have difficulty performing activities of daily living (ADLs), and have difficulty with mobility such as climbing stairs. The impairments and functional limitations may limit activities with peers. Performance of repetitive tasks may also be limited. A child with severe limitations in mobility may benefit from the use of a wheelchair.[5]*

Typical Interventions: *Interventions are used to educate the child and family on compensatory strategies, pain management, maintenance or restoration of range of motion and/or muscle strength, and maintenance of endurance and function.[6] Resistive exercise can benefit the child with JRA. Not only can it increase strength, endurance, and aerobic capacity, but it can also enhance the immune system's functioning.[7] It is important to take into consideration the severity and particular manifestations of the disorder before initiating a physical therapy program. The child's response to the program determines the progression of the interventions.[3]*

General Outcomes: *By adulthood, only 20% of children with JRA have significant limitations that hinder independent function.[8]*

POINTS TO REMEMBER

JRA

Two distinct peaks exist in JRA, initially in the 1- to 3-year-old age group and again in the early teenage years. There are three types of JRA that are grouped according to clinical presentation during the first 6 months of the illness.

1. Pauciarticular—Most common. Involves four or fewer joints.
2. Polyarticular—Involves five or more joints. Hands may be involved.
3. Systemic—Least common. Preceded by an illness with a fever.

Resistive exercises, if appropriate, can be beneficial.

ARTHROGRYPOSIS

Arthrogryposis is classified as a hereditary disorder of fibrous tissues. The term arthrogryposis describes a condition of congenital contraction of joints in flexion. It usually occurs independently of other anomalies, but can be associated with *arachnodactyly* (long and slender feet and hands) and/or premature union of the bones of the skull. Noted pathologic changes include thick, inelastic articular capsules and atrophic muscle fibers with fibrosis and fatty infiltration.[9]

Arthrogryposis multiplex congenita is a special form of the disorder in which a congenital stiffness of one or more joints is associated with a hypoplasia of the attached muscles. It is the result of incomplete fibrous ankylosis. Dislocation of the hips and of other joints is common. This disorder appears sporadically, yet familial cases have been seen.[9] The child presents with the upper extremities internally rotated and the lower extremities externally rotated. The elbows and knees, which appear cylindrical, are usually ankylosed in extension. Fixation of the knees in flexion may also occur. The wrists and fingers are flexed and clubfeet are usually present. There may be groups of muscles that are absent or undeveloped, and the skin appears thickened.

Medical Treatment

Orthopedic surgery is used to correct major joint anomalies. Less invasive treatment consists of massage, passive movement, and gradual correction of various deformities by splints and casting.

Physical Therapy

Practice Pattern: *Impaired Joint Mobility, Motor Function, Muscle Performance, and Range of Motion Associated with Connective Tissue Dysfunction*

Safety Issues: *Joint dislocations are common.*

Common Impairments: *The most common impairments are joint stiffness, contracture, and muscle weakness.*

Functional Limitations: *The child may have difficulty with mobility, ambulation, and performing ADLs.[5]*

Typical Interventions: *Gentle stretching, splinting, and total body positioning are important in order to decrease the degree of joint contracture and improve or maintain postural alignment. Strength and flexibility should be developed and maintained. The child may benefit from the use of a standing frame, braces, or crutches. Often, a wheelchair as well as other adaptive devices must be utilized for mobility to accomplish ADLs. Compensatory movement strategies may be taught to help the child become more independent.[5,8]*

General Outcomes: *Often, developmental delays are seen due to decreased mobility.*

CANCER OF THE MUSCULOSKELETAL SYSTEM

There are three primary bone or soft tissue malignant tumors that occur in children. All three are rare. *Osteosarcoma* is a tumor of the bone that affects adolescent boys about one and a half times more often than it affects girls. It is the most common primary malignant bone tumor in children. The primary tumor is usually located at the epiphysis or metaphysis of areas where maximum long bone growth occurs. The tumor occurs most commonly in the femur followed by the tibia and then the humerus, but any bone can be involved. Genetic factors have been identified in some studies, but to date the cause is unknown.[10] Clinically, the tumor usually presents as pain or a swollen area most commonly around the knee. Pathologic fractures may occur, and usually some types of gait disturbances are present. Plain film radiographs, radionucleotide bone scans, and/or magnetic resonance imaging (MRI) scans of the bone involved should be performed. Chest radiograph or computed tomography (CT) scan helps to diagnosis pulmonary metastasis, which may occur. A biopsy is also essential for determining actual tumor or tissue type.

Ewing sarcoma is another primary bone tumor that is a nonosseous, small, round cell tumor that is extremely malignant. It has usually metastasized at the time of diagnosis. There is a known chromosomal abnormality associated with this tumor, which has two spikes of occurrence. Young children and adolescents are the two most common groups.[10] Unlike osteosarcoma, systemic symptoms such as fever, weight loss, and fatigue occur much more commonly, and the femur and pelvis are the most common sites.

Rhabdomyosarcoma is the most common soft tissue tumor of children and arises primarily from skeletal muscle but can arise in any tissue. There are two peaks of occurrence. The first is between 2 and 6 years of age, and then again in adolescence. The initial peak is associated with more visceral tumors of the prostate, vagina, and bladder, as well as the head and neck. The later peak is more likely to produce tumors of the trunk, extremities, or male genitourinary tract. The clinical picture varies with the site of presentation. In the extremities and trunk, painful masses may be present.

Medical Treatment

Chemotherapy is started as soon as confirmation of osteosarcoma is made by biopsy. This provides tumor shrinkage, and in most cases, a decrease in micrometastatic disease. Limb-sparing surgery has become more common due to the increase in the survival rate over the last 10 to 15 years.[11] These procedures attempt to resect tumors, implant prostheses, and perform bone grafting to maintain mobility of the patient to the greatest degree possible. Amputation may still be necessary in some cases. Physical rehabilitation is imperative after amputation, and is important with any type of limb-sparing surgery.

Chemotherapy is vital to the treatment of Ewing sarcoma, especially because metastasis has generally already occurred. Patients with tumors located in the distal extremities have the best prognosis.[10] Local radiation is used to treat the primary tumor area after surgical removal. Without metastatic disease, 40% to 70% of children have long-term survival.[10] In children younger than 11 years, Ewing sarcoma is usually a curable tumor. Local treatment for the primary tumor includes surgical resection, usually with limb salvage.[11]

Medical treatment of rhabdomyosarcoma consists of tissue sampling or biopsy that is needed for definitive diagnosis. Histopathology also helps to determine the mortality rate. A combination of chemotherapy, surgery, and radiation is used to treat rhabdomyosarcoma. The prognosis is generally determined by location and histopathology of the tumor. The most important determinant of outcome is the extent of metastasis at the time of diagnosis.

Physical Therapy

Practice Pattern: *Primary Prevention/Risk Reduction for Skeletal Demineralization*

Safety Issues: *Individuals undergoing chemotherapy or radiation therapy should not exercise within 2 hours of the treatment.[12] Caution must be used with application of modalities. Monitoring of laboratory values should be done to ascertain the patient's ability to participate in therapeutic exercises.*

Common Impairments: *Impairments vary with disease progression, but the most common impairments include pain, decreased range of motion, and fatigue.[8]*

Functional Limitations: *ADLs may be difficult to perform. Gait deviations may be noted as weight bearing becomes limited.*

Typical Interventions: *A therapeutic exercise program including active-assisted range of motion and isometric exercises is important to implement in early stages. Weight bearing and gait training should also be addressed.[13] Swimming is an alternative activity during early stages of recovery when weight bearing is minimal for those who are not immunosuppressed.[14]*

General Outcomes: *Outcome depends on progression and medical management of the disease. Lung metastases result in a poorer prognosis.[10,15] Independent functioning is usually not limited until late stages of the disease.*

POINTS TO REMEMBER

Cancer

There are three primary bone or soft tissue malignant tumors that occur in children:

1. Osteosarcoma—Most commonly in the femur.
2. Ewing sarcoma—Extremely malignant. Commonly found in pelvis and femur.
3. Rhabdomyosarcoma—The most common soft tissue tumor of children that arises primarily from skeletal muscle.

Check hemoglobin (>8 gm/dL), hematocrit (>25%), and platelet count (>10,000) for appropriateness of exercise. Refer to the oncology department for individual guidelines. Should not exercise within 2 hours of chemotherapy or radiation.

CLUBFOOT (TALIPES EQUINOVARUS)

There are several etiologies of clubfoot, including congenital, teratologic, or positional.[16] A clubfoot is a deformity of the foot and also the entire lower extremity. The congenital form of clubfoot is usually a single birth abnormality. Positional clubfoot is just that—a normal foot that has been held in an abnormal position in utero—whereas a clubfoot relating to a teratology

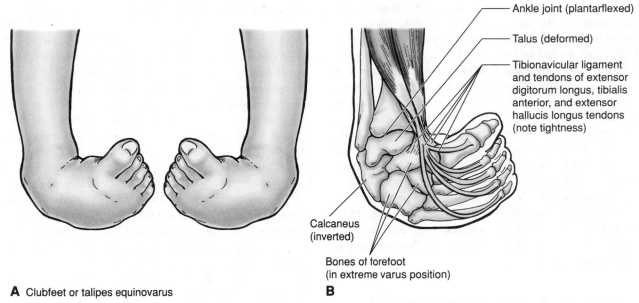

A Clubfeet or talipes equinovarus   **B**

Ankle joint (plantarflexed)

Talus (deformed)

Tibionavicular ligament
and tendons of extensor
digitorum longus, tibialis
anterior, and extensor
hallucis longus tendons
(note tightness)

Calcaneus
(inverted)

Bones of forefoot
(in extreme varus position)

Figure 3-1 ■ Clubfoot (talipes equinovarus). (From Moore KL. *Clinical Oriented Anatomy*, 4th ed. Baltimore: Lippincott Williams & Wilkins; 1999)

is usually present with other abnormalities such as neuromuscular disorders and arthrogryposis multiplex congenita. Although the actual cause of clubfoot is unknown, it has been associated with a single autosomal dominant gene. Most clubfeet are congenital. About 75% of cases are present without other congenital abnormalities.[16] There are varying degrees of congenital clubfoot with regard to rigidity of the foot, calf atrophy, and mild hypoplasia of the tibia, fibula, and bones of the foot. It occurs in a 2:1 male/female ratio, and is bilateral in 50% of cases.[16]

The infant with clubfoot presents with a hindfoot equinus, hindfoot varus, a forefoot adductus, and variable degrees of rigidity (Fig. 3-1). These presentations are due to the fact that the talonavicular joint is medially dislocated. Calf and foot atrophy are more obvious in the older child than in the infant, and are secondary to the neuromuscular etiology of clubfoot.

Medical Treatment

Conservative treatment is always attempted before surgical correction is suggested. Conservative treatment would involve taping, malleable splinting, and serial casting in an attempt to obtain normal positioning of the foot. Taping and malleable splints are especially used for premature infants until they gain enough weight to allow for casting. Serial casting is used most frequently. If normal foot positioning is not successful by 3 months of age, surgical intervention is indicated. Surgical intervention generally accomplishes a complete soft tissue release that corrects all the components of the clubfoot deformity. Successful long-term results can be obtained in 75% of

cases.[16] In cases of extrinsic muscle imbalance of neuromuscular etiology, further surgical intervention may be necessary.

CONGENITAL METATARSUS ADDUCTUS

Congenital metatarsus adductus is a common problem found in infants and young children. It occurs equally in boys and girls and is bilateral in 50% of patients.[16] It is more common in the first-born child than in later children because of the molding effect of the uterus and abdominal wall. Ten percent of metatarsus adductus cases are associated with developmental dysplasia of the hip.[16] Clinically, these children appear with a forefoot that is adducted and occasionally supinated. The hind foot and mid foot are normal. The lateral border of the foot is convex, and the base of the 5th metatarsal appears prominent. The medial border of the foot is concave, and there is an increased space between the first and second toes. The great toe is held in a greater varus position. The forefoot flexibility can vary from flexible to rigid. The gait of a child with an uncorrected metatarsus adductus is in-toed. Shoe fitting and shoe wear are also difficult and abnormal.

Medical Treatment

There are three classifications of forefoot flexibility, and treatment is recommended according to the severity of the congenital deformity. *Type I* deformity presents with a flexible foot that can be actively positioned into the abducted position. This positioning can be elicited by stimulating the peroneal musculature by stroking the lateral border of the foot. This type of deformity does not need treatment. *Type II* deformity presents with a foot that can be corrected to the neutral position by active and passive techniques. This foot can be given a trial use of corrective shoes such as straight or reversed-last shoes. Shoes are typically worn for 22 hours daily. If the condition has improved in 4 to 6 weeks, treatment can be continued. If no improvement occurs, serial casting is indicated. Casting should gradually correct the deformity within 4 to 6 weeks. *Type III* deformities cannot be corrected because of the rigidity of the foot. This foot is treated with serial casts that are changed at 1- to 2-week intervals. Usually, correction is accomplished in 4 to 6 weeks, depending on the child's age and severity of the deformity. Casting should be started before the child is 8 months old.

Physical Therapy for Clubfoot and Congenital Metatarsus Adductus

Practice Pattern: *Impaired Joint Mobility, Motor Function, Muscle Performance, and Range of Motion Associated with Connective Tissue Dysfunction*

Safety Issues: *If splinting or casting is used, maintenance of circulation and skin integrity are necessary.*

Common Impairments: *Decreased range of motion in the forefoot is present as well as poor alignment.*

Functional Limitations: *The child may show limitations or impairments in ambulation. The gait pattern typically presents with in-toeing.*

Typical Interventions: *Mild cases usually do not require physical therapy interventions as resolution occurs on its own. Stretching, strengthening exercises, and corrective shoes may be used to treat moderate cases. Manipulation and serial casting are required to treat severe cases. These techniques are then followed by corrective-shoe wearing and gait training.*[5,16,17]

General Outcomes: *If treated appropriately, most children have good results in functional outcomes.*

P O I N T S   T O   R E M E M B E R

Metatarsus Adductus

There are three classifications of forefoot flexibility that are treated according to the severity of the congenital deformity:

Type I—Forefoot flexible beyond neutral. No intervention necessary.

Type II—Forefoot flexible to neutral. Intervention includes corrective shoes.

Type III—Forefoot cannot be corrected to neutral. Intervention includes serial casting.

DEVELOPMENTAL DYSPLASIA OF THE HIP

Developmental dysplasia of the hip joint (DDH) is a disorder describing an abnormal development or dislocation of the hip. The hips of infants can be easily dislocated during vaginal deliveries. Because this abnormality is not always congenital, it is referred to as developmental. There are two major classifications of DDH. The first is known as *typical* and occurs in infants who are neurologically normal. The second is known as *teratologic* and occurs with an underlying neuromuscular disorder. The teratologic form of DDH obviously develops in utero.

The most common form of DDH is the typical form. Physiologic and mechanical factors influencing the development of DDH are numerous. In 20% of infants with DDH, there is a positive family history.[16] There is usually a generalized ligamentous laxity, due to normal maternal estrogen and other normal circulating pelvic relaxation hormones of pregnancy. More female infants present with the disorder than male infants, as well as first born infants.[16] The breech presentation positioning in utero seems to be the single most important contributor to the development of DDH. In this presentation, the fetal pelvis is positioned in the maternal pelvis, resulting in extreme hip flexion and limitation of hip motion. Stressed hip flexion causes the lax capsule and ligament teres to stretch further with a consequential uncovering of the femoral head. This hip position as well as decreased motion results in an abnormal development of a cartilaginous acetabulum.

There is also an association of congenital muscular torticollis in about 14% to 20%, and metatarsus adductus in about 1% to 10% of children with DDH.[16] If either of these two conditions are present in the infant, careful evaluation of the hips is mandatory. The most common physical finding in an infant with DDH is a positive *Barlow test*—the most important test to determine an unstable or dislocatable hip. In performing the Barlow test, the examiner moves the infant's hip joint into 90 degrees of flexion and then applies a gentle downward pressure while adducting the extremity. If the hip joint subluxes or is dislocatable, the joint play is easily felt. The *Ortolani test* is also used in the examination. This test reduces an already dislocated hip joint. In performing the Ortolani test, the examiner flexes then abducts the hip joint. Relocation is felt as a "clunk" as the femoral head moves into the acetabulum. A positive Ortolani test is likely in a 1- to 2-month-old infant, because it takes about this length of time for true dislocation to occur. There is also potential limitation of hip abduction indicated by soft tissue contractures, an asymmetric number of thigh skin folds, and a shortening of an extremity that can be indicative of proximal displacement of the femoral head. A positive *Galeazzi sign* (with the infant supine and the hip joints flexed to allow the feet to rest on the bed, uneven knee levels are observed), absence of normal knee flexion contracture, or frog leg positioning may also be present.

Medical Treatment

Medical treatment of the condition is dependent on the child's age at diagnosis. Obviously, the desired outcome is a stable hip, resulting in normal growth and development as the child ages. Usual treatment involves double or triple diapering in neonates. This is started after the hospital examination of the infant identifies the unstable hip. The diapering allows maintenance of the hip in the position of flexion and abduction for about 1 to 2 months. This positioning maintains the reduction of the femoral head and allows for tightening of the ligaments and stimulation of normal growth and development of the acetabulum. Treatment is continued until there is clinical stability of the hip as well as radiographic measurements that are normal.

Between 1 and 6 months of age, a Pavlik harness is used (Fig. 3-2). This harness places the hips in flexion and abduction by flexing the hips >90° and providing gentle abduction. This position induces femoral head growth toward the acetabulum. Spontaneous relocation of the femoral head usually is accomplished in 3 to 4 weeks. The Pavlik harness is approximately 95% successful in dysplastic or subluxated hips and is about 80% effective in true dislocations.[16]

Surgical closed reduction is the major form of treatment for an infant from 6 to 18 months of age. Hip *spica casting* is used to immobilize the hip in the flexed and abducted position. If during closed reduction the hip shows residual instability, an open reduction may be performed. After an infant is 18 months of age, open reduction followed by pelvic and or femoral osteotomy is usually needed to correct the problem.

Physical Therapy

Practice Pattern: *Impaired Joint Mobility, Motor Function, Muscle Performance, and Range of Motion Associated with Connective Tissue Dysfunction*

Safety Issues: *When the child is not immobilized, the hip may sublux or dislocate easily until anatomic structures become more stable. The harness should not be placed in >120-degree hip flexion as the vascular supply to the femoral head may be compromised in this position.[5]*

Common Impairments: *The most common impairment is in mobility because the child has restricted motion with bracing.*

Functional Limitations: *Exploration of environment and motor development may be delayed due to immobilization.[8]*

Typical Interventions: *The primary goal of physical therapy is to improve stability of the hip. Immobilizing the hip in a 100-degree flexion and approximately 30-degree abduction will properly position the head of the femur in the acetabulum. This positioning must be continued (approximately 3 to 9 months) until anatomic structures become more stable and do not allow subluxation or dislocation with typical movement. It is important to strengthen musculature around the hip to aid in support.[8]*

General Outcomes: *DDH is reversible without complications if properly treated within the first few weeks of life.[18] Sometimes*

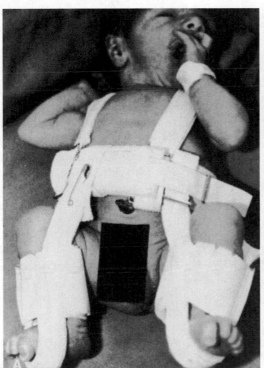 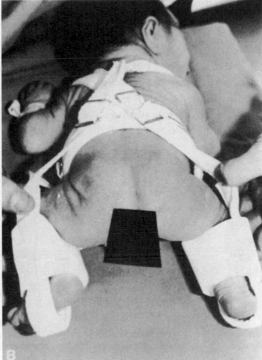

Figure 3-2 ■ Pavlik harness. Toddler with a Pavlik harness that holds the hip joint in flexion, abduction, and external rotation. (From Tecklin JS. *Pediatric Physical Therapy,* 3rd ed. Baltimore: Lippincott Williams & Wilkins; 1999)

surgery is required to secure the femoral head in the acetabulum. In either case, the outcome is favorable. If left untreated, many problems such as back and hip pain, scoliosis, degenerative joint disease, and antalgic gait may develop.[8]

FRACTURES .

Fractures are common childhood injuries. Due to the difference in bone make-up at various stages of growth and development in children and adolescents, healing and treatment vary according to bone age and maturation. The immature bone of children has preosseous cartilage, *physis* (growth plate), and a thick, strong periosteum that produces cartilage in a rapid and copious fashion. Because of its porosity, pediatric bone is stronger than adult bone in that it can absorb more energy before becoming fractured. The remodeling or healing of fractures is affected by three main factors. Foremost, the child's age is important. The younger the child, the greater the potential for remodeling due to rapid new bone formation and periosteal resorption, which occurs in younger children. The location of a fracture in relation to a joint is important in fracture healing due to the fact that physis usually has a greater growth and healing potential. Fractures adjacent to a physis have the greatest amount of remodeling if the fracture is in the plane of

motion of that joint. Fracture remodeling is not effective in fracture displacement or deformity that is not in the plane of joint motion of diaphyseal fractures, malrotation, and intra-articular fractures that are displaced.[16]

Fractures in children generally heal quickly due to the increased metabolic rate of the periosteum and overall increased growth potential of children. Pediatric fractures are usually classified into two categories due to the fact that children have immature bones and, therefore, the physis can be involved in various ways when a fracture occurs. Non-epiphyseal fractures can be classified into four subgroups. The first is complete, which includes spiral, transverse, oblique, or comminuted fractures, or a through-and-through fracture where both sides of the bone are broken. This is the most common type of fracture. The second is the greenstick or incomplete bone fracture with fracture on the tension side of the bone and a bend deformity on the opposite side. The third type of fracture is a buckle or torus, resulting from compression of the bone involved, usually occurring in the metaphyseal area in young children. The fourth type of fracture is a bowing or traumatic bend deformity of the bone without actual fracture.

Epiphyseal fractures occur in approximately 20% of all fractures in the pediatric population.[16] The upper extremity is involved two times as often as the lower. The distal radius is the most common site followed by the distal tibia. The Salter-Harris classification has been used for decades to describe epiphyseal injuries, and remains a standard for orthopedists (Fig. 3-3). There are five groups or types described. By using this classification, orthopedists can predict healing, prognosis, and risk for early physeal closure, which could eventually cause growth discrepancies. Treatment is also dictated by this classification.

Medical Treatment

Most pediatric fractures are treated by closed methods of reduction and/or casting, splinting, etc. Indications for surgical intervention include an unstable fracture, displaced

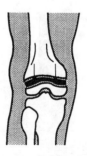 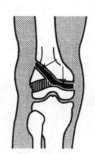 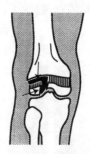 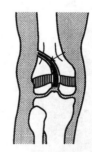 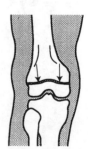

I	II	III	IV	V
Fracture through the physis	**Fracture through physis and metaphysis**	**Fracture through physis and epiphysis**	**Fracture through physis, metaphysis, and epiphysis**	**Fracture through physis with compression**

Figure 3-3 ■ Salter-Harris classification of physis fractures. (From Erkonen WE. *Radiology 101. The Basics and Fundamentals of Imaging.* Baltimore: Lippincott Williams & Wilkins; 1998: 256)

intra-articular fracture, displaced epiphyseal fracture, open fracture, or a fracture that occurred in a traumatic event causing multiple injuries. Anatomic alignment is the goal of surgery so that normal growth of the bone may continue. Internal fixation devices are removed as soon as possible to prevent incorporation into the bone and to prevent physical damage. On occasion, such as in open extremity fractures in conjunction with burns, vascular or nerve damage, and in pelvic fracture, external fixation is used. Pain associated with fractures can be treated with narcotics for severe pain.[19] Patients are gradually weaned to the NSAIDs and acetaminophen as the fracture healing progresses. Radiographs (typically two views) are used in the diagnosis and management of the fracture (Box 3-1, Reading Radiographs). Stress fractures may not be readily apparent on radiographs in the acute stage.

Physical Therapy

Practice Pattern: *Impaired Joint Mobility, Muscle Performance, and Range of Motion Associated with a Fracture*

Safety Issues: *Weight-bearing status must be maintained, and proper use of assistive devices may be necessary for ambulation. If splinting or casting is used, maintenance of circulation and skin integrity are necessary.*

Common Impairments: *Pain, decreased range of motion, and decreased muscle strength of the involved body part typically present.*

Functional Limitations: *ADLs and play may be limited.*

Typical Interventions: *Pain management, gait training, and cast care are common. If non-weight bearing in the lower extremity is needed, pediatric walkers are generally used with children younger than 6 years.*

General Outcomes: *Fracture of a physis may result in growth disturbances.[5]*

BOX 3-1
Tips When Reading a Radiograph

- The way in which the beam passes through the body gives you an orientation to what will be seen on the film. The film is white. Exposure to the x-rays turns the white film black. The denser a body part, the more it absorbs x-rays, leaving the film white.
- The greater the distance between the anatomy and the film, the greater the magnification.
- In posterior/anterior (P/A) radiographs, the x-ray beam passes P/A through the back to front, where the plate is against the patient's chest.
- In anterior/posterior (A/P) radiographs, the x-ray beam passes A/P through the patient's chest to the back, which is against the plate.
- Portable radiographs are usually A/P because they are commonly used when the patient cannot stand.
- Fat on radiographs appears black. Fat on an MRI appears white. This is one way to distinguish CT (x-ray) from MRI (magnetic field).

When examining an image:

1. R and L refer to the patient's right or left. Hold the film with the R in your left hand. You are looking at the patient. Make sure it is head up!
2. Know if the radiograph is an A/P or P/A view. This will give you a picture in your head of how the patient is presented in the radiograph.
3. Look at the whole radiograph in a systematic manner: top to bottom, moving clockwise, or whatever system you choose. Look at the anatomy and identify obvious abnormalities.

Modified from Erkonen W. *Radiology 101: The Basics and Fundamentals of Imaging.* Philadelphia: Lippincott, Williams & Wilkins; 1998.

POINTS TO REMEMBER

Fractures

Pediatric fractures are usually classified into two categories, involvement of the epiphysis and noninvolvement of the epiphysis. Healing takes between 6 and 8 weeks. Significant localized pain and the inability to weight bear are cardinal signs of a fracture.

LEGG-CALVE-PERTHES DISEASE

Because of how the blood supply exists in the hip joint, it is more vulnerable to trauma, septic arthritis, and other damage to the vascular system in general. This vulnerability is due to the fact that the femoral head or capital femoral epiphysis (CFE) and femoral neck are intracapsular, but the blood supply lies on the outer surface of the femoral neck.

Legg-Calve-Perthes disease (LCPD) is also known as *avascular necrosis* and is an idiopathic process that is caused by a disruption of the blood supply to the femoral head. It is bilateral in 20% of children and more common in boys at about a 5:1 ratio.[9] The onset of the disease is between 2 and 12 years, and clinically presents with mild, intermittent pain in the thigh or a noticeable limp. The classic description of LCPD is a "painless limp." Early signs of the disease include antalgic gait, mild restriction of motion of the hip in abduction and external rotation, muscle spasm, proximal thigh atrophy, and a mild shortness of stature. Long-term complications of the disease include osteoarthritis of the hip joint in adulthood. This complication depends mainly on the age of clinical onset and degree of femoral head deformity. A later onset of the disease has a greater risk for this complication.

Medical Treatment

The medical treatment for LCPD revolves around prevention of femoral head deformity and secondary osteoarthritis. It is a self-limiting, self-healing disorder. Treatment is essentially consistent with the containment concept, which uses the acetabulum as a mold to maintain the shape of the femoral head by reossification. This process is used in children 5 years old or older when more than one half of the CFE is involved. Abduction casts and orthoses are used noninvasively, whereas surgical proximal femoral varus osteotomy with or without derotation and pelvic osteotomies to redirect the acetabulum to contain the femoral head in the position of weight bearing is a more aggressive approach. The long-term results of surgical containment are generally effective.[16]

Physical Therapy

Practice Pattern: *Impaired Joint Mobility, Motor Function, Muscle Performance, and Range of Motion Associated with Connective Tissue Dysfunction*

Safety Issues: *Proper positioning of the femoral head in the acetabulum is important and can be maintained with hip joint abduction.*

Common Impairments: *Decreased range of motion, muscle weakness, and pain are usually present.*

Functional Limitations: *Ambulation and ADLs involving the lower extremity may be difficult depending on the severity of the disease.*

Typical Interventions: *Stretching and range of motion exercises along with the use of devices such as splints and braces will help keep the hip joint in the desired alignment. Weight bearing will be determined by the severity of the disease and dictate the appropriate gait-training activities. Aquatic therapy may also be beneficial to the child.*[5,8,20]

General Outcomes: *The prognosis is directly related to the child's age of onset, femoral head deformity, and adherence to the physical therapy program.*[8,21,22] *Children younger than 6 years have shown improvement despite what interventions were used. Children 6 to 9 years of age usually have a good prognosis with containment, including splinting, bracing, and casting. Children older than 9 years typically do not benefit from containment therapy, thus corrective surgery may be required.*[21,22]

MUSCULAR DYSTROPHY

Several common categories of muscular dystrophy have been identified. All have been genetically linked and vary in the age of onset of symptoms.

Duchenne Muscular Dystrophy

Duchenne muscular dystrophy (DMD) is a sex-linked recessive trait found in 20 to 30 of 100,000 boys.[9] The disease is a result of the genetic absence of a large protein called dystrophin, causing abnormal muscle fiber degeneration and regeneration. Age of onset of symptoms is about 3 years, and it commonly appears as an inability to keep up with other children of the same age group (i.e., running, walking, climbing stairs) and difficulty rising from the floor. *Gower's maneuver,* the process of "climbing up the legs," is used to get to the rising position. Contractures of the heel cords and iliotibial bands are apparent by age 6 years. Toe walking is associated with a lordotic posture. Loss of muscle strength is progressive with predilection for proximal limb muscles and the neck flexors. Lower extremity involvement is more severe than upper extremity involvement. Between 8 and 10 years of age, the boy needs braces to assist in walking. Joint contractures and limitations of hip flexion, as well as knee, elbow, and wrist extension, are made worse by prolonged sitting. By 12 years of age, most boys are confined to a wheelchair. By 16 years of age, the upper extremities are almost totally immobilized. Death occurs usually because of pneumonia caused by progressive respiratory muscle failure, or congestive heart failure secondary to cardiac muscle failure from cardiomyopathy. Intellectual impairment in DMD is common. It appears to be nonprogressive and affects verbal ability more than performance.

Becker Dystrophy

Becker dystrophy is also a sex-linked muscular dystrophy arising from a mutation of the same gene locus as DMD, presenting very similarly. The onset of symptoms is usually later than DMD, and progresses at a slower rate. The actual genetic defect results in inadequate production of dystrophin in either amount or molecular structure. Proximal muscle wasting, especially of the lower extremities, is prominent. As the disease progresses, weakness becomes more generalized. Facial muscle weakness is not a feature. Hypertrophy of muscles, particularly in the calves, is an early, prominent finding. By definition, patients with Becker dystrophy walk beyond age 15, whereas those with DMD are using a wheelchair usually by age 12. Patients with Becker dystrophy survive into the fourth or fifth decade. Intellectual impairment may occur, but is not as prevalent as in DMD. Cardiomyopathy is also present and may result in heart failure.

Limb Girdle Dystrophy

Limb girdle dystrophy (LGMD) is actually a syndrome representing approximately 15 different disorders. Boys and girls are equally affected, with the age of onset of the syndrome ranging from late in the first decade to the fourth decade.[9] Children with LGMD usually present clinically with progressive weakness of the shoulder and pelvic girdle musculature. Respiratory dysfunction may occur due to weakness of the diaphragm; cardiomyopathy is usually present. Intellectual function is unaffected. The symptoms progress slowly so that the patient is wheelchair dependent with no capacity for movement of the extremities by mid-adult life. Presently, there are five autosomal dominant and 10 autosomal recessive forms of LGMD.[23]

Facioscapulohumeral Dystrophy

Facioscapulohumeral dystrophy (FSH) is a form of muscular dystrophy that has an onset in childhood or young adulthood. It has an autosomal dominant inheritance pattern.[23] In most cases, facial muscle weakness is the initial manifestation, and the patient appears with mild *ptosis* (drooping eyelid), inability to pucker the lips, or smile. There is a decrease in facial expression due to overall muscle weakness. Loss of scapular stabilizer muscles makes upper extremity elevation difficult. Scapular winging is present with abduction and forward movement of the upper extremities. Biceps and triceps muscles may be severely affected with relative sparing of the deltoid muscles. Weakness is worse in wrist extension than in flexion. Weakness in most patients is restricted to the facial, upper extremity, and distal lower extremity muscles. In 20% of patients, weakness evolves to affect the pelvic girdle muscles. Wheelchair dependency can result.[9] Children with FSH do not usually have involvement of other organ systems.

MEDICAL TREATMENT

Medical treatment for DMD includes the use of glucocorticoids (such as prednisone), which can significantly slow the progression of the disease for up to 3 years. Due to the side effects of the medication, especially weight gain, it can be difficult to tolerate for some children. The benefit of glucocorticoids has not been adequately shown in Becker dystrophy, FSH, or LGMD.[9]

Medical treatment of all the muscular dystrophies should include supportive care, including ambulatory aids when necessary. Stretching of contractures should be attempted, but may be difficult. Scapular stabilization to address scapular winging may help in FSH, but probably will not improve function. Management of cardiomyopathy and arrhythmias with digoxin, beta-blockers, diuretics, and appropriate anti-arrhythmic medications depending on the type of arrhythmia present is necessary in order to prolong the life span. Labile hypertension should be controlled with appropriate antihypertensives in FSH.

PHYSICAL THERAPY

Practice Pattern: *Impaired Muscular Performance*
Safety Issues: *Approach exercise carefully as strenuous exercise may break down muscle fibers.*[24]
Common Impairments: *Muscle weakness, decreased endurance, poor posture, and contractures occur in all forms of muscular*

dystrophy; however, the musculature involved varies with each form.[5,8,25]
Functional Limitations: *The most functional limitation will be seen in ADLs, transfers, and ambulation.*[25]
Typical Interventions: *Stretching, exercise (moderate intensity), the use of orthoses, and environmental modifications are essential in the preservation of function.*[26] *Strenuous exercises or activities should be avoided. Aquatic therapy as well as electrical stimulation may be beneficial as well as the appropriate adaptive devices.*[5,25,27,28] *Power mobility is appropriate at the later stages of DMD.*
General Outcomes: *Most children with muscular dystrophy lead reasonably normal lives with the eventual use of assistive devices and environmental adaptations. Their life span is slightly less than normal.*[8] *Those with DMD typically live to be approximately 25 years of age with ventilatory assistance.*[5] *Those with Becker dystrophy typically cease in ambulation around 27 years of age; death occurs at approximately 42 years.*[5] *Those with LGMD and FSH have a more normal life span as progression of the disorder is much slower and less severe than that of DMD or Becker dystrophy.*[5]

POINTS TO REMEMBER

Muscular Dystrophy

Several common categories of muscular dystrophy have been identified. All have been genetically linked and vary in the age of onset of symptoms.

Exercise is essential in the preservation of function. Strenuous activities may cause muscle fibers to break down and, therefore, should be avoided.

OSTEOGENESIS IMPERFECTA

Osteogenesis imperfecta (OI) is considered an inherited disorder of connective tissue. The most complete data on mutations of heritable disorders of connective tissue are available for this particular disease. OI causes a generalized decrease in bone mass or osteopenia. This, in turn, makes the bones brittle. The most severe forms of OI end in death in utero or at birth. After birth, the course of the patient with mild to moderate OI is more variable. Some patients appear normal at birth and gradually become worse with age. Others develop multiple fractures in infancy and childhood, improve after puberty, and develop fractures again later in life. Women with OI are more prone to fracture with pregnancy and after menopause.

There are varying degrees of congenital abnormalities associated with OI, and four classifications developed by Sillence are commonly used.[9] *Type I* is the mildest form of OI. It is an autosomal dominant trait as far as inheritance pattern. Most patients have distinctly blue sclera, whereas others have abnormal dentition and hearing loss. Some patients have mild bone fragility. *Type II* is the lethal form in utero or shortly after birth.

Types III and *IV* are intermediate in severity between types I and II. Blue sclera is absent or only slight in infancy and become white in adults. There is a high incidence of hearing loss in both groups, and abnormal dentition exists in some, but not all patients. Type III differs from type IV in that bone fragility tends to become worse with age.

The incidence of OI type I is 1 in 30,000.[9] Type II has a reported incidence of 1 in 60,000.[9] In type I OI, physical activity may be limited or the symptoms may be so mild that no disability is apparent to the patient. Radiographs may show a mottled appearance of the skull due to irregular ossification. In type II OI, bones are so fragile that massive injuries occur in utero or at birth during delivery. In types III and IV, multiple fractures from minor injuries where stress can occur cause deformity of varying degrees. Kyphoscoliosis can cause difficulty with respiration and lead to pulmonary infections. In all forms of OI, bone mineral density is decreased, yet the fractures in all types of OI appear to heal normally.

In order to properly diagnosis OI, other causes of pathologic fractures must be excluded, including battered child syndrome, nutritional deficiency, and malignancy. The absence of superficial bruising aids in diagnosis of OI over battered children syndrome. Radiographs usually reveal a decrease in bone density.[23] Genetic testing and evaluation can also be performed and is used to screen family members at risk and for prenatal diagnosis in type I OI.

Medical Treatment

Medical treatment is geared toward the degree of severity of OI. Those patients with a mild form of the disorder will need little treatment after puberty. More severely affected children will need a multidisciplinary approach to the disease, including surgical management of fractures and skeletal deformities, vocational education, and physical therapy. Fractures, if small and minimally displaced, can be treated with splints and traction followed by casting. Counseling and support for patients and families is imperative in successful treatment of OI. There are support groups that exist to help the physician in providing this type of care.

Physical Therapy

Practice Pattern: *Primary Prevention/Risk Reduction for Skeletal Demineralization*

Safety Issues: *Children with OI require gentle handling as bones may fracture extremely easily.*

Common Impairments: *The child with OI may have hypermobile joints, muscle atrophy, and scoliosis. Developmental delay of motor skills is frequently observed.[8]*

Functional Limitations: *The child with OI often displays delayed development of motor skills. Independent ambulation may also be difficult.*

Typical Interventions: *Therapeutic exercise is recommended for strengthening muscles and building bone density. Gentle*

passive range of motion, straight plane stretching, and resisted strengthening exercises should be performed with caution. Aquatic therapy and activities may be beneficial. Braces, walkers, and other assistive devices may also be helpful.[5,8,29]

General Outcomes: *The best predictors of ambulatory status are disease type and the ability to sit by 9 or 10 months of age.[30,31] A large percentage of children with types I and IV OI are ambulatory (functional or household) without the use of braces or assistive devices; about half are independent community ambulators. Approximately 50% of patients with type III depend on power mobility. Bone mineral density appears to be an indicator of long-term functional outcome.[32] Children with types I and IV live reasonably normal lives.[30,31]*

POINTS TO REMEMBER

OI

OI is considered an inherited disorder of connective tissue. There are four types:

Type I—Mildest form with some bone frailty.

Type II—Severe form. Death in utero or from injuries at birth.

Type III—Intermediate form. Moderate severity. Bone fragility tends to become worse with age. Progressive deformities.

Type IV—Variable, usually milder than type III.

Therapeutic exercises are indicated for muscle strengthening and activities that build bone density. Gentle passive range of motion and stretching should be performed with caution.

SCOLIOSIS

Scoliosis is a condition that is generally of unknown causes and describes the abnormal spinal alignment in the anterior/posterior (A/P) or frontal plane. There are several categories of scoliosis that are determined by the etiology of the disorder. The *idiopathic* or unknown form of scoliosis occurs in healthy, normal children. It occurs slightly more often in girls. Girls are more likely to require treatment than boys. A small percentage of children with idiopathic scoliosis have other family members with the condition.[16] It is a disorder that can occur from birth through adolescence, and is usually treated according to the corresponding age group at which it is discovered. It is more common in adolescents, who make up the majority of cases of idiopathic scoliosis.[16] The right thoracic curvature is the most common pattern of the disorder. It is probable that adolescent scoliosis has its origin in the younger years, i.e., ages 4 to 10, but is usually not diagnosed or even screened for by primary care physicians until adolescence.

The *congenital* form of scoliosis originates from abnormalities of vertebral formation during the first trimester of in utero development. Congenital scoliosis is classified as either partial or complete failure of vertebral formation that results in a wedge-shaped vertebra or hemivertebra. There can also be a mixed pattern present. Other bone, neural, visceral, and soft tissue abnormalities of the skeleton may occur in conjunction with this form of scoliosis.

The *neuromuscular* form of scoliosis is commonly associated with many neuromuscular disorders. It is the form of scoliosis that progresses continuously after the scoliosis begins and can become a serious problem. The scoliotic deformity usually is dependent on the progression of the underlying neuromuscular disorder. Nonambulatory patients tend to have longer curvatures often involving the cervical spine as well as the thoracic and lumbar spines. Lung function and sitting balance can be affected secondary to the degree of curvature.

Medical Treatment

The medical treatment of scoliosis varies with the etiology and the severity of the deformity. In idiopathic scoliosis, no treatment is necessary for nonprogressive deformities. There is a higher risk for progression of the abnormalities in girls and also when the onset of this disorder occurs in the younger child.[16] Treatment is either with truncal orthosis or surgery, depending on the degree of curvature. Progressive curves between 25 and 45 degrees in a skeletally immature patient are managed by an orthosis. Curvatures >45 degrees require surgery.

In congenital scoliosis, due to the variability of the vertebral anomalies, the progression of the curvature is variable. Seventy-five percent of children and adolescents will demonstrate progression until skeletal growth stops.[16] Rapid curve progression occurs during rapid growth phases, i.e., before 2 years of age and after 10 years of age. Early diagnosis and treatment are essential in congenital scoliotic curvatures. Spinal fusion without instrumentation, i.e., metal rod placement, is the most commonly used surgical procedure.

In neuromuscular scoliosis, the treatment is geared toward preventing progression of the deformity, which can ultimately lead to functional loss. Orthotic management is usually not effective, and surgical stabilization is used in most cases. Instrumentation is used to stabilize the spine and distribute the connective forces necessary to maintain function of the nonambulating patient in a more comfortable upright sitting position without external support.

Physical Therapy

Practice Pattern: *Impaired Posture*
Safety Issues: *If surgery was performed to correct the curvature, postoperative precautions are necessary. Caution must be taken during mobility with new orthoses for balance. If braced, check for skin integrity.*

Common Impairments: *Postural alignment, decreased range of motion, and pain are most commonly impaired.*
Functional Limitations: *Limitations may be seen in ADLs and vary with severity of the curve and the amount of pain.*
Typical Interventions: *Postural training and core stabilization are used in the management of scoliosis. The primary goal of the treatment program is to prevent progression of the curve that could lead to problems with cardiopulmonary function. The postural training program should include stretching of the concave side and strengthening of the convex side. Spinal orthoses may be recommended.[8] Physical therapy intervention, in conjunction with bracing, sounds logical and may improve spinal flexibility and general health, but the efficacy of bracing and exercise, especially for idiopathic scoliosis, is still questionable.[33]*
General Outcomes: *Depending on the severity of the curve, most children with only the diagnosis of scoliosis lead relatively normal lives.*

SLIPPED CAPITAL FEMORAL EPIPHYSIS

Slipped CFE (SCFE) is the most common hip disorder occurring in adolescents. The etiology is unknown, but mechanical factors are what actually cause the slippage of the femoral epiphysis. Four clinical groups are used to classify the various forms of SCFE. It can also be classified as stable or unstable. *Group I* is known as the preslip and is defined as a wide physis without slippage of the CFE. The adolescent usually experiences mild discomfort, and physical examination is usually normal. Preslips are seen in many cases in the opposite hip of an adolescent with a previous SCFE. In this group, the CFE is stable. *Group II* is known as acute and is defined as a sudden onset of slippage without trauma, presenting with severe pain and inability to weight bear. In this group, the CFE is unstable. *Group III* is known as acute or chronic and is defined as an epiphysis slip that occurs acutely on an existing chronic slip. Pain, limp, and out-toed gait are usually present for several months before the acute slip. Trauma may play a part in the acute slippage. In this group, the CFE is unstable. *Group IV* is the most common group. It is known as the chronic group and is defined as a several month history of pain, limp, and out-toed gait. Symptoms usually get worse as the slip increases. The femoral neck and CFE are contiguous and the adolescent is able to walk. In this group the CFE is stable.

Medical Treatment

Medical treatment is geared toward minimizing the degree of the slippage and the following potential complications. Most techniques are surgical procedures that actually stabilize the hip joint and the deformity by the degree of slippage present in the adolescent. Methods that are used are internal fixation with pins or screws, open or closed bone graft epiphysiodesis, and osteotomies of the femoral neck or subtrochanteric regions.[16] A nonsurgical method is immobilization in a hip spica cast for less severe cases of SCFE.

Physical Therapy

Practice Pattern: *Impaired Joint Mobility, Motor Function, Muscle Performance, and Range of Motion Associated with Connective Tissue Dysfunction*

Safety Issues: *Caution should be taken not to stress the joint postoperatively, until healed. If splinting or casting is used, maintenance of circulation and skin integrity is necessary.*

Common Impairments: *Pain in the groin, thigh, or knee; decreased range of motion; and antalgic gait with the involved lower extremity held in more external rotation.*

Functional Limitations: *Decreases in mobility and in the ability to perform ADLs.*

Typical Interventions: *Range of motion, strengthening of the uninvolved extremities, use of an assistive device, environmental modifications if necessary.*

General Outcomes: *When properly treated, children with SCFE lead relatively normal lives; however, degenerative processes resulting in premature onset of arthritis may affect functional mobility as adults.*

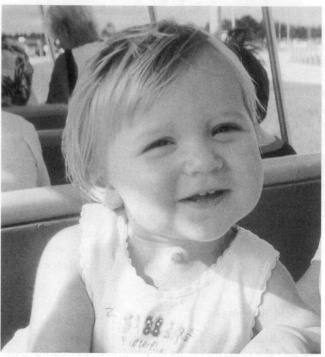

Figure 3-4 ■ Torticollis. Child with torticollis resulting from shortening of the right SCM muscle resulting in lateral flexion to the right and rotation to the left. (From Oatis CA. *Kinesiology: The Mechanics & Pathomechanics of Human Movement.* Baltimore: Lippincott Williams & Wilkins; 2004)

 P O I N T S   T O   R E M E M B E R

SCFE

Four clinical groups are used to classify the various forms of SCFE. It can also be classified as stable or unstable.

Group I—Known as the preslip and is stable. Defined as a wide physis without slippage of the epiphysis.

Group II—Known as acute and is unstable. Defined as a sudden onset of slippage without trauma.

Group III—Known as acute or chronic and is unstable. Defined as an epiphysis slip that occurs acutely on an existing chronic slip.

Group IV—The most common group. It is known as the chronic group and is stable. Defined as a several month history of pain, limp, and out-toed gait.

Degenerative processes resulting in premature onset of arthritis may affect functional mobility in adulthood.

TORTICOLLIS (WRY NECK)

Torticollis describes a disorder that involves shortening of one of the sternocleidomastoid (SCM) muscles. It may be a primary abnormality, known as muscular torticollis, or secondary to a CNS disorder or upper cervical spine abnormalities. The primary abnormality is known as congenital torticollis or wry neck (Fig. 3-4). The head of the child is tilted toward the side of the contracture, and the chin is turned toward the opposite side. A significant resistance is encountered when an attempt is made to try to correct the positioning manually. A firm mass may also be palpable in the involved SCM muscle.

Several etiologies of the primary disorder include in utero malposition, birth trauma, hereditary factors, and SCM muscle compartment syndrome. In secondary torticollis, several etiologies including CNS mass lesions, local head and neck infections, and abnormalities of the cervical spine are included.

Medical Treatment

Medical treatment of the disorder initially involves determining any secondary causes and treating these appropriately. Increasing range of motion of the neck and correcting any cosmetic problems that may be present are ultimate goals of medical treatment. Conservative treatment includes range-of-motion exercises of the head and neck, which involve stretching the restricted muscles several times daily. This treatment is used in children younger than 1 year with no other underlying medical problems. More aggressive treatment is surgical intervention to release all the restricting tissue that is affecting the SCM muscle and other neck structures. This intervention is followed by physical therapy within 2 weeks.

Physical Therapy

Practice Pattern: *Impaired Posture*

Safety Issues: *The physical therapist should be aware that cervical subluxation is common in this population.[16,34] Use of modalities to relax the soft tissues is a precaution due to the age of the infant.*

Common Impairments: *The most common impairments include a decreased range of motion and poor posture.[8,16,35] Flattening of the skull may be noticed.*

Functional Limitations: *No functional limitations should be expected early. If the imbalance persists, rolling may be impaired.*

Typical Interventions: *A positioning program, passive range of motion, and facilitation of active range of motion. The involved side should be gently stretched, and the uninvolved side should be strengthened through active movements. The use of a cervical collar or helmet may also be beneficial.[5,35–37] Active and passive range of motion should be monitored. If resolution of the impairment is not evident, diagnostic imaging may be indicated.*

General Outcomes: *When properly treated with conservative methods, most cases of torticollis resolve within 1 year; however, surgery may be required in a small percentage of cases. Those cases poorly managed or untreated often display permanent deformity and asymmetrical position and shape of the head.[8,16,35]*

■ Physical Therapy Practice Pattern: Neuromuscular

ASSOCIATED MOVEMENT DISORDERS

The following clinical presentations categorized as associated movement disorders are seen in a variety of diseases mentioned throughout this chapter. They are listed here for easy reference.

Dystonia

Dystonia is classified as a *hyperkinetic movement disorder* and is described as hyperkinetic, slow, twisting motions which are involuntary and can result in abnormal postures and repetitive movements.[38] Dystonia is a nearly continuous deviation of posture in one or more joints. It may occur in proximal or distal limbs or an axial structure. Dystonia is present during attempted voluntary movement. It is also associated with the abnormal spread of activation to muscles other than those required to perform the attempted movement. This is known as "overflow." A unique characteristic of dystonia is that it can often be slowed or lessened by tactile or proprioceptive input. Dystonic tremor may be present.[39] It resembles an essential tremor in its characteristic succession of rapid dystonic movements.

The dystonias are classified by age of onset (i.e., childhood vs. adult), region of the body involved, and etiology. *Primary dystonias* are syndromes in which the actual dystonic movement is the only clinical manifestation of the disease. The major childhood syndrome in this group is idiopathic torsion dystonia (ITD) or Oppenheim dystonia. It is an autosomal dominant disorder affecting mainly Ashkenazy Jewish families in >90% of all cases.[9]

Secondary dystonias are largely caused by drugs and other environmental factors. External factors producing dystonia are cerebral trauma, peripheral nerve injury, cerebral hypoxia, some infectious and postinfectious states, and toxic exposures to manganese, cyanide, and 3-nitroproprionic acid.[38]

Hypertonicity

Hypertonicity, or increased muscle tone, may be evident as spasticity. *Spasticity* is defined as the resistance determined by the angle and velocity of motion.[9] It is most often seen in corticospinal tract disease or disease of the upper motor neuron. Cerebral vascular accidents are the most common cause of damage to the corticospinal tract. Tumors, trauma, infections, demyelinating syndromes, and metabolic and degenerative diseases also injure the corticospinal tract.

Hypotonicity

Hypotonicity, or decreased muscle tone, is most commonly due to lower motor neuron or peripheral nerve disorders. There is a multitude of lower motor neuron diseases that can be present with hypotonicity in infants and children, including muscular dystrophy, polio, spinal muscular atrophy (SMA), diphtheria, myositis; and metabolic, endocrine, and mineral disorders.[9] Peripheral nerve disease can also present with hypotonicity, including Guillain-Barre syndrome (GBS); vitamin E, vitamin B_1, and vitamin B_{12} deficiencies; toxins; and collagen vascular disease, to name a few.[9]

Rigidity

Rigidity is defined as an increase in muscle tone with resistance to passive stretch throughout the range of motion of a muscle. It affects the extensor and flexor muscles equally. Rigidity occurs with certain extrapyramidal disorders and is seen in hypokinetic movement disorders.

PHYSICAL THERAPY

Practice Pattern: *Movement disorders can be associated with a variety of practice patterns, for example: Impaired Motor Function and Sensory Integrity Associated with Nonprogressive Disorders of the CNS—Congenital Origin or Acquired in Infancy or Childhood*

Safety Issues: *There is an increased risk of joint subluxation, dislocation, and lack of normal postural control. Appropriate supervision should be provided with movement activities.*

Common Impairments: *Increased or decreased range of motion, lack of joint stabilization, and muscle weakness may be noted. Common impairment in motor control.*

Functional Limitations: *The child may have developmental delays, especially in motor function.*

Typical Interventions: *Handling, positioning, range of motion, therapeutic exercise, splints, orthotics, use of assistive technology, and functional training may be effective. Dystonia can be addressed by the use of positioning devices.*

General Outcomes: *Management of increased muscle tone is often addressed with medications or surgery. Therapeutic handling and positioning techniques offer transient effects and should be followed by strengthening exercise and the promotion of function. Hypotonia can be addressed through therapeutic exercise and splinting for joint protection.*

ATTENTION DEFICIT HYPERACTIVITY DISORDER

Clinically, children with Attention Deficit Hyperactivity Disorder (ADHD) present as being inattentive, easily distracted, and overactive, and they display a degree of impulsivity that interferes with everyday functioning in school and at home. This impulsive nature is exhibited as the inability to control a reaction or response to a situation. Acting without thinking and inability to complete one task before moving on to another are also symptoms. Children with ADHD are easily distracted by environmental stimuli and are unable to focus on the task at hand, especially in a situation such as the classroom. Overactivity may or may not be present. ADHD is more likely to occur in boys with a 4:1 male predominance. Constant motion is the descriptive term most consistent with an overactive child. Some of these movements include body rocking, tapping fingers, swinging of the lower extremities, climbing, and/or running around a room with some body part always in motion. The classifications that presently exist for ADHD are the impulsive overactive type, the inattentive type, and the mixed combination forms.[40]

Physical examination is usually normal. Psychological evaluation often aids in making an accurate diagnosis, as some degree of neurologic and behavioral immaturity is normally present in children, especially boys. Parental inadequacies in controlling the behavior of the child, due to poor or lacking parenting skills, may contribute to the appearance of ADHD-like behaviors that must be distinguished from true ADHD before medical treatment begins.

Medical Treatment

Medical treatment of ADHD combines medication and environmental interventions in addition to psychological, emotional, and educational treatments. Treatment is truly a team approach, involving the patient, physician, parents, teachers, and often times a psychologist to assist in behavioral and emotional issues. All of these factors must be addressed before proper responses to pharmacologic treatment are actually seen. The medications used to treat ADHD are thought to have their neuropharmacologic effects on dopaminergic neurons in the brain stem reticular activating system. The majority of these medications are psychostimulants that allow the child to focus in on appropriate behavior and control the hyperactivity. Methylphenidate and dextroamphetamine are commonly used along with amphetamine mixed salts (Adderall), which is available in an extended release form for longer bioavailability. Atomoxetine (Strattera) is the only non-controlled medication available for treatment of ADHD. These medications have multiple side effects, including sleep and appetite disturbances, elevation of heart rate and blood pressure, rebound overactivity, and irritability on withdraw of the medication.[41]

Physical Therapy

Practice Pattern: *Impaired Neuromotor Development*

Safety Issues: *Avoid activities that result in overstimulation and fatigue.*

Common Impairments: *Children often display a decreased attention span, hyperactivity, and clumsiness, and are often impulsive.[5,42] They may present with proximal muscle weakness, mild impairments in postural control, and an inability to attain higher-level gross motor skills that require increased coordination and attention.*

Functional Limitations: *Limitations of higher-level motor skills and completion of ADLs may be noted.*

Typical Interventions: *Family education is important in the management of ADHD. The child's daily routine should be consistent with expectations clearly defined. Rules should be clear, simple, and concise.[42] Therapeutic exercise and functional training may be beneficial.*

General Outcomes: *Research shows that 50% of all children diagnosed with ADHD grow to be productive adults within society.[42]*

AUTISM

Autism is viewed as a spectrum of disorders that range from mild to severe. The prevalence in society ranges from 0.7 to 4.5 in 10,000 children.[40] The etiology of the spectrum of disorders is unclear, and the clinical disorders in general have been associated with a multitude of different causes. Clinically, children with an autistic disorder present as being unable to relate to other people, including their own parents. In infancy, the autistic child may be noticeably unattached to his parents or caregivers, he may lack or display a delay in the development of a social smile, or may be developmentally normal until regression of developmental milestones are noticed around age 2 years. These are especially common with regard to speech and other communicative abilities. The young child may appear to be socially inept or withdrawn around other children and adults who attempt to interact with him. He may appear cold or aloof, rarely making eye contact, if at all. The autistic child may spend hours in solitary play activity. Compulsive routines and/or ritualistic behaviors can be completely absorbing to the child. Disruption by a parent or other caregivers can cause tantrums and rage-like reactions. Some of these behaviors include head banging, teeth grinding, and rocking. A decreased responsiveness to painful stimuli and environmental stimuli are noted; in severe cases, self-mutilation is usually seen. Developmental speech patterns are abnormal and, if present at all, usually consist of nonsense rhyming, repetition of a spoken word or sentence referred to as *echolalia*, and other abnormal language forms. The intelligence quotient (IQ) of these children is difficult to measure with conventional testing, but the prognosis is much better for a child who has a higher intelligence level and is able to communicate more effectively by age 5 years.

Medical Treatment

Because the etiology is unclear in the autism spectrum disorders, medical treatment is geared toward early intervention by initially making an appropriate diagnosis, then intensively treating the child with speech therapy to improve communication skills and interventions aimed at improving cognition, social–emotional skills, and behavior.[41,43] Interventions that include the parent appear to have a positive outcome for children with autism.[43] Therapy and support groups are important for family members as autism can affect the entire dynamic make-up of the family.

Physical Therapy

Practice Pattern: *Impaired Neuromotor Development*

Safety Issues: *It is important not to disrupt the routines previously established by the child and his family as the child may not deal well with such changes.*[44]

Common Impairments: *The child may not be able to adequately communicate (verbally, nonverbally, or both), may have difficulty with gross and fine motor skills and exhibit proximal muscle weakness, and may present with decreased endurance.*

Functional Limitations: *The lack of communication may result in learning disabilities as well as limited social interaction. Limitations of higher-level motor skills and completion of ADLs may be noted.*

Typical Interventions: *Family education is essential when working with children who have autism. A multidisciplinary program should be customized to the individual needs of the child. An integral part of therapy is behavior modification.*[44]

General Outcomes: *The probability of the child to fulfill an independent and functioning role within society as an adult depends upon the developmental level and extent of communicative skills.*[44]

BEHAVIORAL DISORDERS

There are four pervasive developmental disorders identified in the *Diagnostic and Statistical Manual of Mental Disorders, Fourth Edition, Text Revision* (DSMIV-TR).[40] The first, autism, was discussed previously. The remainder of the disorders in this category are Rett disorder, childhood disintegrative disorder, and Asperger syndrome. This group of disorders includes conditions that consist of delays in the development of social, communication, and behavioral skills. Children with these disorders often show particular and intense interest in a small range of activities, resist any type of change, and do not respond appropriately to the external social environment. These disorders are usually first seen early in life and become persistent, causing continued dysfunction.

Rett Disorder

Rett disorder appears only to be found in girls. It is characterized by normal development for about 6 months, with stereotyped hand movements, a loss of purposeful motions, decreasing social interaction, poor coordination, and decreasing language use. The cause is unknown and likely to be genetic in origin, although this is yet to be determined.

The stereotypic hand movements can be hand wringing, licking or biting the fingers, and tapping or slapping the fingers. The head circumference growth slows down, and microcephaly develops. The child loses all ability to speak and understand speech. Social skills plateau at about a 6- to 11-month developmental age level. Poor muscular coordination and an apraxic gait, which is stiff and unsteady, develop.

In 75% of all children affected with this disorder, seizures can occur.[40] An additional feature is the appearance of irregular respiration with episodes of hyperventilation, apnea, and breath holding, which seem to be intentional as none of these symptoms occur during sleep. As the disorder progresses, muscle tone may increase from an initial hypotonic condition to spasticity and then rigidity. Children with this disorder usually require a wheelchair for mobility by 10 years of age with muscle wasting, rigidity, and little to no language ability. Children with Rett disorder may live into adulthood.

MEDICAL TREATMENT

Medical treatment for Rett disorder is symptomatic only. Medications in the form of anticonvulsants are usually needed to control seizures. Behavioral therapy, in addition to medications such as risperidone (Risperdal), usually helps to control self-injurious behaviors and helps to regulate the breathing irregularities. Risperidone, a serotonin dopamine antagonist in the category of an atypical antipsychotic, is used most frequently.

Childhood Disintegrative Disorder

Childhood disintegrative disorder is characterized by marked regression in several areas of functioning after 2 years of normal development. It is also called Heller syndrome. In most cases, the age of onset is between 3 and 4 years of age. The etiology is as yet unknown. In some cases, the child may show signs of restlessness, increased activity levels, and anxiety before the loss of function occurs. This disorder is noted for a loss of communication skills, onset of stereotyped movements, and compulsive behaviors often seen in autistic children, as well as regression of reciprocal interactions in social situations. Symptoms of anxiety are common, and regression of skills, such as bowel and bladder control, motor control, and play, are also common. These children often develop seizure disorders.

MEDICAL TREATMENT

Because of the clinical similarity to autism, the treatment of this disorder includes the same components used in the treatment of autism. Seizures are controlled with oral anticonvulsant agents such as those previously mentioned.

Asperger Syndrome

Asperger syndrome is characterized by severe, sustained impairment in social interaction and restricted, repetitive patterns of behavior, interests, and activities. There are no significant delays in language, cognition, or appropriate self-help skills as there are in the other disorders in this category. Social impairment usually presents with markedly abnormal nonverbal communication gestures, the failure to develop peer relationships, lack of social or emotional reciprocity, and impaired ability to express pleasure in another persons' happiness. These children show no language delay, no significant cognitive delay, and no adaptive impairment.[45]

MEDICAL TREATMENT

Behavior therapy geared toward the patient's level of adaptive functioning is used. Some of the same techniques used for autistic disorder are usually beneficial in Asperger syndrome with severe social impairment. Medication is usually not beneficial for the primary symptoms of this disorder.

PHYSICAL THERAPY: BEHAVIORAL DISORDERS

Practice Pattern: *Impaired Neuromotor Development*
Safety Issues: *Child may be prone to injury to self or others.*

Common Impairments: *Impairments are variable. Majority includes communication and social skills. Some children with Asperger syndrome may have delayed motor skills and impaired coordination.*[45]
Functional Limitations: *Variable. May involve limits in ADLs and instrumental ADLs (IADLs).*
Typical Interventions: *The most important intervention in the management of a child with a behavior disorder is parent, family, and team education. Goals of the intervention and expectations should be clearly outlined. Adhering to a set schedule and working with the child's interest are important components of intervention for a child with Asperger syndrome.*
General Outcomes: *Based on identification of the underlying cause of the behavior. Consistent and uniform response to identified behavior is important for an effective outcome. Children with Asperger syndrome can improve with maturation and are able to live independent lives.*[45]

BRACHIAL PLEXUS INJURY

A brachial plexus injury is considered an injury due to birth trauma. Generally, the brachial plexus is injured during vaginal delivery when excessive traction is placed on the neck of the infant. This trauma may produce paresis or complete paralysis, depending upon the degree of force placed and the nerve root(s) involved. Phrenic nerve palsy may occur after damage to the 3rd, 4th, and 5th cervical nerves. This deficit can be deadly in that it may result in diaphragmatic elevation and paralysis leading to respiratory distress.

Several types of brachial plexus injuries have been identified including *Erb-Duchenne paralysis*, which occurs after damage to the 5th and 6th cervical nerves during delivery. The infant is able to painlessly adduct and internally rotate the upper extremity and pronate the forearm. The infant is usually unable to abduct or externally rotate the upper extremity at the shoulder, or supinate the forearm. The hand grasp is normal; there is no Moro (or startle) reflex on the affected side.

Klumpke paralysis occurs due to injury of the 7th and 8th cervical nerves and the 1st thoracic nerve. This results in a paralyzed hand. Horner's syndrome (ptosis and contraction of the pupil of the ipsilateral eye) can occur if the sympathetic nerves at these levels are affected also. With damage to the 5th, 6th, 7th, and 8th cervical nerves and 1st thoracic nerve, there is complete upper extremity paralysis.

Medical Treatment

Initial medical treatment is conservative and depends on the degree of paralysis of the upper extremity. Avoidance of contractures is foremost in treatment and positioning to do so along with active and passive range-of-motion exercises. If deficits persist or are severe, nerve-grafting surgical procedures may be used to correct these deficits so that the greatest range of motion of the upper extremity is obtainable.

Physical Therapy

Practice Patterns: *Impaired Joint Mobility, Motor Function, Muscle Performance, Range of Motion, and Reflex Integrity Associated with Spinal Disorders; Impaired Peripheral Nerve Integrity and Muscle Performance Associated with Peripheral Nerve Injury*

Safety Issues: *Caution should be taken not to further stretch the brachial plexus during therapeutic interventions and handling.*

Common Impairments: *Decreased sensation, motor control and range of motion, which could ultimately result in contracture, are common. The muscles of the shoulder and posterior upper trunk can be paralyzed with injury.*[5]

Functional Limitations: *Various functional limitations may result due to the extent of the injury and the rate of nerve regeneration. Difficulty may be expressed with bilateral tasks due to neglect of the involved extremity.*[5]

Typical Interventions: *Immobilization and positioning as well as passive range of motion are imperative in order to prevent contractures and promote normal joint development.*[16,46,47] *Gentle massage may be used for relaxation of tight musculature prior to range-of-motion exercises.*[16] *Parent/caregiver and family education is also important.*

General Outcomes: *The outcome is directly related to the severity of the injury; a more severe injury results in a poorer prognosis.*[16] *The best indicator of recovery is active extension in the upper extremity by 3 months of age. Spontaneous recovery has been shown to occur within 4 to 9 months; however, recovery could take as long as 4 years.*[5]

BRAIN TUMORS

Primary brain tumors are second only to leukemia in occurrence of malignant disease in children. Approximately nine different types of primary brain tumors have been identified overall and can occur at any time between 2 and 5 months of age through 12 years of age in various parts of the brain. Symptomatology with regard to the tumor is particular to the area of the brain in which it originates and develops.[16]

Two peculiarities exist in primary brain tumors that develop in children. First, childhood brain tumors are usually derived from embryonic cells. Second, they are usually located in the posterior fossae of the brain (i.e., cerebellum, mid-brain, and brain stem areas). The majority of childhood tumors, therefore, are classified as infratentorial tumors. Supratentorial tumors do exist in children, but with a lower incidence of occurrence.

Unfortunately, the clinical presentation of a child with a primary brain tumor is vague and nonspecific.

As the tumor grows and intracranial pressure increases (and as it potentially affects cranial nerve function), a brain tumor is usually considered in the differential diagnosis. Headache is one of the symptoms that may be indicative of increased intracranial pressure due to tumor growth. Headaches that occur at night or with waking in the morning, worsen with straining to urinate/defecate or with coughing, are intermittent, and gradually increase with frequency and intensity are highly suggestive of an intracranial tumor etiology and must be investigated. Vomiting without nausea, usually occurring with waking, and strabismus with double vision are also signs of increased intracranial pressure and possible brain tumor. Head tilt is seen due to compensation for loss of binocular vision and is also associated with extraocular muscle weakness. Ataxic gait can be associated with a cerebellar tumor or a brain stem tumor. A Babinski sign, hyperreflexia, spasticity, or loss of dexterity may also indicate a brain stem tumor. Seizures, personality changes, changes in school performance, and change in hand preference are also seen with tumors of the cortex.

A detailed history, physical examination with emphasis on the neurologic areas and the visual field, and fundi examination are essential to aid in the diagnosis. An MRI of the head is necessary for absolute diagnosis of a primary brain tumor. A CT scan is also used, but may be less absolute in diagnosis because of its poor imaging quality of the posterior fossae area of the brain due to thicker bone overlay. A spinal tap is usually performed to aid in the differential diagnosis of the tumor and to obtain cerebrospinal fluid (CSF) to rule out metastasis.

Medical Treatment

Medical treatment involves the administration of corticosteroids, which are usually used as soon as possible after a tumor is discovered in order to reduce the degree of edema caused by the tumor. This in turn reduces the associated symptoms such as headaches, vomiting, and other neurologic deficits caused by the tumor. Anticonvulsants are used to control seizures associated with cortical tumors, and are usually initiated as soon as possible. Carbanazepine (Tegretol), phenobarbital, and phenytoin (Dilantin) are commonly used anticonvulsants in the pediatric population.[19] Radiation therapy is used more than any other treatment for primary pediatric brain tumors. Treatment of malignant tumors in children is aggressive. Neurosurgical techniques are also used to obtain tissue for diagnosis, reduce the size of the tumor, or completely excise the tumor if it is within a good location to do so. Chemotherapy is being used more often for primary pediatric brain tumors, usually in conjunction with radiation. It is being used specifically with medulloblastoma and with infants on whom radiation may be more detrimental than beneficial.[16]

Physical Therapy

Practice Pattern: *Impaired Motor Function and Sensory Integrity Associated with Progressive Disorders of the CNS*

Safety Issues: *Vital signs must be closely monitored before, during, and after treatment.[8] Signs and symptoms of increased intracranial pressure may include irritability, lethargy, projectile vomiting, and blurred vision. Caution must be used with application of modalities.*

Common Impairments: *A child may present with fatigue and abnormal muscle tone. Cognitive, visual, and verbal impairments may be present. Decreased mobility and weakness result from neuromuscular and cardiopulmonary impairments.*

Functional Limitations: *Mobility and ADLs may be difficult to complete independently.*

Typical Interventions: *Positioning and range-of-motion exercises are initiated when the child is stable. Strengthening exercises are also useful.[8] Therapeutic exercise to increase endurance and interventions to improve independence with ADLs may also be appropriate.*

General Outcomes: *In most cases, younger patients have a greater disability and, thus, a poorer prognosis.[16]*

POINTS TO REMEMBER

Signs of Increased Intracranial Pressure

Signs and symptoms of increased intracranial pressure may include:

- Headache
- Double vision
- Projectile vomiting
- Nausea
- Lethargy

CEREBRAL PALSY

The term cerebral palsy (CP) is used to describe a group of nondegenerating neurologic disabilities caused by a variety of factors. These factors may occur developmentally in utero, via injuries prenatally, or injuries in the perinatal period. The result is abnormal motor function often accompanied by a seizure disorder and mental retardation in 25% of the children.[16] The incidence is believed to be 4 in 1,000 live births.[16] Causes of CP include developmental anomalies, congenital infections, perinatal trauma, cerebral infarction, metabolic disorders in the perinatal period, hypoxia–ischemia in the premature and full-term infant, hypoglycemia, hyperbilirubinemia, and thromboembolic events.

Several patterns of CP can be classified according to clinical manifestations. The first is *spastic diplegia*. Children with spastic diplegia are typically low-birth-weight infants.[16] Spastic diplegia is related to cerebral asphyxia with or without intraventricular hemorrhage (IVH). The presentation of this category is an infant with spasticity of the lower extremities more so than of the upper extremities and of one hemibody more than the other. The child may have increased deep tendon reflexes and a Babinski reflex. Seizures, language problems, learning disabilities, and mild-to-moderate cognitive impairment can occur with this form of CP. The second category is *spastic quadriplegia*. Children with spastic quadriplegia are usually also low-birth-weight infants with severe asphyxial insults. The presentation of this category is an infant with spasticity in all four extremities, seizures, and feeding difficulties. Scoliosis and other orthopedic problems are more common in this type of CP. The third category is *spastic hemiplegia*. The previously described etiologic scenarios are common with this category, but other etiologies include cerebrovascular accidents, such as embolism or vascular malformations. Cognitive abilities may be normal because only one side of the brain is involved. Motor impairments and language processing dysfunction are usually present and can be severe. The fourth category is *athetoid*, which presents with hypotonia, choreoathetosis, and the development of dystonic movements later in life. Hearing impairment and motor speech disorders are more common in this category of CP. There are fewer seizures and more normal cognitive function in this form than in other forms of CP.

Medical Treatment

Medical treatment is geared toward the severity and presentation of deficits of the individual child. Medical management of seizures is usually accomplished with anticonvulsive medications and monitoring of blood levels of these medications until optimal control is obtained. Baclofen, especially via pump administration, has been used for the management of severe muscle spasticity.[48] Orthopedic surgery may be necessary for severe contractures or abnormalities that may limit movement or ambulation. Increasing the functional capabilities of these children to their maximum capacity is accomplished with physical and occupational therapy. Gearing educational situations to maximize the intellectual capabilities of these children is also imperative.

Children with CP thrive best in a situation where there is a supportive family environment. The family members should be educated to assist in the care of the child emotionally and physically. Support groups are available for the family members and are highly recommended due to the demanding and exhausting care that most children with CP require.

Physical Therapy

Practice Pattern: *Impaired Motor Function and Sensory Integrity Associated with Nonprogressive Disorders of the CNS—Congenital Origin or Acquired in Infancy or Childhood*

Safety Issues: *May be difficult to handle due to poor postural control and excessive use of extension posturing. Adequate supervision with movement activities is necessary due to impairments in this area.*

Common Impairments: *Impairments vary with the type of CP expressed. Common deficiencies include decreased range of motion, muscle weakness, abnormal muscle tone, poor muscle control, decreased mobility, and abnormal posture. Cognitive impairments and developmental delays may also be present.[5,8,49]*

Functional Limitations: *The most common limitations are with ADLs and mobility. Because of these limitations, the child may experience limited social interaction.[8]*

Typical Interventions: *Providing strategies and parental education for everyday activities such as feeding, bathing, and playing are important in order to develop parental confidence in the management of the child.[5,16] The primary goals are to prevent contractures and promote function. These goals may be achieved by range-of-motion exercises, stretching, and relaxation techniques. Exercises to promote postural control and positioning techniques such as splinting and serial casting may be used to improve joint alignment. The use of orthotics and assistive devices, as well as learning compensatory strategies, may help to promote independence in the child.[8] Therapeutic exercises with appropriate levels of resistance may improve muscle strength and ambulation skills.[50] Endurance activities should also be promoted.*

General Outcomes: *The potential for functional ambulation is dependent on achievement of developmental milestones. If the child can sit independently by 2 years of age, it is probable that the child will ambulate in the future. Functional ambulation may not be achieved if walking has not occurred by 8 years of age. Ambulation potential is the greatest for children with a spastic hemiplegic and athetoid presentation, followed by spastic diplegic, then quadriplegic presentations.[8] A normal life span can be expected for the majority of children with mild-to-moderate cases of CP.[51] Respiratory disease is the leading cause of death in adults with CP.[52]*

CEREBRAL VASCULAR ACCIDENTS

Intracranial/Intraventricular Hemorrhage

Several forms of intracranial hemorrhage (ICH) can occur in infancy and childhood. In the fetus and neonate, ICH may result from trauma or anoxia. During delivery, traumatic hemorrhage is not as common as it used to be due to the advancement in obstetric and pediatric management. In prolonged labor, breech deliveries, precipitate deliveries, or mechanical interference with delivery may actually cause traumatic ICH. In premature infants, intracerebral hemorrhages and intraventicular hemorrhages (IVHs) are more common.[16] IVH diagnoses are aided by the use of ultrasound or CT scan and are graded based on the anatomic distribution of the hemorrhage. Grade I is used for bleeding that is confined to the germinal matrix or <10% of the ventricle. Grade II includes bleeding into the lateral ventricles (approximately 50%). Grade III includes >50% bleeding into the ventricle with ventricular distention. Grade IV includes evidence of periventricular hemorrhage.[16]

Symptoms of ICH/IVH can be present at birth or appear soon after delivery. Failure to exhibit normal movement, decreased Moro (and/or startle) reflex, poor muscle tone, lethargy, and, in severe cases, irregularity of the respirations, are common symptoms. In premature infants, symptoms may not occur until day 2 or 3 of life. Symptoms of apnea episodes, paleness, cyanosis, vomiting, convulsions, decreased muscle tone, and paralysis are common initial presentations. A CT scan is necessary to make a definitive diagnosis of an intracranial bleed in a neonate. A lumbar puncture is helpful in diagnosing a subarachnoid bleed. When intracranial bleeding is severe, the child will become comatose. In cases of recurrent minor episodes of bleeding, there may be symptoms of headaches and focal seizures leading to a severe bleed.

Rarely do symptoms from aneurysms occur until early adulthood. If a rupture of an aneurysm does occur in a child, the presentation is an acute, severe headache, which could occur in a well child. Coma usually occurs quickly. Hemiparesis is common with rupture of a middle-cerebral-artery aneurysm. Cerebral artery angiography is also needed for definitive diagnosis of a ruptured intracranial aneurysm.

MEDICAL TREATMENT

Treatment of the neonate with an ICH/IVH involves as little physical handling as possible. Incubator care with continuous observation, excellent ventilation, and temperature control is imperative. Anticonvulsant drugs are used to control seizures. Vitamin K oxide should be administered, and fresh blood is indicated in the presence of hemorrhagic disease of the newborn. Dexamethasone or mannitol may be indicated for treatment of increased intracranial pressure, especially if the infant's condition is rapidly deteriorating. In infants and children with cerebral hemorrhage due to arteriovenous (AV) malformations, surgery may be necessary, depending on the location of the lesion. Gamma-knife surgery or actual excision may be possible. In intracerebral aneurysms, surgical ligation or clipping of the aneurysm, depending on the location of the lesion, is indicated. Bleeding may recur up to many years later in survivors.

PHYSICAL THERAPY

Practice Pattern: *Impaired Motor Function and Sensory Integrity Associated with Progressive Disorders of the CNS*

Safety Issues: *Vital signs must be monitored before, during, and after treatment.[8] Signs and symptoms of increased intracranial pressure may include irritability, lethargy, projectile vomiting, and blurred vision.*

Common Impairments: *The child may present with poor muscle tone, fatigue, and altered consciousness. Motor and cognitive problems as well as seizures may be noted.*[16]

Functional Limitations: *Poor muscle tone may hinder the child's ability to feed, as sucking may be impaired.*

Typical Interventions: *Positioning, range of motion, stretching, and strengthening exercises may be appropriate. Techniques to promote motor control, oral motor skills, compensatory strategies, and the use of adaptive devices will aid in improving function.*

General Outcomes: *A poor prognosis is correlated with persistent and/or progressive hydrocephalus.*[16] *The more severe the IVH, the more severe the impact on development. Children with Grades I and II tend to have less severe impairments than those with Grades III and IV.*[53]

Cerebral Vascular Occlusion

Various forms of cerebral vascular occlusions can occur. These may be either thrombotic or embolic if arterial in nature, or thrombotic or thrombophlebitic if venous in nature.

CEREBRAL ARTERIAL OCCLUSION

Cerebral arterial occlusion is uncommon overall in childhood, but occurs with increased frequency in the 1- to 3-year-old age group. It is due to thrombosis or embolism in the internal carotid or middle cerebral artery. Thrombosis in the intracranial portion of the internal carotid artery can be caused by inflammation of the vasculature by infection of the tonsils, cervical lymph nodes, or trauma locally. Systemic illnesses such as sickle cell anemia, lupus, and cyanotic heart disease can cause arterial occlusions in childhood. In infants younger than 2 years who have had congenital heart disease, *polycythemia* (an increase in the number of red blood cells), and/or iron deficiency, cerebral arterial occlusion can be common. In an older child, cerebral embolism is possible in association with congenital heart disease.

Clinical signs and symptoms of a cerebral arterial occlusion resemble those seen with a stroke in an adult. These stroke-like symptoms may be preceded by a febrile illness in a child. The symptoms of hemiparesis may occur suddenly or over a several hour time frame. Focal or generalized seizures can occur frequently in the acute phase, and if the dominant hemisphere is affected, aphasia can occur. There is usually no increased intracranial pressure, and CSF remains normal. Recurrent seizures are common, especially following acute hemiplegia in infancy. Many children who had a cerebral arterial thrombosis have mild intellectual impairment and behavioral abnormalities.

CEREBRAL VENOUS THROMBOSIS

Cerebral venous thrombosis usually occurs due to complications from severe dehydration and extension of local infection into cerebral veins. The occluded venous system is classified into three categories: sagittal sinus thrombosis, lateral sinus thrombosis, and cavernous sinus thrombosis.[9] *Sagittal sinus thrombosis* is rare and is a complication of severe dehydration, especially in infants with diarrhea. Cerebral swelling can occur, which causes increased intracranial pressure, stupor, coma, dilated scalp veins, and bulging anterior fontanelle. There can be a widespread hemorrhagic infarct of the brain. Symptoms also include seizures and quadriparesis. *Lateral sinus thrombosis* is rare today as it is usually a complication of untreated otitis media. Symptoms include chills, fever, and a slow onset of intracranial pressure with the sequelae of that event. *Cavernous sinus thrombosis* usually follows infection of the face, orbit, or nasal sinuses. Again, with aggressive antibiotic therapy this condition has become much less common. The infection spreads through anastomoses of the facial vein with the ophthalmic veins, which drain directly into the cavernous sinuses. Symptoms of high fever, malaise, and paralysis of the ocular muscles can develop.[54]

Medical Treatment

Medical treatment of cerebral arterial occlusion is directed toward underlying etiologies of the occurrence. Infectious processes must be treated aggressively with IV antibiotics. Seizures must be brought under control with anticonvulsant medications. Usually, this is done acutely with IV forms of the medication, and recurrent seizures usually are maintained under control with oral formulations.

The prognosis for speech recovery is good with the aid of speech therapy. There is usually some residual hemiparesis, and spasticity can develop within weeks. Physical therapy is needed to obtain as much function as possible.

Treatment of cerebral vein thrombosis includes aggressive IV antibiotics to treat the underlying infectious cause. Localized collections of pus should be drained surgically. If intracranial pressure becomes a problem, it should be treated with mannitol or dexamethasone IV immediately to prevent future sequelae.[54]

Physical Therapy

Practice Pattern: *Impaired Motor Function and Sensory Integrity Associated with Nonprogressive Disorders of the CNS*

Safety Issues: *There may be a decrease in balance, therefore, increasing the risk of falling.*

Common Impairments: *The location and extent of damage determines the level of impairment. The most common impairments include decreased range of motion, strength, and sensation, as well as difficulty with motor control and speech.*[8]

Functional Limitations: *Independence with ADLs may be lost. Decreased mobility and ability to communicate also hinder independent functioning.*

Typical Interventions: *Positioning, range of motion, stretching, and strengthening may be appropriate. Tech-*

niques to promote motor control and learning, compensatory strategies, and the use of adaptive devices will aid in improving function. Aerobic training has also been shown to be beneficial.[8]

General Outcomes: Currently there is no evidence in the literature that a child who has sustained an ischemic stroke will make a better recovery than an adult.[55] In the adult population, physical therapy is most helpful 6 to 18 months poststroke. Prognosis depends on the location and extent of the hemorrhage with functional recovery good in most cases.[8]

CHARCOT-MARIE-TOOTH DISEASE

Charcot-Marie-Tooth Disease is an inherited peripheral nerve disease in children. It is also known as hereditary motor sensory neuropathy and is a polyneuropathy with presenting symptoms of foot deformity, weakness, and wasting of distal limb muscles beginning in the preschool years.

On examination, the child presents with high arched feet and weakness of foot dorsiflexors. Symptoms include paresthesia and "tripping." There can be a broad spectrum of presentation of the disease symptoms. Usually, progression is slow over years and decades. Type I is a demyelinating disease, whereas Type II is a neuronal form. Both are inherited as autosomal dominant.[23] Type I is more severe in its debilitating symptoms than Type II.

Medical Treatment

Specific medical treatment with regard to medications is not available. Early surgery for a child is not indicated due to progression of the disease over time. Braces to keep the feet in dorsiflexion can improve function.

Physical Therapy

Practice Pattern: Impaired Neuromotor Development
Safety Issue: Decreased balance may present.
Common Impairments: Distal muscle weakness, decreased endurance, and decreased proprioception.
Functional Limitations: The child may show decreased ambulation as well as decreased performance in higher level gross motor skills.
Typical Interventions: Interventions to preserve function and minimize orthopedic deformity, range of motion, stretching, splints, and orthotics are used. Skin care is also important.
General Outcomes: Since progression is slow, it may take years or even decades to notice effects of the disease. Members of the same family may present with severe weakness so that the use of a wheelchair for mobility may be necessary, whereas others only have mild foot deformities. Those with Type I have a poorer prognosis as this type is more debilitating.[23]

DEPRESSION

Depression can appear in children of all ages. The essential features of major depression are similar in children, adolescents, and adults with the presentation of these features modified to coincide with the age experience and maturity level of the patient.[56] These disorders are more common in childhood and adolescents than previously thought. Depression in preschool children is rare, i.e., <0.3% in the community setting.[40] About 2% of school-age children are thought to have a major depressive disorder, and about 5% of adolescents are thought to have this disorder in the community.[40] Among hospitalized patients, 20% of children and 40% of adolescents have a major depressive disorder.[40] There does seem to be a familial link with depression and all mood disorders. Children with one parent with depression double his or her risk of developing depression. With two parents the risk of developing depression quadruples before age 18 years compared with the risk of a child with two unaffected parents.[40]

Major depressive disorder may be insidious and difficult to diagnosis initially. It may be diagnosed only after a child has several years of hyperactivity, separation anxiety symptoms, and intermittent symptoms of depression. According to the DSM IV-TR, the diagnostic criteria for a child or adolescent experiencing a major depressive episode must have at least 5 of the 13 symptoms for a period of 2 weeks, and there must be a change from previous functioning.[40] Among the necessary symptoms are either a depressed or irritable mood, or loss of interest or pleasure. Other symptoms from which the other four criteria are taken are daily insomnia or hypersomnia, daily fatigue or loss of energy, psychomotor agitation or retardation, feelings of worthlessness or guilt, diminished ability to think or concentrate, recurrent thoughts of death, and a failure to make expected weight gains. These symptoms must produce social or academic impairment.

A major depressive episode in a prepubertal child is likely to be manifested by somatic complaints, psychomotor agitation, and mood-congruent hallucinations. Anhedonia, or loss of enjoyment of life, is also frequent. In adolescents, anhedonia is even more common. Negativism, frank antisocial behavior, and use of illicit drugs and alcohol are also very common. Feelings of restlessness, grouchiness, aggression, sulkiness, reluctance to cooperate with family events, withdrawal from social activities, and a desire to leave home are also symptoms. Adolescents may not care about their personal appearance, show increased emotional lability (especially in rejection in love relationships), and school problems are also common.

Children and adolescents diagnosed with major depressive disorder usually have difficulty with peer relationships, family relationships, and school performance due to difficulty with concentration, slow thinking, lack of motivation, and fatigue. Depression in a child may be misdiagnosed as a learning disorder. Learning problems secondary to depression are corrected rapidly after a child's recovery from a depressive episode.

The mean length of an episode of a major depressive disorder in a child or adolescent is about 9 months. Probability of recurrence is 40% by 2 years and 70% by 5 years.[40] A young age of onset and multiple comorbid disorders predict the poor long-term prognosis. Children who live in family environments with chronic conflict are more likely to relapse.

Medical Treatment

Hospitalization may be necessary if the child or adolescent is suicidal. Hospitalization may also be needed if the child or adolescent has a co-existing substance abuse disorder.

Cognitive behavioral therapy is very helpful as an interventional treatment for moderate to severe depression in children and adolescents.[56] Cognitive behavioral therapy attempts to enhance problem-solving abilities and social interactions, and it also helps to correct maladaptive beliefs. Relaxation techniques are also shown to be helpful for treatment in mild to moderate depression. Modeling and role-playing techniques can be used to improve problem-solving skills.

Medications considered first line in therapy for a major depressive disorder are the serotonin reuptake inhibitors (SSRIs). These have been shown in controlled, double-blind studies to have efficacy in children and adolescents.[40] Some recent reports of increased rates of suicide with children on various SSRIs early on are considered controversial and have led to very close monitoring of these groups of patients when initiating any antidepressant medications. Medications are started at very low doses and increased very slowly, and the patient is carefully monitored, especially during the early phases of medication initiation. The available SSRIs used in childhood and adolescents include fluoxetine (Prozac), sertraline (Zoloft), paroxetine (Paxil), and citalopram (Celexa). Bupropion (Wellbutrin) has stimulant properties as well as antidepressant efficacy and has been used in children and adolescents with both ADHD and depression.

Family education and involvement in the treatment of the child or adolescent with depression is imperative. A depressed child's psychosocial function may be impaired for long periods even after the depressive episode has resolved. The family must be present for support and assistance before and after the occurrence.

Physical Therapy

Practice Pattern: *Can be associated with a variety of practice patterns. One example would be Primary Prevention/Risk Reduction for Loss of Balance and Falling*

Safety Issues: *Depression is a medical diagnosis. Care should be taken not to label sadness or grief with this diagnosis.*

Common Impairments: *Deconditioning may develop. The child may have difficulty performing motor tasks.*

Functional Limitations: *The child may be limited in ADLs and IADLs.*

Typical Interventions: *Interventions will be determined by the practice pattern. Injury prevention, education, aerobic training, endurance, and relaxation techniques may be appropriate.*

General Outcomes: *Depression is treatable. The length of a depressive episode for a child is approximately 9 months with a high probability of recurrence.[40] Existing comorbidities and family environments with persistent conflict predict a poorer long-term prognosis.*

DEVELOPMENTAL COORDINATION DISORDER

Developmental Coordination Disorder (DCD) is defined in the DSM IV-TR as a condition characterized by low performance in daily activities that require coordination, usually below what is expected for the age and intellectual level of the child.[40] The disorder may present early as the inability to achieve motor milestones such as sitting, crawling, and walking. Symptoms of clumsy gross and fine motor skills may be present; bumping into things, dropping things, and tripping may be noted by the parent or caregiver. Normal coordination is not met for the age group and, thus, elementary school children may be unable to bike ride, run, skip, and hop, whereas a middle school child may do poorly in team sports, such as soccer and baseball. Fine motor skills including using forks and spoons, buttoning buttons, zipping zippers, using scissors, and styling hair may be difficult for these children. Social difficulties with peers often occur due to these problems.

Studies show that perinatal problems such as prematurity, low birth weight, and hypoxia may contribute to this disorder.[40] Children with DCD are at higher risk for language and learning disorders. Older children may have academic problems and poor peer relationships.

Medical Treatment

The treatment of DCD usually involves versions of sensory-integration (SI) programs and modified physical education. SI programs consist of physical activities that increase awareness of motor and sensory function, gearing to the specific difficulties a child may have. Language and learning disorders should be dealt with through individual speech therapy and specialized evaluation and treatment of the learning disabilities. Emotional problems associated with rejection by peers and low self-esteem need to be addressed individually with a psychologist or therapist. Parental counseling may help reduce parental guilt and anxiety about the disorder, as well as assist parents in coping with their child more effectively.

Physical Therapy

Practice Pattern: *Primary Prevention/Risk Reduction for Loss of Balance and Falling*

Safety Issues: *There may be an increased risk of falling.*

Common Impairments: *The most common impairments are clumsiness, delayed motor skills, impaired sensory integration, and difficulty performing motor tasks.*

Functional Limitations: *The child may be limited in ADLs and IADLs.*

Typical Interventions: *Interventions often involve a team approach. Therapeutic exercise, balance training, coordination activities, agility training, postural control activities, and functional activities may be appropriate.*

General Outcomes: *The outcome depends on the degree of severity. Lack of coordination may continue.*

DOWN SYNDROME

The correct terminology for Down syndrome is *Trisomy 21*. It is the most common autosomal chromosomal abnormality that exists in the human species. The incidence of this abnormality is about 1 in 700 live births, and the risk increases as the maternal age increases.[23] The majority of children with Down syndrome have a *trisomy* with an extra 21 chromosome present in all cells of the body. About 5% of children with Down syndrome have a translocation of the 21st chromosome with the extra chromosome being attached to another chromosome.[23] Clinically, children with Down syndrome with translocation trisomy and simple trisomy appear the same.

Congenital heart disease occurs in almost 40% of children with Down syndrome.[23] In particular, these defects are potentially endocardial cushion defects, atrial septal defect (ASD), ventricular septal defect (VSD), or Tetralogy of Fallot. Also, there is noticeable smaller stature, developmental delays, craniofacial abnormalities including a small mid-face, upturned nose, epicanthal folds, brachycephaly, flat occiput, speckled iris, and palpebral fissures that slant to the midline. Other clinical findings that may be present in Trisomy 21 are an exaggerated space between the first and second toe, short broad feet, digits and hands, with a single palmar crease. Smaller stature than peer group is always present, and intelligence levels usually have a wide range of abilities present. The mean of intellectual ability is usually below the normal range. Hypotonia and hyperextensible joints are considered major abnormalities in these patients. Gastrointestinal (GI) abnormalities may also be present.

Medical Treatment

Medical treatment of Down syndrome or Trisomy 21 is geared toward helping the patient function as normally as possible according to his abilities. Also, the goals are to medically and/or surgically treat any problems that may arise from congenital abnormalities. GI and cardiac abnormalities may necessitate surgical repairs. Small sinuses may lead to recurrent sinus infections. Severe periodontal disease is a potential problem, and close dental monitoring of these patients is imperative. There is a statistically increased risk for leukemia and hypothyroidism that necessitates the early diagnosis and treatment of these diseases. Children with Down syndrome may be mainstreamed into the regular school system with special education classes when needed. Some may need more intense help with ADLs.

Physical Therapy

Practice Pattern: *Impaired Neuromotor Development*

Safety Issues: *Due to the hypermobile nature of the joints of a child with Down syndrome, atlantoaxial instability (AAI) could be a potential problem. Any activities that produce a direct downward force on the cervical spine should be avoided.[8] Be aware of any cardiopulmonary impairments.*

Common Impairments: *The most common impairments are seen in developmental delay and mental retardation. The child also has hypotonia and hypermobile joints, which may result in decreased postural control. Decreased oral motor skills and respiratory compromise may also be present.[8]*

Functional Limitations: *There are many musculoskeletal and orthopedic complications that are a direct result of soft tissue laxity and muscle hypotonia. These, along with cognitive impairments may limit ADLs. Children with Down syndrome may not fully participate in childhood games and play activities due to joint instability, especially AAI.[8]*

Typical Interventions: *The small nasal bridge and poor oral motor tone of an infant with Down syndrome make feeding a difficult task. Physical therapists working with such infants can educate the family in proper positioning that will make feeding more efficient. Therapeutic exercise and a strengthening program are also important to help stabilize hypermobile joints and promote the acquisition of developmental skills. Improving aerobic capacity and respiratory health could also be beneficial.*

General Outcomes: *Life expectancy of an individual with Down syndrome has significantly increased with better health management, allowing many children with Down syndrome to live well into the fourth and fifth decade. Median life expectancy is 49 years.[57] Many individuals can perform ADLs, with some capable of IADLs. Some level of assisted living may be required.*

EPILEPSY AND SEIZURE DISORDER

There is a broad spectrum of clinical presentations of epileptic seizure disorders. Classification of these disorders considers the age of onset, the etiology, and the association of seizure types. *Generalized tonic-clonic seizures* are the most common childhood seizures.[16] This form of epilepsy is believed to be idiopathic. These types of seizures may occur alone or in combination with other types of seizures, and can occur at any time in childhood or infancy. Clinically, the seizure presents abruptly with myoclonic jerks. An *aura,* or subjective symptoms that precede the seizure, may or may not occur. Consciousness and loss of posture occur next, followed by tonic stiffening and upward deviation of the eyes. Diaphoresis, hypertension, pupillary dilation, and pooling of secretions frequently occur as well. Clonic jerks follow the tonic phase, and then a brief tonic phase is repeated. A *postictal* (postseizure) state follows with flaccidity and incontinence possible. Irritability and headache are common as the child regains consciousness. Febrile and post-traumatic seizures fall into the category of primary generalized tonic-clonic seizures.

Generalized tonic-clonic activity of ≥30 minutes is considered *status epilepticus.* This state can cause actual brain damage whereas brief seizures are not believed to cause any brain damage. In a status epilepticus state, reductions in cortical partial pressure of oxygen, which can cause irreversible brain damage, occur. The mortality rate is approximately 5%.[16] About 25% of children experiencing status epilepticus have etiologies such as meningitis or encephalitis as an infectious cause, or acute anoxia from brain trauma, electrolyte disorders, or congenital malformations.[16] Status epilepticus can also be caused by abrupt discontinuation of anticonvulsant medications or high fever.

Partial seizures make up about 40% of seizures in children.[16] Simple partial seizures arise from a specific anatomic focus in the brain. Location of this focus specifies the overall clinical symptoms presented during the seizure, i.e., motor, autonomic, and sensory phenomenon. Consciousness is not impaired in this type of seizure. In complex partial seizures, the clinical abnormalities are similar to simple partial seizures, but consciousness is impaired. Abnormal CT findings can include cerebral hemisphere tumors, arterial venous malformation, agenesis of the corpus callosum, focal atrophy, medial temporal sclerosis, cortical dysplasia, and brain tumors. Genetic factors also play a role in partial seizures. The symptoms of partial seizures are diverse and may include vertigo, flashing lights, spots in the visual fields, altered depth perception, changes in smell such as a detection of an unpleasant odor, uncontrolled laughing, or lip smacking. Tachycardia, increased GI motility, or uncontrolled shivering may be possible.

Benign focal epilepsy usually begins between the ages of 5 and 10 years. The incidence is about 16% of all afebrile seizures in children younger than 15 years.[16] The seizure presentation is usually a focal motor seizure, and it usually occurs only during sleep or upon awakening. Speech and swallowing are impaired in the awakened state, and there is a slight genetic association in this type of seizure disorder. Usually this disorder is self-limiting and disappears in adolescence to early adulthood.

An *absence seizure* is described as a brief loss of awareness of one's surroundings with eye fluttering, rarely persisting for longer than 30 seconds. These types of seizures usually occur after age 5 years and are mild and nonprogressive, with a very low incidence of underlying brain disease or abnormalities.[16]

Myoclonic seizures are characterized by repetitive seizure activity consisting of brief, symmetrical muscle contractions with a loss of muscle tone resulting in a falling or slumping forward.[16,19,21] This seizure can often lead to injury of the mouth and face. It can also be associated with structural brain abnormalities and disease and can occur along with generalized tonic-clonic seizures. Myoclonic seizures can range from the benign type seen in infancy to the progressive type first seen in adolescents.

Infantile spasms appear as brief contractures of the neck, trunk, and arm muscles, followed by a phase of sustained muscle contraction lasting from 2 to 10 seconds. The peak onset is between 4 and 8 months of age. These seizures usually occur in clusters and can occur frequently throughout the day. A majority of infants have a known etiology for these seizures that include metabolic, developmental malformations; syndromes; congenital infections; and encephalopathies. Children with known etiologies usually will be developmentally delayed and have a poor response to medical treatment. The remaining children with this disorder, for which no etiology can be determined, respond well to treatment and can have a normal life.[16]

Medical Treatment

It is important to diagnose any underlying etiology for seizure disorders soon after the first seizure activity occurs. Metabolic testing, CT scan, or MRI along with infectious and poisoning workup should proceed after a careful history and neurologic examination is performed to help point the primary care physician in a direction for testing and diagnosis. When drug therapy is initiated, the goal is to achieve optimal function of the patient with a minimal amount of side effects. A single drug is initially chosen because of the improved incidence of compliance, low cost, and decreased risk of toxicity. Serum blood levels of medications are used to help adjust dosages of medications. About 50% of children are controlled on one drug.[19] Additional medications are only added after therapeutic levels are reached with the first drug.

Contact sports and hazardous physical activities are generally not recommended for children with seizure disorders. Children with generalized tonic-clonic seizures, absence seizures, and certain partial seizures may not require drug therapy beyond 4 years. The risk of reoccurrence is higher when partial seizures occur. Children with myoclonic seizures and atypical absence seizures generally require treatment for life. Children who have neurologic abnormalities, or those who have seizures that were initially difficult to control and have persistently abnormal electroencephalograms (EEG) are at a high risk for recurrence when or if drug therapy is stopped.

Physical Therapy

Practice Patterns: *Children with epilepsy can fall into several practice patterns, for example: Primary Prevention/Risk Reduction for Loss of Balance and Falling, or Impaired Neuromotor Development*

Safety Issues: *The most important thing to do when the child has a seizure is to make sure the environment will not cause harm or injury to the child during the episode. Maintaining an adequate airway may be achieved by rolling the child to his side.[8]*

Common Impairments: *The child may have a loss of confidence due to unpredictable seizure activity. Depression could also result.[8] Learning disabilities may be present.[16]*

Functional Limitations: *The fear of having a seizure at any time or any place may force the child to lead a restricted lifestyle. Children with epilepsy are usually able to participate in organized sports, but this is often discouraged.[8]*

Typical Interventions: *Therapeutic exercise as well as swimming may be implemented for general well-being. These activities should be supervised for safety.[8,16]*

General Outcomes: *Epilepsy does not pose a great danger to life when managed. Chronic epilepsy is more likely when accompanied by neurologic impairment, when the seizures begin before 2 years of age, and when complex partial seizures are predominant.[58]*

FAILURE TO THRIVE

Inadequate growth rate in a young child or infant is termed "failure to thrive." This is a general term with a multitude of etiologies, and it is the diagnosis for 3% to 5% of children admitted to hospitals.[59] There is a wide spectrum of normal in the infant and young child with regard to weight. Growth percentile changes are generally best monitored over time rather than day to day. Wide fluctuations in growth percentiles are not uncommon in normal children. Monitoring of head circumference and height in addition to weight on a growth chart is essential to the primary care physician in order to put into perspective dramatic drops in weight and to determine whether further investigation and/or hospitalization is necessary.

In early infancy, problems with feeding are the main causes of failure to thrive. These are mainly inadequate feeding frequency or amounts, including formula mixing errors or inability to adequately breastfeed. These errors result in a decrease in caloric intake either by ignorance of the caregiver or neglect by the caregiver. A child or infant who is failing to thrive as a result of inadequate caloric intake will drop in weight percentile before dropping in head circumference or height. Other environmental contributors to failure to thrive are maternal depression, either postpartum or major depressive disorder, poor mother–child interaction (which is seen frequently when the mother is very young), poor feeding techniques, or in a social environment full of stress and lack of social support.

Organic causes of failure to thrive include an inability to adequately suck, swallow, or chew. This situation can be caused by a CNS pathology or neuromuscular disease. Maldigestion and malabsorption due to Cystic Fibrosis (CF), celiac disease, and/or chronic diarrhea, as well as poor nutrient utilization as in renal failure, and/or inborn errors of metabolism may also present as failure to thrive. Chronic vomiting or increased intracranial pressure may also cause failure-to-thrive symptoms. Elevated metabolic rate due to thyrotoxicosis, cancer, inflammatory bowel disease, and chronic disease, as well as regurgitation (such as in gastroesophageal reflux disease [GERD]) or hiatal hernia and fetal alcohol sysdrome, may also present as failure to thrive.[59]

Medical Treatment

A careful history and physical examination of the infant or child is usually the most beneficial toward leading the practitioner in the direction of a particular test or diagnostic procedure that eventually leads to the underlying etiology for failure to thrive. Outpatient attempts at monitoring caloric intake are usually undertaken before the infant or child is hospitalized.

Maintaining a detailed diary of feedings by caregivers including frequency, volume of feedings, and consistency of stools and vomitus is a reasonable initial outpatient plan of care. If the child continues to lose weight within several weeks, hospital admission is necessary because of the absolute need to maintain adequate nutrition for brain development and growth. On admission, the child is fed the appropriate number of calories and monitored as to the weight gain. If the child fails to gain weight, an organic cause is more of a possibility and the child should be aggressively worked-up and appropriately treated. If the child does gain weight while in the hospital, major steps potentially involving social services should be taken to support the home environment as well as to closely monitor the nutritional intake of the child. A nutritional support team or dietitian and a behavioral or a developmental specialist should also be consulted while the child is hospitalized in order to continue outpatient care. Frequent follow-up visits to the primary care physician are imperative for close monitoring of weight and progress.

Physical Therapy

Practice Pattern: *Impaired Neuromotor Development*

Safety Issues: *A special diet may be given to the child. It is necessary to measure caloric intake to ensure proper nutrition.*

Common Impairments: *The most common impairment is physical growth retardation, measured by anticipated weight and height for age. Difficulty swallowing or reflux may be associated with the diagnosis.[59]*

Functional Limitations: *Children who have been malnourished often have developmental delays, emotional problems, and poor social skills.*

Typical Interventions: *Therapeutic exercise, developmental activities, postural control, oral motor training, and parent education are common.*

General Outcomes: *Prognosis varies depending on the severity of the malnutrition and the quality of the parent–child relationship.[60]*

GUILLAIN-BARRE SYNDROME

Guillain-Barre syndrome (GBS) is considered an autoimmune neuromuscular disease that has a characteristic sudden onset of paralysis. In over ⅔ of cases of GBS, a viral infection precedes the symptoms by 1 to 3 weeks.[9] Typically, the acute infectious process is respiratory or GI. GBS has a rapid progression of evolving areflexic motor paralysis. Some cases present with sensory disturbance. The usual pattern is an ascending paralysis, which may be first noticed with "rubbery legs." Weakness of the lower extremities evolves over hours to a few days and is usually accompanied by tingling dysesthesias. The legs are usually more affected than the arms; facial diparesis is present in 50% of patients.[9]

Most patients require hospitalization because of the involvement of the lower cranial nerves and the difficulty with handling secretions and maintaining an airway;

there is about a 30% chance of needing ventilatory assistance at some point in the disease.[9] Pain is another common feature of GBS. The most common type is a deep aching pain in the weakened muscles. Back pain involving the entire spine and dysesthetic pain in the extremities is common due to involvement of the sensory nerve fibers. There are several subtypes of GBS that are recognized and distinguished by body areas and nerves involved. In the worsening phase of GBS, most patients require monitoring in the critical care setting, especially of cardiovascular status, vital capacity, and performance of chest physical therapy.

Diagnosis of GBS is made by recognizing the pattern of rapidly evolving paralysis with areflexia, absence of fever or other systemic symptoms, and the characteristic antecedent illness. Required criteria for the diagnosis of GBS include four important findings. Progressive weakness of two or more limbs due to neuropathy, and a disease course of <4 weeks duration are the first two criteria. Areflexia must be present, and all other disease etiologies must be excluded to meet all requirements for GBS.[9] Supportive criteria for the diagnosis of GBS include mild sensory involvement, absence of fever, a typical CSF profile (i.e., acellular with an increased protein level), and facial nerve or other cranial nerve involvement. Also included are the presence of relatively symmetrical weakness, and electrophysiologic evidence of demyelination.[9]

Medical Treatment

Medical treatment should be initiated as soon as possible after diagnosis. About 2 weeks after the first motor symptoms appear, immunotherapy is no longer effective. Either high-dose intravenous immunoglobulin (IVIg) or plasmapheresis should be initiated. They are equally effective. IVIg is more commonly used due to its ease in administration and safety record. Maximum paralysis usually occurs 1 to 3 weeks after onset. In patients who are treated early in the course of GBS and improve, relapse may occur in the second or third week. Brief treatment with the original therapy is usually effective.

Physical Therapy

Practice Pattern: *Impaired Motor Function and Sensory Integrity Associated with Acute or Chronic Polyneuropathies*

Safety Issues: *Vital signs must be regularly monitored. Respiratory impairment may be present if intercostal muscles are affected. In early treatment, the active or active-assisted exercises performed should be equal to that of the child's muscle strength.[8] Avoid fatigue with exercises or activities.*

Common Impairments: *The child may have pain, decreased range of motion, muscle weakness, lack of motor control, and decreased mobility.*

Functional Limitations: *ADLs are most commonly limited by a decrease in the ability to ambulate.*

Typical Interventions: *Intervention in the early phase of recovery includes maintaining range of motion and breathing exercises. As recovery progresses, aquatic therapy, proprioceptive neuromuscular facilitation, and progressive resistive exercises should be introduced. Gait training may also be necessary.*

General Outcomes: *Recovery without residual impairments is directly related to the length of time for recovery to begin following the period of maximal impairment. Even though most children recover, residual neurologic deficits have been seen in 20% of cases.[61] Assistive devices and orthotics may be required in order to increase function. A child showing continued difficulty with ambulation may benefit from a wheelchair or scooter.[8]*

HYDROCEPHALUS

Hydrocephalus (Fig. 3-5) is a main cause of macrocephaly and is due to an increased production of CSF, a block in the flow of CSF, or impaired absorption of CSF. The choroid plexus of the lateral, third, and fourth ventricles in the brain normally continuously produce CSF. The etiology of hydrocephalus is obstruction of CSF flow anywhere along its course through the brain. Obstructive or internal hydrocephalus is due to a block before the CSF reaches the subacromial space. Extraventricular obstructive hydrocephalus is impairment of absorption of CSF. Hydrocephalus caused by overproduction of CSF without true obstruction is caused by choroid plexus papillomas, which may be present in early infancy.

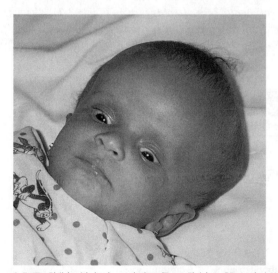

Figure 3-5 ■ Child with hydrocephalus. (From Fleisher GR, Ludwig W, Baskin MN. *Atlas of Pediatric Emergency Medicine.* Philadelphia: Lippincott Williams & Wilkins; 2004)

Clinically, children with hydrocephalus have dilatation of the lateral ventricles resulting in stretching of the corticopontocerebellar and corticospinal pathways. This stretching causes spasticity and ataxia that are present initially in the lower extremities. Distention of the third ventricle can cause compression of the hypothalamus and results in endocrine dysfunction, visual dysfunction from compression of the optic nerves, chiasm, and tracts, and impairment of upward gaze can occur due to compression of the periaqueductal gray matter. Manifestations of increased cerebral pressure can occur slowly over time or acutely. Acute symptoms include headache, vomiting, cranial nerve dysfunction, and coma in rapid sequence. These symptoms usually follow complete obstruction to CSF flow from tumors, infection, or hemorrhage. Gradually forming hydrocephalus results in craniocephaly, scalp vein distention, ataxia, spasticity, papilledema, optic atrophy, and endocrine dysfunction such as growth failure.

Medical Treatment

Treatment of this disorder is medical and surgical. Medications that transiently decrease CSF production may help with the impairment of flow or absorption of CSF following meningitis or subarachnoid hemorrhage.[19] Surgical treatment involves removing any cysts, tumor, or aneurysm which may be obstructive, or placing a shunt to divert CSF to other sites for absorption. The cranial end of the polyethylene tubing shunt, which may or may not have a valve, is usually placed in the lateral ventricles or occasionally in a posterior fossa cyst in certain conditions. The distal end is placed usually in the peritoneal cavity, a ventriculoperitoneal shunt (VP) or atrium of the heart (VA). The shunt itself may become occluded and must be monitored regularly. The patient must also be monitored for possible infection due to shunt placement.

Physical Therapy

Practice Pattern: *Impaired Motor Function and Sensory Integrity Associated with Progressive Disorders of the CNS*

Safety Issues: *Signs and symptoms of shunt malfunctioning (increased intracranial pressure) may include irritability, lethargy, projectile vomiting, and blurred vision.*

Common Impairments: *The child may present with fatigue and spasticity. Cognitive, visual, and verbal deficits may be exhibited.[16]*

Functional Limitations: *There is an increased risk for developmental delay and learning disabilities.[16]*

Typical Interventions: *Therapeutic exercise and functional activities help improve independence.*

General Outcomes: *A poor prognosis is correlated with persistent and/or progressive hydrocephalus.[16]*

MYELOMENINGOCELE

Myelomeningocele is a neural tube deficit that results in a birth defect of the spinal cord and meninges. It occurs at an incidence of 1:1,000 births and generally is a lesion that involves multiple unfused vertebrae with a meningocele (meninges only) or myelomeningocele (meninges and spinal cord).[16] Infants with myelomeningocele usually also have hydrocephalus due to *Arnold Chiari malformation,* which is defined as a prolapse or displacement into the foramen magnum of the medulla and cerebellum of varying degrees. The fourth ventricle is thus obstructed causing hydrocephalus.

Diagnosis is possible in utero by finding high maternal serum α-fetoprotein levels. This test is usually followed by performing fetal ultrasonography and amniocentesis to confirm the elevated α-fetoprotein and acetylcholinesterase levels. Clinical presentation is an infant with severe neurologic deficits that correlate with the level of the neural tube defect. Thoracic lesions are associated with the poorest presentation neurologically. Loss of bowel or bladder function, paralysis, and loss of sensation are common with some degree of bowel and bladder dysfunction in all of these patients. Mental functioning is usually normal if there are no CNS anomalies. Functional movement is related to the level of involvement.

Medical Treatment

Medical treatment of infants with myelomeningocele includes multiple surgical procedures to improve the appearance of neurologic defects caused by the lesion. The spinal defect is corrected by closing the skin over the open spinal level or levels. Hydrocephalus is treated by a VP shunting procedure to reduce fluid and intracerebral pressure. Intermittent bladder catheterization may be necessary for a poorly functioning bladder. Physical therapy is necessary to improve overall mobility and ambulation potential and may include bracing of the lower extremities to promote ambulation. This neural tube defect may be prevented by supplementation of folic acid early in the pregnancy.

Physical Therapy

Practice Patterns: *Impaired Motor Function and Sensory Integrity Associated with Nonprogressive Disorders of the CNS—Congenital Origin or Acquired in Infancy or Childhood*

Safety Issues: *This population has predisposition to fractures and hip dislocation, so range-of-motion exercises should be performed with caution.[62] Children with myelomeningocele also have a high tendency to be allergic to latex; therefore, toys and utensils containing latex should be avoided.[63] The physical therapist should also be aware of the signs of hydrocephalus shunt malfunction.[8,16]*

Common Impairments: *The child with myelomeningocele may display sensory and/or motor disturbances depending upon the location and severity of the lesion. The most common impairments include flaccidity of lower extremities, absence of deep tendon reflexes, postural abnormalities, and incontinence of the bowel and/or bladder.[8,16] Although children with myelomeningocele show normal intelligence, there is a high incidence of learning disabilities as well as seizure disorders.[16,64]*

Functional Limitations: *The ability to ambulate, play, and perform ADLs varies with the location and severity of the lesion.*

Typical Interventions: *Child and family education is essential. Gentle range-of-motion exercises may be performed with the lower extremities. Therapeutic exercises that include strengthening and endurance activities are appropriate. Adaptive equipment may be recommended depending on the level of disability.[8] Mobility training via assisted ambulation or wheelchair is important to promote a good quality of life.[64] Having a lesion below L3, an IQ ≥80, absence of lower extremity contractures, and having normal strength in the quadriceps muscles are strongly associated with independence in self-care.[64]*

General Outcomes: *Functional ambulation depends on the location and severity of the lesion (Table 3-1). The majority of children with sacral or lumbosacral lesions reach functional ambulation; about half of those with higher lesions*

TABLE 3-1 Spina Bifida and Mobility Expectations			
Spinal Segment	**LE Movement**	**Possible Orthotic**	**Ambulation**
T12	Absent	HKAFO	Exercise only
L1–2	Hip flexion, adduction	HKAFO, RGO, KAFO	Short distances in house
L3–4	Knee extension	KAFO, AFO	Household with limited community
L4–5	Knee flexion, DF, hip abduction	AFO	Household with limited community
S1	Foot eversion strong knee flexion, hip extension	Shoe orthotic or none	Community
S2–3	PF	Shoe orthotic or none	Community

LE, lower extremity; AFO, ankle, foot orthosis; KAFO, knee, ankle, foot orthosis; HKAFO, hip, knee, ankle, foot orthosis; RGO, reciprocal gait orthosis.

reach ambulatory status, but require braces and other assistive devices.[16] A good prognosis for ambulation is if the child can walk by 7 years of age. The child most likely will not ambulate if walking has not occurred by 7 to 9 years of age.[65,66] It is common for ambulation to decline around 12 years of age. Children with myelomeningocele continue physical therapy services when they reach adulthood in order to manage secondary complications including pain, musculoskeletal deformities, and pressure ulcers. There is a high incidence of depression in this population due to poor social interaction.[8]

SPINAL CORD INJURY

Spinal cord injury may occur during normal vaginal delivery when the infant is in the cephalic or breech presentation. With excessive rotational force at the C3–4 level or longitudinal force at the C7–T1 level, spinal cord injuries can occur. Fractures of vertebrae are not as common and may cause direct damage to the spinal cord that can result in transection of the cord and permanent damage, hemorrhage, edema, and neurologic dysfunction such as complete flaccid paralysis, absent deep tendon reflexes, and absence of response to painful stimuli below the affected spinal level. Painful stimuli may elicit reflex flexion of the legs. Infants may appear flaccid, apneic, and/or asphyxiated, and eventually will develop bowel and bladder problems. Traumatic spinal cord injury can occur at any age throughout life including childhood and adolescence. Most injuries occurring after birth are due to trauma.

The uppermost level of the spinal cord lesion can be localized by segmental signs corresponding to abnormal motor or sensory innervation by an individual cord segment. Hyperalgesia or hyperpathia fasciculations, muscle atrophy, or a diminished or absent deep tendon reflex may be noted. With severe and acute transverse lesions of the spinal cord, the limbs may initially be flaccid rather than spastic. This is known as "spinal shock" and usually lasts for several days, rarely for weeks. It can be mistaken for extensive damage to many segments.

The disability associated with irreversible spinal cord damage is determined primarily by the level of trauma. Upper cervical cord trauma may be fatal. It can produce quadriplegia and weakness of the diaphragm. The diaphragm is innervated by C3–5 (remember: "C3,4,5 keep you alive"). The key cervical segments for upper extremity movements are the following: C5, elbow flexion (biceps), C6, wrist extension (extensor carpi radialis), C7, elbow extension (triceps), C8, finger flexion (flexor carpi ulnaris), and T1, finger abduction (interossei). In the thoracic spine, trauma is localized by the sensory level on the trunk and midline where back pain is present. Lower extremity weakness and disturbance of bowel and bladder

function accompany the paralysis. Trauma to T9–10 paralyzes the lower, but not the upper abdominal muscles. If the lumbar spine is damaged at the L2–L4 levels, paralysis in flexion and adduction of the hip (iliopsoas and adductors), weak knee extension (quadriceps), and obliteration of the patellar reflex occurs. Trauma to L5–S1 paralyzes the movement of the foot and ankle (plantarflexion), flexion at the knee (hamstrings), and extension of the hip (gluteus maximus), and obliterates the Achilles reflex (S1). Sacral and conus medullaris trauma can cause at the S3–S5 levels bilateral *saddle anesthesia* (loss of sensation around the anus, perineum, and inner thighs) and severe bowel and bladder dysfunction. At S2–S4, the anal and bulbocavernosus reflexes are absent whereas muscle strength is largely preserved.

Medical Treatment

Immediate neurosurgical consultation should be obtained after trauma to assess the benefit of depressurization of the affected spinal levels or stabilization of vertebral fractures. Acute posttraumatic treatment will involve the use of IV glucocorticoids to reduce edema of the affected tissues. There are currently no treatments available to promote repair of injured spinal cord tissue; after 6 months, the prognosis is poor for recovery. There are experimental procedures being investigated now that are promising, including use of factors that influence reinnervation by axons of the corticospinal tract, local injection of stem cells, and nerve graft bridges that promote reinnervation across spinal cord lesions.[9]

Development of a rehabilitative plan that faces the reality of the degree of trauma, while caring for the medical and psychological complications of the injury are necessary and should be primary goals of treatment. Many of the usual symptoms associated with medical illnesses, especially pain, may be lacking due to the trauma. Inability to maintain normal body temperature can produce recurrent fever. Detrusor muscle spasticity can be treated with medication. Intermittent catheterization may be needed if the sphincter muscle fails to relax during bladder emptying. Bladder areflexia due to spinal shock or lower sacral trauma is also treated by catheterization. Bladder paralysis and dysfunction and recurrent catheterization predispose the patient to chronic urinary tract infections. These need to be checked routinely, especially with the onset of an acute fever. Bowel regimens and disimpaction are necessary for most patients with the goal to evacuate the colon at least twice weekly to prevent colonic distention and obstruction.

If the patient has had a high cervical cord trauma, artificial ventilation may be necessary. With severe respiratory failure, tracheal intubation followed by tracheotomy provides tracheal access for ventilation and suctioning. Phrenic nerve pacing may aid some patients with trauma at C5 or above.

Patients with acute cord injury are at high risk for venous thrombosis and pulmonary embolism. During the first 2 weeks, compression devices of the calves are used along with anticoagulation medications. If paralysis is persistent, anticoagulation should be continued for 3 months.[23] Prophylaxis against decubitus ulcers should be done by frequent positional changes in the chair or bed, use of special mattresses and cushions, and padding over pressure areas. Muscle spasticity is helped with medications and is used at bedtime for nocturnal leg cramps, if present.

Physical Therapy

Practice Pattern: *Impaired Motor Function, Peripheral Nerve Integrity, and Sensory Integrity Associated with Nonprogressive Disorders of the Spinal Cord*

Safety Issues: *The physical therapist must be cognizant of the signs and symptoms of orthostatic hypotension (e.g., dizziness, blurred vision, syncope), respiratory and cardiovascular complications, and autonomic dysreflexia (e.g., headache, sweating, blurred vision).[8] The proper medical attention should be sought if any of these conditions arise.*

Common Impairments: *The child may show a decrease in range of motion, strength, and mobility. Respiratory impairment will be present with high thoracic and cervical injuries.*

Functional Limitations: *Depending on the level and location of the lesion, the child may have difficulty performing ADLs and independent ambulation.*

Typical Interventions: *Therapeutic exercise including range of motion and strengthening exercises should be introduced. Regular position changes should be encouraged in order to prevent the development of pressure ulcers. Functional electrical stimulation may be used to re-educate innervated muscles. Orthotics or the use of a wheelchair may be recommended to improve mobility.[8]*

General Outcomes: *Functional outcome depends on the location of the lesion and whether the child has a complete or incomplete lesion of the spinal cord. Many children with lower level spinal cord injuries live relatively functional lives with the appropriate assistive devices.*

SPINAL MUSCULAR ATROPHY

The spinal muscular atrophies (SMA) are a group of three related autosomal recessive, selective lower motor neuron diseases with onset from intrauterine life to late childhood. The genetic defect causes extensive loss of the large motor neurons. In general, the earlier in life that the process starts, the more rapid the progression of the symptoms.

Infantile SMA (SMA I) is also known as Werdnig-Hoffman disease and has the earliest onset. It may be apparent before birth by decreased fetal movements late in the third trimester. Infants are alert at birth, but are weak, hypotonic, and "floppy," and lack muscle stretch reflexes. These infants usually progress to flaccid quadriplegia with bulbar palsy, respiratory failure, and death by 1 year of age.

Chronic childhood SMA (SMA II) begins within 6 months to 6 years of age and may progress rapidly, slowly, or with a rapid initial start that develops into a plateau phase. Infants present with progressive weakness, especially in the proximal muscle groups. There is decreased spontaneous movement, "floppiness," or hypotonicity. The legs tend to lie in a frog-legged position, with the hip abducted and knees flexed. The intercostal muscles are weak, although the diaphragm muscles are spared, which creates a paradoxical breathing pattern. Muscle atrophy is usually severe, and head control is lost. With time, the legs stop moving altogether, and children play with toys put in their hands only. Facial expression gradually decreases, and there is an increase in gurgling and drooling. Fasciculations can be seen in the tongue when the child is sleeping. With the decline of respiratory muscles, breathing becomes shallow and rapid and abdominal accessory muscles are used. The mental functioning of the child remains normal with bright open and mobile eyes because extraocular muscle function remains intact. Normal social and interactive functioning remains intact also.

Juvenile SMA (SMA III) is also known as Kugelberg-Welander disease. It begins in late childhood with proximal weakness of the legs. It usually progresses slowly over decades. Children with SMA III may survive into adulthood. Normal social and language skills are also present.

Medical Treatment

Because of the similarities of the symptoms of SMA to those of primary myopathies such as Limb Girdle Dystrophy, it is often necessary to obtain muscle biopsies for evidence of denervation. No true effective treatment for SMA exists. Symptomatic therapy is directed toward aiding in oxygenation and preventing aspiration. Respiratory infections should be treated aggressively and early with appropriate antibiotics, pulmonary toilet, oxygen, and physical therapy. Artificial ventilation may become necessary to continue respiratory function. Symptomatic therapy is also used to prevent scoliosis and therefore aid in respiratory functioning and for minimizing contractures. A team approach can be used to maximize social, language, and intellectual skills. The team approach should involve the school system, parents, patients, physicians, occupational therapists, speech therapists, and physical therapists.

Physical Therapy

Practice Pattern: *Impaired Motor Function and Sensory Integrity Associated with Progressive Disorders of the CNS*

Safety Issues: *Pressure ulcers and other skin problems could be prevented by frequently changing position. Secondary conditions such as fractures and scoliosis often develop.[8]*

Common Impairments: *These may include decreased range of motion, strength and mobility, atrophy, abnormal muscle tone, and fatigue.[8] Respiratory impairment may be present.*

Functional Limitations: *ADLs, especially feeding, and ambulation are frequently limited.*

Typical Interventions: *Positioning and splinting may be used to maintain or improve range of motion. Therapeutic exercise and a strengthening program should be incorporated into treatment. Airway clearance techniques (percussion and postural drainage) may be an appropriate intervention. Orthotics and assistive devices may be recommended.[8]*

General Outcomes: *Functional outcome depends on the type of SMA and the age of onset. Poorer prognosis is directly related to earlier age of onset and more rapid progression of muscle weakness. Type I is the most severe with the poorest prognosis; death usually occurs within 6 months. At some point, children with Type III usually do ambulate; however, use of a wheelchair is often required by mid-adulthood.[67]*

 P O I N T S   T O   R E M E M B E R

SMA

SMA I—Werdnig-Hoffman disease. Infants usually progress to flaccid quadriplegia with bulbar palsy, respiratory failure, and death by 1 year of age.

SMA II—Chronic childhood SMA begins within 6 months to 6 years of age and may progress rapidly or slowly. Mental functioning remains normal.

SMA III—Kugelberg-Welander disease begins in late childhood with proximal weakness of the legs. It usually progresses slowly over decades. These children may survive into adulthood.

TRAUMATIC BRAIN INJURY

There is a broad spectrum of symptoms and sequelae associated with traumatic brain injury. The most common etiologies for trauma are motor vehicle accidents, sports, recreation-related injuries, and child abuse.

The most common form of brain injury is known as a concussion. *Concussion* is a brief period extending seconds to minutes of unconsciousness that occurs immediately following head trauma. Amnesia often follows concussions. Two types of amnesia are described. Retrograde amnesia is the inability to remember events immediately before the trauma. Antegrade amnesia is the inability to form new memories or to remember things that have happened since the accident. The periods of amnesia usually correlate with the severity of the trauma.

The pathophysiology of a concussion is a shearing of the white matter that occurs as the brain is shaken within the cranium that results in a temporary failure of axon conduction. A more severe form of this type of injury is known as a *contusion* or a laceration that actually leads to focal or generalized brain swelling. The more severe form is probable if unconsciousness is longer than 1 hour or if recovery is slow and accompanied by focal neurologic defects.

With trauma to the head, posttraumatic intracranial hemorrhage (ICH) may occur. The location and the severity of the bleed are determined by a skull radiograph and CT scan as soon as possible after the trauma as well as by examining the neurologic status of the patient. This will dictate the course of treatment. An epidural bleed occurs within minutes to hours after trauma to the head. Third cranial nerve (CN III) palsy and contralateral hemiparesis are seen on examination. Surgical evacuation of this bleed may be necessary, and prognosis is good. An acute subdural bleed usually occurs within hours after trauma. Focal neurologic deficits may be seen on examination. Surgical evacuation is needed, and the prognosis is guarded. A chronic subdural bleed may not occur for weeks to months after the trauma. Anemia, macrocephaly, seizures, and vomiting can occur. Subdural taps or subdural shunting may be necessary, and prognosis is good. Intraparenchymal bleeds may present as depressed consciousness and focal neurologic defects. Usually, only supportive care is offered for these patients, and the prognosis is guarded. A subarachnoid bleed presents generally with a stiff neck and a late developing hydrocephalus. Usually, supportive care only is given to these patients, and their prognosis is variable.

An intracranial contusion presents with focal neurologic deficits and brain swelling. Treatment of elevated intracranial pressure with IV glucocorticoids is necessary, and the prognosis is also guarded.

Posttraumatic seizures following head trauma are common. A generalized seizure occurring within seconds of the injury or what is known as an *impact seizure* is considered benign and is not associated with the increased risk of developing epilepsy. Early posttraumatic seizures are seen with severe head injuries, but are not a predictor for the development of late posttraumatic seizures.

Medical Treatment

Children who have been unconscious from a head injury or who have had amnesia after a head injury should be observed in the emergency room for several hours following the occurrence of the event. Occasionally, epidural hemorrhage, other ICH, or a rapid life-threatening increase in intracranial pressure can develop in a child who appears stable for hours following the head trauma. High-risk patients include those with persistent depressed level of consciousness, focal neurologic signs, and depressed skull fractures. CT scan or MRI is the diagnostic study of choice.

Children with more severe head trauma and neurologic deficits should be admitted to the hospital for close neurologic observation. Damage to the brain from trauma is immediate. The goal of treatment is to prevent secondary brain injury from hemorrhage, cerebral edema, and hypoxia-ischemia. Surgical intervention may be necessary to evacuate a specific bleed. IV steroids are used to reduce brain edema and intracranial pressure routinely. In severe cases, artificial ventilation is used to promote oxygenation to the brain.

Children who experience a concussion without neurologic deficits have a good prognosis. Children with contusions for the most part make good recoveries even if neurologic signs continue for weeks after the event. Poor memory and slowing of motor skills are most common. There is usually a decrease in the cognitive skills, behavior changes, and attention deficit. Poor prognostic features include a Glasgow Coma Scale score of 3 to 4 on admission with no improvement in 24 hours, persistent plantar reflexes, and absent pupillary light reflexes.[16] A team approach consisting of the primary care physician, physical therapist, behavior specialist, and occupational therapists are necessary for maximizing recovery potential for children who sustained a head trauma.

Physical Therapy

Practice Pattern: *Impaired Motor Function and Sensory Integrity Associated with Nonprogressive Disorders of the CNS—Congenital Origin or Acquired in Infancy or Childhood*

Safety Issues: *There is an increased risk for seizures in children with traumatic brain injury; the physical therapist must be aware of how to deal with an episode if it were to occur during a treatment session. Cognitive impairments may require increased attention to safety during activities.*

Common Impairments: *The child with a traumatic brain injury may experience decreased attention span, memory loss, muscle weakness, and decreased mobility.*

Functional Limitations: *Muscle weakness leads to decreased head, neck, and trunk control that could result in swallowing dysfunction. Gait deviations may also be present. ADL's and AOL's could be limited.*

Typical Interventions: *Therapeutic exercise including range of motion and strengthening should be implemented. Positioning and relaxation techniques may also be useful. Orthotics and assistive devices may be recommended to improve independent function.[8]*

General Outcomes: *The primary determinants of outcome are the severity of the injury and length of the loss of consciousness (LOC).[8]*

■ Physical Therapy Practice Pattern: Cardiovascular/Pulmonary

ASTHMA

Asthma is a condition that involves reversible obstruction of large and small airways due to the body's overreaction to various immunologic and nonimmunologic stimuli. The incidence of asthma has increased worldwide within the last 10 years. Asthma is considered the most common chronic disease in children and certainly is the most common cause of emergency room visits, hospital admissions, and school absenteeism in childhood. Eighty to 90% of children have their first episode of asthma symptoms by 4 to 5 years of age.[16]

Reactive airway disease, or bronchial hyperreactivity, is the hallmark of asthma for which children carry a genetic predisposition to the disease.[9] There are multiple triggers of asthma, including sensitivity to seasonal and perennial allergens, viral respiratory infections, as well as bacterial infection of the larger airways.[23] A number of environmental triggers can instigate asthma symptoms, including cigarette smoke, cold air, air pollution, and solvents. Exercise can trigger asthma in exercise-induced asthma by increasing exposure of airways to cool, dry air. Aspirin and nonsteroidal anti-inflammatory medications can also trigger asthma and must be avoided by some patients.

Symptoms including wheezing, persistent cough, dyspnea, tachypnea, and chest pain are common during acute exacerbation of asthma. A history of persistent undiagnosed cough is treated as asthma until proven otherwise. This includes a night cough, exercise-induced cough, and a cough after cold air exposure or laughter. In a progressive asthma attack, expiratory wheezes, tachypnea, tachycardia, cyanosis, use of accessory muscles of respiration, decreased breath sounds with diaphoresis, and inability to speak will occur. Unless quickly and properly treated, an acute asthma attack can be fatal. Three major pathologic occurrences cause the airway obstruction in asthma, including smooth muscle contraction, production of mucus, and mucosal edema.

Diagnosis of asthma can usually be made via pulmonary function testing, including Methacholine-Challenge testing, which is performed via spirometry and is useful in evaluation of small and large airway function. It is also very good at diagnosing airway hyperreactivity. This testing is usually reserved for more cooperative children older than 5 years of age. Skin testing and RAST (radioallergosorbent testing) are helpful in identifying environmental triggers.

Medical Treatment

Medical treatment is geared toward reversal of the symptoms of the disease and the prevention of recurrence of the symptoms. Included in this treatment is allowing the patient to maintain normal activity levels as well as exercise. Prevention of hospitalization is also a goal of therapy. These goals are accomplished via medication, education, and avoidance or control of triggers inducing asthma flare-ups. Peak flow monitoring is used to assess and monitor lung function objectively and aids in overall treatment of the disease. This monitoring can be done at home, and even by very young children.

Asthma is a disease that involves the entire family with regard to education and environmental control measures (such as cigarette smoking, wood burning stoves, kerosene heaters, household animal dander). Medication used to treat asthma is geared toward anti-inflammatory therapies in patients with chronic asthma such as inhaled corticosteroids. Other anti-inflammatory medications are taken daily to achieve and maintain control of persistent asthma. Prevention of symptoms is the goal. Systemic corticosteroids are used in long-term therapy to gain prompt control of the disease and also to manage severe persistent asthma. It is possible to prevent disease progression with their early use. Inhaled β-2 agonists such as albuterol (Proventil) are used and preferred for the relief of acute symptoms. They are known as the "escape inhalers" and should not be used more than several times weekly for chronic maintenance. Longer acting inhaled β-2 adrenergic agents such as salmeterol xinafoate (Serevent) are not used acutely, but help control nighttime cough and chronic asthma symptoms in general. Aerosolized versions of these medications are administered via nebulizer with exacerbation of the disease. Leukotriene antagonists such as zafirlukast (Accolate) or montelukast (Singulair) are used as adjunctive medications even in very young children to help control the symptoms of asthma, especially those triggered by allergens.

Physical Therapy

Practice Patterns: *Impaired Aerobic Capacity/Endurance Associated with Deconditioning; Impaired Ventilation, Respiratory/Gas Exchange, and Aerobic Capacity/Endurance Associated with Airway Clearance*

Safety Issues: *Take bronchodilator 20 minutes before exercise. Exercise-induced asthma may develop 5 to 15 minutes after initiating strenuous exercise. Cyanosis or difficulty breathing for a period of 20 minutes without change requires immediate medical attention. Long-term use of corticosteroids can increase risk of fractures.*

Common Impairments: *The most common impairment is shortness of breath.*

Functional Limitations: *The child may not be able to fully participate in endurance activities or sports, depending on the trigger.*

Typical Interventions: *The most important intervention is patient education and reinforcement of self-management. Relaxation and breathing techniques (diaphragmatic and pursed-lip breathing) may aid in easing the attack. Children with asthma usually have a good response to swimming and other water activities.[8]*

General Outcomes: *Asthmatic symptoms may fade as the child grows; however, only 25% of children completely 'outgrow' the condition. Uncontrolled asthma as an adult may lead to chronic obstructive pulmonary disease (COPD) and other severe respiratory conditions.[8]*

POINTS TO REMEMBER

Asthma

Take bronchodilator 20 minutes before exercise. Exercise-induced asthma may develop 5 to 15 minutes after initiating strenuous exercise. Cyanosis or difficulty breathing for a period of 20 minutes without change requires immediate medical attention.

BRONCHOPULMONARY DYSPLASIA (CHRONIC LUNG DISEASE)

Bronchopulmonary dysplasia (BPD) is a complication of respiratory distress syndrome (RDS) in neonates. In most neonates, BPD develops following mechanical ventilation for RDS that may have been complicated by patent ductus arteriosus or pulmonary interstitial emphysema. Oxygen concentrations >40% are toxic to the neonatal lung, and mechanical ventilation with high peak pressures can produce barotrauma with prolonged need for ventilation over 2 weeks. Also, infants weighing <1,000 grams require mechanical ventilation for poor respiratory drive in the absence of RDS. These particular scenarios are prone to the development of BPD. The clinical appearance of BPD is oxygen dependence, compensatory metabolic alkalosis, *hypercapnia* or increased arterial CO_2 tension, pulmonary hypertension, and the development of right-sided heart failure. Increased airway resistance with reactive airway bronchoconstriction is usually present. Fluid retention due to chest retractions and right-sided heart failure can occur.

Medical Treatment

Neonates with BPD can require treatment with mechanical ventilation for many months. Ventilator settings are kept as low as possible to reduce oxygen toxicity and barotrauma. Tracheotomy may be indicated to reduce the risk of subglottic stenosis. Dexamethasone therapy may be used to reduce inflammation, improve pulmonary function, and promote ventilator weaning. When increased airway resistance with reactive airway bronchoconstriction is present, bronchodilators are used. Fluid retention is treated with fluid restriction and diuretics.

Physical Therapy

Practice Pattern: *Impaired Ventilation, Respiration/Gas Exchange, and Aerobic Capacity/Endurance Associated with Respiratory Failure in the Neonate*

Safety Issues: *Long-term use of corticosteroids can increase risk of fractures. Universal precautions are necessary to decrease risk of exposure to respiratory infection. Closely monitor vitals (especially O_2 saturation) for signs of stress and response to intervention.*

Common Impairments: *Being on ventilation for prolonged periods of time may result in growth retardation and psychomotor deficits.*[16]

Functional Limitations: *Developmental delays may be noted as prolonged ventilation decreases the child's ability to explore his environment to learn.*

Typical Interventions: *Positioning, chest physical therapy, postural drainage (if applicable), and range of motion of thorax are commonly used in the management of BPD.*

General Outcomes: *The long-term prognosis is good for infants who have been weaned off oxygen before discharge from the neonatal intensive care unit (NICU). Prolonged ventilation past the first year of life is indicative of a poorer prognosis.*[16]

Cancer: Leukemia

In the United States, the incidence of leukemia is about 40 per 1,000,000 children under the age of 15 years.[68] The most common form of leukemia is *acute lymphoblastic leukemia* (ALL), occurring in about 75% of children with leukemia.[68] The second most common form is *acute myelogenous leukemia* (AML), occurring in 15% to 20% of children with leukemia.[68] The remainder of the cases represent a multitude of different subtypes. The etiology of the two main forms of leukemia is unknown to date, although some groups of children are considered at higher risk for development of the disease. Examples of these groups would be children exposed to radiation and some chemotherapeutic agents, children with Trisomy 21, and the identical twin of a patient younger than 4 years with leukemia.

The definition of acute leukemia is the malignant transformation and expansion of hematopoietic cells that are blocked at a particular stage of differentiation so that they are not able to progress to more mature forms of the cell. Signs and symptoms of leukemia are results of leukemic cells infiltrating into normal tissues. This infiltration results in bone marrow failure such as anemia, neutropenia, and thrombocytopenia. Tissue infiltration by these leukemic cells can result in cutaneous lesions, lymphadenopathy, liver and spleen enlargement, bone pain, and arthralgia. Common presenting symptoms are anemia causing pallor, petechiae, ecchymosis, fever, anorexia, extremity or joint pain, and malaise. Lymphadenopathy and hepatosplenomegaly are also usually found on physical examination. Neurologic symptoms due to CNS involvement may present as headaches, vomiting, papilledema, and cranial nerve VI palsy.

Laboratory studies are imperative in the diagnosis of leukemia. The usual scenario is abnormal white blood cells and differential counts, anemia, and thrombocytopenia. Some children with ALL may have a normal complete blood count at diagnosis, although on careful evaluation, subtle changes in the peripheral smear will identify an abnormality leading to the diagnosis.[68] It is necessary to obtain a bone marrow biopsy when leukemia is suspected as the definitive diagnosis is made via this partic-

ular test. Precise diagnosis of the type of leukemia is also imperative so that specific therapy can be tailored to that type of leukemia. The severity of the leukemia presentation and the age of the child at diagnosis are the two most important prognostic factors for survival. Other studies have shown that the presence of massive organomegaly and CNS disease may also be important factors leading to a poor prognosis.[68]

MEDICAL TREATMENT

The two most common types of leukemias are treated very differently. In ALL, the therapy involves hydration, treating *hyperuricemia* (increased concentration of uric acid in the blood) to avoid renal failure, and daily oral prednisone treatment. Irradiation is used for mediastinal masses, spinal tumors, or other mass-like lesions. Complete remission is defined as a disappearance of the clinical signs and symptoms of the leukemia that were present on diagnosis, including resolution of the abnormal blood count, and restoration of the bone marrow.

It is also necessary to begin CNS prophylaxis at diagnosis. This treatment should continue after successful remission, because without this prophylaxis about 50% of patients with ALL will develop CNS leukemia.[68] Maintenance therapy or remission treatment must continue for 2 to 5 years in order to totally eliminate all leukemic cells. Combinations of drugs with different modes of activity are used to help prevent the development of drug resistance. Bone marrow transplantation has been used in the second remission if a matched sibling or donor is available.

The treatment for AML is more aggressive from the onset. During the induction phase of treatment, intensive multiagent chemotherapy is used. This intensive treatment produces transient bone marrow aplasia. After this phase, intensive chemotherapy is continued along with bone marrow transplantation if a donor is available.

The prognosis is variable for leukemia. About 70% of children with ALL who are treated with the above-mentioned therapy achieve long-term, disease-free survival. For children at a lower risk (i.e., the younger age group between 1 and 9 years of age with low white blood cell counts), the rate of survival is 85%. Those children with more severe disease have a 60% to 80% survival rate with aggressive therapy.[68] Five-year survival without relapse is considered a cure.

PHYSICAL THERAPY

Practice Pattern: *Impaired Aerobic Capacity/Endurance Associated with Deconditioning*

Safety Issues: *Children undergoing chemotherapy and/or radiation therapy should not exercise within 2 hours of the treatment. The child may be more susceptible to infection due to a decreased immune system function. After chemical treatments, there is an increased risk for spontaneous hemorrhage.*[8]

Check hemoglobin (>8 g/dL), hematocrit (>25%), and platelet count (>10,000) for appropriateness of exercise. Refer to the oncology department for individual guidelines.

Common Impairments: *Impairments vary with disease progression, but the most common impairments include bone pain, decreased range of motion, and decreased endurance. Depression may also result.[8]*

Functional Limitations: *ADLs may be difficult to perform.*

Typical Interventions: *Therapeutic exercise may be used to maintain strength and range of motion. Interventions are modified depending on the fitness level of the patient.*

General Outcomes: *Leukemia may result in death when left untreated. Children treated for leukemia showed a 75% survival rate 5 years after diagnosis.[8]*

CONGENITAL CARDIAC DEFECTS

A wide variety of congenital heart defects and diseases are possible, with the majority of them manifesting symptoms in the neonatal period. These cardiac defects include cyanotic and acyanotic lesions with decreased or increased pulmonary blood flow, respectively. More than 17 different congenital malformation syndromes are associated with congenital heart disease first seen in neonates.[16] Although there is a large variety of possible diagnoses, a majority of infants affected by these diseases have one of seven lesions.[16] These lesions include: hypoplastic left ventricle syndrome; transposition of the great arteries with intact ventricular septum; hypoplastic right ventricle with tricuspid atresia; hypoplastic right ventricle with pulmonary atresia; complicated coarctation of the aorta with ventricular septal defect (VSD); Tetralogy of Fallot; and obstructed total anomalous veins.

Diagnosis of these lesions is made by a thorough history and physical examination, chest radiograph, electrocardiogram (ECG), and echocardiogram. This process alone is usually enough to diagnose without the aid of more invasive testing. Fetal echocardiography is more accurate in diagnosis of the most severe types of congenital cardiac defects such as valve atresia and severe stenosis. It cannot diagnose mild defects such as patent ductus arteriosus or atrial septal defect (ASD), which are normal in the fetus. It can usually diagnose VSD or coarctation of the aorta. Fetal ultrasonography is helpful in the diagnosis of arrhythmias and in following the progression and response to treatment.

The important presenting symptoms of congenital cardiac defects include cyanosis with respiratory distress, which is seen with transposition of the great arteries with or without an intact ventricular septum. This lesion is associated with increased pulmonary blood flow. Cyanosis without respiratory distress can also occur in right heart obstruction due to tricuspid atresia, pulmonary atresia, pulmonary stenosis, and Tetralogy of Fallot. These lesions are associated with decreased pulmonary blood flow. Hypoperfusion can also occur and produces a poor cardiac output. The anatomic cause in this situation is left heart obstruction due to total anomalous pulmonary venous return with obstruction, aortic stenosis, hypoplastic left heart syndrome, or coarctation of the aorta.

Medical Treatment

These congenital cardiac defects are treated with various surgical procedures to correct the lesion enough to improve oxygenation and pulmonary blood flow, increase valve patency, and prevent heart failure.

Physical Therapy

Practice Pattern: *Impaired Aerobic Capacity/Endurance Associated with Cardiovascular Pump Dysfunction or Failure*

Safety Issues: *Palpitations, syncope, and orthostatic hypotension may be present. Closely monitor vitals for signs of cardiac distress and response to intervention*

Common Impairments: *The most common impairments include dyspnea, fatigue, peripheral edema, and decreased endurance. Postoperatively, the child will demonstrate impairments in range of motion secondary to surgical procedure of the chest.*

Functional Limitations: *A decrease in physical activity and developmental delay may result.*

Typical Interventions: *Breathing exercises, chest range of motion, therapeutic exercises, gait training, and energy conservation techniques are appropriate interventions.*

General Outcomes: *Outcomes vary depending on the defect. Surgical intervention has significantly improved the outcome for children.*

CYSTIC FIBROSIS

Cystic fibrosis (CF) is a complex autosomal recessive disorder. It is the most common lethal genetic disorder affecting Caucasians. The gene has been localized to the long arm chromosome seven with >400 different mutations of this specific gene that cause the CF phenotype. Present available testing is able to identify 90% of carriers.[9] The CFTR (CF transmembrane regulator) protein for which the affected gene encodes is involved in chloride conductance. Ninety-nine percent of patients with CF have elevated levels of sweat chloride.[9] The major organs involved in CF are epithelial, and their secretory and absorptive abilities are affected by the disorder. CFTR regulates epithelial chloride and sodium transport. It is unknown as to how exactly abnormal chloride conductants account for the clinical signs and symptoms of CF, but they may reduce the function of airway defenses or allow for bacterial adhesions to airway epithelium. Due to marked impermeability of epithelial tissue to chloride and excessive reabsorption of sodium, the airway secretions are decreased, mucociliary transport is impaired, and airway obstruction occurs. Thus, chronic bronchial infections occur. The symptoms of chronic bronchial infections are cough, sputum production, hyperinflation, bronchiectasis, and eventually, pulmonary insufficiency and death.

Ninety percent of patients with CF have pancreatic insufficiency at birth or in early life as a result of inspissation of mucus in the pancreatic ducts and thus autodigestion of the pancreas.[23] Maldigestion and malabsorption due to pancreatic insufficiency cause steatorrhea (or fatty stools) and vitamin deficiency. Intestinal obstruction is present in 10% of patients at birth due to a meconium ileus, and in older patients intestinal obstruction occurs due to poor digestion and thick mucus. Insulin deficiency can develop, and hypoglycemia could occur.[23]

Diagnosis of CF is made when chloride sweat testing, when performed accurately, is positive on two separate occasions. In addition, the patient must have COPD, exocrine pancreatic insufficiency, or a confirmed family history of classic CF in a sibling or a first cousin.

Medical Treatment

There is no universally acceptable protocol for treatment of CF, but it is imperative that the complex management of this disease be a team effort among the patient, physician, family, and caretakers. It is recommended that the actual treatment of the disease is coordinated by a tertiary referral center where the disease is commonly treated. The approach to care should be aggressive and preventative with efforts to control the progression of lung disease and avoid infection via updated immunizations.

Lung disease is treated by bronchodilators and aerosolized DNAase to clear mucous from the airways and improve function of the bronchial system. Antibiotic therapy to control chronic infection is also necessary, along with the monitoring of pulmonary bacteria flora via sputum cultures. Antibiotic therapy must be aggressive to prevent the progression of lung disease, and patients are frequently hospitalized when needed to treat organisms resistant to oral agents. Pancreatic insufficiency is treated by replacing pancreatic enzymes and by encouraging higher caloric intake than normal. Fat is not withheld from the diet; instead, higher doses of enzymes are added to normalize stools as much as possible. Fat-soluble vitamins are added in twice the normal doses in water-miscible form. The electrolyte loss resulting from the sweat defect is treated by adding more salt to the diet.

Physical Therapy

Practice Pattern: *Impaired Ventilation, Respiratory/Gas Exchange, and Aerobic Capacity/Endurance Associated with Airway Clearance*

Safety Issues: *Malnutrition may occur. The child is at risk for dehydration. Chest physical therapy should not be performed before or immediately following meals due to the associated risk of aspiration.*

Common Impairments: *Impaired ventilation, muscle weakness, decreased endurance, and impaired posture are common.*

Functional Limitations: *ADLs are difficult to perform. Play and social interactions may also be limited.*

Typical Interventions: *Patient education on self-management is imperative and should include relaxation, breathing, and coughing techniques as well as nutrition. Percussion and postural drainage may be performed, if appropriate. A program consisting of stretching, strengthening, and postural training should be implemented. Participation in sports, aerobic, and endurance activities may also have positive results.*[69–71]

General Outcomes: *The median survival rate has drastically improved to 32 years of age; more than half of children with CF live into adulthood.*[72] *Pulmonary failure is the most common cause of death.*

DIABETES

Diabetes is a disease that occurs in children and essentially has two different classifications due to two distinct etiologies. The most common type occurring in childhood is insulin-dependent diabetes mellitus (IDDM) or Type I diabetes, which is actually due to an autoimmune process that destroys the pancreas, causing permanent insulin deficiency. These children will require insulin throughout their lifetime for survival and prevention of acidosis caused by the enhanced production of ketone bodies (*ketoacidosis*). Type II diabetes, or non–insulin-dependent diabetes mellitus (NIDDM), was much less common in children until several years ago. With the incidence of obesity and inactivity dramatically increasing in children in the United States, this form of diabetes has had a dramatic increase. NIDDM results usually from insulin resistance with an inability of the pancreas to maintain adequate compensatory hyperinsulinemia. Much less common are the subtypes of NIDDM resulting from genetic defects of the insulin receptors or inherited abnormalities in sensing of ambient glucose concentration by pancreatic beta cells.[73] Diabetes mellitus is defined by the presence of hyperglycemia and *glycosuria* (urinary excretion of carbohydrates).

Insulin-Dependent Diabetes Mellitus

IDDM (Type 1) is the most common pediatric endocrine disorder. It affects about 1 in 500 children younger than 18 years worldwide. The prevalence in the United States of IDDM is highest in Caucasians and lower in African Americans and Hispanic Americans. There is a genetic component to this disease (about 5% increase in siblings or offspring of patients with diabetes).[73]

Several clinical symptoms of IDDM are *polydipsia* (increased thirst) and *polyuria* (increased urination) due to the dehydration that occurs with increased urine glucose causing osmotic diuresis. Sodium and potassium are lost in addition to large amounts of water. Increase in thirst is the attempt to compensate for increased fluid loss. Weight loss occurs as the loss of ingested calories through glycosuria and ketosis occurs when an increased catabolic state persists.

Diabetic ketoacidosis is defined as arterial blood pH <7.25, serum bicarbonate level <15 meq/L, and ketones present in the serum or urine. This state is potentially fatal in IDDM and can occur in patients who are not regularly controlling their blood sugars with insulin injections, or in those who experience infection concurrently. Patients with diabetic ketoacidosis present with a history of polydipsia, polyuria, nausea, and vomiting. Abdominal pain often occurs and can be severe. Respiratory compensation in the form of tachypnea or rapid breathing occurs, and often there is an acetone or fruity odor to the breath. The mental status can be altered in the form of disorientation or even coma. Elevated serum glucose levels may range from 200 mg/dL to >1,000 mg/dL.

MEDICAL TREATMENT

Medical treatment of IDDM revolves around early detection and appropriate blood sugar monitoring of the disease. Both of these potentially avoid the occurrence of diabetic ketoacidosis. Regular insulin injections are imperative to maintain blood sugar control. A multitude of different insulin preparations exist and are tailored toward the individual child. Very short-acting insulin has an onset of action in 15 to 30 minutes and a peak action at 30 to 90 minutes. Long-acting preparations have an onset of action at 4 to 6 hours and peak action at 8 to 20 hours.[74] These insulins are used in various combinations depending on the individual needs of the child. The most commonly used regimen in school-age children involves two subcutaneous injections daily of intermediate-acting insulin and short-acting insulin. Meals must be kept at a rigid schedule and can be difficult to coordinate around daily activities. Other regimens use multiple injections of short-acting insulin before meals and long-acting insulin at bedtime. This regimen requires multiple injections daily but gives the child more flexibility. Insulin pumps are also an option for older children and adolescents. The pump provides a continuous subcutaneous perfusion of short-acting insulin and allows for tight control of serum blood sugars.

IDDM is a disease that requires long-term management. The families of these patients must be involved in all aspects of the care, including medical, nutritional, and psychosocial issues. It is imperative that the patients and their families learn about the disease process in general, and also the specifics such as meal planning, insulin administration, glucometer testing, and how to handle hypoglycemic episodes.

Non–Insulin-Dependent Diabetes Mellitus

NIDDM (Type II) has increased in prevalence due to the increase in childhood obesity. Obesity and a family history of NIDDM are thought to be risk factors. The most common etiology of this disease is insulin resistance and the inability of the pancreas to maintain compensatory hyperinsulinemia. Genetic subtypes of this form of diabetes can exist but are rare in occurrence.

Differentiation of IDDM from NIDDM is important for proper treatment. A strong family history of NIDDM, *acanthosis nigricans* (excessive axillary pigmentation), and obesity that is noted on physical examination, with absence of antibodies to beta-cell antigens at the time of diagnosis of diabetes, are important factors for the differentiation of the NIDDM. Ketoacidosis can occur but does so much less frequently and usually under conditions of physiologic stress. Serum insulin levels will be elevated in NIDDM also.

MEDICAL TREATMENT

Regaining normal weight for age, height, and frame remains the mainstay in treatment of NIDDM in children. Healthy, nutritious weight loss management is imperative in addition to increasing overall activity levels in order to increase metabolic rate, burn calories, and aid in weight loss. Regular measurement of blood sugars via glucometer at home helps to teach the family and the patient about the effects of diet and exercise on serum blood sugar levels.

Serum glycohemoglobin levels should be determined every 3 months by the primary care physician; this can aid in proper overall long-term management of the diabetic patient. (Glycosylated hemoglobin levels are an average measurement of the serum blood sugar levels over a 3-month time period, and ideal levels are around 6.0%.)

Management of the child or adolescent with NIDDM is also a family affair. The family must make major lifestyle changes in order to help the patient lose weight healthfully and increase activity levels. Because obesity is a combination of nature versus nurture, families of diabetic patients will benefit also from healthier lifestyle choices.

Long-term complications of uncontrolled IDDM and NIDDM are many. As the patient gets older, the complications become more serious and often fatal. Diabetic retinopathy, nephropathy, macrovascular disease, and neuropathy are common complications if blood sugars remain poorly controlled. Some degree of diabetic retinopathy develops in patients with IDDM. Nephropathy usually occurs in 30% to 40% of postpubertal patients with IDDM and leads to sensory, motor, or autonomic deficits.[9] Neuropathy accounts for about 30% of all cases of end-stage renal disease in adults. Macrovascular disease results in myocardial infarction and stroke in a high number of patients with IDDM and NIDDM later on in life.

Research has shown that tight control of blood sugars by frequent glucometer testing, multiple daily insulin injections (or insulin pump) in IDDM, and weight control in NIDDM can substantially reduce the complications and sequelae of diabetes. Current research is geared toward prevention of diabetes in patients known to be at risk.[9]

PHYSICAL THERAPY

Practice Pattern: *Primary Prevention/Risk Reduction for Cardiovascular/Pulmonary Disorders*

Safety Issues: *It is important to monitor glucose levels before and after exercise. The physical therapist should be aware of the signs and symptoms of hyperglycemia (blood glucose >300 mg/dL: symptoms may include a gradual onset, thirst, lethargy, and confusion), hypoglycemia (blood glucose <70mg/dL: symptoms may include a sudden onset, pallor, diaphoretic, tremors, and numbness of the lips), and ketoacidosis (blood glucose >300mg/dL: symptoms may include a gradual onset, hyperventilation, flushed appearance, headache, and increased temperature). Skin care and inspection, especially of the distal lower extremities, is important to prevent open wounds.*

Common Impairments: *Endurance is the most common impairment. If the disease is not appropriately controlled, sensory impairments may develop later in life.*

Functional Limitations: *The child with diabetes should not have any functional limitations if the disease is properly managed.*

Typical Interventions: *The most important aspect of controlling diabetes is child and family education on nutrition and exercise. An exercise program consisting of stretching, strengthening, and endurance activities should be promoted.[75] Aquatic exercise may also prove to be beneficial.[8]*

General Outcomes: *Children taught how to manage their diabetes with diet, medication, and exercise have the potential to live normal lives.[8]*

POINT TO REMEMBER

Diabetes

IDDM is the most common pediatric endocrine disorder. It is important to monitor glucose levels before and after exercise. The physical therapist should be aware of the signs and symptoms of hyperglycemia (blood glucose >300 mg/dL: symptoms may include a gradual onset, thirst, lethargy, and confusion); hypoglycemia (blood glucose <70 mg/dL: symptoms may include a sudden onset, pallor, diaphoretic, tremors, and numbness of the lips); and ketoacidosis (blood glucose >300 mg/dL: symptoms may include a gradual onset, hyperventilation, flushed appearance, headache, and increased temperature).

RESPIRATORY DISTRESS SYNDROME (HYALINE MEMBRANE DISEASE)

The term respiratory distress syndrome (RDS) is used to describe the condition that results from a deficiency of pulmonary surfactant in the fetus and ultimately the neonate. Surfactant is a lipid that prevents atelectasis by reducing surface tension. Infants who are premature (born before 34 weeks) are most at risk for developing RDS. The lower the gestational age, the greater the chance of developing RDS. RDS develops in 60% to 80% of infants born at 28 weeks' gestation or earlier, in approximately 30% of infants born between 32 and 36 weeks' gestation, and rarely in infants brought to term.[16] Other risk factors include male sex, Caucasian race, being the second twin, being an infant of a diabetic mother, asphyxia, delivery of a previous preterm infant with RDS, and hypothermia.[16]

Signs of RDS can develop anytime from immediately in the delivery room in infants 26 to 30 weeks' gestation, to 3 to 4 hours after birth in infants 34 weeks' gestation. Symptoms include grunting, cyanosis, tachypnea, nasal flaring, and intercostal sternal retractions. Atelectasis is seen on chest radiograph.

Medical Treatment

The most important treatment of RDS is prevention of premature birth from either elective cesarean section or premature labor. Prevention of birth asphyxia, cold stress, and hypovolemia reduces the risk of RDS. If premature birth is unavoidable, the administration of corticosteroids to the mother before birth stimulates fetal lung production of surfactant over a 48-hour time period. After delivery, RDS may be prevented by intratracheal administration of synthetic or natural surfactants to infants as well as the administration of oxygen. Mechanical ventilation may be needed in severe cases.

Physical Therapy

Practice Pattern: *Impaired Ventilation, Respiration/Gas Exchange, and Aerobic Capacity/Endurance Associated with Respiratory Failure in the Neonate*

Safety Issues: *Long-term use of corticosteroids can increase risk of fractures. Universal precautions are necessary to decrease risk of exposure to respiratory infection. Closely monitor vitals for signs of cardiac or respiratory distress and response to intervention.*

Common Impairments: *Being on mechanical ventilation for prolonged periods of time may result in growth retardation and psychomotor deficits.*

Functional Limitations: *Developmental delays may be noted as prolonged ventilation decreases the child's ability to explore his environment to learn.*

Typical Interventions: *Positioning, chest physical therapy, postural drainage (if applicable), and range of motion are common.*

General Outcomes: *The long-term prognosis is good for infants who have been weaned off oxygen before discharge from the NICU. Prolonged ventilation past the first year of life is indicative of a poorer prognosis.*

SUDDEN INFANT DEATH SYNDROME

Sudden infant death syndrome (SIDS) refers to the unexpected and unexplained death of an infant younger than 1 year. The peak incidence is at 2 to 3 months of age. In the United States, SIDS is the most common cause of death in an infant between 1 and 12 months of age.[76] There seems to be an increased incidence in the occurrence of SIDS with prematurity, in a sibling of a SIDS victim, maternal drug abuse, maternal cigarette smoking, in male infants, and in infants with preceding upper respiratory infections. SIDS is rare in full-term infants prior to 4 weeks of age or after 6 months of age.[76] No absolute mechanism has been determined for the etiology of SIDS. The pathology of SIDS appears to be acute or chronic hypoxia. Because of the risk of SIDS being three to five times higher in siblings of a SIDS victim, a genetic and/or environmental etiology may be suggested.

Consistent signs and symptoms of SIDS are not conclusive. Usually, no known abnormalities previous to death are present, and the typical presentation is a 2- to 3-month-old child who was previously well, found cyanotic, apneic, or pulseless in the crib.

Medical Treatment

Obviously, due to the increased risk of SIDS in brothers and sisters of victims of the syndrome, monitoring of these children is necessary. Home apnea monitoring has not been found to be preventative in studies that have been done. Studies have shown that infants who sleep in the prone position are at an increased risk for SIDS. Recommendations over the last 10 years have been to have all infants sleep on their backs or sides. This recommendation alone has decreased SIDS by about 50%.[76] Very recent recommendations by the American Pediatric Association (APA) are to have an infant sleep on his back only, due to the instability of the side-sleeping position. Recent long-term surveys done by the APA have shown a decrease in incidence in SIDS with children who use pacifiers. The other recent recommendation by the APA is to have infants sleep in the same room with the parent or parents, but not in the same bed.

SIDS can be a devastating situation for a family. Although child abuse is a potential etiology, inappropriate investigation should be avoided due to the traumatic effect on the family. Intense support psychologically through individual family or group counseling is imperative. SIDS support groups exist nationally for parents and siblings.

Physical Therapy

Practice Pattern: *Primary Prevention/Risk Reduction for Cardiovascular/Pulmonary Disorders*
Safety Issues: *SIDS risks factors include prone sleeping position, sleeping on a soft surface, maternal smoking during* *pregnancy, prematurity, low birth weight, overheating, and male sex.*[76]
Typical Interventions: *Position supine to sleep. Parental education to reduce risk by positioning supine to sleep and making other modifications as appropriate.*
General Outcomes: *SIDS accounts for 35% to 55% of infant deaths between 1 month and 1 year of age.*[76] *Risk of SIDS begins to decline after 4 months of age.*

■ Physical Therapy Practice Pattern: Integumentary

BURNS

Burns are a leading cause of unintentional death in children, second only to motor vehicle accidents.[77] Fire continues to be the major killer of children, and scalding injuries are the most common types of burns that require medical attention in children younger than 4 years. Approximately 18% of burn injuries are a result of child abuse, which emphasizes the importance of history taking and examination of the burn pattern.[77] Burns are classified on the basis of four criteria: depth of injury, percentage of body surface area involved (Box 3-2, Rule of 9s), location of the burn, and association with other injuries. The majority of burns in children occur on the upper extremities, with half of those involving the head and neck.[77]

A first-degree burn is superficially red, painful, and dry. Damage is limited to the epidermis and is commonly seen with mild scald injuries or sun exposure. These types of burns usually heal in 3 to 6 days and leave no scarring.

A second-degree burn is also called a partial thickness burn and involves the entire epidermis and variable portions of the dermis. The burn may be superficially red, painful, and blistering. These types of burns usually heal in 10 to 21 days with little or no scarring. These burns may also be deep dermal, with a pale or yellow color, and painful, resulting from immersion or flames. This type of second-degree burn takes 21 to 28 days to heal with potential scarring.

A third-degree burn is also known as a full thickness burn and involves the destruction of the entire epidermis and dermis. This type of burn requires skin grafting, is usually avascular, and usually has coagulation necrosis. Severe burns are defined as covering >15% of total body surface area or involving the face or perineum. Second- and third-degree burns of the hands or feet or circumferential burns of the extremities are also classified as severe. Included in this category are inhalation injuries causing impaired pulmonary function.

The location of the burn is important in assessing the risk for disability. With partial thickness burns, no resulting disability typically occurs. With full thickness burns, the result is usually some degree of permanent

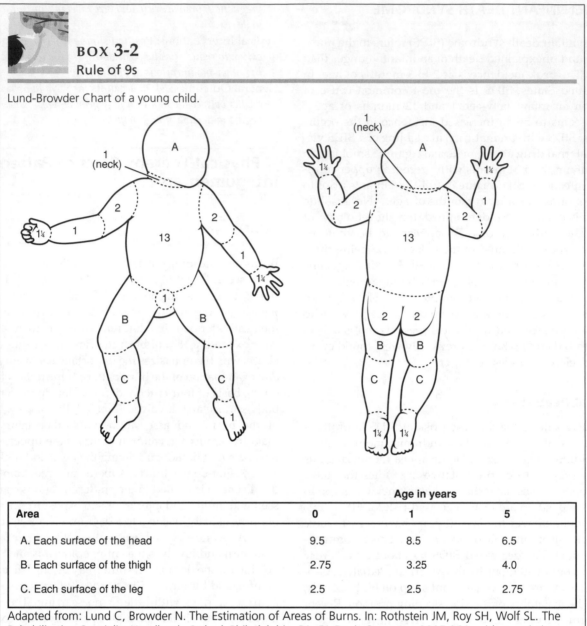

BOX 3-2
Rule of 9s

Lund-Browder Chart of a young child.

	Age in years		
Area	0	1	5
A. Each surface of the head	9.5	8.5	6.5
B. Each surface of the thigh	2.75	3.25	4.0
C. Each surface of the leg	2.5	2.5	2.75

Adapted from: Lund C, Browder N. The Estimation of Areas of Burns. In: Rothstein JM, Roy SH, Wolf SL. The Rehabilitation Specialist Handbook. 3rd ed. Philadelphia, PA. FA Davis Company. 2005:964, with permission.

impairment. Associated injuries such as soft tissue trauma, fractures, and head injuries, and complicating medical problems such as diabetes, heart disease, pulmonary disease, or gastric ulcerations will, in addition to the extent and body surface area involved in the burn, determine whether the child or adolescent is hospitalized. Suspected child abuse or neglect, self-inflicted burns, and psychological illness may necessitate hospitalization also.

Medical Treatment

Prevention is the goal of burn treatment. The majority of all burns occur in the home; therefore, using smoke and fire alarms, escape routes, and fire extinguishers; reduc-

ing hot water temperature to 120°F; and supervising cooking activities are imperative for prevention of this type of injury.

Fluid and electrolyte management is critical to the care of the child who has been significantly burned. IV fluids are provided to maintain blood volume and electrolyte balance throughout hospitalization if necessary. Because the skin is disrupted during burns, there may be an impairment in the child's ability to regulate body heat and to fight off infections. Both of these functions must be monitored during treatment. Burns cause a hypermetabolic response, and children with severe burns should be fed parentally immediately. The hypermetabolic state can also be treated with effective management of anxiety and pain with sedatives and analgesics including narcotic agents. Hypothermia is prevented through maintenance of a neutral thermal environment.

Surgical management is also essential for severe burns. Surgical care involves relieving any pressure on the peripheral circulation by the developing eschar and debridement followed by topical silver sulfadiazine applied to a fine mesh or gauze to cover the burn area. Neosporin ointment can be used if the burns are shallow. Temporary grafting may also be used to cover wounds such as porcine xenografts and artificial bilaminate.[9] For full thickness burns, skin autografting and artificial skin substitutes are required for external closure.[77] Some complications from severe burns may include: cardiac dysfunction treated with *inotropic* agents (which influence the contraction of muscle tissue) and diuretics; contractures treated with physical therapy interventions; renal failure treated with supportive care and dialysis when necessary; anemia treated with blood transfusions; pneumonia treated with appropriate antibiotics; and pulmonary edema treated with diuretics. Burn management and rehabilitation involve a highly specialized team approach to care and are usually performed in specialized burn units located in trauma hospitals and tertiary care centers.

Physical Therapy

Practice Pattern: *Primary Prevention/Risk Reduction for Integumentary Disorders (classification into a practice pattern is determined by the degree of the burn)*

Safety Issues: *Universal precautions are taken to reduce the risk of infection, especially in the acute stage. Care should be taken with skin grafts, which should be immobilized. Active range of motion is initiated after the graft has adhered. Frequent change in body position (every 2 hours) should be done to prevent decubiti formation. If splints are used in the acute phase, they should be checked daily for any signs of skin irritation or impingement that may arise from developing or fluctuating edema.*

Common Impairments: *Pain, range of motion, and mobility are impaired. Sensation may also be impaired.*

Functional Limitations: *Bed mobility, transfers, mobility, and play may be decreased depending on the degree and extent of the burn. ADLs may also be compromised.*

Typical Intervention: *Therapeutic modalities and exercise, including passive and active motion, are utilized to address range, strength, mobility, and endurance impairments. Scar management and pressure garments may be used. Manual interventions should be coordinated with medication regimen.*

General Outcomes: *Depending on the degree and extent of the burn, most children will have a good prognosis; however, lifetime management of scars is imperative.[5,8]*

PRESSURE ULCERS (DECUBITI)

Immobility is the main cause of pressure ulcers, which tend to occur over bony prominences such as the sacrum, ischial tuberosity, greater trochanter, posterior calcaneous, and posterior skull. Mechanical pressure, moisture, friction, and shearing forces all predispose to the development of these lesions.[78]

Pressure ulcers are placed into four categories, depending on their stage of development. *Stage I* ulcers are characterized by a nonblanchable erythema on intact skin. *Stage II* ulcers include the epidermis, dermis, or both. *Stage III* ulcers extend to the subcutaneous tissue, and *stage IV* ulcers involve muscle, bone, and/or supporting tissues.[9]

Medical Treatment

The most important treatment is prevention. Bed rest should be avoided whenever possible. If unavoidable, special mattresses are used to reduce pressure, such as foam mattresses or static air mattresses. When pressure ulcers or decubiti do occur, the treatment depends on the stage of development. For Stage I ulcers, eliminating excess pressure and ensuring adequate hygiene and nutrition are imperative. For the remaining stages of development, the ulcer must stay clean and moist. When saline dressings are used, they should be changed when they are damp and not dry. Synthetic dressings are more effective because they require fewer changes and, therefore, fewer disruptions of the tissue.

Bacterial colonization of pressure ulcers is universal. Swab cultures should not be done, and topical antibiotics should be used only if the ulcer has not healed after 2 weeks of intervention. Cellulitis, osteomyelitis, or sepsis requires systemic antibiotic therapy only after blood culture and wound border biopsy cultures are obtained. Surgical or enzymatic debridement may be required for Stage III and IV ulcers.

Physical Therapy

Practice Pattern: *Primary Prevention/Risk Reduction for Integumentary Disorders (classification into a practice pattern is determined by the stage of the pressure ulcer)*

Safety Issues: *Prevention is the most effective aspect and may be attained by removing the causative factor(s) and alleviating friction. When decubiti are present, universal precautions are followed to reduce the risk of infection.*

Common Impairments: *The child may have limited range of motion and mobility as well as varying degrees of pain that must be managed. Sensation may also be impaired.*

Functional Limitations: *Depending upon the size and location of the pressure ulcer, the child may have difficulty with transfers, ambulation, and completion of ADLs.*

Typical Interventions: *Education on prevention is vital. The management of bowel and bladder function is important to maintain skin integrity in that region. Daily skin inspections also aid in early detection. Weight shifting should be encouraged at least every 15 minutes if the child is capable of doing so on his own. Complete position changes should be made every 2 hours. The use of various therapeutic modalities may aid in debridement and healing. Debridement may include autolytic, enzymatic, mechanical, or sharp debridement, depending on the amount of necrotic tissue. The use of electric stimulation may also aid in the healing process. Adherence to a prescribed diet and/or proper nutrition should be reinforced due to its importance in the healing process.*

General Outcomes: *Comorbidities play a significant role in the healing process of a pressure ulcer. In order for the ulcer to heal, there should be a good blood supply, no medical complications, and no infection, and pressure should be eliminated.[8] Normal wound healing takes 4 to 6 weeks; however, decubiti may take months to heal.*

POINTS TO REMEMBER

Pressure Ulcers

Stage I lesion is an ulcer characterized by a nonblanchable erythema on intact skin.

Stage II lesion consists of an ulcer of the epidermis, dermis, or both.

Stage III lesion is an ulcer that extends to the subcutaneous tissue.

Stage IV lesion involves muscle, bone, and/or supporting tissues.

Prevention of pressure ulcers is the most important intervention.

CASE STUDY

Oscar

History

June. Oscar is an 18-month-old boy who was referred to the physical therapy department by his physician, who was concerned about the developmental delay in the expression of independent ambulation. He was accompanied by his mother and maternal grandmother. Mom reported a normal course of gestation and delivery (vaginal) at 40 weeks. An enlarged liver and spleen were identified in Oscar shortly after birth, but the cause is unknown. He has undergone several blood tests to determine the cause. These tests involved repeated drawing of blood from the soles of his feet. The child's development has been reported to be somewhat delayed. Mom reports that Oscar rolled at 6 months, sat independently at 8 months, crawled at 12 months, pulled to stand at 13 months, cruised along furniture at 15 months, and took an independent step at 16 months. Mom reports that he is very sensitive to touch on the soles of his feet. He does have a history of frequent ear infections and had tubes placed in his ears at 15 months of age. His growth has been unremarkable. He has had all the appropriate immunizations to date. There is no family history of delayed walking or genetic syndromes.

System Review

Cardiovascular/pulmonary: Heart rate and respiratory rate were unremarkable. Oscar does have a history of pneumonia when he was 6 months old. Broad chest and protruding abdomen are noted, which is consistent with the hepatosplenomegaly.

Musculoskeletal: Muscle tone appears low normal upon palpation. Body is symmetrical. No visible muscle atrophy noted.

Neuromuscular: Oscar does withdraw his foot to light touch on the sole of his foot, both on the left and right. He will weight bear through his lower extremities in supported stance. His hearing and vision appear intact and functional.

Integumentary: Subcutaneous nodules were palpated in the area of the anterior knee. These nodules (five in all) were firm and did not appear to cause pain or discomfort with palpation. Fusiform swelling was noted in the knee joints only.

Communication: Oscar was able to follow one-step commands, and he is verbal and visually attentive. He responds appropriately to social interaction with the therapist.

Tests and Measures

There was no noticeable increase in resistance to passive stretch with passive movement (spasticity). The muscle tone appeared to be low normal throughout his trunk and extremities.

Range of motion of the trunk and extremities was within normal limits and symmetrical throughout. Hip, knee, and ankle range was also within normal limits for both active and passive motions. His spine appeared straight upon visual examination. The integrity of the hip, knee, and ankle joints was age appropriate and symmetrical.

Oscar displayed protective extension in all directions and equilibrium reactions to displacement in sitting in all directions. He did take five steps independently in a pattern that is typical of a toddler who is learning to walk. His upper extremities were held in a medium guarded position. He was unable to rise from the floor without upper extremity assist. With assistance of his upper extremities, he uses a half kneel to rise to stance leading with his right. He does not assume or maintain a full squat. He will reciprocally crawl for short distances (5 feet). He will crawl up three steps and will attempt to climb up on furniture.

DIAGNOSIS

The expression of developmental skills denotes impairment in muscle strength and a functional limitation in the movements that would be expected for a child at his age.

PRACTICE PATTERN

Pattern 5B: Impaired Neuromotor Development. Consult with the physician regarding findings and concerns over the fusiform swelling and nodules found in the anterior aspect of the knees. Oscar had adequate strength to walk, but refused to take more than five steps for some other reason, possibly discomfort. After five steps, he would not fall or show signs of muscle fatigue, he would simply sit down in a controlled fashion. Oscar was attentive and interested in his environment. The presence of hepatosplenomegaly, ability to walk but stopping after a certain distance, fusiform swelling of the knees, and presence of subcutaneous nodules were suspicious. There is more to his diagnosis than muscle weakness that was impairing his function. The physician agreed with my concerns.

INTERVENTION

Physical therapy was recommended once a week for 4 weeks to address Oscar's sensitivity to light touch on the soles of his feet and his proximal muscle weakness, and to promote independent ambulation for 20 feet over level surfaces. Parent would be independent in a home exercise program to promote independent ambulation. His hypersensitivity on the soles of his feet, proximal muscle weakness, and possible decrease in endurance were his obvious impairments to his ability to walk.

After 1 month of treatment, Oscar's mother demonstrated independence in the home exercise program. Oscar was able to tolerate touch to the soles of his feet 50% of the time. He was able to stand alone for 10 seconds and ambulated 7 feet before stopping. These were improvements in his level of impairment and functional limitation, but the cause was still unknown. Physical therapy was recommended for one time per month to continue to promote the acquisition of age-appropriate gross motor skills through home programming and to monitor his progress.

Two months later, Mom reported that Oscar was falling daily. His physician had been notified. His falls were not controlled and have resulted in lacerations and contusions to his forehead and face. Physical therapy was increased to once a week to address this impairment. Intervention strategies were implemented to promote safety with movement and to promote proximal muscle strength, which had shown signs of decreasing. This was noted by his inability to use a half kneel when rising to stance with upper extremity assistance, and by a decrease in the length of time he could stand alone (now 7 seconds). The physical therapist recommended the use of a protective bicycle helmet during ambulation.

One month later, Oscar was diagnosed with an autosomal recessive genetic disorder of metabolism. Cholesterol and other lipids within the cell are impaired in their ability to be metabolized, leading to the accumulation of these lipids in various organs and joint spaces (the nodules in the knee). The disease is characterized by hepatosplenomegaly and progressive neurologic degeneration (falling), resulting in severe disability and death.

DIAGNOSIS

Pattern 5E: Impaired Motor Function and Sensory Integrity Associated with a Progressive Disorder of the CNS

INTERVENTION

Physical therapy is provided weekly with interventions now incorporating more compensatory strategies with the focus of maintaining function, given the progressive nature of his disease. Emphasis on promoting and maintaining pulmonary health and to provide for family education and support are added for long-term management.

The goal of therapy is to maintain Oscar's quality of life, minimize secondary complications, promote comfort, and provide family/caregiver support. The use of medications, therapy, and respite care for the mother, are utilized for this purpose.

Reflection Questions

1. What health factors in Oscar's history could be associated with his initial diagnosis of Impaired Neuromotor Development?
2. What additional tests or measurements could be utilized in the patient management process now that Oscar has been diagnosed with a progressive disease?
3. Identify the difference between interventions to promote function and interventions to maintain function given the progressive nature of Oscar's disease. How could the maintenance of function be captured in the physical therapy documentation?

SUMMARY

A diagnosis is a collection of signs and symptoms that categorizes children into specific groups, aiding in the selection of interventions and clarifying possible outcomes. In the field of medicine, a diagnosis is based primarily on the child's pathology. Performing an examination and making a diagnosis is one of the most important aspects in patient management and allows the physician to implement an appropriate course of treatment. The physical therapist also makes a diagnosis through the examination process. Information on impairments and functional limitations is obtained, which results in a diagnosis reflected by the Guide to Physical Therapist Practice Patterns. This diagnosis also aids in the selection of appropriate interventions and assists the physical therapist in predicting the outcome of physical therapy services. Even though the physician and physical therapist independently make a diagnosis using the same process of decision making, both are looking at their specific dimension of the child. Generally, the physician examines the body's systems and cellular activities, whereas the physical therapist examines the body's ability to move and function. Working together allows the team to see a clearer picture of the child and hopefully develop a more appropriate plan of care.

REVIEW QUESTIONS

1. You are working at the local elementary school. One of the parents informs you that she thinks her son is autistic, but the physician disagrees. Her son is 7 years old and has difficulty paying attention in class. A primary clinical sign seen in children with autism is the child's inability
   a. to relate to others, specifically his parents.
   b. to attend to one task for more than 5 minutes.
   c. to perform coordinated movements with his upper extremities.
   d. to use complete sentences when speaking.

2. You are performing musculoskeletal screenings in a preparticipation activity at the local high school. You are aware that although rare, osteosarcoma does occur in adolescents. Pain and impairment in movement without a precipitating injury or known cause would be reason to refer to a physician for further study. Osteosarcoma can occur in any bone but is most common is which of the following?
   a. Radius
   b. Pelvis
   c. Femur
   d. Lumbar spinal vertebrae

3. You are examining a 3-month-old infant who presents with metatarsus adductus, Type III. Of the following, which would be the most appropriate intervention for this infant?
   a. Do nothing. The malalignment will correct itself by the time the infant begins walking.
   b. Stretch the foot beyond the neutral position, holding at the end range for 15 seconds. Instruct the mother to perform 10 stretches daily.
   c. Use corrective shoes to address the malalignment.
   d. Use serial casting to address the malalignment.

4. You are working with a 2-month-old infant who has DDH. He is using a Pavlik harness to encourage the femoral head to grow toward the acetabulum. The position of the hip joints should be maintained in which of the following?
   a. Hip extension to neutral with 30-degree abduction.
   b. Hip flexion at 100 degrees with 30-degree abduction.
   c. Hip extension to 10 degrees with 10-degree adduction.
   d. Hip flexion <90 degrees with 0-degree adduction.

5. Upon your examination of a 5-year-old boy, you notice that in order for him to rise from the floor, he assumes a modified plantargrade position and "walks" his hands up his legs. This is indicative of proximal muscle weakness and is termed
   a. a Gower maneuver.
   b. an Ortolani test.
   c. a Galeazzi sign.
   d. a positive Barlow test.

6. Caleb is a 4-month-old boy who presents with muscular torticollis, with his head tilted to the left and rotated to the right. The most appropriate intervention at this time would be which of the following?
   a. Nothing, this type of torticollis resolves without intervention.
   b. Active movement to the right.
   c. Active movement to the left.
   d. Passive stretching to midline.

7. Jason is an ambulatory 7-year-old boy who has CP. He presents with spasticity (Ashworth +2) in his right upper extremity and in both of his lower extremities. His deep tendon reflexes in the knee and ankle are +3 bilaterally and there is a positive Babinski reflex noted. Given this information, you can tell that Jason presents with which pattern of CP?
   a. Spastic diplegia
   b. Spastic hemiplegia
   c. Spastic quadriplegia
   d. Athetoid

8. In your examination of the skin integrity of your 12-year-old patient, who sustained a complete spinal cord injury, you note an area that is nonblanchable erythema of intact skin on the posterior aspect of his left calcaneus. This pressure ulcer would be classified as which of the following?
   a. Stage I
   b. Stage II
   c. Stage III
   d. Stage IV

9. John is your patient on 8 North of the hospital, which is the neurosurgical unit. He is status post VP shunt placement secondary to hydrocephalus. You are the substitute physical therapist for the day. Upon entering his room, you notice that John has a decreased level of alertness. You arouse him and begin asking him how he is feeling today. He reports that he has had a sudden onset of a severe headache and is "seeing double." What should you do next?
   a. Have him breathe deeply and focus his gaze to an object across the room. Reassess in 10 minutes to see if he is capable of participating in physical therapy.
   b. Evaluate the integrity of the cranial nerves. You suspect involvement of cranial nerves III, IV, and VI. Document your findings and continue with the plan of care for the day.
   c. Notify nursing. You are concerned that he may have increased intracranial pressure.
   d. Proceed with physical therapy, taking precautions that he is safe with transfers and ambulation activities, secondary to his visual impairment.

10. Children with spina bifida are at risk of developing a prolapse of the cerebellum and medulla into the foramen magnum. This condition is referred to as
    a. meningomyelocele.
    b. hydrocephalus.
    c. an Arnold Chiari malformation.
    d. sacral sparing.

REFERENCES

1. Guccione A. Physical therapy diagnosis and the relationship between impairments and function. *Phys Ther J.* 1991;71:499–503.
2. Drnach M. Complementing the MD Diagnosis. *Physical Therapy Products Magazine.* 2005;16:28–32.
3. Miller ML, Cassidy JT. Juvenile Rheumatoid Arthritis. In: Behrman RE, Kliegman RM, Jenson HB, eds. *Nelson Textbook of Pediatrics,* 16th ed. Philadelphia: W.B. Saunders Co.; 2000.
4. Bekkering WP, ten Cate R, van Suijlekom-Smit LW, et al. The relationship between impairments in joint function and disabilities in independent function in children with systemic juvenile idiopathic arthritis. *J Rheumatol.* 2001;2834:1099–1105.
5. Campbell S, Vander Linden D, Palisano R. Physical therapy for children. Philadelphia: W.B. Saunders Co.; 2000.
6. Cakmak A, Bolukbas N. Juvenile rheumatoid arthritis: physical therapy and rehabilitation. *South Med J.* 2005;98:212–216.
7. Velazquez V, Fisher NM, Venkatraman JT, et al. The effect of a lower extremity resistance exercise rehabilitation program on TNF and TNF receptors in juvenile arthritis. *Annual Scientific Meeting of the Association of Rheumatology Health Professionals and the American College of Rheumatology,* Boston, November 16, 1999.
8. Goodman C, Boissonnault W, Fuller K. *Pathology: implications for the physical therapist.* Philadelphia: W.B. Saunders Co.; 2003.
9. Kasper DL, Fauci AS, Longo DL, Braumald E, Littauser S, Jameson JL. *Harrison's Principles of Internal Medicine,* 16th ed. New York: McGraw-Hill; 2005.
10. Arndt CA. Neoplasms of bone. In: Behrman RE, Kliegman RM, Jenson HB, eds. *Nelson Textbook of Pediatrics,* 16th ed. Philadelphia: W.B. Saunders Co.; 2000.
11. Krajbich I. Lower-limb deficiencies and amputations in children. *J Am Acad Orthop Surg.* 1998;6:358–367.
12. Gerber L, Augustine E. Rehabilitation management: restoring fitness and return to functional activity. In: Harris J, Lippman M, Morrow M, et al., eds. *Diseases of the Breast.* Philadelphia: Lippincott; 2000;1001–1007.
13. Gudas SA. Rehabilitation of pediatric and adult sarcomas. *Rehabil Oncol.* 2000;1833:10–13.
14. Pfalzer L. Exercises for patients with disseminated cancer, APTA Newsletter 1987;5:5–7. American Physical Therapy Association.
15. Salter RB. *Textbook of Disorders and Injuries of the Musculoskeletal System,* 3rd ed. Baltimore: Williams & Wilkins; 1999.
16. *Nelson Textbook of Pediatrics,* 15th ed. Philadelphia: W.B. Saunders Co.; 1996.
17. Faulks S, Luther B. Changing paradigm for the treatment of clubfeet. *Orthop Nurs.* 2005;24:25–30.
18. Malvitz TA, Weinstein SL. Closed reduction for congenital dysplasia of the hip: functional and radiographic results after an average of thirty years. *J Bone Joint Surg* 1994;76:1777–1792.
19. *Manual of Pediatric Therapeutics,* 5th ed. Boston: Little, Brown and Company; 1998.
20. Tecklin JS. *Pediatric Physical Therapy,* 3rd ed. Philadelphia: Lippincott, Williams & Wilkins; 1999.
21. Carney B, Minter C. Nonsurgical treatment to regain hip abduction motion in Perthes disease: a retrospective review. *South Med J.* 2004;97:485–488.
22. Herring J, Kim H, Browne R. Legg-Calve-Perthes Disease. Part II: prospective multicenter study of the effect of treatment and outcome. *J Bone Joint Surg.* 2004;86-A:2121–2134.

23. Goldman L, Bennett JC, eds. *Cecil Textbook of Internal Medicine,* 21st ed. Philadelphia: W.B. Saunders Co.; 2000.
24. Petrof BJ, Shrager JB, Stedman HH, Kelly AM, Sweeney HL. Dystrophin protects the sarcolemma from stresses developed during muscle contraction. *Proc Natl Acad Sci U S A.* 1993;90:3710–3714.
25. Nair KP, Vasanth A, Gourie-Devie M, et al. Disabilities in children with Duchenne muscular dystrophy: a profile. *J Rehabil Med.* 2001;33:147–149.
26. Lovering R, Porter N, Bloch R. The muscular dystrophies: from gene to therapies. *Phys Ther.* 2005;85:1372–1388.
27. Deerling MB. Physical therapy management of muscular dystrophy. Middletown, Ohio: The Parent Project for MD Research, 2001. In: Goodman C, Boissonnault W, Fuller K. *Pathology: implications for the physical therapist.* Philadelphia: W.B. Saunders Co.; 2003.
28. Pourmand R, ed. *Neuromuscular Diseases, Expert Clinicians' Views.* Woburn, MA: Butterworth-Heinemann; 2001.
29. Rauch F, Glorieux FH. Osteogenesis imperfecta. *Lancet.* 2004;363:1377–1385.
30. Daly K, Wisbeach A, Sanpera I, Fixsen JA. The prognosis for walking in osteogenesis imperfecta. *J Bone Joint Surg Br.* 1996;78:477–480.
31. Engelbert RH, Uiterwaal CS, Gulmans VA, Pruijs H, Helders PJ. Osteogenesis imperfecta in childhood: prognosis for walking. *J Pediatr.* 2000;137:397–402.
32. Huang R, Ambrose C, Sullivan E, Haynes R. Functional significance of bone density measurements in children with osteogenesis imperfecta. *J Bone Joint Surg.* 2006;88-A:1324–1330.
33. Lenssinck ML, Frijlink AC, Berger MY, Bierman-Zeinstra SM, Verkerk K, Verhagen AP. Effect of bracing and other conservative interventions in the treatment of idiopathic scoliosis in adolescents: a systematic review of clinical trials. *Phys Ther.* 2005;85:1329–1339.
34. Slate RK, Posnick JC, Armstrong DC, et al. Cervical spine subluxation associated with congenital muscular torticollis and craniofacial asymmetry. *Plast Reconstr Surg.* 1993;91:1187–1195.
35. Luther B. Congenital muscular torticollis. *Orthop Nurs.* 2002;2133:21–28.
36. Karmel-Ross K, Lepp M. Assessments and treatment of children with congenital muscular torticollis. In: Karmel-Ross K, ed. *Torticollis: Differential Diagnosis, Assessment and Treatment, Surgical Management and Bracing.* New York: The Haworth Press; 1997:21–69.
37. Jacques C, Karmel-Ross K. The use of splinting in conservative and post-operative treatment of congenital muscular torticollis. In: Karmel-Ross K, ed. *Torticollis: Differential Diagnosis, Assessment and Treatment, Surgical Management and Bracing.* New York: The Haworth Press; 1997:81–91.
38. Bhidayasiri R. An overview of dystonia, part I: classification and diagnosis. *CNS News,* July 2005, (7:7).
39. Bhidayasiri R. Recurrent facial twitches. *CNS News,* October 2005, (7:10).
40. *Kaplan & Sadolck's Synopsis of Psychiatry,* 9th ed. Philadelphia: Lippincott, Williams & Wilkins; 2003.
41. Holzman D. Autism. *CNS News,* September 2005, (7:9).
42. Daruna J, Dalton R, Forman MA. Neurodevelopment dysfunction in the school-aged child: attention deficit hyperactive disorder. In: Behrman RE, Kliegman RM, Jenson HB, eds. *Nelson Textbook of Pediatrics,* 16th ed. Philadelphia: W.B. Saunders Co.; 2000.
43. Levy S, Kim A, Olive M. Interventions for young children with autism: a synthesis of the literature. *Focus Autism Other Dev Disabl.* 2006;21:55–62.

44. Dalton R, Forman MA. Pervasive developmental disorders and childhood psychosis: autistic disorder. In: Behrman RE, Kliegman RM, Jenson HB, eds. *Nelson Textbook of Pediatrics,* 16th ed. Philadelphia: W.B. Saunders Co.; 2000.

45. Schnur J. Asperger syndrome in children. *J Am Acad Nurse Pract.* 2005;17:302–308.

46. Price A, Tidwell M, Grossman JA. Improving shoulder and elbow function in children with Erb's palsy. *Semin Pediatr Neurol.* 2000;73:44–51.

47. Ramos LE, Zell JP. Rehabilitation program for children with brachial plexus and peripheral nerve injury. *Semin Pediatr Neurol.* 2000;7:52–57.

48. Bhidayasiri R. An overview of dystonia, part II: treatment. *CNS News,* September 2005, (7:9).

49. Campbell SK. Decision making in pediatric neurologic physical therapy. New York: Churchill Livingstone; 1999.

50. Morton J, Brownlee M, McFadyen A. The effects of progressive resistance training for children with cerebral palsy. *Clin Rehabil.* 2005;19:283–289.

51. Singer RB, Strauss D, Shavelle R. Comparative mortality in cerebral palsy patients in California. *J Insur Med.* 1998;30:240–246.

52. Strauss D, Cable W, Shavelle R. Causes of excess mortality in cerebral palsy. *Dev Med Child Neurol.* 1999;41:580–585.

53. Gardner M. Outcomes in children experiencing neurologic insults as preterm neonates. *Pediatr Nurs.* 2005;31:448–456.

54. Bhidayasiri R. A case of cerebral venous and sinus thrombosis. *CNS News,* September 2005, (7:9).

55. Hartel C, Schilling S, Sperner J, Thyen U. The clinical outcomes of neonatal and childhood stroke: review of the literature and implications for future research. *Eur J Neurol.* 2004;11:431–438.

56. Depression in children and adolescents. In: Hazell P, ed. *Clinical Evidence,* 4th ed. London: BMJ Publishing Group; 2000.

57. Yang Q, Rasmussen SA, Friedman JM. Mortality associated with Down's sysdrome in the USA from 1983 to 1997: a population-based study. *Lancet.* 2002;359:1019–1025.

58. O'Donohoe NV. *Epilepsies of Childhood,* 3rd ed. Oxford, U.K.: Butterworth-Heinemann; 1994.

59. Bauchner H. Children with special needs: failure to thrive. In: Behrman RE, Kliegman RM, Jenson HB, eds. *Nelson Textbook of Pediatrics,* 16th ed. Philadelphia: W.B. Saunders Co.; 2000.

60. Iwaniec D, Sneddon H, Allen S. The outcomes of a longitudinal study of non-organic failure-to-thrive. *Child Abuse Rev.* 2003;12:216–226.

61. Dunn D. Chronic regional pain syndrome. *AORN J.* 2000;72:422–423.

62. Hinderer KA, Hinderer SR, Shurtleff DB. Myelodysplasia. In: Campbell SK, ed. *Physical Therapy for Children,* 2nd ed. Philadelphia: W.B. Saunders Co.; 2000;621–671.

63. Gunther KP, Nelitz M, Parsch K, et al. Allergic reactions to latex in myelodysplasia: a review of the literature. *J Pediatr Orthop B.* 2000;933:180–184.

64. Schoenmakers MA, Uiterwaal CS, Gulmans VA, Gooskens RH, Helders PJ. Determinants of functional independence and quality of life in children with spina bifida. *Clin Rehabil.* 2005;19:677–685.

65. Asher M. Factors affecting the ambulatory status of patients with spina bifida cystica. *J Bone Joint Surg.* 1983;65:350–356.

66. Findley T. Ambulation in adolescents with myelodysplasia: early childhood predictors. *Arch Phys Med Rehabil.* 1987;68:518–522.

67. Russman BS, Buncher CR, White M, et al. Function changes in spinal muscular atrophy II and III. The DCN/SMA group. *Neurology.* 1996;47:973–976.

68. Crist WM, Smithson WA. The leukemias: leukemia. In: Behrman RE, Kliegman RM, Jenson HB, eds. *Nelson Textbook of Pediatrics,* 16th ed. Philadelphia: W.B. Saunders Co.; 2000.

69. Cystic Fibrosis Foundation (CFF). Clinical practice guidelines for cystic fibrosis. Bethesda, MD: 1997.

70. Cystic Fibrosis Foundation (CFF). An introduction to chest physical therapy. Bethesda, MD, 1997.

71. Fiel SB, Palys B, Sufian B, et al. Growing older with CF: a handbook for adults. Brussels, Belgium: Scienta Healthcare Education, Solvay Pharmaceuticals; 1997.

72. Mahadeva R, Webb K, Westerbeek RC, et al. Clinical outcome in relation to care in centers specializing in cystic fibrosis: cross sectional study. *BMJ.* 1998;316:1771–1775.

73. Spelling MA. Diabetes mellitus in children: diabetes mellitus. In: Behrman RE, Kliegman RM, Jenson HB, eds. *Nelson Textbook of Pediatrics,* 16th ed. Philadelphia: W.B. Saunders Co.; 2000.

74. Murphy JL, ed. *Monthly Prescribing Reference.* New York: Hay Market Media Publication; August 2005.

75. Loganathan R, Searls Y, Smirnova I, Stehno-Bittel L. Exercise-induced benefits in individuals with type I diabetes. *Phys Ther Rev.* 2006;11:77–89.

76. Hunt CE. Unclassified disorders: sudden infant death syndrome. In: Behrman RE, Kliegman RM, Jenson HB, eds. *Nelson Textbook of Pediatrics,* 16th ed. Philadelphia: W.B. Saunders Co.; 2000.

77. Antoov AY, Donavan MK. Burn injuries. In: Behrman RE, Kliegman RM, Jenson HB, eds. *Nelson Textbook of Pediatrics,* 16th ed. Philadelphia: W.B. Saunders Co.; 2000.

78. Barker LR, Burton JR, Ziene PD, eds. *Principles of Ambulatory Medicine.* Philadelphia: Lippincott, Williams & Wilkins; 1998.

Additional Online Resources

The Arthritis Foundation at http://www.arthritis.org/
The National Osteonecrosis Foundation at
   http://www.nonf.org
Muscular Dystrophy Association at http://www.mdausa.org
National Scoliosis Foundation at http://www.scoliosis.org
National Institute of Neurological Disorders and Stroke at
   http://www.ninds.nih.gov
The Dystonia Foundation at http://www.dystonia-foundation.org
Children and Adults with Attention Deficit/Hyperactivity
   Disorder at http://www.chadd.org
Autism Society of America at http://www.autism-society.org
International Rett Syndrome Association at
   http://www.rettsyndrome.org
The National Center on Birth Defects and Developmental
   Disabilities at www.cdc.gov/actearly
United Cerebral Palsy at http://www.ucp.org
National Stroke Association at http://www.stroke.org
Charcot-Marie-Tooth Association at
   http://www.charcot-marie-tooth.org
National Mental Health Association at
   http://www.nmha.org/children/children_mh_matters/
   depression.cfm
National Down Syndrome Society at http://www.ndss.org
Epilepsy Foundation at http://www.epilepsyfoundation.org
Guillain-Barre Syndrome Foundation International at
   http://www.gbsfi.com/about.html
The Hydrocephalus Association at
   http://www.hydroassoc.org
National Spinal Cord Injury Association at
   http://www.spinalcord.org
National Resource Center for Traumatic Brain Injury at
   http://www.neuro.pmr.vcu.edu

Asthma and Allergy Foundation of America at
   http://www.aafa.org
American Lung Association at http://www.lungusa.org
Association of Cancer Online Cancer Resources at
   http://leukemia.acor.org
The Children's Heart Institute at
   http://www.childrenheartinstitute.org
Cystic Fibrosis Foundation at http://www.cff.org
National Diabetes Education Program at
   http://www.ndep.nih.gov/diabetes/youth/youth_FS.htm

Acute Respiratory Distress Syndrome Clinical Network at
   http://www.ardsnet.org
American Sudden Infant Death Syndrome Institute at
   http://www.sids.org

Website: *National Cancer Institute at www.cancer.gov*
Website: *Osteogenesis Imperfecta Foundation at www.oif.org*
Website: *Spina Bifida Association at www.sbaa.org*
Website: *Muscular Dystrophy Association at www.mdausa.org*

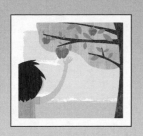

PART II

PRACTICE SETTINGS

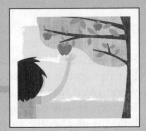

CHAPTER **4**

Providing Services in the Clinical Setting: Neonatal Intensive Care Unit and Inpatient

Tasia Bobish and Meg Stanger

LEARNING OBJECTIVES

1. Understand the philosophy that shapes the structure of the Neonatal Intensive Care Unit (NICU) and acute inpatient facility.
2. Understand the general influences that affect the decision-making process of the health care staff and parents in the hospital setting, including the NICU.
3. Understand the typical presentation and behaviors of a preterm infant and be able to differentiate those behaviors from the typical presentation and behaviors seen in a full-term infant.
4. Describe the role of physical therapy in the NICU.
5. Construct some common goals that the physical therapist may prescribe for an infant in the NICU.
6. Identify the general criteria used to transition a patient out of the NICU or hospital setting.
7. Understand the general considerations for a pediatric inpatient.
8. Identify patients with particular diagnoses that may need special considerations.

The practice of physical therapy with children is provided in a variety of settings with a unique perspective of the role of the physical therapist depending on the setting and the circumstances of the child and family. Unlike other patient populations, pediatrics always involves a parent or guardian who is intimately involved in the care, well-being, and decision making of the patient; the child. As in other patient populations, a variety of professionals and paraprofessionals are frequently involved in the delivery of a variety of services in each setting. This chapter will identify the general role and practice of the physical therapist in a neonatal intensive care unit (NICU) and in a pediatric inpatient acute care hospital. It will present a brief overview of the development and philosophies of these facilities and the unique external factors that influence the delivery of services in these settings. It introduces one of the practice settings in which physical therapists provide services to very young children, which may be the first contact a family has with a physical therapist.

THE PRACTICE ENVIRONMENT: THE HOSPITAL

In the 1700s and 1800s, early hospitals in the United States were charitable organizations focused on caring for the physically sick as well as protecting the public from those who had either physical or mental illness. Individuals with financial means obtained the services of a physician or nurse in their homes. Families without financial resources or the ability to care for their family members sent them to hospitals where they were isolated from the public, with visitation restricted. This isolation may have helped to curb the spread of disease in the general public, but not in the hospital building. Hospitals in the 1800s were overcrowded and offered limited health care.[1] Physicians saw the importance of this separation and isolation, but also the opportunity to study, teach medical students, and practice skills on a population brought together in one place, the hospital.[1] A transformation from care to cure had begun.

As with the development of the profession of physical therapy, hospitals were also transformed by wars, epidemics, and federal legislation. The growing need to care for individuals disabled by war or infected by influenza or poliomyelitis led to a greater need for facilities to aid them. In the 1900s, the development of private third-party payment systems, the rapid expansion of hospitals, facilitated by the *Hill-Burton Hospital Construction Act of 1946*, and the passage of *Title XVIII of the Social Security Act,* Medicare (which includes financial supplements for medical student education), were major factors that led to the structure and function of hospitals today.

Another important factor that played a role in shaping the delivery of health care is the treatment-oriented approach to illness found in the United States. In the United States, the development of health care was influenced by the attitude that the body is a machine that can be fixed. Treatment is provided with an aim to cure the person of illness or disease. This attitude is reflected in the sophisticated technology used to maintain life or prolong it, more so than in preventing or living with a long-term illness or disability.[1] This influence can be seen today in the intensive care provided to the infant who is born prematurely or to the elderly person whose life is dependent on cardiopulmonary machines.

POINTS TO REMEMBER

Influences on Hospital Development

Three major influences on the development of hospitals were:

The development of third-party payment systems for health care;

Congressional passage of the Hill-Burton Hospital Construction Act of 1946, and;

The creation of Medicare.

The growth, development, and utilization of hospitals also brought about new issues. With the increasing utilization of hospitals came the need to address issues of infection control to curb the spread of diseases *within* the hospital building, the need to protect the information about the people who were admitted to the hospital, and the need to provide a certain level of quality care to all people who received a service from the hospital. These identified factors, as well as others, reflect the growing influence of external agencies and legislation on the delivery of services in the acute care hospital.

Standard Precautions

The U.S. Department of Health and Human Services, Centers for Disease Control and Prevention (CDC), publishes guidelines on the standard precautions that should be taken to reduce the risk of transmission of microorganisms from infectious materials that apply to all patients receiving care in a hospital, regardless of the patient's diagnosis or infectious status.[2] These *standard precautions* include procedures for hand washing; the use of personal protective equipment (PPE) such as gloves, masks, gowns, and eye protection; the use of patient care equipment; procedures for the routine care, cleaning, and disinfection of equipment, furniture, and other environmental surfaces; the use of linens; the handling of blood and procedures to follow if inadvertently exposed to blood or injury due to needles, scalpels, or other sharp instruments; and the placement of patients who are infectious.

POINTS TO REMEMBER

Standard Precautions

Standard precautions include procedures for:

Hand washing,

The use of PPE,

The use of patient care equipment,

The use of linens,

The handling of blood or bodily fluids, and

The placement of patients who are infectious.

For more information, access the CDC website at www.cdc.gov.

Three of the more common infections encountered in the acute care hospital today are *methicillin-resistant staphylococcus aureus* (MRSA), *vancomycin-resistant enterococcus* (VRE), and *clostridium difficile* (C. diff).

Patients with prolonged hospital stays and heavy antimicrobial therapy are at an increased risk for acquiring MRSA, which frequently colonizes in the nose, axilla, groin, and/or wound sites, including burns. The most common mode of transmission is by contact. Droplet/contact precautions are used for patients infected with MRSA. The patient is placed in a private room or with a roommate who also is infected with MRSA. Everyone who enters the room should don a mask. Gloves should be worn if the patient will be touched, and a gown should be worn if there is a possibility of clothing coming in contact with the patient or anything in the patient's room. If the patient must walk in the hallway she must wear a mask, gloves, and a gown. The patient should avoid common areas such as the activity room, cafeteria, or gift shop. Any equipment (e.g., walker, cuff weights) or testing tools (e.g., goniometer, tape measure, stethoscope) used with the infected patient must be disinfected after use.

VRE is a bacterium that colonizes in the gastrointestinal tract. Patients with prolonged hospital stays and antimicrobial therapy are at risk for acquiring VRE. The most common mode of transmission is by contact. Contact precautions are used for patients infected with VRE. The patient is placed in a private room or with a roommate who also is infected with VRE. Everyone who enters the room must wear gloves if the patient will be touched and a gown if there is a possibility of clothing coming in contact with the patient or anything in the patient's room. The patient can walk in the hallway as long as she is wearing gloves and a gown. Ideally, if physical therapy is provided in the department, it should be at the end of the day and away from other patients. All equipment (e.g., parallel bars, mat table) or testing tools used with the infected patient must be disinfected after use.

C. diff is a bacterium that colonizes in the large bowel or colon. It releases a toxin that causes diarrhea and abdominal pain. Patients who had abdominal surgery or are receiving antibiotics or chemotherapy are at an increased risk for acquiring C. diff. The most common mode of transmission is by contact. Contact precautions are used for patients infected with C. diff. The patient is placed in a private room or with a roommate who also is infected with C. diff. Everyone who enters the room must wear gloves if the patient will be touched and a gown if there is a possibility of clothing coming in contact with the patient or anything in the patient's room. If the patient must walk in the hallway, she must wear gloves and a gown. The patient should avoid walking in common areas. As with other infectious diseases, all equipment or testing tools used with the infected patient must be disinfected after use.

The patient not only needs protection from contagious organisms, but also from the misuse or inappropriate disclosure of personal information. It is not only respectful of the patient's privacy but is also the law.

POINTS TO REMEMBER

MRSA, VRE, C. diff.

MRSA: Droplet/Contact Precautions. MRSA grows in the nose (and other places). Wear mask, gloves, and gown. Avoid walking patient in hallways.

VRE: Contact Precaution. VRE grows in the gut. Wear gloves and gown. Patient can walk in hallway if wearing gloves and gown.

C. diff: Contact Precautions. Colon-Diarrhea. Wear gloves and gown. Avoid walking patient in hallways.

Always disinfect all surfaces and equipment after working with an infected patient.

Health Insurance Portability and Accountability Act (HIPAA)

The purpose of the *Health Insurance Portability and Accountability Act* of 1996 (HIPAA) was to simplify the administrative procedures within the health care system and to move toward full electronic claims transactions. HIPAA also includes rules to protect the privacy and security of the exchange of individually identifiable health information.[3] Patient information that is exchanged among providers must be de-identified, and only the minimum information necessary is exchanged. Patients or guardians must sign consents for release of information among some care providers. For example, a physical therapist working in a hospital cannot call the school physical therapist who may be treating that child on her return to school without a signed consent from the parent. HIPAA applies to all government health plans, managed care plans, and many private health plans, as well as health care providers such as hospitals, ambulatory care centers, home care agencies, and durable medical equipment suppliers. Federal legislation is one way to influence the behavior of health care providers; voluntary accreditation by a group of one's peers is another way.

POINT TO REMEMBER

HIPAA

Always check the chart for signed authorization to release information *before* providing information to anyone.

Accreditation

Most hospitals are voluntarily accredited through an external organization such as the *Joint Commission on Accreditation of Healthcare Organizations* (JCAHO) or the *Commission on Accreditation of Rehabilitation Facilities* (CARF; see Chapter 5). A facility with a JCAHO and/or CARF accreditation has demonstrated that they have met the standards for patient care issued by the accrediting agency that represents a body of their peers. Facilities are accredited for a period of time, typically 2 to 3 years, must regularly submit predetermined data to maintain their accreditation, and must be reaccredited after the 2- to 3-year period. Accreditation standards generally address patient safety, quality of patient care, patient satisfaction, and performance measurement. Accreditation reports are available to the public for review.

The mission of JCAHO is to continuously improve the safety and quality of care provided to the public through the provision of health care accreditation and related services that support performance improvement in health care organizations.[4] Almost half of the JCAHO standards are related to patient safety issues such as staffing levels and competency, medication use, infection control, use of restraints, fire safety, and safety of medical equipment, to name a few. In 2002, JCAHO issued the first set of national patient safety goals, with updates to the pool of goals each year. Accredited facilities must adhere to the national goals and are held accountable to demonstrate compliance. For example, the first set of national goals placed a strong emphasis on proper patient identification to address the incidences of procedures occurring to the wrong patients. Each facility determines its procedures and protocols for adherence to the various standards, including staff education and knowledge of the various procedures. Physical therapists are an integral part of the delivery of patient care services and must adhere to their facility's standards.

The Joint Commission has also taken measures to insure that medical errors and events are reported and analyzed, that new procedures are implemented after analysis, and that the information learned is shared with other organizations to improve patient safety nationally. Steps have been taken legislatively to create a nonpunitive environment and limit the damage from civil law suits when a health care worker makes a report.

Beginning in 2006, all JCAHO surveys for accreditation are unannounced, meaning that the surveyors can present themselves at the facility at any time. They will follow identified patients through the patient care process and talk with hospital personnel as the patient moves through her day and scheduled procedures. All hospital personnel, including physical therapists, must be aware of the standards and policies of their facility and be comfortable discussing those procedures with a surveyor. After an accreditation survey, a hospital is provided with a score and a detailed report from the commission. Joint Commission quality reports contain information on accredited health care organizations and are available to the public.

Another key component of JCAHO is the inclusion of performance measures for comparison among health care facilities. The performance measures are referred to as the ORYX initiative. The ORYX acronym does not have any meaning, but the ORYX performance measures must be data-driven and statistically valid indicators that will provide performance information for the organization. The performance data are available for comparison among other heath care organizations and for review by outside stakeholders. A physical therapist needs to be aware of her facility's ORYX initiatives and how her role impacts the data collected and ultimately the facility's performance.

The control of infections, the protection of information, and the push to demonstrate quality care are done to promote the health and wellness of the patient and to improve the health care that is provided in the hospital setting. These factors influence the provision of services at all levels of the organization.

POINT TO REMEMBER

JCAHO

The mission of JCAHO is to continuously improve the safety and quality of care provided to the public through the provision of health care accreditation and related services that support performance improvement in health care organizations.

THE NEONATAL INTENSIVE CARE UNIT

In the acute care hospital, there may be a variety of levels of care for providing services to a pediatric patient. For a newborn, this could be a NICU; for a child, a pediatric intensive care unit (PICU), or a cardiac intensive care unit (CICU). For less critical care infants and children, it would be a regular room in an acute hospital.

The population of infants in the NICU is made up primarily of infants who were born prematurely, before 37 weeks' gestation, and who may or may not have additional complicating factors. The NICU may also have full-term infants who had difficulties during delivery or who had problems within the first few days of their lives. In the United States, there are three levels of neonatal care. *Level I* is a basic newborn nursery. These nurseries service infants who are healthy, born close to full term, and who may have minor short-term issues, such as jaundice. *Level II* is an intermediate care nursery. These nurseries are located in regional hospitals. In general, the infants requiring this level of care are born at >32 weeks' gestation and weigh >1,500 grams. The nurseries are staffed by specially trained personnel who can care for infants who require IV antibiotics, IV feedings, nasal or oral tube feedings, supplemental oxygen, or phototherapy for hyperbilirubinemia. It can be the first place to which an infant with intermediate health issues is transferred, or it can serve as a step down from the NICU for infants with more serious difficulties.[5,6] *Level III* nurseries are NICUs or special care nurseries, usually located at major medical centers. They are staffed with neonatologists and neonatal nurses. Infants at these facilities are medically fragile due to prematurity, serious congenital or genetic disorders, or a medical condition, such as sepsis. Level III nurseries vary in the type of services they provide, but in general, they provide *incubators* to help the infants to maintain the proper body temperature, mechanical ventilation, a number of imaging techniques (i.e., computed tomography [CT], magnetic resonance imaging [MRI], and echocardiography), pediatric surgical specialists, and pediatric anesthesiologists to perform major surgery. Extracorporeal membrane oxygenation (ECMO) and surgical repair of serious congenital cardiac malformations that require cardiopulmonary bypass are only offered at a few NICUs.[5,6]

POINTS TO REMEMBER

Three Levels of Neonatal Care

Level I: Basic newborn nursery
Level II: Intermediate care nursery with specially trained staff
Level III: NICUs have specialized staff such as neonatologists and neonatal nurses.

Regardless of the level of care, having an infant or a child with acute medical needs can be extremely stressful for a family. This can be magnified when intensive care is needed to save the life of a newborn. Several health care providers will be providing services throughout the day, and incorporating parents who may be fatigued, stressed, and emotionally sensitive. Each provider should be aware of the goals of intensive care. In the NICU, the overall goals are to reduce the total noxious load to which an infant is exposed, streamline procedural techniques, restructure the physical environment to reduce light and noise levels, and through handling and positioning promote sensorimotor maturation and development.[7] NICUs utilize (a) organization of the care provided to minimize noxious stimuli, (b) containment or positioning strategies to optimize motor development and provide comfort to the infant, and (c) nonnutritive sucking with or without sucrose to facilitate the infant's comfort. They integrate the infant's family so that they will bond with their infant and carry over optimal handling and care of the infant after discharge.[7]

The particular philosophy of a NICU and how it is implemented varies from place to place, but the general philosophy in recent times is to be patient and family centered. Care of the infant is individualized. Medical needs of the infant take priority, but an attempt is made to address these needs in the least stressful way for the infant and parents. The least stressful way is chosen because conservation of an infant's energy is often a prime goal. Anything that needlessly stresses an infant wastes what precious energy she has, and can lessen the chance of survival. To this end, light and noise are reduced. Soothing music may be played. Maintenance of a steady body temperature is a goal. Attempts are made to put the infant on a regular sleep schedule where care is clustered during the infant's awake time and the infant is allowed periods of uninterrupted sleep. Positioning and handling of the infant is utilized to reassure and relax the infant, promote normal shaping of the infant's head, and encourage the infant's overall development. When appropriate, pain relief is given to the infant. Research indicates that an infant who receives developmentally supportive care experiences fewer ventilator days, earlier discharge, and an improved developmental outcome.[8]

From the beginning, parents are involved in the examination process and in the provision of certain interventions. In some ways, the needs of the family are to be considered equal to the needs of the infant. Parents must be given a time to grieve for the birth of their normal infant that did not occur, but then must be given time to bond and attach with the infant they have. They should be supported as they learn to correctly read what their infant's behaviors are telling them. Parents should also be taught what to expect from their infant and given confidence in the handling and management of their infant before the discharge to the home. This is a new undertaking for a family with an infant with medical needs or a premature infant.

POINTS TO REMEMBER

Overall Goals of the NICU

Maintain life.
Promote maturation and development.
Streamline procedural techniques to allow the infant to rest and grow.
Reduce noxious stimuli to the infant.

Examination

The examination of the newborn begins with a review of the medical record and an observation of the infant in her crib or incubator. (See Appendix A for an example of a developmental evaluation form.) Any medical diagnoses should be noted as they may impact the evaluation or subsequent interventions. Box 4-1 contains some common medical diagnoses and the related symptoms that can be seen in infants in the NICU. The medical record may also contain the infant's *Apgar scores* taken at the time of birth. The total Apgar score is derived from an examination of the newborn's heart rate, respiratory effort, muscle tone, reflex irritability, and color, each rated a 0, 1, or 2, at 1 and 5 minutes after birth. The Apgar score is not used as an indicator of the need for resuscitation; rather, it may be used to examine an infant's response to resuscitative measures. In term and preterm infants, the Apgar score remains a valuable predictor of infants who will need ongoing support in the immediate postpartum period and those who are at higher mortality risk in the neonatal period.[9] In addition, information on the infant's weight and vital signs should also be noted. The average birth weight of an infant ranges from 5.5 to 8.8 pounds, heart rate ranges from 120 to 160 beats per minute, respiratory rate ranges from 20 to 60 breaths per minute, and axillary body temperature can range from 36.3°C (97.3°F) to 36.9°C (98.6°F).

BOX 4-1
Common Diagnoses and Symptoms in Infants in a NICU:[18,62]

Apnea is cessation of respiration of ≥20 seconds. It is frequently complicated by cyanosis, pallor, hypotonia, or bradycardia. It is inversely related to gestational age.

Bradycardia is a heart rate <100 beats per minute.

Bronchopulmonary dysplasia (BPD) is a chronic lung condition that is the result of an initial, acute lung injury that is treated with prolonged exposure to oxygen and prolonged mechanical ventilation.

Failure to thrive (FTT) is a failure to gain weight as expected, which may be due to the infant not being given enough food; or the infant not being able to take in, retain, or utilize enough calories to gain weight.

Gastroesophageal reflux (GER) is gastric acid regurgitation into the lower third of the esophagus; it may interfere with feeding. In severe cases, it can cause an aversion to feeding that may result in FTT.

Intraventricular hemorrhage (IVH) is bleeding that occurs around the lateral ventricles in the brain. It is rated from I through IV: I being the mildest and IV the most severe. Infants most at risk for it are those born before 32 weeks' gestation.

Necrotizing enterocolitis (NEC) is acute intestinal necrosis. Preterm infants are at higher risk, especially very LBW infants, although roughly 10% of the cases occur in infants who are full term. It is treated in a variety of ways, occasionally requiring surgery for removal of a section of intestine.

Patent ductus arteriosus (PDA) occurs when the fetal ductus arteriosus fails to close spontaneously after birth, resulting in the mixing of the blood of the two ventricles of the heart. It is common in preterm infants, but uncommon in full-term infants. If it does not resolve spontaneously, surgery may be needed.

Periventricular leukomalacia (PVL) occurs when white tissue (motor tracts) around the lateral ventricles is damaged. Spastic diplegic cerebral palsy is the most common diagnosis associated with it.

Respiratory distress syndrome (RDS) is also referred to as hyaline membrane disease. It is caused by immature lungs and lack of surfactant. Mortality from RDS has been reduced by antenatal administration of steroids, surfactant replacement therapy, and improved mechanical ventilation.

Retinopathy of prematurity (ROP) is exclusively found in premature infants. It occurs when blood vessels of the eyes grow abnormally, and as a result the retina may detach. A contributing factor is thought to be exposure to high concentrations of oxygen.

Seizures manifest differently in the neonate because of the immaturity of the brain. They may manifest as repetitive lip smacking or chewing, repetitive eye blinking, generalized clonic movements, or apneic episodes.

POINTS TO REMEMBER

Birth Weight

Macrosomia—weighing ≥4,000 grams.
Normal birth weight—2,500 (5.5 lb) to 3,999 grams (8.8 lb).
Low birth weight (LBW)—1,500 (3.3 lb) to 2,500 grams (5.5 lb).
Very LBW—<1,500 grams (3.3 lb).

POINTS TO REMEMBER

Vital Signs

Axillary temperature of preterm infants ranges from 36.3°C (97.3°F) to 36.9°C (98.6°F) and for term infants 36.5°C (97.7°F) to 37.5°C (99.5°F).
Preferred heart rate is 120 to 160 beats per minute.
Preferred respiratory rate is 20 to 60 breaths per minute.

The examination continues with a systems review and the application of appropriate tests and measurements. A systems review takes into account the status of the infant's various systems, in particular the respiratory system, which may be impaired and which can dramatically impact what can or cannot be done with the infant at this time. Observation of and gentle interaction with the infant should be done, taking note of the clinical signs present. Prior to handling the infant, the physical therapist should consult with the infant's nurse. Coordination of care is important in order to minimize the disturbance of the infant, allowing for proper rest for growth and development. A conversation with the nurse will also provide information on the current status of the infant and any additional tests or procedures that were done or are being planned for that day. It may also aid in determining the reason or need for the physical therapy referral or in identifying the expectation of the referral source, which will aid in the evaluation.

Before the physical therapist begins to handle the infant, he should take note and be aware of the unique equipment in use in the NICU (Fig. 4-1).[10] Some of the more common equipment that may be found includes an *incubator*. Many NICU infants cannot maintain their body temperatures within a safe range. A safe range for axillary temperature is between 36.5°C to 37.5°C (97.7°F to 99.5°F) for term infants, and 36.3°C to 36.9°C (97.3°F to 98.6°F) for preterm infants. Sweating may occur in a term infant, but generally is not present in infants of less than 36 weeks' gestation. An incubator provides an environment that can regulate a preterm infant's body temperature. The goal in controlling the temperature of the environment is to minimize the energy expended to maintain a "normal" body

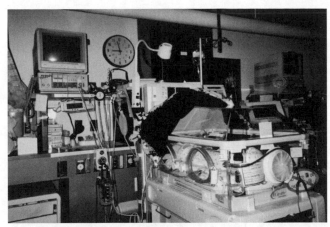

Figure 4-1. ■ The neonatal intensive care unit (NICU) environment. The neonatal intensive care environment can be intimidating. The amount of equipment that is used to maintain life can overshadow the presence of the infant. Being familiar with the variety of lines, monitors, and alarms provides a level of competence when providing services, and guides the interventions selected. Note the blanket on top of the incubator. It is used to shield the infant from the overhead light, which is one way to control sensory stimulation.

temperature, which in these fragile infants can be a source of stress. Newborns rarely shiver and must rely on *thermogenesis* (production of body heat by the breakdown of brown fat) to produce the necessary heat.[11] There are open incubators or radiant warmers for the infant who will receive frequent medical care. There are closed incubators or Isolettes for infants who need help with maintaining body temperature, but need only sporadic medical care. *Infant cribs* are used for larger or older infants in whom maintaining a safe body temperature is no longer a concern.

In addition to the vital sign monitors, an infant may also have a *pulse oximeter*. This device monitors the concentration of oxygen attached to hemoglobin in the infant's peripheral circulatory system. It typically is attached to the hand or foot of the infant, and the alarm will go off if the oxygen level reading goes below 90%. The sensor is sensitive to movement, so it is not unusual for it to go off if the infant moves or is moved. If this occurs, observe the infant and other instruments to determine the state of the infant. If in doubt, call the infant's nurse. *Transcutaneous peripheral oxygen and carbon dioxide monitors* measure the concentration of oxygen or carbon dioxide through the skin. The readings are more accurate than those from the pulse oximeter but less accurate than blood chemistry.

Intravenous lines or IVs can be used to administer medication, fluids, volume expanders, blood products, and parenteral nutrition.[12] The sites for the IV placement in infants are veins in the head, arms, hands, legs, or feet. A *central line* is an IV line inserted into a larger vein than a regular IV. It is placed in the chest, neck, arm, or groin. It is used to deliver medicines or *total parenteral nutrition* (TPN: nourishment provided by a

nongastrointestinal route). A PICC (peripherally inserted central catheter) line is a type of central line that is put in the arm and threaded from there into a larger vein in the body close to the heart. *HICKMAN* catheters and *BROVIAC* catheters are common types of central lines inserted into the jugular vein (neck) or subclavian vein (chest). *HICKMAN* and *BROVIAC* are registered trademarks of C.R. Bard, Inc., and its related company, BCR, Inc.[13,14]

Ventilators are also found in the NICU. There are several different ways an infant can be ventilated. The simplest is a bag and mask that fits over the infant's mouth and nose that can be used to ventilate an infant for a short period of time. *Continuous positive airway pressure* (CPAP) is used to assist in maintaining end-expiratory lung volume in infants who can breathe for themselves. For an infant who cannot maintain breathing on her own, mechanical ventilation incorporating an endotracheal tube may be used.

After the equipment and current monitor readings are identified, an observation of the infant is appropriate. The results of a physical therapist's examination will be greatly affected by how awake, sleepy, or upset the infant is during the process.[15-17] Generally, there are six states of infant behavior:

Deep Sleep *(State 1): The infant demonstrates no spontaneous movement. The eyes are closed and there is no eye movement noted. Breathing is regular. There is a relaxed expression on the infant's face.*
Light Sleep *(State 2): The infant has random movements. There is eye movement under closed eyelids (rapid eye movement [REM]) and irregular abdominal breathing, and intermittent sucking movements are noted.*
Drowsy *(State 3): The infant displays variable movement. The eyelids flutter. There is a delayed response to sensory stimuli. The infant may have facial grimacing, fussing, or whimpering. Respiration is more rapid and shallow.*
Quiet Alert *(State 4): The infant displays minimal movement. The eyes are open. The infant focuses and holds her attention on a source of stimulation and processes information.*
Active Alert *(State 5): The infant is very active and aroused. The infant may fuss, but does not cry. Respiration is irregular.*
Crying *(State 6): The infant has a robust cry. Respiration is rapid, shallow, and irregular.*

Relative to the full-term infant, the preterm infant will spend less time in Deep Sleep, Quiet Alert, and Active Alert states. This enables the infant to conserve energy and maintain homeostasis. Quiet Alert is the optimal state for learning. Right after a full-term infant is born, she is in a state of quiet alert, which aids in the bonding of the infant to the parent. The sleep patterns of a preterm infant who is 40 weeks postconception are not as well organized as those of a full-term newborn. By 44 to 48 weeks postconception, preterm and full-term infants who are exposed to proper fluctuation of light will develop a sleep–wake rhythmicity. Diurnal rhythm is necessary for growth hormone secretion and for neuronal maturation.[15]

Observation of the infant will also provide additional pertinent information. Full-term infants are born in what is called *physiological flexion*. This can be observed as the infants maintain a posture of extremities being flexed, and the body posture is relatively symmetrical. If an extremity is passively flexed, then extended, then released, it springs back into a flexed posture. Full-term infants randomly move their arms, legs, and head in the supine position. Their range of motion may temporarily lack full extension in the shoulders, elbows, hips, and knees. The range of motion of the feet can be affected for an extended period of time by how the infant was positioned in utero. Infants generally demonstrate the following reflexes: tonic neck, Moro, Galant, gag, suck, swallow, palmar grasp, and plantar grasp. Their sensory systems are generally intact at birth, except for vision. At birth, newborn infants are able to see an object that is 8 to 10 inches from their face and prefer looking at the human face. They also have periods of being awake and alert, although the length and frequency of those times vary with the individual infant.[15,18]

Preterm births account for 12% of all births in the United States.[19] Roughly 1.3% of all births are of infants who weigh <1,500 grams (3.3 lb) when they are born.[20] They are different than full-term infants. Preterm infants may have trouble with maintaining physiologic homeostasis (maintaining a steady body temperature), a steady heart rate, respiration rate, blood pressure, and blood oxygenation level. They may have trouble calming themselves. Their extremities are not held in as much flexion as a full-term infant's. The more preterm an infant, the more extended her extremities are held. This can have a later effect on the infant's posture and movement patterns even without neurologic insult. Their range of motion generally is greater, because there is not the flexor bias that develops in the third trimester and their muscle tone is lower than what is found in a full-term infant. There is also a paucity of movement noted. Preterm infants demonstrate fewer reflexes depending on their gestational age, and their sensory systems are less well developed. (Hearing begins around 23 to 24 weeks' gestation.) Visually, they have more difficulty attending or tracking. Preterm infants have fewer and shorter periods of being awake and alert or they may have none. In general, as gestational age decreases, the above differences become more pronounced.[21]

A general examination of the infant's *range of motion* should be performed, taking into consideration the gestational age of the infant. There are certain diagnoses that are associated with reduced mobility, i.e., developmental dysplasia of the hip, arthrogryposis multiplex congenita, and achondroplasia. The resting position of the feet may cause some concern. The positioning of the feet of infants can be affected by how they were positioned in utero. The only time that the range of motion of the feet should be a concern is when a foot does not have full passive range of motion, as seen in conditions such as talipes equinovarus (clubfoot) or metatarsus adductus.

The infant's *muscle tone* can also be examined. At <28 weeks' gestational age, the infant is flaccid with an overall extended, flat body posture. At 32 weeks' gestational age, flexor muscle tone begins to develop in a foot-to-head pattern.[18] The following are three tests utilized to examine an infant's muscle tone:

Heel to Ear—*The infant's foot is grasped and taken towards the infant's ear. In a typical full-term infant, the foot will go to approximately the level of the chest or shoulder. The closer the foot comes to the ear, the lower the muscle tone. Close approximation of the heel to the ear is also associated with a preterm infant.*

Popliteal Angle—*The infant's leg is flexed until the thigh rests against the infant's abdomen. The physical therapist then grasps the infant's foot and extends the infant's knee until firm resistance is met. In a typical full-term infant, the angle at the knee joint is about 90 degrees. An angle greater than that indicates low muscle tone. A greater angle is also seen in the preterm infant.*

Scarf Sign—*This examines muscle tone in the shoulder girdle. The physical therapist takes the baby's hand to the opposite shoulder like a scarf. In a typical full-term infant, the hand does not go past the shoulder and the elbow does not cross the midline of the chest. The more it does, the more hypotonic and preterm the infant.*[15]

Muscle Tone

At less than 28 weeks' gestation, the infant is flaccid. At 32 weeks' gestational age, flexor muscle tone begins to develop in a foot-to-head pattern. Examining the heel-to-ear distance, popliteal angle, or scarf sign can be used to examine an infant's muscle tone.

In addition to muscle tone, the infant's *reflexes* are also examined.[15,16,22–24] Although there is general agreement on what reflexes are present in a full-term infant, there is some disagreement over when they present in the preterm infant.[24] Therefore, the gestational levels given in the following reflexes should be taken as estimates. Even reflexes that are present at 28 weeks' gestational age will not be as easily elicited as those in the full-term infant, even when the preterm infant reaches 40 weeks' postconception age.[18] The usefulness of testing for reflexes may also be debated. The asymmetric tonic neck reflex (ATNR), rooting, and suck–swallow reflexes are a few of the primitive reflexes that are relevant to a physical therapy examination and may provide a better understanding of the treatment protocols used with preterm infants. The ATNR can interfere with visual tracking and bringing the hands to midline, and may influence the development of orthopedic deformities (e.g., head molding, hip subluxation, scoliosis). Rooting and the suck–swallow reflex can interfere with the infant's ability to feed. Swallowing begins at 12 weeks' gestation, but not until 32 to 37 weeks' gestation does the infant begin to coordinate swallowing with sucking. Therefore, no bottle-feeding or breastfeeding will be attempted with an infant until around 34 weeks' gestational age. Additional examination of primitive reflexes can be performed to provide some information on the maturation of the central nervous system (CNS). See Box 2-3 in Chapter 2 for a listing of additional primitive reflexes.

The *sensory systems* of the infant are also included in the examination. The following sensory systems are presented in the order in which they mature.[18,25] The younger the preterm infant, the less sensory input she will tolerate, and the more multisensory input should be avoided. Touch or *tactile sense* is the first sense to develop. It begins at 8 to 10 weeks' gestational age. Full-term and older, more stable preterm infants typically enjoy being held and carried. More stable preterm infants have shown increased weight gain and improved muscle tone with tactile input. However, in the more fragile preterm infant, most handling is related to medical or nursing procedures. Because of this, very young and fragile preterm infants have demonstrated unfavorable responses to tactile stimulation. Gentle touch has been shown to have the least adverse effect.[26] Types of tactile input that may be seen in the NICU are kangaroo care and cobedding of multiples. *Kangaroo care* or skin-to-skin holding began in 1981 and consists of mothers holding their infants beneath their clothing, upright on their chest so that there is skin-to-skin contact. Cobedding of multiples is when infants that are twins or higher multiples are put for a time in the same bed. Both types of tactile input have been shown to have beneficial effects on the infants. There is some concern with cobedding of multiples of increasing an infant's chance for infection, but it has not been documented.[15]

The *vestibular system* is functioning at 28 weeks' gestational age. Rocking and swinging are calming to full-term and stable preterm infants. The sense of taste or *gustation* in full-term infants is developed, and these infants have shown a preference for sweet tasting liquids. Pacifiers that are dipped in sucrose water and given to infants have been shown to reduce crying and facilitate hand-to-mouth activity, and have been used during and after painful procedures to reduce distress and crying.[27]

Fetuses begin *hearing* at 22 to 24 weeks' gestational age. At <30 weeks' gestational age, the fetus will respond to sound by showing an avoidance reaction.[18] When born, full-term infants are able to distinguish the voice of their mother, father, and siblings, or a story repeatedly read to them in utero.[28] In response to a sound, an infant may change motor activity, smile, grimace, become alert, cry, cease to cry, or stop sucking. The ability to habituate to a sound indicates an intact CNS. Rhythmic sounds quiet and soothe infants.[15]

Visual development of the eyes begins 22 days after conception, but the eyelids fuse at 10 weeks and do not open until 26 weeks into the pregnancy. How wide the eyelids open is a function of maturation. At 32 weeks' gestational age, an infant can briefly focus on an object 6 to 9 inches from her face. At 33 weeks, she can horizontally track, and by 35 weeks she can vertically track. By 38 weeks' gestational age, an infant can visually fixate on an object.[18] Even in a full-term infant, vision is not fully developed at birth. Full-term newborns are able to distinguish light and dark, but it takes another 6 months to develop better visual acuity. She can see an object that is within 8 to 10 inches of her face, and can recognize her mother's face.

Systems Development

The following systems are presented in the order that they mature:

    Tactile
    Vestibular
    Gustation
    Hearing
    Vision

BOX 4-2
Standardized Tests Appropriate for the Neonatal Intensive Care Unit

Alberta Infant Motor Scales (AIMS)
Assessment of Preterm Infant's Behavior (APIB)
Bayley Scales of Infant Development, Second Edition (BSID)
Brazelton's Newborn Behavior Assessment Scale (NBAS)
NICU Network Neurobehavioral Scale (NNNS)
Neurobehavioral Assessment of the Preterm Infant (NAPI)
APIB, NNNS, NAPI were designed for preterm infants or high-risk newborns.[16]

Appropriate *developmental tests* and measurements can also be done as part of the examination and evaluation. Box 4-2 contains a list of some tests and measurements with good reported validity and reliability used by physical therapists in a NICU.

It is important to remember throughout the examination that full-term infants spend their last 3 months developing *motor skills* in a quiet, dark, essentially gravity-free environment with dynamic circumferential boundaries at all times. The womb keeps them in a flexed, generally symmetrical position. Because of the elasticity of the womb, they may extend their head and extremities, but the womb will push them back into flexion. In contrast, depending on when they are born, preterm infants develop their motor skills in a world of noise, light, gravity pulling them into extension, and primitive reflexes making them asymmetrical. Add on top of that the possibility of endotracheal intubation, mechanical ventilation, IVs, central lines, and periodic episodes of pain as procedures are done, and it is no wonder, even if a preterm infant is born without a medical problem, that she will develop differently than a full-term infant.[29]

Looking at it neurologically, infants are born with an excess of neural connections. The first couple of years are spent pruning those connections. The pathways that the infant/toddler uses are strengthened and become dominant. The pathways that are not used are weakened or disappear.[30] It is easier for an infant in utero, where gravity is eliminated, to move in multiple directions. In contrast, the preterm infant who is not as strong or healthy as the full-term infant has to deal with the effect of gravity. As a result, she moves less, her head is pulled to one side, and her extremities, unless supported otherwise, are pulled into abduction, extension, and external rotation.[29] The asymmetry, the increased extension, and the decrease in movement lead to different neural pathways being developed in the preterm versus the full-term infant even if corrected for age.

How infants are positioned can affect motor development. This can be seen even in normal, full-term infants.

Full-term newborns, when laid supine, will have their head to one side, usually the right. If their position is varied, this has no detrimental affect on motor development. However, as a result of the recommendation to have infants sleep supine to prevent Sudden Infant Death Syndrome (SIDS), there has been an increased incidence in full-term infants of *brachycephaly*, where the infant's head is flatter in the back with a bald spot, and there is forward displacement of the ipsilateral ear, forehead, and maxilla.[31] If such an effect can be seen in full-term infants, then positioning can have even more of a detrimental effect on preterm infants, whose heads are softer and thinner, who lack the strength of the full-term infant to counter gravity, and who may be attached to equipment that pulls the head to one side. In the NICU, infants are frequently placed supine for monitoring and access purposes. As stated, having the head chronically to one side can affect the shape of the head. Secondary to this, ipsilateral tightness in the sternocleidomastoid muscle can occur. Preferential head turning can result in dominance of a hand too early, and eventually even an asymmetric gait pattern.[31]

Another head shaping that may occur in very preterm infants is *dolichocephaly*. Dolichocephaly occurs when the head of the infant becomes unusually narrow from side to side, and elongated from front to back, as a result of positioning. It does not affect cognitive function, but cosmetically can result in the infant looking different.

The uncorrected supine posture of the upper extremities in preterm infants in the NICU consists of adducted scapula and retracted, externally rotated shoulders. This results in their arms being out to the side in a "W" position. The impact of this posture is that the hands are not in the visual field of the infant and there is less hand-to-mouth time (which hinders desensitizing the oral area and developing self-calming skills) and less playing of the hands in midline. If the infant is not placed in a prone position, or spends too little time in a prone position, shoulder girdle stability may be impaired. The problem perpetuates itself, in that the infant will fuss whenever placed in a prone position, because she is unable to prop up on her arms. The long-term effect may result in an infant who is less likely to roll, crawl, or use her arms to transition from one position to another. It can also lead to the utilization of unusual movements, such as back arching and scooting on the head to achieve mobility. Along with the gross motor skills, lack of shoulder girdle stability has an adverse effect on fine motor control.[31]

The uncorrected supine posture of the lower extremities in preterm infants in the NICU consists of the *frog leg position*. In this position the hips are abducted and externally rotated, and knees are flexed. This can result in a delay in crawling and walking. It may also result in an increased probability of toe-walking and persistent out-toeing in the gait pattern.[31] Although nothing can be done to make the preterm infant's existence the same as that of an infant in utero, attention to the preterm infant's positioning can lessen the effects of having been born early.

One area that should not be overlooked in the examination is *pain.* Younger preterm infants display a less vigorous and less robust response to pain. They are less likely to cry. Because of this, in the past, it was felt that young preterm infants did not perceive pain as well as did full-term infants, nor did they remember the pain, so little was done to ameliorate it. However, recent research has shown that the absence of response might only indicate the depletion of response capability and not lack of pain perception.[32] The pain response in preterm infants does exist, but it is more subtle. In a study on extremely LBW infants (≤1,000 grams), they displayed extensor movements, such as finger splaying and leg extension, when exposed to pain. In these infants, the incidence of arching, squirming, startling, and twitching did not increase with painful procedures, and thus were not thought to be pain indicators.[33] Even in cases where there is an absence of behavioral signs, infants have shown physiologic signs such as elevated vital signs and decreased oxygenation following painful stimuli.[34,35]

Pain puts stress on an infant's system. NICUs have strategies to help infants cope and recover from painful clinical procedures that are unavoidable in this setting. The strategies are both pharmacologic and nonpharmacologic. Pharmaceuticals utilized are opioids; local anesthetics such as lidocaine and acetaminophen; and anti-inflammatory drugs. Nonpharmacologic methods are *swaddling* (wrapping with a blanket snugly so that limb movement is restricted) or other forms of containment, holding, skin-to-skin contact (kangaroo care), and nonnutritive sucking on a pacifier with or without sucrose.[36,37]

Nonnutritive sucking with sucrose has been the subject of many studies. Sucrose is an effective way to relieve an infant's pain and can be given by itself or on a pacifier. This has been the most widely studied intervention for infant pain management. Sucrose is also associated with statistically and clinically significant reductions in crying after a painful stimulus.[38] The following are a few scales that have been developed to rate pain in infants:

(CRIES) Neonatal Postoperative Pain Measurement Score[39]
Premature Infant Pain Profile (PIPP)[40]
Neonatal Infant Pain Scale (NIPS)[41]
Neonatal Pain, Agitation, and Sedation Scale (N-PASS)[42]

P O I N T S T O R E M E M B E R

Pain Response

In the absence of behavioral signs of pain, infants may show physiologic signs, such as elevated vital signs or decreased oxygen saturation, following a painful stimulus. Nonnutritive sucking with sucrose on the pacifier is an effective way to relieve an infant's pain.

Evaluation and Plan of Care

After gathering information during the examination, the physical therapist makes an evaluation of the infant based on the identified impairments or risks, and what long-term consequences may be associated with the identified impairments or risks. This process will direct the physical therapist to appropriate goals and interventions to incorporate into the infant's plan of care.

The first and foremost goal is to do no harm. An infant in the NICU can be very medically fragile and may have difficulty maintaining body homeostasis. Her vital signs can change dramatically in a short period of time, and she may not show the signs that a healthy, full-term infant would when she is tired or overstimulated. Therefore, the physical therapist, throughout the session, should monitor the infant's vital signs and be alert to any subtle signs that indicate fatigue or intolerance. The general goals of intervention are to provide education to the caregivers on positioning and handling in order to promote appropriate development, and to facilitate the acquisition of an adequate suck for food intake and the promotion of growth.

P O I N T S T O R E M E M B E R

General Goals of Physical Therapy

Do no harm.
Provide education on handling and positioning to promote overall development.
Promote sucking.

Interventions to address these goals may include the purposeful and skilled interaction of the physical therapist with the infant and with other individuals involved in the infant's care. These interactions should help to promote appropriate musculoskeletal development, sensory organization, and maturation of the neuromotor system. This is done through appropriate handling, the controlled presentation of sensory stimuli, and through proper total body positioning.

Changes in *positioning* are needed to counter the development of skull deformity and musculoskeletal malalignment that can occur from maturation-related hypotonia, combined with the positioning restrictions placed on the infant due to certain medical procedures, such as prolonged ventilation, in which symmetric midline postures are difficult to maintain. Prolonged positioning can lead to asymmetric flattening of the skull and secondary torticollis. Shoulder retraction frequently accompanies supine positioning with the head to one side. This combination can result in impairments in active cervical range of motion, early preference in the use of one hand, decreased shoulder stability, and a decreased use of both hands in midline activities.

The goal of positioning is to optimize body alignment. This includes a neutral alignment of the neck and trunk and a semiflexed, midline orientation of the extremities. Positioning can incorporate the use of commercial positioning products, blanket rolls, and/or gel pillows to compensate for the infant's immature motor system and the pull of gravity. An infant responds well when her body posture and movements are supported within the containment boundaries of rolls, a swaddling blanket, or other positioning aids. Body containment can increase the infant's sense of security, promote self-regulation, decrease stress and energy expenditure, enable the infant to deal with stress, and promote physiologic homeostasis. However, the infant should not be completely immobilized. Even with swaddling, some movement should be possible with the tension from any lines, monitor leads, and endotracheal or nasogastric tubes avoided or minimized. Besides the physical boundaries provided by positioning aids, a physical therapist can provide comforting boundaries such as holding the infant's hand(s), holding her arms against her body, or placing a hand on the trunk while doing physical therapy.

In the supine position, commercial positioning products or rolled blankets are used to surround the infant and keep the infant's body symmetrical and slightly flexed. The physical therapist should keep the upper and lower extremities adducted toward the body, the shoulders slightly rolled forward, and the feet inside the boundaries. The infant's neck should be kept in a neutral position; not hyperextended or hyperflexed. If the infant is on mechanical ventilation, it is optimal to have the infant's head in midline, if possible (Fig. 4-2). Swaddling an infant in a blanket when supine reduces extraneous movements, maintains the limbs in a flexed position, and provides warmth and a sense of security to the infant. Keeping an infant calm conserves the infant's

energy, which is critical in young preterm infants. However, as an infant's motor system matures, swaddling may be too limiting to her voluntary movements.[31]

An infant's position should be changed a minimum of every 2 to 4 hours. Other positions the infants can be placed in are prone, side lying, and supported sitting. The prone position promotes flexion and can be done with or without positioning aids. The prone position in itself provides boundaries that are comforting to the infant. It improves breathing and sleep, lowers energy use, and gives the infant a better overall physiologic status.[43] The physical therapist can place a blanket roll under the infant's chest or along the length of the trunk to encourage the shoulders to round forward and to relieve some of the pressure on the knees of the flexed legs. Although the American Academy of Pediatrics recommends only supine sleeping for healthy infants, prone positioning is safe and appropriate in a NICU setting.[44]

Side lying is the easiest position for the infant to bring her hands to her face and play with her hands in midline. It also counters the abducted lower extremity posture often assumed in the supine position. A blanket roll or positioning aid can be placed behind, and in front of, the infant to keep the infant in side lying and to slightly separate the legs. The top hip should be slightly ahead of the bottom hip.

The infant can be placed in a supported sitting or semireclining position, if it can be tolerated. For supported sitting, the infant can be placed in an infant seat, which may rock or vibrate, or in an infant swing. No matter what the position, the physical therapist must take care to try and keep the infant symmetrical, in some flexion, and in no way medically compromised. Although positioning is important, it is secondary to the medical stability of the infant.[31]

Positioning is an important concept for the physical therapist to include in parent education so that it is continued when the infant is discharged to home. In addition, before discharge, the infant should be conditioned to sleep in a supine position for carryover at home. Proper positioning helps to optimize motor development, improve muscle tone, minimize positional deformity, and improve physiologic stability, and it comforts the infant.[31]

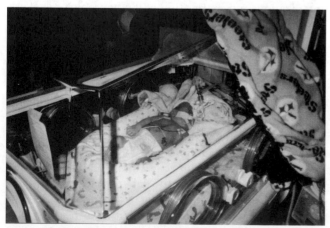

Figure 4-2. ■ The infant. Note the use of a roll to provide a boundary for the infant (Max) and to promote flexion and adduction of his extremities.

> ### POINT TO REMEMBER
>
> **Infant Positioning**
>
> How an infant is positioned can affect motor development. An infant should be positioned in supine, prone, and side lying, if and when appropriate.

The presentation of *sensory stimuli* is important in the NICU. In general, the younger and sicker the preterm infant, the more likely she is to be overwhelmed by sensory input.[16] The infant's state of behavior, sensory threshold, physiologic homeostasis, and stress cues must be taken into consideration.[15] Therefore, it is initially recommended that the physical therapist minimize and control the sensory input presented to the infant, and pay attention to the infant's responses to help guide the delivery of the interventions.

The preterm infant is more likely to be overstimulated than understimulated in the NICU; therefore, the physical therapist may want to begin his interactions with the infant with the lights dimmed and minimal noise, and speak with a soft voice, paying close attention to the infant's response. Negative responses by the infant can be seen in an increase or decrease in respiration or heart rate, irregular respirations, episodes of apnea, a drop in oxygenation level of the blood, a change in skin color, spitting up, vomiting, tremors, a change in muscle tone, frowning, grimacing, eye closing, sneezing, or coughing.[15] Positive responses are seen as a minimal change in respiration, heart rate, and oxygenation level of blood, smiling, maintaining eye contact, and appearing relaxed.[15] The physical therapist wants to protect the preterm infant from sensory overload, but provide enough stimulation to promote maturation of the sensorimotor system and promote the infant's ability to self-calm.

The tactile, vestibular, and proprioceptive systems are functioning in the preterm infant. All of these systems can provide input that is either soothing or arousing, depending on the state and maturation of the infant, and how the sensory input is provided. Swaddling can help with motor organization and self-regulation, and may be an appropriate initial intervention with a preterm infant. If the infant is not swaddled, soothing inputs to her in the supine position can include gentle, but firm whole-hand touching on the infant's chest or head, holding the infant's arms in against her body, or holding the infant's hands. The side lying and prone positions in themselves can be soothing to the infant, and may be more calming if a caregiver's hand is placed on the infant's buttocks or back. In side lying, the infant will have an easier time bringing her hand to her mouth, which can aid in self-calming. The prone position provides a constant, deep proprioceptive/tactile input. Holding the infant against the caregiver's chest and slowly rocking can also be calming to the infant.

As the preterm infant matures, other styles of sensory input can be tried. Stroking or patting has a positive effect on a physiologically stable infant, but may not on a physiologically unstable infant.[15] Sometimes older preterm infants may respond well to infant seats that swing or vibrate. Faster rocking or gentle jostling may be too much sensory input. It is best to start out with a single mode of sensory input: tactile, vestibular, or proprioceptive. As the preterm infant matures, multisensory input may be introduced.

Another sensory technique that is used with infants is massage. Massage has been shown to have beneficial effects such as weight gain, more active alert periods, and more mature orientation, habituation, and motor activity when performed on stable preterm infants.[45–47] Again, it is necessary to evaluate how the infant physiologically responds to the intervention. Massage stimulates nerve pathways and can increase hypothalamic activity and the production of the growth hormone somatotropin, which aids in the myelinization of nerves.[45]

In the process of providing sensory stimuli that are positively received by the preterm infant, it is anticipated that the infant will sort, order, and eventually put all the individual sensory inputs together into an integrated concept of the body. Besides developing useful perceptions in the infant, sensory stimuli contribute to the emotional and physiologic health of the infant, and when taught to the caregivers, can promote bonding and improve the long-term developmental outcome of the infant.[48]

Handling of the infant is used to facilitate movement and promote physical activity. Daily physical activity has been shown to improve bone growth and development in LBW preterm infants.[49] Physical therapy interventions may include techniques to encourage the development of the flexor muscles throughout the infant's body and promote midline orientation of the head and extremities. It is important to remember when handling an infant in the NICU to support her head and keep the extremities in flexion. Slow and gentle passive movements aid in the maintenance of a calm and steady behavioral state and help the infant to maintain control. Vigilant monitoring of the infant for negative responses to handling is necessary to avoid sensory overload.

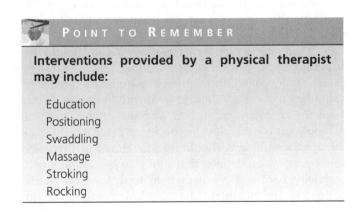

POINT TO REMEMBER

Interventions provided by a physical therapist may include:

Education
Positioning
Swaddling
Massage
Stroking
Rocking

TRANSITIONING

An infant historically has remained in the NICU until she reached a preset weight of 5 to 5½ pounds. Today several additional factors are considered which may include: the ability of the infant to coordinate sucking, swallowing, and breathing; to demonstrate a consistent pattern of weight gain; and to maintain normal body temperature when clothed in a bed with normal ambient temperature. Additional factors are the presence of active parental involvement and an established schedule of follow-up physician visits.[50]

From the NICU, an infant may be discharged to a Level II nursery, to a transitional facility, or to home. If an infant is to be discharged home, a home physical therapy program may be appropriate and should be demonstrated, explained, and illustrated by the physical therapist to the parents. The long-term goals of the home program should be clear and understood. Even if the infant is referred to an early intervention program after discharge, parental involvement and how the parents handle their infant are critical to the infant's development.[51]

Most infants who have been in a NICU will be scheduled for follow-up visits in a multidisciplinary developmental clinic for the first year or more.[52] Extended follow-up visits are necessary as there has been little success in predicting outcomes of infants from assessments in their first 6 months.[52,53] Many infants in the NICU, if not discharged out of the unit into a regular bed in the hospital, may be referred to an early intervention program (Chapter 6).

THE INPATIENT, ACUTE CARE

In the inpatient pediatric acute care hospital, the overall goals are similar to those in the NICU: to maintain life; to promote health; to maintain, restore, or minimize the loss of function; to minimize the negative aspect of the experience on the patient; and to control pain. In the inpatient hospital, the patient is often assigned a particular physician, nurse, and physical therapist, as well as other healthcare professionals. Often playrooms are available in certain areas of the hospital. Parents are generally present and may accompany the patient to the physical therapy department for treatment.

There are a variety of reasons a child might be admitted to an acute hospital setting. They can range from a fever, to a femur fracture, to traumatic brain injury secondary to a car accident, to treatment for cancer, to the need for an organ transplant. Because of the range of diagnoses, it is difficult to be specific as to what a physical therapist should and should not do. However, there are some general guidelines that apply to the examination and delivery of services that would apply to any pediatric patient in the hospital. The physical therapist should work to minimize the fear and stress of the patient. The following are suggestions on how a physical therapist or a physical therapy department might do this during the examination or delivery of services.

- A physical therapist should take a few minutes to introduce himself, explain what he does, and why he is there to see this particular child/patient.
- Generally a pediatric patient may feel safer if her parents, or other people she is familiar with, are allowed to stay with her during the session.
- A physical therapist should try to achieve goals through age-appropriate activities.

- Allow the patient to choose, or offer a choice of activities.
- Try to have the same physical therapist see the patient each session.
- See if there is a time of day that is better for the patient. For example, the patient may routinely take a nap in the afternoon, or feel more energetic in the morning. Ask the parent what they feel would be a good time of day.
- Repeating some of the same activities each session may give the patient a feeling of predictability, which may be comforting and reduce her anxiety.

POINT TO REMEMBER

Acute Care

The goal of acute care is to medically stabilize the patient and then begin the process of rehabilitation, which typically includes some level of mobility.

Examination

An examination is done prior to the initiation of physical therapy services. It consists of history, systems review, and tests and measurements that are appropriate for the individual patient. (See Appendix B for an example of a gait evaluation form used with inpatients.) A chart review and communication with the patient's nurse should be a routine aspect of the physical therapist's examination and treatment process in the hospital. In acute care, the patient's status can change quickly. Additional services, medical tests, and other professionals also are involved in the care of the patient, and are scheduled at various times during the patient's stay. Coordination of care is an important aspect of services in this setting. If possible, the pediatric patient's parents or guardian should be present during the examination. If they are not available, a timely review of the evaluation with them would be appropriate.

In the hospital the patient is typically limited not only by pain, but also by medical procedures, such as surgery, that have been implemented during this current admission. Performing a standardized test beyond the typical tests and measurements used in a physical therapy evaluation could be time consuming and inappropriate, given the shorter length of stay and the ability of the acutely ill patient to participate in this environment. The physical therapist should consider the use of a standardized test based on the ability of the patient to participate and the value of the results obtained with regard to intervention decisions or outcome management.

There are a variety of standardized tests and measurements that can be applicable in the acute care setting. A quick and reliable test may be more appropriate based on the expected decreased endurance of the patient in this setting. The *Functional Independence Measure for Children* (WeeFIM), as described in Chapter 1, is one such standardized test that may be appropriate.[54] This test measures a child's disability and the level of assistance required in daily activities, or burden of care for the caregiver. It can be done at admission and discharge with the scores used as an outcome measurement. In addition, the *Functional Reach Test*, which is commonly used with the adult population, has also been found to be reliable (interrater [$r = 0.98$], intrarater [$r = 0.83$], and test-retest [$r = 0.75$]) in the pediatric population without disabilities.[55,56] This dynamic balance test examines forward weight shift, reaching, and postural control using both feet, as opposed to other one-legged balance tests. Admission and discharge scores of appropriate children could be used to note changes in balance skills. The *Timed Up and Go test* (TUG) is another quick and practical test of functional mobility.[57] A modified version of this test, that was designed for adults, has been shown to be reliable with children, with and without disabilities, as young as 3 years of age.[58] All children in the study were able to walk independently with orthoses or assistive devices such as walkers or crutches. Reliability was high, with an intraclass correlation coefficient (ICC) of 0.89 (without disabilities) and 0.99 (with disabilities) within session, and 0.83 for test-retest reliability. The TUG has also been shown to be responsive to change over time, providing another possibility for an outcome measurement.[58]

POINT TO REMEMBER

Choosing a Standardized Test

The physical therapist should consider the use of a standardized test based on the ability of the patient to participate and the value of the results obtained with regard to intervention decisions or outcome management.

In addition to mobility and functional skills, the patient's level of *pain* should be measured. A pediatric patient who has just undergone surgery, who is undergoing treatment for cancer, or who has sustained a fracture of a bone may be very anxious about what kind of pain she is going to feel during the physical therapy session. In an acute care hospital, pain relief may be addressed in a variety of ways, from *patient-controlled analgesia* (PCA; personally administered dosages of pain medication into IV lines that are time limited), to pain medication administered through epidural catheters or IV lines, to oral medication. Before beginning physical therapy, the physical therapist should check with the patient's nurse to obtain information on what pain medication the patient is receiving and the schedule for delivery of the medica-

tion. A bolus of pain medication can be given through a PCA system right before physical therapy. Pain medication can be given through an IV line that should take effect within approximately 10 minutes of administration, but has a limited duration of approximately 30 minutes. Oral pain medication may take at least 30 minutes before the effects are felt by the patient, but it generally maintains its analgesic effect for several hours. The physical therapist should try to time the examination or delivery of interventions for when the pain medication is most effective.

POINT TO REMEMBER

Pain Medications

IV medications generally take effect within 10 minutes. Oral medications generally take at least 30 minutes to have an effect.

To determine the patient's level of pain, have her rate her pain before, during, and after physical therapy. There are a number of pain scales that have been shown to provide valid self-reports in children[59,60] (Box 4-3). If medically cleared, the physical therapist may have the patient actively help with her transitions during physical therapy as the patient may perceive less pain if she is in control of the movements. The physical therapist should reassure the patient that the activity will be done slowly, if appropriate, and will be kept within her level of pain tolerance.

Part of the examination could also include information gained from *diagnostic imaging*. Although the interpretation of diagnostic imaging is beyond the scope of education of a physical therapist, understanding diagnostic imaging and the fundamental relationship to anatomy will aid the physical therapist in understanding the extent of the medical diagnosis, medical interventions, and prognosis of the patient. The information will also aid in the evaluation of the patient by the physical therapist and assist in the patient management process. It

BOX 4-3
Pediatric Pain Assessments

Faces Pain Rating Scale[63]
Visual Analogue Scale (VAS)[64]
Color Analogue Scale (CAS)[65]
7-point Faces Pain Scale (FPS)[66]

BOX 4-4
Reading Diagnostic Images

1. Identify if the film is a CT, MRI or radiograph.
2. Orient the film appropriately. Identify specific anatomy. Right or left on the film refers to the patient's right or left.
3. Look at the whole image for obvious anatomic abnormalities. When looking at a CT scan of the brain, look for symmetry. Is the skull intact? Bleeding in the brain, outside the vascular system, will often appear initially as a white blob.
4. Do a systematic review. You may begin at the lower left hand corner of the image and study it in a clockwise manner; begin proximal and study to the distal images; or review it in a cephalo-caudal manner.

Adapted from Erkonen W, Smith W. *Radiology 101. The Basics and Fundamentals of Imaging*, Second ed. Philadelphia, PA: Lippincott, Williams & Wilkins; 2005.

can also aid in patient education, if appropriate, and provide additional information on the patient's condition and prognosis for functional recovery. Box 4-4 lists one way to examine diagnostic images. Knowing anatomy is fundamental in this process.

Passing x-rays through a film produces plain *radiographs,* often called x-rays. The film is white, and turns black as it is exposed to x-rays. The more the body's tissue or object in the body absorbs the x-rays, the whiter the image on the film. CT (or CAT) scans produce images by using x-rays, detectors, and computers. CT scans are often used to visualize anatomy in slices. Using x-rays and working like radiographs, which take a picture of the entire area, CT scans "slice" the area into pieces allowing for a more refined examination of the anatomy. MRIs are produced by using magnetic fields, radiofrequency waves, and computers to create images of anatomy. MRIs are used best to visualize soft tissues. One way to help distinguish between CT scan images and MRIs is to note that fat on radiographs (CT scans) appears black, whereas fat on MRIs appears white.

Evaluation and Plan of Care

When the examination is complete, the physical therapist evaluates the information and makes a diagnosis based

POINT TO REMEMBER
CT or MRI?
Fat on radiographs (CT scans) appears black.
Fat on MRIs appears white.

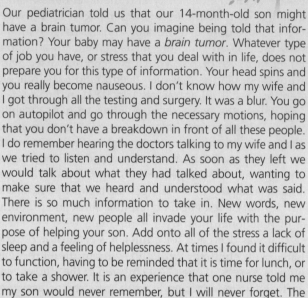
PARENT PERSPECTIVE
BAD NEWS

Our pediatrician told us that our 14-month-old son might have a brain tumor. Can you imagine being told that information? Your baby may have a *brain tumor*. Whatever type of job you have, or stress that you deal with in life, does not prepare you for this type of information. Your head spins and you really become nauseous. I don't know how my wife and I got through all the testing and surgery. It was a blur. You go on autopilot and go through the necessary motions, hoping that you don't have a breakdown in front of all these people. I do remember hearing the doctors talking to my wife and I as we tried to listen and understand. As soon as they left we would talk about what they had talked about, wanting to make sure that we heard and understood what was said. There is so much information to take in. New words, new environment, new people all invade your life with the purpose of helping your son. Add onto all of the stress a lack of sleep and a feeling of helplessness. At times I found it difficult to function, having to be reminded that it is time for lunch, or to take a shower. It is an experience that one nurse told me my son would never remember, but I will never forget. The hospital staff are wonderful people; they saved my son's life.
—A Dad

on the information obtained. This diagnosis guides the physical therapist in the selection of interventions, goals, and outcomes for this particular patient.

Physical therapy goals in an acute care setting are not the same as those in a rehabilitation hospital. Physical therapy is not the main reason the child was admitted to the hospital, so generally the goal is to maintain or minimize loss of function during the child's stay. If the child is in need of rehabilitation services, she will be transferred to a rehabilitation hospital, or she will be referred for outpatient physical therapy services when medically appropriate. The primary goal in the acute care hospital is to promote the optimal amount of independence and mobility given the medical status of the patient. Many times the goal is to get the patient up out of bed and (if possible) walking as soon as possible. As in the NICU, the physical therapist integrates the following five elements of patient management: examination, evaluation, diagnosis, prognosis, and intervention.

POINTS TO REMEMBER
Physical Therapy Goals in Acute Care
Physical therapy goals in an acute care setting are not the same as those in a rehabilitation hospital. Physical therapy is not the main reason the child was admitted to the hospital, so generally the goal is to maintain or minimize loss of function during the child's stay.

Communication, coordination, and documentation are the most important physical therapy interventions in the acute care setting. A patient's status can change quickly. It is important for the physical therapist to review the patient's medical record for current, up-to-the-minute information on the health status of the patient. What are the patient's current vitals or laboratory values? This information will aid in the determination of the type and intensity of the physical therapy intervention, if appropriate at this time. Laboratory values, such as hemoglobin (Hgb), hematocrit (Hct), and platelet count (as examples), should be evaluated to determine if the patient should be expected to perform specific intensities of exercise. If any laboratory values are abnormal for the patient's age, the physical therapist should determine the effect that that value would have on the patient's ability to participate in the physical therapy session, and alter the intervention as appropriate. The presence of a fever (>98.6°F or >37°C) will also affect the patient's ability to participate. Additional questions could include: What are the current orders of the physician or specialist? Were there any medical tests recently done or anticipated in the next few hours? Are there any restrictions associated with the medical test, such as wearing of a cervical collar until the cervical spine has been cleared by radiograph, or bed rest following a lumbar puncture? Were there any recent test results that identified an infection or the presence of an infectious disease? This information can be found documented in the patient's medical record, but for the most up-to-date information, it is recommended to talk to the patient's primary nurse before beginning physical therapy. The primary nurse will know exactly what is happening to the patient at all times and will help with the coordination of services that are provided. The patient may be scheduled for a radiograph within the next 30 minutes, or she may have just completed a session with the occupational therapist and requires a rest before proceeding with the next service.

When the documentation has been reviewed and the care coordinated, the patient is seen and a systems review is again done to evaluate the current status of the patient and to determine if the anticipated interventions are appropriate. *Patient-related instruction* is an important intervention in this environment. Because of the possible fluctuations in the patient's ability to learn and perform motor tasks, the risk of injury, and the rapid recovery that can also be expected, repeated reviews of safety precautions, movement restrictions, use of assistive devices, and the importance of patient involvement in daily exercises or activities is necessary. The patient, as well as her parents, may not be in the optimal state to learn or assimilate new information and apply it consistently. Parents are under a lot of stress when their child is hospitalized. Prioritizing and understanding information can be a challenge. Repeated review and positive reinforcement of the rehabilitation process should be part of every physical

BOX 4-5

An Example of Common Physical Therapy Procedural Interventions Applied to the Acute Care Setting

Therapeutic exercise
Aerobic capacity/endurance activity
Balance and coordination training
Body mechanics for bed mobility and transfers
Gait training/stair negotiation
Muscle strengthening
Functional training in self-care
ADL training
   Dressing
   Using the toilet
   Washing face/combing hair/brushing teeth
Device/equipment training
   Using crutches/walker
   Using orthotics
Injury prevention
Manual therapy techniques
   Range of motion
   Joint mobilization
Airway clearance techniques
   Postural drainage
   Percussion
   Coughing techniques
   Breathing exercises
Integumentary repair and protection

therapist's protocol for patient and family interaction in the acute care setting.

Procedural interventions used in the acute care setting can include the variety of those provided by physical therapists as listed in the *Guide to Physical Therapist Practice*.[61,62] These can range from airway clearance techniques to therapeutic exercise. Box 4-5 lists some examples of procedural interventions. Intervention can include activities in a physical therapy department where additional equipment is available. If the patient is able to leave the unit, physical therapy intervention in the department or gym may provide access to mat tables, parallel bars, modalities, and steps that are not easily accessed on the unit. The application of modalities to decrease pain or increase range of motion can be applied prior to strengthening exercises to allow for a more efficient execution of the exercise. Exercises using resistance as well as aerobic and endurance training through use of a treadmill or stationary bicycle are also commonly seen in the physical therapy department.

 POINT TO REMEMBER

Physical Therapy Interventions

Communication, coordination, and documentation are the most important physical therapy interventions in the acute care setting.

With children who have sustained lower extremity or pelvic fractures or have undergone orthopedic surgery on a leg, the physical therapist is often asked to teach the child to walk with crutches or a walker. As a general guideline, it is recommended that children who are younger than 6 years, have coordination difficulties, or are fearful of walking be taught to ambulate with a walker. The main limitation of using a walker is that it cannot be used on stairs, and a child will ambulate at a slower rate. A young child who is using a walker can be taught to go up and down stairs on his buttocks, or an adult can carry him. Children who are 6 years old or older and do not have coordination issues are taught to use axillary crutches. Crutches can assist a child to negotiate stairs, although it is always recommended to use a railing, if available, with the crutches.

POINT TO REMEMBER

When to Use a Walker Instead of Crutches

As a general guideline, it is recommended that children who are younger than 6 years, have coordination difficulties, or are fearful of walking, be taught to ambulate with a walker.

Transitioning

When the patient is medically stable, the medical staff may consider discharge from the acute care hospital to home or another setting, such as a rehabilitation hospital. When discharge comes close for the patient, it is the role of the physical therapist in this setting to give input as to whether further physical therapy services are needed for the patient and, if so, whether an in-house rehabilitation facility or an outpatient facility is recommended. Generally, when the patient is medically stable, the health care team would decide if the patient's current impairments and functional limitations require a certain level of professional input to achieve a prior level of functioning or rehabilitation. Can the parents adequately manage the impairments or functional limi-

POINTS TO REMEMBER

Discharge Criteria

The patient is symptomatically stable.
The patient's current impairments and functional limitations are adequately managed with the assistance of a knowledgeable caregiver (at home: parent; at a rehabilitation hospital or outpatient clinic: physical therapist).
Follow-up visits have been coordinated and scheduled.

tations, or do the limitations require the skilled intervention and knowledge of rehabilitation professionals? Is the patient appropriate for outpatient services, or will she require placement in a rehabilitation hospital? When these issues have been determined, the nurse is typically in charge of making sure that all follow-up visits have been made with the appropriate providers and the family.

■   C A S E   S T U D Y   ■

Joann

Inpatient. Status: post posterior spinal fusion. Medical diagnosis: Scoliosis, status post (s/p) Posterior Spinal Fusion (PSF) with bone graft.

Joann is a 14-year-old girl who has a medical diagnosis of a 40° right thoracic adolescent idiopathic scoliosis (AIS). The scoliosis was corrected surgically through the placement of Herrington rods and spinal fusion using a bone graft from the right iliac crest. Presently, Joann is s/p surgery day one. She is in pain, which limits her motion, and is lethargic secondary to anesthesia.

Impairments: She is unable to perform bed mobility without assistance, transition to sit independently, or ambulate independently secondary to pain and decreased endurance.

Functional limitations: Her limitations impair her from exploring her environment, and at present from going back to school (disability).

Systems Review

Cardiovascular/Pulmonary: From medical record, hematocrit (Hct) 35%; hemoglobin (Hgb) 15 g/dL. Body temperature is 37°C. Patient is on 2 L of oxygen via nasal cannula. From monitor, blood pressure = 120/80; respiration rate = 12; pulse = 84 beats per minute regular. Pulse oxygen is 97%.

Neuromuscular: Gross sensation to touch intact in the lower extremities. Patient is on IV morphine, PCA.

Musculoskeletal: Gross range of motion of upper extremities is within functional limits (WFL). Gross lower extremity active movement is limited secondary to pain. Supine posture is unremarkable. Patient is 5 feet 4 inches tall and weighs 135 pounds.

Communication: Not impaired.

Integumentary: No prior surgery to low back reported. Surgical wound dressed. No leakage noted.

Test and Measures

Patient is alert and oriented ×3. Her mother is present. Parent reports that Joann lives at home with both parents and two younger siblings. Parent reports that there are five steps to get into the house and another 12 to go to the second floor that contains Joann's bedroom and the only bathroom in the house. There is a handrail on the right. The school that Joann attends is a single-story building.

Joann reports no episodes of urination. She has not been out of bed since surgery. She has not taken any food by mouth since before surgery. She complains of feeling lightheaded and nauseous, but no episodes of emesis. Joann rates pain 7/10 in her back and right hip, in the area of the iliac crest. Sensation to light touch and sharp/dull discrimination is intact along the dermatomes L3 to S1.

Leg lengths appear equal. In supine the legs are externally rotated equally.

No edema noted in the lower extremities.

Capillary refill time is <3 seconds in both feet.

Bilateral upper extremity strength is 5/5 in upper trapezius, middle deltoids, biceps, and triceps muscles. Grip strength is symmetrical bilateral with appropriate cocontraction of the muscles that cross the wrist joint noted. Bilateral lower extremity ankle dorsiflexion and plantar flexion strength are 5/5. Other manual muscle test (MMT) deferred secondary to patient's report of pain with hip and knee movements when supine.

Limitations in trunk range of motion secondary to pain and postsurgical precautions. Pain in back increases to 9/10 when transitioning supine to sit. Pain decreases when in stance. Pain is localized to the back and right hip with no radiation reported.

Impairments:

Pain

Impaired joint mobility

Decreased range of motion

Decreased endurance

Limited independence in activities of daily living (ADL)

Diagnostic Pattern: Impaired Joint Mobility, Motor Function, Muscle Performance, and Range of Motion Associated with Bony and Soft Tissue Surgery

GOALS

1. Patient will transition supine to sit with minimal assistance to allow her to function in her home with the assist of one parent.
2. Patient will transition sit to stand independently to allow her to rise from a toilet.
3. Patient will ambulate 200 feet over level surfaces within 1 day in order to allow her to access rooms in her home.
4. Patient will ascend and descend 15 steps with the assist of a handrail in order to access the second floor of her house.
5. Caregiver will be able to verbalize precautions to excessive spine movements during the healing phase of surgery in order to decrease the risk of injury to the surgical site.

PHYSICAL THERAPY INTERVENTIONS

Patient Education:

1. Education regarding the effects of morphine on feeling lightheaded, dizzy, and nauseous.
2. Deep breathing and pursed-lipped breathing exercises will aid in pain management.

3. The importance of deep breathing for pain management and walking to aid in gastrointestinal mobility. When moving, do not hold your breath.
4. Reinforced log rolling and use of upper extremities to move from side lie to sit with proper breathing. Movement initially will cause some discomfort, but when up and walking she should feel better and the pain will subside.

Aerobic Capacity/Endurance; Body Mechanics; Muscle Performance; Gait:

Elevate the head of the bed (HOB) to 60 degrees for 10 minutes to allow for her to adjust to the upright position.

Have her move to the edge of the bed (EOB) then place her feet on the floor.

Assist her to transition sit to stand. After standing, Joann should keep her eyes open and focus on breathing.

Begin ambulation with moderate assist (two points of contact on the patient). Measure distance in feet, noting standard tiles on hospital floor are typically 1 foot long.

Return to room and sit upright in chair for at least 1 hour.

Provide additional pillows to the back of chair to allow for a more upright posture.

Caregiver Education:

Instruct family or nurse in proper guarding or assistance of Joann to transition her sit to stand or sit to supine safely.

TREATMENT

Second visit in the afternoon, repeat morning activities. Increase endurance and add step-ups or stair climbing.

OUTCOMES

Patient has met 4/4 (100%) of the goals stated in her initial evaluation. Parents (caregivers) were able to verbalize precautions to excessive movement of the spine. Patient is safe to discharge to home with her parents. Physician will release to return to school.

Reflection Questions

1. Often patients who undergo spinal stabilization via autographs have pain at the donor site postsurgery. Joann had significant pain at the donor site. How do you think this may affect her rehabilitation?
2. How would the interventions differ if the scoliosis were due to a nonmalignant tumor or an asymmetry in muscle tone?
3. If Joann remains on IV pain medications, ascending and descending 12 stairs would be limited secondary to the IV pole and pump. What alternate therapeutic exercises can be incorporated into her program to promote stair negotiation?

SUMMARY

The physical therapist plays an important role in both the NICU and the pediatric acute care hospital. In the NICU, the physical therapist provides a valuable service in caregiver education, positioning and handling of the infant, facilitation of oral motor development, prevention of impairments, and encouragement of sensorimotor development. When the infant is medically stable and demonstrates a consistent pattern of weight gain, and the parents are competent in the care of the infant, the infant may then be discharged home. If additional ongoing medical care is needed, the infant may be transferred to the inpatient unit. Any physical therapist who plans on working with infants and families in the NICU should be competent to deal with the variety of unique experiences and specialized skills needed in this practice setting.

In the acute care hospital, the physical therapist can help minimize the effects of the hospitalization on the pediatric patient's motor skills and function during her hospital stay. The primary goal of physical therapy in this setting is to promote recovery and optimal independence, including mobility, given the current medical status of the patient. When the patient is medically stable, the physical therapist plays a key role in the recommendation of future physical therapy services, through either an outpatient or inpatient rehabilitation setting.

REVIEW QUESTIONS

1. Which of the following infants would be considered to be born prematurely?
   a. Amanda, who was born at 41 weeks' gestation.
   b. Bert, who was born at 38 weeks' gestation.
   c. Caleb, who was born at 36 weeks' gestation.
   d. All of the above.
2. Maria was born weighing 3 pounds 8 ounces. She would be considered:
   a. Within the normal range of birth weight
   b. LBW
   c. Very LBW
   d. Macrosomal
3. You are performing an examination of an infant born at 28 weeks' gestation. During the examination, which of the following would provide you with the best information regarding the infant's tolerance to your tests and measurements?
   a. Monitoring increases in heart rate and respiratory rate and decreases in oxygen saturation.
   b. Monitoring the infant's ability to attend by noting her eye movements and ability to maintain a gaze.
   c. Monitoring the amount of time that you perform any one test or measurement. Limiting your tests to 60 seconds will allow the infant to sufficiently rest between tests.
   d. Performing the necessary tests and measurements as the infant allows, or until the infant cries, which will tell you that the sensory input is too much for her.
4. Which of the following states of infant behavior would be the optimal state for infant learning?
   a. The infant is randomly moving with noted eye movement under closed eyelids. Irregular abdominal breathing is noted.

b. The infant displays variable movement with a delayed response noted to sensory stimuli when presented. The infant is demonstrating facial grimacing.
   c. The infant displays minimal movement. Eyes are open, and the infant appears to be looking at an object in the incubator.
   d. The infant is very active and aroused. She may be fussy but does not cry. She looks briefly at the objects in her incubator.
5. Which of the following positions would be the optimal position to facilitate an infant's hands to midline and hands to mouth when in an incubator?
   a. Prone
   b. Supine
   c. Side lie
   d. Supported sitting
6. You receive a referral to evaluate an infant in the hospital's NICU. After review of the medical record, which of the following should you do next?
   a. Consult with the infant's nurse to coordinate care in order to minimize the disturbance of the infant.
   b. Perform a systems review on the infant.
   c. Provide the infant with a pacifier soaked in sucrose to minimize the discomfort and stress from the examination.
   d. Begin your examination of the infant noting the state of behavior before, during, and after the evaluation is completed.
7. Your patient has undergone a posterior spinal fusion and is now 1 day postoperative. Physical therapy has been ordered to get the patient out of bed and ambulating. She is on an IV of morphine for pain. The nurse gives her a bolus of morphine via IV. How much time will elapse before the patient will experience the effects of the medication?
   a. The patient should experience pain relief immediately.
   b. The patient should experience pain relief within 10 minutes.
   c. The patient should experience pain relief within 30 minutes.
   d. The patient should experience pain relief within 45 minutes.
8. As a general rule, a child who is nonweight bearing through his lower extremity can be taught to use axillary crutches for gait training if he is at least how old?
   a. 2 years of age
   b. 4 years of age
   c. 6 years of age
   d. 8 years of age
9. You are working on the medical-surgical floor of the hospital. Your next patient is in isolation due to VRE infection. Which of the following PPE would most likely be needed with this type of infection?

a. Mask
b. Mask and gloves
c. Gloves and gown
d. Mask, gloves, and gown

10. You are physical therapist A and are planning a discharge from the inpatient hospital for a 7-year-old patient. This patient was admitted to the hospital and had a dorsal rhizotomy for the management of spasticity. The physical therapist from the rehabilitation hospital (physical therapist B) calls you for an update on the discharge process and background information on the patient. Of the following, which would be the most appropriate thing to do?

a. Discuss with physical therapist B the current status of the patient and what information that patient and his family have already received and what he will need.
b. Check the patient's medical chart to see to whom the family authorized the release of information. Do not discuss anything with physical therapist B until you get consent from the family to do so.
c. Do not discuss anything with physical therapist B, even if you have the family's consent. Discharge information is only given out by the nurse.
d. You can discuss with physical therapist B only the patient's name and current medical status and the planned date of discharge. All other information will have to be provided by written report.

Developmental Evaluation Form

PATIENT PROFILE
DEVELOPMENTAL

PHYSICAL THERAPY DEPARTMENT
FORM NO. 7500-DF357A (REV. 9-97)

LOCATION:
- ☐ Fifth Avenue
- ☐ North
- ☐ South
- ☐ East
- ☐ _____

PATIENT NAME

UNIT NUMBER

BIRTH DATE

Addressograph Plate Area

- ☐ Inpatient
- ☐ Outpatient
- ☐ SDS Pre-Op
- ☐ SDS Post-Op
- ☐ Initial Evaluation
- ☐ Discharge Summary

PATIENT HISTORY

EVALUATION

GENERAL OBSERVATIONS

BEHAVIORAL STATE

PROM   Upper Extremities   Lower Extremities
  WFL except for:

Neck / Trunk

TONE   Upper Extremities   Lower Extremities
  WNL except for:

Neck / Trunk

KEY (ASHWORTH SCALE MODIFIED)

0 = Hypotonic, 1 = Normal, 2 = Slight Increase in resistance through part of range, 3 = More marked resistance through most of range
4 = Considerable increase in resistance; passive movement is difficult, 5 = Rigid in flexion and / or extension, FI = Fluctuating tone

SENSORY

REFLEXES

Rooting	Palmar grasp	Asymmetrical tonic neck		Protective ext. downward (LE)
Moro	Plantar grasp	Tonic labyrinthine		Protective ext. forward (UE)
Traction	Spontaneous stepping	Tonic labyrinthine		Protective ext. sideward (UE)
Crossed Extension	Landau	Positive support (WB) UE		Protective ext. backward (UE)
Flexor withdrawal	Head righting	Positive support (WB) LE		

KEY: NL = normal for age, + = present, ± = equivocal, ↑ = obligatory, A = asymmetry, - = absent

PATIENT NAME	UNIT NUMBER

EVALUATION (continued)
DEVELOPMENTAL SKILLS
Supine
Sidelying
Prone
Sitting
Standing
Transitions / Mobility
EQUIPMENT
HANDLING / POSITIONING INSTRUCTION
ASSESSMENT
PLAN
GOALS
RECOMMENDATIONS

SIGNATURE PHYSICAL THERAPIST	DATE

Department of Physical Therapy. Children's Hospital of Pittsburgh. Pittsburgh, PA. 2007, with permission.

Gait Evaluation Form Used with Inpatients

GAIT TRAINING ASSESSMENT

PHYSICAL MEDICINE DEPARTMENT
FORM NO. 7500-DF2018A (10-97)

LOCATION:
☐ Fifth Avenue
☐ North
☐ South
☐ East
☐ _____

PATIENT NAME

UNIT NUMBER

BIRTH DATE

Addressograph Plate Area

☐ Inpatient   ☐ SDS Pre-Op   ☐ Initial Evaluation
☐ Outpatient   ☐ SDS Post-Op   ☐ Discharge Summary

PATIENT HISTORY

HOME SITUATION

	YES	NO		YES	NO
Parent/guardian supervision at all times	☐	☐			
Stairs to enter (#) _____	☐	☐	Railing	☐	☐
Stairs to bed/bathroom _____	☐	☐	Railing	☐	☐
Stairs at school _____	☐	☐	Railing	☐	☐
Prior use of device _____	☐	☐	Other home equipment		

EVALUATION

GENERAL OBSERVATIONS

ROM/POSTURE   Within functional limits except for:

STRENGTH   Within functional limits except for:

FUNCTIONAL MOBILITY   WB Status: R / L   LE   NWB   TDWB   PWB   WBAT   Other: _____

Assistive device: Crutches   Walker   Other: _____

	Independent	Supervision	Contact Guard	ASSIST Minimal	ASSIST Moderate	ASSIST Maximal
TRANSFERS: Bed to / from Wheelchair						
Sit to / from Stand						
AMBULATION: Level surface (Distance _____)						
Stairs (#____ Rail _____)						
☐ On buttocks ☐ Parent demonstrates safe guarding						

ASSESSMENT

HOME SITUATION
Safe for discharge home at above status
Would benefit from further gait training due to:
☐ Poor balance   ☐ Poor coordination   ☐ Pain   ☐ Decreased strength   ☐ Poor endurance   ☐ Parent unavailable

GOALS (to be achieved by discharge)
☐ Patient will transfer   bed to / from wheelchair   sit to / from stand _____
☐ Patient will ambulate _____ feet _____ on level surfaces with walker / crutches, _____ weightbearing _____
☐ Patient demonstrates safe and appropriate guarding and assistance
☐ Patient will be provided with written instructions regarding proper use of device with prescribed weightbearing status
☐ Patient will be provided with home exercises and demonstrate good technique of such to address ROM / strength deficit(s)

PLAN

☐ See BID in Physical Therapy department for: transfer / gait training
☐ Patient discharged from Physical Therapy
☐ Recommend outpatient Physical Therapy after cast / hardware removal to increaase patient's strenth, ROM, and function

SIGNATURE

PHYSICAL THERAPIST'S SIGNATURE   DATE

Department of Physical Therapy. Children's Hospital of Pittsburgh. Pittsburgh, PA. 2007, with permission.

REFERENCES

1. Sultz H, Young K. *Health Care USA. Understanding Its Organization and Delivery*, 4th ed. Boston: Jones and Bartlett; 2004.
2. The U.S. Department of Health and Human Services, Centers for Disease Control and Prevention. Standard Precautions. Excerpted from Guidelines for Isolation Precaution in Hospitals (January 1996). Date last modified April 1, 2005. Available at: http://www.cdc.gov/ncidod/dhqp/gl_isolation_standard.html. Accessed April 29, 2006.
3. Health Insurance Portability and Accountability Act of 1996. Public Law 104-191.
4. JCAHO Standards 2005. Available at: http://www.jointcommission.org/. Accessed May 12, 2006.
5. Vergara E. Historical evolution of the neonatal therapist's role. In Vergara E, ed. *Developmental and Therapeutic Interventions in the NICU*. Baltimore, MD: Paul H. Brookes; 2004.
6. Agency for Healthcare Research and Quality (AHRQ). Excerpted from National Guideline Clearinghouse. Bibliographic source: Stark AR, Couto J. Levels of neonatal care. *Pediatrics*. 2004;114(5):1341–1347. [47 references] Available at: http://www.guideline.gov/summary/summary.aspx?view id=1&doc_id=5986. Accessed March 12, 2007.
7. Bozzette M, Kenner C. The neonatal intensive care unit environment. In: Kenner C, McGrath JM, eds. *Developmental Care of Newborns & Infants: A Guide for Health Professionals*. St. Louis, MO: Mosby; 2004.
8. Hendricks-Munoz K, Predergast C, Caprio M, et al. Developmental care: the impact of Wee Care developmental training on short-term infant outcome and hospital costs. *Newborn Infant Nurs Rev*. 2002;2:39–45.
9. Niermeyer S, Clarke S. Delivery room care. In: Merenstein GB, Gardner SL, eds. *Handbook of Neonatal Intensive Care*, 5th ed. St. Louis, MO: Mosby; 2002.
10. Vergara E. Physical context, equipment, environment stressors, and sources of support in the NICU. In: Vergara E, ed. *Developmental and Therapeutic Interventions in the NICU*. Baltimore, MD: Paul H. Brookes; 2004.
11. Blake W, Murray J. Heat balance. In: Merenstein G, Gardner S, eds. *Handbook of Neonatal Intensive Care*, 5th ed. St. Louis, MO: Mosby; 2002.
12. Heiss-Harris G. Common invasive procedures. In: Verklan MT, Walden M, eds. *Core Curriculum for Neonatal Intensive Care Nursing*, 3rd ed. St. Louis, MO: Elsevier Saunders; 2004.
13. March of Dimes. Common NICU Equipment. Available at: http://www.marchofdimes.com/prematurity/21278–11032.asp. Accessed March 12, 2007.
14. KidsHealth. Nemours Foundation. When Your Baby's in the NICU. Available at: http://kidshealth.org/parent/system/ill/nicu_caring.html. Accessed March 12, 2007.
15. Gardner S, Goldson E. The neonate and the environment: impact on development. In: Merenstein G, Gardner S, eds. *Handbook of Neonatal Intensive Care*, 5th ed. St. Louis, MO: Mosby; 2002.
16. Vergara E. Developmental capabilities of preterm and low birth weight infants. In: Vergara E, ed. *Developmental and Therapeutic Interventions in the NICU*. Baltimore, MD: Paul H. Brookes; 2004.
17. Brazelton T. *Neonatal Behavioral Assessment Scale. Clinics in developmental medicine: No. 50*. Philadelphia: Lippincott, Williams & Wilkins; 1973.
18. Long T, Toscano K. Pediatric conditions. In: Long T, Toscano K, eds. *Handbook of Pediatric Physical Therapy*, 2nd ed. Philadelphia: Lippincott, Williams & Wilkins; 2002.
19. Hoyert DL, Mathews TJ, Menacker F, et al. Annual summary of vital statistics: 2004. *Pediatrics*. 2006;117(1):168–183.
20. Kochanek K, Martin J. Supplemental Analyses of Recent Trends in Infant Mortality. U.S. Department of Health and Human Resources. Centers for Disease Control and Prevention. 2007. Available at: http://www.cdc.gov/nchs/products/pubs/pubd/hestats/infantmort/infantmort.htm. Accessed March 13, 2007.
21. Larsen P, Stensaas S. PediNeuroLogic Exam: A Neurodevelopmental Approach. Newborn > Normal. Available at: http://library.med.utah.edu/pedineurologicexam/html/newborn_n.html. Accessed March 12, 2007.
22. McGrath G. Neurologic development. In: Kenner C, McGrath J, eds. *Developmental Care of Newborns & Infants: A Guide for Health Professionals*. St. Louis, MO: Mosby; 2004.
23. Vergara E. Developmental capabilities of full-term NICU infants. In: Vergara E, ed. *Developmental and Therapeutic Interventions in the NICU*. Baltimore, MD: Paul H. Brookes; 2004.
24. Iannelli V. keepkidshealthy.com. A Pediatrician's Guide to Your Children's Health and Safety. Available at: http://www.keepkidshealthy.com/newborn/newborn_reflexes.html. Accessed March 12, 2007.
25. Lutes L, Graves C, Jorgense K. The NICU experience and its relationship to sensory integration. In: Kenner C, McGrath J, eds. *Developmental Care of Newborns & Infants: A Guide for Health Professionals*. St. Louis, MO: Mosby; 2004.
26. Harrison L. Research utilization: handling preterm infants in the NICU. *Neonatal Netw*. 1997;16:65–69.
27. Barr R, Quek V, Cousineau D, et al. Effects of intra-oral sucrose on crying, mouthing, and hand-to-mouth contact in newborn and six-week-old infants. *Dev Med Child Neurol*. 1994;36:608–618.
28. DeCasper A, Fifer W. Of human bonding: newborns prefer their mother's voices. *Science*. 1980;208:1175.
29. Sweeney J, Gutierrez T. Motor development chronology: a dynamic process. In: Kenner C, McGrath J, eds. *Developmental Care of Newborns & Infants: A Guide for Health Professionals*. St. Louis, MO: Mosby; 2004.
30. Van Heijst J, Touwen B, Vos J. Implications of a neural network model of sensori-motor development for the field of developmental neurology. *Early Hum Dev*. 1999;55:77–95.
31. Hunter J. Positioning. In: Kenner C, McGrath J, eds. *Developmental Care of Newborns & Infants: A Guide for Health Professionals*. St. Louis, MO: Mosby; 2004.
32. Walden M, Franck L. Identification, management, and prevention of newborn/infant pain. In Kenner C, Lott JW, eds. *Comprehensive Neonatal Nursing: A Physiologic Perspective*, 3rd ed. St. Louis: W.B. Saunders; 2003.
33. Grunau R, Holsti L, Whitfield M, et al. Are twitches, startles, and body movements pain indictors in extremely low birth weight infants? *Clin J Pain*. 2000;16:37–45.
34. Craig K, Whitfield M, Grunau R, et al. Pain in the preterm neonate: behavioral and physiological indices. *Pain*. 1993;52:287–299.
35. Stevens B, Johnston CC, Horton L. Factors that influence the behavioral pain responses of premature infants. *Pain*. 1994;59:101–109.
36. Walden M, Jorgensen K. Pain management. In: Kenner C, McGrath JM, eds. *Developmental Care of Newborns & Infants: A Guide for Health Professionals*. St. Louis, MO: Mosby; 2004.
37. Agarwal R, Hagedorn M, Gardner S. Pain and pain relief. In: Merenstein G, Gardner S, eds. *Handbook of Neonatal Intensive Care*, 5th ed. St. Louis, MO: Mosby; 2002.
38. Stevens B, Taddio A, Ohlsson A, et al. The efficacy of sucrose for relieving procedural pain in neonates: a systematic review and meta-analysis. *Acta Paediatr*. 1997;86:837–842.
39. Krechel S, Bilder J. CRIES: a new neonatal post-operative pain measurement score: initial testing of validity and reliability. *Paediatr Anaesth*. 1995;5:53–61.

40. Stevens B, Johnston C, Petryshen P, et al. Premature infant pain profile: development and initial validation. *Clin J Pain*. 1996;12:13–22.

41. Lawrence J, Alcock D, McGrath P, et al. The development of a tool to assess neonatal pain. *Neonatal Netw*. 1993;12:59–66.

42. Hummel P, Puchalski M. Establishing initial reliability & validity of the N-PASS: Neonatal Pain, Agitation, and Sedation Scale. Poster presentation at Association for Women's Health, Obstetric, and Neonatal Nursing (AWHONN) 2002 National Convention, Boston, MA, June 23–26.

43. Vergara E. Elements of neonatal positioning. In: Vergara E, ed. *Developmental and Therapeutic Interventions in the NICU*. Baltimore, MD: Paul H. Brookes; 2004.

44. Lockridge T, Taquino L, Knight A. Back to sleep: is there room in that crib for both AAP recommendations and developmentally supportive care? *Neonatal Netw*. 1999;18:29.

45. Field T. Infant massage therapy. In Goldson E, ed. *Nurturing the Premature Infant*. New York: Oxford University Press; 1999.

46. Browne J. Considerations for touch and massage in the NICU. *Neonatal Netw*. 2000;19:61.

47. Dieter J, Field T, Hernandez-Reif M, et al. Stable preterm infants gain more weight and sleep less after five days of massage therapy. *J Pediatr Psychol*. 2003;28:403–411.

48. Turnage-Carrier C. Caregiving and the environment. In: Kenner C, McGrath J, eds. *Developmental Care of Newborns & Infants: A Guide for Health Professionals*. St. Louis, MO: Mosby; 2004.

49. Moyer-Mileur L, Brunstetter V, McNaught T, et al. Daily physical activity program increases bone mineralization and growth in preterm very low birthweight infants. *Pediatrics*. 2000;106:1088–1092.

50. American Academy of Pediatrics. Hospital Discharge of the High-Risk Neonate. Proposed Guidelines. *Pediatrics*. 1998;102:2:411–417.

51. Cameron DC, Maehle V, Reid J. The effects of an early physical therapy intervention for very, preterm, very low birth weight infants: a randomized controlled clinical trial. *Pediatr Phys Ther*. 2005;17:107–119.

52. Allen M, Donohue P, Porter M. Follow-up of the NICU infant. In: Merenstein G, Gardner S, eds. *Handbook of Neonatal Intensive Care*, 5th ed. St. Louis, MO: Mosby; 2002.

53. Aylward GP, Pfeiffer S. Correlation of asphyxia and other risk factors with outcome: a contemporary view. *Dev Med Child Neurol*. 1989;31:329–340.

54. Guide for the Uniform Data Set for Medical Rehabilitation. (Wee FIM^sm). Guide to the WeeFIM. Version 1.5. Buffalo, NY: Research Foundation—State University of New York; 1991.

55. Duncan P, Weiner D, Chandler J, et al. Functional reach: a new measure of balance. *J Gerontol Med Sci*. 1990;45: 192–197.

56. Donahoe B, Turner D, Worrell T. The use of functional reach as a measurement of balance in boys and girls without disabilities ages 5 to 15 years. *Pediatr Phys Ther*. 1994;6: 189–193.

57. Podsiadlo D, Richardson S. The Timed 'Up and Go Test': a test of basic functional mobility for frail elderly persons. *J Am Geriatr Soc*. 1991;39:142–148.

58. Williams E, Carroll S, Reddihough D, Phillips B, Galea M. Investigation of the timed "Up and Go" test in children. *Dev Med Child Neurol*. 2005;47:518–524.

59. O'Rourke D. The measurement of pain in infants, children, and adolescents: from policy to practice. *Phys Ther J*. 2004;84:560–570.

60. Bulloch B, Tenenbein M. Validation of 2 pain scales for use in the pediatric emergency department. *Pediatrics*. 2002;110:e33.

61. American Physical Therapy Association. *Guide to Physical Therapist Practice*, 2nd ed. Alexandria, VA: Rev. American Physical Therapy Association; 2003.

62. Vergara E. Medical management of high-risk infants. In: Vergara E, ed. *Developmental and Therapeutic Interventions in the NICU*. Baltimore, MD: Paul H. Brookes; 2004.

63. Wong D, Hockenberry-Eaton M, Wilson D, et al., eds. *Nursing Care of Infants and Children*, 2nd ed. St. Louis, MO: Mosby; 1991.

64. McGrath P, deVeber L, Hearn M. Multidimensional pain assessment in children. In: Fields H, Dubner R, Cervero F, eds. *Proceedings of the Fourth World Congress on Pain*. New York: Raven Press; 1985.

65. McGrath PA, Seifert CE, Speechley KN, et al. A new analog scale for assessing children's pain: an initial validation study. *Pain*. 1996;64:435–443.

66. Bieri D, Reeve RA, Champion GD, et al. The Faces Pain Scale for the self-assessment of the severity of pain experienced by children: development, initial validation, and preliminary investigation for ratio scale properties. *Pain*. 1990;41:139–150.

Additional Resources

Sweeney J, Heriza C, Reilly M, et al. Practice guidelines for the physical therapist in the neonatal intensive care unit (NICU). *Pediatr Phys Ther*. 1999;11:119–132.

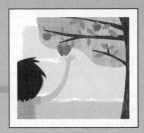

C H A P T E R **5**

Providing Services in the Clinical Setting: Rehabilitation and Outpatient

Meg Stanger

LEARNING OBJECTIVES

1. Understand the various factors, including legal, regulatory, family, and patient presentation that influence decision making in the rehabilitation setting.
2. Discern the differences in service delivery between inpatient and outpatient rehabilitation settings.
3. Understand the role and responsibilities of the physical therapist as part of a comprehensive rehabilitation team.
4. Delineate appropriate tests and measures and interventions to be utilized in the rehabilitation setting.
5. Determine and justify need for assistive and adaptive devices to augment the rehabilitation process.
6. Recognize the role of the physical therapist in transitioning the patient through the rehabilitation setting to school and/or community facilities.

This chapter will discuss the provision of physical therapy services in both the inpatient and outpatient pediatric rehabilitation settings. Topics will include regulatory standards, expected patient outcomes, reimbursement, and service delivery that can impact clinical decision making. Patient care discussions will address decision making regarding use of orthotic devices, assistive technology, and transition to home and the relevance of physical therapy carryover in the home environment.

The rehabilitation setting includes children of varying ages and diagnoses. The types of children and diagnoses seen in a rehabilitation setting may range from those children with a congenital or chronic diagnosis such as cerebral palsy to children who were growing and developing typically until they sustained an injury or were diagnosed with a disease process. An inpatient rehabilitation unit would typically include children who sustained a traumatic brain injury (TBI), spinal cord injury, near-drowning occurrence, multiple orthopedic injuries, juvenile rheumatoid arthritis, pain syndromes, or burns or children who may have had surgery to remove a newly diagnosed brain tumor. Other children may have a chronic diagnosis such as cerebral palsy and may be admitted to the unit for intensive rehabilitation following orthopedic surgery, a dorsal rhizotomy procedure, or the implantation of a pump for intrathecal baclofen.

The child and the family can be at various stages in the acceptance process of a diagnosis or may be dealing with the possibility of death or a significant change in the child's ability to function. Some families will be able to identify very clear and precise goals, whereas others may only identify broad goals such as "I want him to do everything he could do before the accident" or "I just want him to have everything he needs to be healthy."

THE PRACTICE ENVIRONMENT

Many inpatient pediatric rehabilitation hospitals were started 80 to 100 years ago as places to care for children with disabilities resulting from the polio epidemic or congenital orthopedic diagnoses. They were often initially funded by a local wealthy family and established in country or seaside settings away from the overcrowded and industry-polluted cities. Over the past several decades, many of these independent facilities have become fully accredited rehabilitation hospitals that are part of a larger, university-affiliated medical system.

An inpatient rehabilitation unit may be a smaller unit within a larger pediatric acute care medical center, or it may be a freestanding facility that receives patients from the surrounding community hospitals. Outpatient facilities may be community-based satellites of a large medical system or freestanding units. Outpatient centers may also be part of a national or state pediatric rehabilitation network such as the Easter Seal Societies and United Cerebral Palsy Centers. In addition, a physical therapist may establish a freestanding private practice. Access to each of these environments is determined by state licensure laws, reimbursement regulations, and procedures unique to each facility. There are many federal and state laws that affect the delivery of health care in a variety of settings.

The Federal Government

The Department of Health and Human Services (DHHS) is the government's primary agency that is responsible for protecting the health of all Americans and for providing health services to identified populations. DHHS includes >300 services or programs covering a variety of topics (such as improving maternal and child health, preventing child abuse and domestic violence), as well as medical and social science research. DHHS manages these activities through operating divisions such as the National Institutes of Health, the Food and Drug Administration, the Centers for Disease Control and Prevention, the Centers for Medicare & Medicaid Services (CMS), and the Administration for Children and Families, and the National Center for Medical Rehabilitation Research (NCMRR), to name a few. Box 5-1 lists the research initiatives of NCMRR.

In addition, Congress has passed several significant pieces of legislation that influence the delivery of health care. Each chapter of this book highlights some of the significant pieces of legislation as they pertain to the chapter's practice setting. Some of the more applicable laws that pertain to the rehabilitation and outpatient setting include the *Technology-Related Assistance for Individuals with Disabilities Act* of 1988 (PL 100-407) also referred to as the Tech Act, The Americans with Disabilities Act (ADA), the Patient Self-Determination Act of 1990, and the Health Insurance Portability and Accountability Act, also known as HIPAA (1996).

POINT TO REMEMBER

DHHS

DHHS is the government's primary agency that is responsible for protecting the health of all Americans. Additional information about DHHS is available at www.hhs.gov.

The Tech Act recognizes that technological advances would benefit individuals with disabilities and aims to provide states with federal funding to implement technology assistance programs.[1] *Assistive technology* is defined as "any item, piece of equipment or product system, whether acquired commercially off the shelf, modified, or customized, that is used to increase, maintain, or improve the functional capabilities of individuals with disabilities" (Section 3a(2)). Assistive technology ranges from low-tech devices such as walkers or bath seats to high-tech equipment such as powered mobility systems and communication devices with various methods of switch activation. In addition, the law defines assistive technology services as evaluation, selection of the device, and training in the use of the device.

The *Americans with Disability Act of 1990* (ADA) of 1990 prohibits discrimination and ensures equal opportunity for individuals with disabilities in employment, public transportation, public accommodations, and telecommunications.[2] The physical therapist working in a rehabilitation setting should assist the child and family with the development of goals that will prepare for transition to an accessible work and living environment as a young adult. See Chapter 10 for more information on the ADA.

BOX 5-1
The National Center for Medical Rehabilitation Research Initiatives

- Improving functional mobility.
- Promoting behavioral adaptation to functional losses.
- Assessing the efficacy and outcomes to medical rehabilitation therapies and practices.
- Developing improved assistive technology.
- Understanding whole-body system responses to physical impairments and functional changes.
- Developing more precise methods of measuring impairments, disabilities, and societal and functional limitations.
- Training research scientists in the field of rehabilitation.

From Research Plan for the National Center for Medical Rehabilitation Research. National Institute of Child Health and Human Development. National Institutes of Health. U.S. Department of Health and Human Services. Public Health Service. NIH Publication No. 93–3509. March 1993.

The Patient Self-Determination Act requires health care facilities that participate in Medicare and Medicaid to give adult individuals information regarding the hospital's policies on advance directives and the patient's right to accept or refuse treatment should the adult patient become incompetent during the hospitalization.[3] This Act defines an *adult patient* as a person 18 years old or older. Therefore, any pediatric rehabilitation facility that provides services to young adults must adhere to these regulations often thought to pertain to only adult facilities. Patients older than 18 years have the right to consent to treatment, refuse treatment, and to formulate advance directives regarding the health care provided. The two most common types of advance directives are (i) a living will, and (ii) a designated durable power of attorney. One purpose of this law is to address the confusion and ambiguity that may arise when an adult patient becomes incompetent during the hospitalization. Clear, written instructions help in the decision-making process in the event of the occurrence of this type of situation. If the patient is younger than 18 years, a parent or legal guardian must provide the necessary consent for treatment and is responsible for the decisions if a grave situation arises during the hospitalization.

HIPAA includes rules to protect the privacy and security of exchange of individually identifiable health information.[4] Patient information that is exchanged among providers must be de-identified, and only the minimum information necessary is exchanged. The adult patient, or parents or adult guardian of a minor, must sign consents for release of information before that information is shared. For example, a physical therapist working in a rehabilitation center cannot call the physical therapist in another outpatient clinic and discuss a patient without a signed consent. HIPAA applies to all government health plans, managed care plans, and many private health plans as well as health care providers such as hospitals, ambulatory care centers, home care agencies, and durable medical equipment suppliers.

In addition to federal laws and regulations, most rehabilitation hospitals are accredited through an external organization such as the *Joint Commission on Accreditation of Healthcare Organizations* (JCAHO) and/or the *Commission on Accreditation of Rehabilitation Facilities* (CARF) (see Chapter 4 for additional information on JCAHO). The mission of CARF is to promote quality, value, and optimal outcomes of services through accreditation that centers on enhancing the lives of the persons served.[5] CARF accreditation signifies that the facility has demonstrated a commitment to continually enhance the quality of their services and to focus on the satisfaction of the patients served. Examples of values of quality of service are the inclusion of the patient in the design of the service plan, the individualization of services to meet the patient's unique needs, the satisfaction of patients with the services they have received, and the use of data from a continuous performance improvement system to manage the quality of services delivered to patients.

A key element of CARF's strategic plan is to enhance the use of outcomes management as part of a continuous quality performance improvement system. An outcome management system is utilized to measure the performance of a program, both internally over time and with external peers, and to monitor the results of patient outcomes. The information obtained from outcomes measurement is utilized by the organization to manage and improve its programs and to benchmark its programs with similar programs across the country.

POINT TO REMEMBER

Accreditation

JCAHO and CARF accreditation is voluntary. CARF emphasizes satisfaction of the consumer, individualized services to each consumer, and the monitoring of patient outcomes through functional assessments.

In addition to the federal government and nationally recognized accreditation agencies, state governments also enact laws and regulations that influence the delivery of health care services in their state.

The State Government

Each state has a *Physical Therapy Practice Act* that governs the role of physical therapists and physical therapist assistants. Physical therapists can release aspects of their interventions to other professionals and caretakers to insure continuity of care. In the rehabilitation setting, physical therapists will often instruct nursing personnel in positioning and transfer techniques, range-of-motion exercises, and donning and doffing of orthotic devices to provide continuity of care for the patient (see Chapter 1 for more information on State Practice Acts).

States also have specific regulations and laws to protect children from *physical or sexual abuse or neglect*. Physical or sexual abuse and negligent treatment of a child younger than 18 years are clearly defined in the Child Abuse Prevention and Treatment Act of 1974 (Public Law 93-247).[6] Regulations vary from state to state but generally require that any case of suspected child abuse or neglect be reported to the appropriate personnel. Failure to report a case of suspected child abuse or neglect may result in a fine, imprisonment, and/or suspension or revocation of a physical therapist's professional license.

A physical therapist working in care outpatient rehabilitation setting may be the first health professional to see signs of abuse or neglect (refer to Box 5-2, A and B). In this setting, the physical therapist will see patterns of attendance and compliance. During routine outpatient treatment

BOX 5-2
Signs and Symptoms

A. Signs and Symptoms of Neglect

Poor hygiene (soiled clothing, body odors, minimal evidence of routine bathing. May see frequent diaper rash).

Frequent cancellations, "no-shows," or missed appointments.

Lack of compliance with follow-through or home program.

Poor nutrition (child is frequently hungry, underweight, pale, or showing signs of malnourishment).

Lack of follow-through with other medical appointments or treatments.

Poor dental care with evidence of caries.

B. Some Signs and Symptoms of Physical Abuse

Frequent and unexplained bruises, welts, hematomas, etc.

Burns on trunk or extremities (including small burns from cigarettes).

Bony fractures (often may have conflicting cause of injury).

Internal injuries.

POINTS TO REMEMBER

Reimbursement

Reimbursement differs significantly from the inpatient to the outpatient setting. Many third party payers will reimburse for inpatient rehabilitation at a predetermined rate regardless of the individual services provided. Outpatient services are typically billed on a fee-for-service basis.

interventions, the physical therapist may typically have the child remove some clothing, revealing bruises, burns, or welts. The physical therapist is considered a mandatory reporter and is obligated by law to report such occurrences (for more information, see Chapter 13).

Physical therapists also need to be aware of the state's laws that affect *reimbursement issues* (see the Medicaid section in Chapter 10). Reimbursement differs significantly from the inpatient to outpatient setting. In many states, the third party payers have not adopted the Diagnosis-Related Group (DRG) system for inpatient pediatric rehabilitation that is utilized in the acute care and adult rehabilitation settings. However, prior to a child's admission to a rehabilitation unit, a contract for services or individual negotiations that determine a set price per day or length of stay have been determined. This means that the third party payer will reimburse the facility a predetermined rate regardless of the individual services provided or adaptive equipment supplied to the child. Most third party payers will reimburse a medical equipment vendor separately for high end or high-tech assistive technology items such as wheelchairs and communication devices.

Outpatient services are typically billed as a fee for service related to the service performed and the time the physical therapist spent with the patient. Payment may be dependent upon contractual agreements between a provider or facility and the third party payer. Chapter 14 discusses in further detail the reimbursement for physical therapy services and some of the basic billing knowledge needed by a physical therapist to bill accurately and productively.

THE INPATIENT REHABILITATION UNIT

When the patient in an acute care hospital is medically stable, the medical staff may consider discharge from the hospital to home or another setting, such as a rehabilitation hospital. Many general rehabilitation hospitals require that the patient be medically stable in order to participate in rehabilitation. There must be reason to believe that the patient has not met his full level of independence and has the potential to benefit from rehabilitative services. The patient should also be able to tolerate several hours of therapy service a day and have the need for more than one type of rehabilitation service, such as physical therapy, occupational therapy, or speech therapy.

Inpatient rehabilitation provides an intensive comprehensive interdisciplinary approach to the restoration of function for children and adolescents who have sustained injuries or undergone surgical procedures that impact their activity and participation levels compared to their baseline level of function. An inpatient rehabilitation unit can be a freestanding facility or a specialized unit within an acute care hospital. CMS criteria for admission to an inpatient rehabilitation hospital include medical stability and the ability to tolerate a minimum of 3 hours of rehabilitation therapy per day for at least 5 days per week. CMS also classifies hospitals as inpatient facilities by the "75%" rule that requires that patient diagnoses fall into certain diagnostic groups.[7] The majority of the patients seen in most pediatric rehabilitation facilities do not fall under the Medicare diagnosis rulings. Pediatric inpatient rehabilitation hospitals generally follow the CMS criteria for number of hours of therapy as part of their admission criteria, as well as for the patient to be medically stable and have the potential to benefit from interdisciplinary rehabilitation services.

The multidisciplinary inpatient rehabilitation team includes physicians, nurses trained in rehabilitation, dieticians, occupational therapists, physical therapists, speech pathologists, psychologists, social workers, and orthotists. The team is led by a pediatric physiatrist, pediatrician, orthopedist, or neurosurgeon, but this varies among facilities. Other physician subspecialists will be requested for consultation as needed. The child's family and caregivers are an integral part of the team throughout the rehabilitation process. Multidisciplinary teams will function differently among rehabilitation facilities. Some teams may work as an interdisciplinary team or even a transdisciplinary team at times, wherease in other facilities the team will remain a multidisciplinary team with each discipline working separately on its own goals. In the ideal scenario, the team will work as an interdisciplinary team with all members aware of and striving toward the same goals.

Weekly multidisciplinary conferences or *care-coordination conferences* are held on most rehabilitation units. These conferences serve as quick updates for the entire team regarding the patient's progress, plans for discharge, teaching and equipment that is needed prior to discharge, and status of caregivers competency with carryover of care at home. Typically, updates are also provided on the child's functional status. An identified team member, often the physician or the social worker, will meet with the patient and/or family to review the conference findings and plan of care.

Certain inpatient rehabilitation units specialize in one type of patient population such as TBI or spinal cord injury, and have the appropriate staff to meet the unique needs of patients with these specific diagnoses. Regardless of the specialty, admission to an inpatient rehabilitation unit would be followed by an examination and evaluation of the patient.

POINT TO REMEMBER

Common Admission Criteria for Inpatient Rehabilitation

Patient:

- is medically stable
- has not reached full potential for independence
- has the potential to benefit from therapy services
- is able to participate in 3 hours of therapy a day
- is in need of more than one rehabilitative service

Examination

When a child is transferred to an inpatient rehabilitation unit, either from another facility or from within an acute care hospital, an initial examination is performed to determine the child's baseline and to develop a plan of care. In an interdisciplinary setting, much of the initial history can be gathered from the child's medical record rather than by asking the parent or caregivers the same questions repeatedly. Important information to obtain prior to examining the child includes the child's diagnosis and mechanism of injury, if pertinent; surgical procedures performed; precautions to be followed due to infection, medical instability, and/or surgical procedures; current medications; and level of function prior to the recent admission. If a child has a chronic diagnosis, such as cerebral palsy, past medical and surgical history can provide very pertinent information.

POINT TO REMEMBER

Initial Evaluation

For the initial evaluation of a child on an inpatient rehabilitation unit, much of the initial history can be gathered from the child's medical record rather than by asking the parent or caregivers the same questions repeatedly.

Many children admitted to an inpatient rehabilitation unit present with significant medical issues and/or significant impairment in levels of arousal and alertness. These children may have multiple leads connected to monitors that continuously record their vital signs. They may also have a tracheostomy with or without ventilator support, a gastrostomy tube for nutrition, a peripheral IV line or a central IV line. (Chapter 4 discusses in further detail equipment commonly seen in the acute care setting.) Safe practice would be to complete the initial examination at the child's bedside and progress to the gym area as appropriate from a patient safety standpoint.

An initial *review of systems* should include the child's heart rate and oxygen saturation levels (if they are monitored) and blood pressure readings. The integrity of the child's skin should be examined as well as skin color and healing scars. Some children will be transferred to the rehabilitation unit with casts for fracture management or for the purpose of improving joint range of motion (ROM); skin color and temperature of the distal casted extremity should be closely monitored. Observation of the child's position is also important. Is the child relaxed in bed? Is he exhibiting abnormal postures that may indicate underlying abnormal muscle tone or movement disorders? Could these abnormal postures lead to skin breakdown and/or further joint ROM issues?

The initial examination will vary from child to child but will include muscle performance, both muscle tone and strength as well as voluntary control of movement, ROM, pain, neuromotor development, and gait. A standardized assessment tool to assist with goal development and to monitor outcomes will be required in most inpatient rehabilitation facilities that are CARF accredited. Box 5-3 lists tests and measures frequently utilized in a rehabilitation setting. A brief description of key components of the tests and measures are presented at the end of this section with specific references to commonly encountered diagnoses on an inpatient pediatric rehabilitation unit.

BOX 5-3
List of Tests and Measures

Developmental Assessments:

Bruinicks-Oseretsky II (BOT II)
Peabody Developmental Motor Scale

Balance Assessments:

Berg Balance Test for Pediatrics

Functional Assessments with National Database for Outcome Measurement:

Focus on Therapeutic Outcomes (FOTO)
Gross Motor Function Measure (GMFM*)
PEDI
Functional Independence Measure, pediatric version (WeeFIM)

Timed Assessments:

Timed-Up-and-Go (TUG)
Timed Up and Down Stairs (TUDS)
Walk tests: 30-second test, 2- or 6-minute walk tests

*National database not available; designed for children with cerebral palsy.

POINT TO REMEMBER

The Initial Examination

The initial physical therapy examinations may vary depending on the requirements of the inpatient unit and the unique characteristics of the child, but each initial evaluation should include basic information on muscle performance, muscle tone and strength, as well as voluntary control of movement, ROM, pain, neuromotor development, and if applicable the gait pattern.

Children who have sustained a TBI may demonstrate impaired *levels of arousal and attention*. The level of coma may be monitored using several criterion-based scales; progression from a lower number to a higher number is indicative of improvement. The Glasgow Coma Scale (GCS) is a standardized tool that is used to evaluate a patient's responses in eye opening, motor activity, and verbal responses.[8] A pediatric version of the GCS, the Pediatric Coma Scale (PCS), has been developed for children 9 to 72 months old with norms for specific age groups.[9]

The Rancho Los Amigos Level of Cognitive Function Scale (Rancho Scale) is frequently used during inpatient rehabilitation to rate cognitive and behavioral function and to guide interventions.[10] A specific test to assess orientation post TBI has been designed for children: the

Children's Orientation and Amnesia Test (COAT).[11] The COAT asks questions that children would know and has been found to be reliable for children 4 to 15 years of age. Other members of the team will complete in-depth examinations to determine communication abilities and the ability to attend to tasks and solve problems. This information will be shared at the multidisciplinary meetings to determine consistent methods of communication, behavior management, improving memory, etc.

The initial examination should include information on current *assistive and adaptive devices* used by the child or his family. These devices will most likely change over the course of the admission and may be a focus of the intervention for some children. Many children with a chronic diagnosis will have assistive devices that they use very well to improve their function and independence. If a surgical procedure has been performed, they may need assistance to use the device again or to progress to another type of assistive device. Parents can provide valuable input as to what they may need help with at home and what devices have been tried and unsuccessful in the past.

Adaptive devices for function at home and school may become a significant focus of the interventions provided during the admission for children with a newly acquired diagnosis. Most children with a new diagnosis, such as a spinal cord injury, will not have adaptive devices at home. The initial examination will need to determine the accessibility of the child's environment to assist with recommendations prior to discharge.

POINT TO REMEMBER

Assistive Devices

Many children with a chronic diagnosis will have assistive devices and techniques for mobility that they use very well. If possible, ask them to demonstrate and show you how they use the equipment.

Children will often be admitted to the rehabilitation unit with *orthotic, protective, and/or supportive devices* that they received in the acute care setting (refer to Appendix A for a description of orthotic devices). Mechanical ventilators, endotracheal tubes, and gastrostomy tubes (G-tubes) are frequently encountered on a rehabilitation unit. A review of the medical record and communication with the nursing and physician staff will detail the child's ventilator settings, respiratory status, and ability to be weaned from the ventilator for periods of time during the day.

Children who have sustained a TBI may be admitted to the unit with orthotic devices or serial casts to maintain or improve their ROM. Children who have had a spinal fusion after a spinal cord injury may wear a thoracic lumbar sacral orthosis (TLSO) to protect the spine until the fusion is stable. Children who have had orthopedic procedures such as a femoral osteotomy or adductor tendon lengthening may also utilize positioning devices, such as abductor wedges. Pressure wraps or pressure garments may be worn continuously or for specific time periods during the day (for children with skin grafts secondary to severe burns). Whatever the device, it is important to know if the device can be removed safely for the therapy session, how often and for how long the device should be worn, and whether the physical therapist will be expected to make recommendations to change or progress the device.

POINTS TO REMEMBER

Orthotics

Orthotic devices are often used to immobilize a body part or to provide support while the body is healing. Understand the purpose of the orthotic device and when or if the orthotic device may be removed before beginning an examination or interventions.

Evaluation of *pain* should be completed for all children, but specific attention should be given to those children who had surgery recently, who sustained a fracture, or who are admitted with a diagnosis associated with pain such as hemophilia, arthritis, etc. A variety of pain scales are available for use with children and adolescents dependent upon their age and cognitive abilities. Refer to Box 5-4 for a list of common pediatric pain scales. Children older than 8 years are usually able to rate their pain using the typical 0 to 10 numbered Visual Analog Scale.[12] Younger children are able to rate their pain with a less abstract system than one using numbers, and may benefit from use of specifically designed pediatric pain scales that make use of faces, colors, or "ouchers."[13–15] Pain assessment for all patients during the initial examination should also include questions about pain during activity or movement, waking from sleep secondary to pain, what alleviates the pain, and what medications or other interventions may be currently used for pain management.

POINTS TO REMEMBER

Pain

Children older than age 8 years are usually able to rate their pain using the typical 0 to 10 numbered Visual Analog Scale. Younger children need a less abstract method.

The *integrity of the skin* should be examined in all children, but special attention should be given to those patients with limited or absent voluntary movement or patients with limited or altered sensation, as is seen with

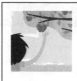

BOX 5-4
Pain Scales

For Infants and Toddlers:

CRIES Scale: 0 to 6 months (acronym for the components that include crying, requirement of oxygen, increase in vital signs, expression, and sleepless)
FLACC Scale: >6 months (acronym for the components that include face, legs, activity, cry, consolability)

For Preschoolers and Young Elementary Ages:

Color Analog Scale
FACES (Wong-Baker Faces Pain Rating Scale)
Ouchers Scale

For Children ≥8 Years:

Visual Analog Scale

a spinal cord injury. As mentioned earlier, the skin of any child wearing orthotic devices or casts should also be inspected for color and integrity. Scar formation in children who have been transferred from a burn unit needs to be examined for continued healing and potential impediment of joint motion.

Children with a neurologic diagnosis, whether chronic or recently acquired, will exhibit some type of secondary movement disorder. The *muscle tone* of children with a movement disorder is often affected resulting in spasticity, dystonia, athetosis, chorea, ataxia, myoclonus, and/or tremors. Children often exhibit more than one movement disorder. Spasticity and dystonia are frequently seen in children with cerebral palsy or in children who have sustained brain injuries. Tremors may be seen in children who have sustained a brain injury or in children with brain tumors. Ataxia is typically seen in children with a brain tumor, after an infectious process, or after a head injury.

Spasticity is typically graded clinically using the Ashworth scale or Modified Ashworth scale[16,17] (Table 5-1). These are both ordinal scales, but the Modified Ashworth scale includes an additional rating at the lower end of the scale to render the scale more discrete. The scales are not meant to be summed but rather to grade muscle groups individually. Both of these scales require moving a joint passively through the ROM at a standard speed and then rating the resistance on a five- or six-point scale, respectively. Therefore, it must be remembered that both of these scales are a measure of hypertonia and not a true measure of spasticity. (The Taskforce on Childhood Motor Disorders defines *spasticity* as "hypertonia in which one or both of the following signs are present: (i) resistance to externally imposed movement increases with increasing speed of stretch and varies with the direction of joint movement; (ii) resistance to externally imposed movement rises rapidly above a threshold speed or joint angle.)[18]

TABLE 5-1 Ashworth Scales[16,17]

Ashworth Scale	Modified Ashworth Scale
1 No increase in muscle tone	0 No increase in muscle tone
2 Slight increase in tone, giving a "catch"; affected part is moved in flexion or extension	1 Slight increase in muscle tone, manifested by a catch and release or by minimal resistance at the end of the ROM
3 More marked increase in tone; passive movements difficult	1+ Slight increase in muscle tone, manifested by a catch, followed by minimal resistance throughout the remainder of the ROM (less than half)
4 Considerable increase in tone; passive movements difficult	2 More marked increase in muscle tone through most of the ROM, but affected part(s) move easily
5 Affected part rigid in flexion or extension	3 Considerable increase in muscle tone, passive movement difficult
	4 Affected part(s) rigid in flexion or extension

Note: ROM, range of motion.

A comparison of the Ashworth and the Modified Ashworth scales showed that the inter-rater reliability was better for the Ashworth Scale.[19] Most of the disagreement with the Modified Ashworth scale included the additional rating at the lower end of the scale that may impact the reliability. Several studies investigating only the Modified Ashworth scale found the scale to be more reliable for upper extremity muscle groups, especially the elbow flexors more than for the lower extremity.[17,20,21] These studies included adults and adolescents, in whom it may be more difficult to reliably move the larger (and heavier) lower extremity than the upper extremity through the joint motions. The Ashworth scales are quick and simple to administer, can be utilized with children with cognitive impairments, and do not require specialized equipment.

One of the disadvantages of the Ashworth scales is that they do not truly measure spasticity as they only measure passive movement at a single speed. The Modified Tardieu scale assesses the resistance to passive stretch after an initial "catch" or resistance is felt and at varying speeds.[22] The scale also incorporates the joint angle when resistance to passive stretch is encountered (Table 5-2). Minimal studies have examined the reliability or validity of the modified Tardieu scale with children. However, one study found poor reliability among testers and over sessions in a small sample of children with hemiplegic cerebral palsy.[23]

TABLE 5-2 Tardieu Scale[22]

Velocity of stretch:

V1: As slow as possible (slower than the natural drop of the limb under gravity).

V2: Speed of the limb segment falling under gravity.

V3: As fast as possible (faster than the rate of the natural drop of limb under gravity).

V1 measures the passive range of motion (PROM); only V2 and V3 are used to rate the spasticity.

Quality of the muscle reaction (X):

0–No resistance throughout the course of the passive movement.

1–Slight resistance throughout the course of the movement, no clear "catch" at a precise angle.

2–Clear catch at a precise angle, interrupting the passive movement, followed by release.

3–Fatigable clonus (<10 seconds when maintaining the pressure) appearing at a precise angle.

4–Non-fatigable clonus (>10 seconds when maintaining the pressure) at a precise angle.

Angle of muscle reaction (Y):

Measured relative to the position of minimal stretch of the muscle (corresponding to angle zero) for all joints except hip, where it is relative to the anatomic resting position.

The importance of examining both spasticity and dystonia is to determine their severity and the implications for the development of secondary musculoskeletal deformities such as contracture of soft tissue structures, hip subluxation/dislocation, and torsional bony deformities. The information will aid in grading the severity of the movement disorder and in determining the deforming or imbalanced forces.

The Fahn-Marsden scale has been used to grade dystonia in adults.[24] The Barry-Albright Dystonia (BAD) scale is a modification of the Fahn-Marsden scale that was designed for use with children, including those with cognitive impairments.[25] The BAD scale consists of a five-point ordinal scale that rates the dystonia present in eight areas of the body. The BAD scale has been shown to have very high inter-rater and intra-rater reliability for the total score; the inter-rater reliability decreases slightly when comparing individual body area scores.[22]

POINTS TO REMEMBER

Rating Muscle Tone

1. The Ashworth scale and the Modified Ashworth scale are clinical measures of hypertonia.
2. The Ashworth scale appears to be more reliable than the Modified Ashworth scale.
3. Both of these scales measure an impairment, and scores do not necessarily correlate to function.[26]
4. The Modified Tardieu scale attempts to measure resistance to passive stretch at varying speeds, but reliability with children has yet to be determined.
5. The BAD scale is a reliable clinical measure of dystonia in children.

Along with muscle tone, joint ROM is also examined. Although the goniometric techniques used to measure active or passive ROM in children and adults are similar, age-related differences exist. Reliability studies of the use of goniometry in children are present in the literature and should guide physical therapists in their use of goniometric measures to document ROM. Several researchers have investigated the reliability of goniometric measurement in children with Duchenne muscular dystrophy and in children with cerebral palsy. High intra-rater reliability was present in those studies, but inter-rater reliability was shown to be variable throughout the studies.[27,28] When measuring ROM in children, the most reliable results are obtained when the same examiner evaluates changes in ROM over time. As with adults, variations of 0° to 5° do not necessarily signify change, but could be equated to error and variability.

Testing of *muscle strength* will vary depending upon the age and size of the child. Muscle strength testing will help to identify muscle activity in specific muscle groups of a child with a spinal cord injury and will assist with developing intervention programs for those children who have undergone soft tissue lengthening procedures. (Refer to the outpatient examination section later in this chapter for a more in-depth discussion of muscle strength testing in children.)

Testing of *cutaneous sensation* is especially important for children with a spinal cord injury. Testing techniques do not differ from those used with adults; however, very young children may have difficulty understanding the directions or expectations. Any identified impairments in cutaneous sensation will assist with determining appropriate transfer techniques to use, what motions to avoid, position changes, and patient education for skin care.

The initial examination after admission to the inpatient rehabilitation unit should include a *standardized measure* of the child's functional abilities. This standardized measure will help to depict how various impairments are impacting the child's activity level and ability to participate in his community setting upon discharge. This functional measure will be monitored periodically throughout the admission and at discharge by the multidisciplinary team involved in the child's care. Standardized functional tests and measures also serve as the outcome data monitoring required by regulatory agencies to monitor patient outcomes and for benchmark data with other facilities nationally (Box 5-3).

There are a small number of nationally recognized outcomes database systems available that will allow a user facility to monitor patient outcome data and benchmark nationally for a pediatric rehabilitation population that encompasses a variety of diagnoses. Those outcomes database systems are the Focus on Therapeutic Outcomes (FOTO), Pediatric Evaluation of Disability Inventory (PEDI), and Uniform Data System for Medical Rehabilitation (UDSMR).[29–31] UDS uses the pediatric version of the Functional Independence Measure (WeeFIM) for the pediatric rehabilitation population.[32]

Focus on Therapeutic Outcomes, Inc., is a national outcomes database company that includes a pediatric outcomes measure and database. The pediatric outcomes program includes a functional evaluation, parent satisfaction survey, child health related quality of life survey (CHQ), and resource utilization across disciplines. The functional evaluation is referred to as the Functional Rehabilitation Evaluation of Sensori-Neurologic Outcomes (FRESNO). The FRESNO contains 196 items across five domains: self-care, motor, communication, cognition, and socialization and is used with children and adolescents from 0 to 18 years of age.[33] Reliability and validity studies are small but have demonstrated high inter-rater reliability of 0.87 to 0.97 for the five content domains. Strong concurrent validity was also demonstrated, as was evidence of construct validity as a developmentally sensitive outcome measure.[33]

The PEDI was designed for the functional evaluation of children between 6 months and 7.5 years of age, but can be used for older children if their abilities are less than those of a 7.5-year-old child. Function is measured in three content domains: (i) self-care, (ii) mobility, and (iii) social function. Functional performance also includes the level of caregiver assistance needed to complete a skill such as eating or toilet transfers, and records the environmental modifications and equipment required to complete the functional skill. The test can be completed by professionals familiar with the child's functional abilities or through parent interview. The PEDI takes approximately 45 to 60 minutes to complete in its entirety, including the 197 items on the functional scales and the 20 items on the caregiver assistance and modification scales. Intra-rater reliability has been shown to be high for both the functional scales and the caregiver assistance scales. Inter-rater reliability for the functional scales ranges from 0.95 to 0.99, with decreased reliability noted for specific items, such as household chores, that are often not observed in the clinic setting.[30,34] Inter-rater reliability has been found to be variable and lower than intra-rater reliability, with parent or clinicians who are with the child throughout the day providing higher scores for assistance than clinicians who may only see the child for short time frames.[34] The PEDI has been found to be sensitive to changes in function in an inpatient pediatric population with an acquired brain injury.[35]

The WeeFIM is the pediatric version of the Functional Independence Measure used in adult rehabilitation and includes a functional assessment and survey of parent satisfaction at discharge and resource utilization efficiency. The WeeFIM is a minimum data set and consists of 18 items that measure independence in functional skills across the domains of self-care, mobility, and cognition. The test is designed for use among children and adolescents 6 months to 21 years of age who exhibit a functional or developmental delay. The test is administered by direct observation or caregiver interview and can be completed in 10 to 15 minutes.[31] Ottenbacher et al.[36] found stability in WeeFIM scores across age ranges. This study demonstrated high reliability among raters and over time by the WeeFIM subscale scores with intraclass correlation coefficients (ICC) of 0.87 to 0.98. High reliability with an ICC of 0.98 for data collected in person compared to over the phone was also demonstrated.

All inpatient rehabilitation facilities should be using an outcome measure to monitor change over time with patients. Ideally, the test is one with a national database to allow for benchmarking and improvements in quality of care. The three tests discussed above are all discipline-free assessments, therefore lending themselves for use in an interdisciplinary or transdisciplinary inpatient setting. The WeeFIM is a faster test to administer due to the limited data set. However, some clinicians may voice concerns that the WeeFIM is not sensitive to small changes in function due to the limited data set.

Functional assessments are not meant to replace other evaluation tools, so other measures such as developmental evaluations, balance tests, and timed tests may also be used to complete the examination and develop a plan for intervention. Thomas-Stonell and colleagues[37] investigated the responsiveness of nine outcome scales on the World Health Organization's domains of activity and participation (see Chapter 1: ICF model). They evaluated 33 children (mean age 12.5 years) who had sustained TBIs, and found that the PEDI had a ceiling effect, with 70% of children achieving the maximum score by discharge. This study found the WeeFIM and the CHQ to be consistently the most responsive, followed by the Gross Motor Function Measure (GMFM) (refer to Chapter 1 for an explanation of the GMFM). The combination of the WeeFIM or CHQ, GMFM, and the American Speech-Language Hearing Association National Outcomes Measure System captured all of the improvements cited by parents and clinicians.

After all of the necessary examination information is obtained, an evaluation and diagnosis are made to facilitate the development of a plan of care.

POINTS TO REMEMBER

Standardized Measurements

The initial examination to the inpatient rehabilitation unit should include a standardized measurement of the child's functional abilities to be used as an outcome measurement and to monitor the progress of the child throughout the inpatient stay. Ideally, the test should be one that has a national database to allow for benchmarking with other programs.

Evaluation

Synthesis of the examination findings must also include the parent's and/or child's goals and the living situation to which they will be returning upon discharge. A return to a home environment with all rooms on one level and a parent present 24 hours a day will have different functional expectations than a return to a home environment that has a full flight of stairs to enter and no parent or caregiver present during the day. The physical therapist's evaluation will be incorporated with those of the other disciplines to provide a unified plan of care that will be presented to the patient and family and carried out in some form by all staff members.

In an inpatient rehabilitation setting, the plan of care is developed through an interdisciplinary team. Many times this will occur at a regularly scheduled care coordination conference, often called a "staffing" or "*rounds*," during which patient progress is reviewed and progress and impediments toward discharge are discussed. The plan of care is ideally an interdisciplinary document that includes the patient's functional level based on standardized testing, goals with expected outcomes, estimation of length of time to achieve the goals, disciplines involved in the care of the patient and their frequency of intervention, and the interventions to be provided to achieve the goals. The plan of care is updated at regular intervals and serves as the template for discharge planning. Ideally the family and patient (if applicable) are involved in the development of the plan of care, which helps serve as a means to understand when to expect the patient to be discharged, where they will be discharged, the patient's level of functional independence expected at discharge, and equipment and environmental modifications that may be needed in the home or school environment.

Physical therapists need to understand their role in the interdisciplinary team. Each member should be working toward previously agreed upon functional goals and not primarily amelioration of identified impairments. Team members are aware of all of the patient's goals and interventions and help to carry over those interventions during their interactions with the patient and the family. For example, communication may be a significant activity limitation, and the physical therapist must be able to understand and carry out the communication strategies implemented by the speech pathologist to insure continuity of care for the patient.

POINTS TO REMEMBER

Role of the Interdisciplinary Team

Physical therapists should understand their role in the interdisciplinary team. Each member should be working toward the agreed upon functional goals and not primarily amelioration of identified impairments.

INTERVENTION

The safe return of a child to his home environment at the maximal level of independence should be the driving force behind all interventions. Interventions will be determined by the goals and expected outcomes in the plan of care, and should focus on improving function. Depending upon the extent of injuries sustained by the patient and procedures performed, there may be impairments that were identified on the examination that will interfere with accomplishing the functional goals. Remediation of impairments and improving the patient's functional status are addressed through interventions described in the *Guide to Physical Therapists Practice*.[38] Physical therapists would use these procedures and techniques in the rehabilitation setting just as they would in another setting. A few key elements of interventions that are typically emphasized in the rehabilitation setting are briefly discussed below.

POINT TO REMEMBER

Interventions

Physical therapy interventions will depend on the patient and/or family goals, which should be related to the safe return of the child to his home environment, at the maximal level of independence.

Effective *communication* with the patient, family, and other members of the multidisciplinary team is essential to efficiently achieve optimal outcomes for the patient and to provide high levels of satisfaction for both the patient and family. Communication begins at the time of admission when identifying goals with the family and/or patient and extends through to the examination and daily therapy sessions. Time must be taken to explain the interventions and the patient's responses and progress in the plan of care. Communication extends to all team members and includes formal reporting at care conferences, consultations and instruction with other disciplines, reporting outcomes, and progress toward discharge. At some point the physical therapist will need to communicate with professionals in the patient's home community such as school personnel, durable medical equipment vendors, or physical therapists in an outpatient setting closer to the child's home.

During intervention sessions with a patient, the physical therapist will often carry over plans implemented by other disciplines to optimize the care provided to the patient. Children who are recovering from a traumatic head injury may exhibit confusion or even aggressive behavior, whereas others will have limited methods of communicating their needs. A psychologist or behavior specialist may implement a structured program to be followed by all personnel and family members to provide consistent methods of dealing with inappropriate behavior, whereas the speech pathologist may outline basic methods of communication responses to expect from the child in response to simple questions. To insure consistency for the child, the physical therapist must understand and seek information from other disciplines involved in the care of the child.

In some rehabilitation units the physical therapist may serve as the case manager for a patient and will need to *coordinate care* throughout the hospital stay including follow-up after discharge. Case management, or case coordination, is a skill that often requires mentoring before a physical therapist is fully competent to collaborate among team members and facilitate an optimal outcome for the patient.

Instruction to other team members and caregivers is crucial for carryover of goals throughout the day. Areas of patient instruction often include ROM exercises, donning and doffing of splints, positioning in bed and/or a wheelchair, and transfer techniques. These activities can also be taught to family members to increase their involvement in their child's care and to assist with preparation for discharge.

Therapeutic exercise is a large category of interventions used by physical therapists, with many of the techniques utilized in other settings applicable to the rehabilitation setting. Increasing ROM, improving strength, and increasing endurance for a specific skill or movement is often a focus of intervention for children who have sustained a traumatic injury or undergone a surgical procedure. Children who have sustained a severe brain injury often initially present to the rehabilitation unit with joint contractures requiring long-term interventions such as dynamic splinting or serial casting. Serial casts are most commonly applied to the ankles to increase dorsiflexion motion and to the elbows or wrists to improve extension ROM. Impairments may need to be addressed, but functional skills should also be addressed simultaneously. Developmental activities for younger children, balance and gait training, and endurance activities are all interventions used in inpatient rehabilitation.

Functional training is another frequently utilized intervention in the rehabilitation setting. Most current theories of motor development emphasize the multiple subsystems required for movement to occur. Those subsystems include the musculoskeletal, neuromuscular, sensory, and cognitive with an emphasis on an opportunity to practice the desired skill. For functional training activities to be effective, the impairments in the subsystems must also be addressed or compensated.

Functional training begins from the time of admission to decrease the activity limitations that may be present at the time of discharge. Early functional training includes bed mobility and transfers and should be carried out by all team members. For functional training to be effective for the patient, communication among staff and with the family, as well as practice throughout the day for the child, is important. For example, if the child is working on sit-to-stand maneuvers for strengthening or as a component of a transfer, this skill should be practiced not only during the therapy session, but each time the child transfers in and out of bed, from the toilet, etc.

POINT TO REMEMBER
Impairments
Impairments should be identified and addressed, but functional skills should also be addressed simultaneously.

In order to optimize a child's function or aid in the recovery process, sometimes it is necessary to *prescribe or fabricate certain devices or equipment*. At the beginning of the inpatient admission, some children will require serial casting and/or orthotic devices to improve and then maintain specific joint ROM needed for later functional skills. Children who have had a surgical procedure may exhibit ROM that is improved from their preoperative baseline and may require reassessment of the appropriateness of their current orthotic devices. The physical therapist will be asked to provide input as to what type of orthotic device is indicated for the child to promote optimal joint alignment, preserve joint motion and integrity, and promote function. A chart on the basic types of orthotic devices can be found in Appendix A.

A crucial piece of the ongoing discharge planning is determining what *adaptive and assistive devices* will be needed in the discharge environment to promote optimal safe function for the child and ease of care for caregivers. Ordering of adaptive and assistive devices, often referred to as *durable medical equipment* by third party payers, involves coordination with multiple team members and the caregivers. Adaptive and assistive devices that may be needed prior to safe discharge range from bath and toilet seats to power wheelchairs and lifts for transfers in the home environment.

A home visit by one or two members of the team is an essential piece of prescribing and ordering assistive devices and equipment for the home. The home visit provides crucial information as to what type of equipment will work in the home and what devices are necessary for safety. The parents are an integral part of the team as they are the ones who will be using the equipment with the child on a daily basis. Prior to discharge of the patient, the family should receive equipment that is needed for a safe and appropriate discharge to the home. The family should be fully trained in the use of the equipment with their child, including direct observation by team members.

OUTCOMES

Outcomes are based on the goals that were established at admission and reassessed throughout the inpatient episode of care. Goal development can be difficult as there are minimal predictive data for the pediatric rehabilitation population. Severity of the brain injury is a predictor for morbidity. More severe injuries, indicated by length of time the child is unconscious, result in greater cognitive and behavioral deficits that are linked to independence with ambulation.[39] Dumas and colleagues investigated the predictive value of several variables in the recovery of ambulation in children who had sustained a TBI.[40] For their study, ambulation was defined as "being able to walk indoors without an assistive gait device, support, guarding or supervision for balance on level surfaces." Absence of lower extremity hypertonicity was the strongest predictor of recovery of ambulation by the time of discharge. Severity of injury and lower extremity injury were also factors that helped in predicting the ability of the child to ambulate. This type of information can be very useful to the clinician in developing realistic goals and expected outcomes.

Outcomes are also based on the data from functional assessments such as the WeeFIM, and provide the clinician with individual patient outcomes and outcomes by diagnostic groupings for the facility and the nation.

When the child in an inpatient rehabilitation hospital has reached his potential, demonstrated by meeting all the goals of the program or by a lack of progress toward those goals, the team may consider discharge to home. This may include a referral for outpatient services if necessary. Some of the factors that may influence this decision are: the ability of the child to perform his activities of daily living (ADLs) with minimal or moderate assistance from a caregiver; the services required are on a less intense basis than inpatient rehabilitation; and the family is able to manage the child's care and medical needs in the home environment. Discharge from an inpatient program often involves the transition of rehabilitation services to an outpatient and/or school setting in the child's community.

POINTS TO REMEMBER

Common Discharge Criteria for Inpatient Rehabilitation

The patient:

- has reached his full potential for independence or can achieve this on an outpatient basis.
- no longer requires the comprehensive services of inpatient rehabilitation.
- is able to be cared for at home.
- can access the level of rehabilitation services on an outpatient basis.

THE OUTPATIENT REHABILITATION SETTING

Criteria for admission to an outpatient program will vary among facilities, but most require that at a minimum the child is medically stable and has the potential to benefit from outpatient services. Individual facilities may have specific admission criteria related to age or diagnosis, and many will have policies that allow for discharge of the patient for attendance failures or a lack of demonstrated progress over a specified period of time. The ultimate goal of rehabilitation is to have the child reach his full potential for independence regardless of the setting. For some individuals, this may occur within a defined period of time associated with healing and a return to a preinjury physiologic state. For other individuals, this may

occur and reoccur over a lifetime as the person with a chronic disability moves through episodes of care associated with the management of a chronic disability.

Outpatient physical therapy services are not a substitute for school based or early intervention services that address the needs of the child and family in a different context. School-based physical therapy is mandated by educational law that entitles eligible students to receive services related to their education and support the student's individual education plan. Early intervention services are also provided under educational law, to eligible families and their child to aid the family in meeting their individual goals in accordance with the individual family service plan. Although the interventions provided by the physical therapist may be similar across these settings, the role and intent for the provision of physical therapy services is different.

Outpatient rehabilitation is typically less intensive than an inpatient approach but is directed at a specific activity limitation for a defined episode of care. An outpatient facility may be an outpatient department or satellite center of a pediatric hospital, a freestanding, nonprofit organization such as United Cerebral Palsy or Easter Seal Society, or a freestanding private practice. The practice setting will determine the other disciplines that may also provide services and the types of multidisciplinary care that may be available. A private practice may only offer physical therapy services or may offer other rehabilitation services such as occupational therapy. Most of the other types of organizations mentioned will provide multidisciplinary services that are center based. Age ranges and diagnoses served may vary among facilities, with some organizations offering specialty services or expertise in specific diagnostic areas. Some smaller private practices may limit their patient referrals to those with orthopedic diagnoses only, whereas others may specialize in children with neurologic disorders. Many larger facilities, especially those associated with a hospital, will serve children across a wide age range with varying diagnoses.

Outpatient physical therapy services differ from those provided in an inpatient rehabilitation setting in several key areas. An obvious difference is that the child is now living at home. The home is certainly the ideal environment for the child, but now he is suddenly not available for physical therapy whenever the physical therapist is available. Physical therapy appointments are dependent upon the parent or caregiver's ability to transport the child, parent work schedules, school hours if the child is in school, and the schedules of siblings in the home. In the home, the child is under the care and decision making of the parent; in the inpatient setting, a team of professionals is involved in the child's care as well as the parent. The parent often initiates outpatient physical therapy services and is the driver of the frequency of those services during the child's outpatient episode of care.

The patient's initial entry into outpatient services will vary among states depending upon direct access regulations and state practice acts. Many states will require a prescription for outpatient physical therapy either at the onset of services or within a defined time period after the initiation of services. As in other settings, the initial visit to an outpatient facility would include an examination and evaluation of the child.

POINT TO REMEMBER

Outpatient Rehabilitation

Outpatient rehabilitation is typically less intensive than an inpatient approach but is directed at a specific activity limitation for a defined episode of care.

Examination

Much of the same information that is gathered for the inpatient evaluation is obtained when seeing the patient for the first time as an outpatient. Some of the most important initial information to obtain from the parent and/or child is to determine why they are present for the examination. This information can be obtained with questions such as: What brings you here? What are your concerns? What would you like to be able to do that is difficult for you right now or what would you like your child to be able to do that he is having difficulty with right now? Does your child have any pain? These types of questions will help drive the tests and measures you select and immediately involve the parent or child in the evaluation process and ultimately in the plan of care to be developed.

Answers to the questions above will assist with prioritizing and organizing the examination. For example, if a parent states that their child is getting bigger and they can't continue to lift the child anymore, you may start by observing the parent transfer the child. Observation may lead you to decide that you need to look at joint mobility and muscle power as the child seems to weight bear on his legs in a flexed posture. The examination should not be a listing of every impairment or body structure and then progress to examining the child's functional skills. Instead, the functional goals should lead the physical therapist to investigate impairments that may be impeding progress toward a specific goal or activity.

A frequent impairment that is often encountered in physical therapy is limitation in *joint ROM*. Although the goniometric techniques used to measure active or passive joint ROM in children and adults are similar, several factors must be kept in mind when assessing ROM in children. Age-related differences exist in ROM values in adults, infants, and young children. For example, a 6-month-old child will exhibit residual flexion contractures of the hips secondary to intrauterine positioning.

Muscle length tests should also be included in the overall joint motion examination. Specific tests and their procedures do not differ from standard procedures used with the adult population; however, several tests may be used more frequently in pediatrics. Hip flexor muscle length is examined using the Thomas test or the prone hip extension test. Hamstring length is usually examined in adults using the straight leg raise test; however, the passive knee extension test (PKE) is commonly used with pediatric patients. The PKE can be used in the presence of a knee flexion contracture; therefore, it is useful for children who present with involvement of multiple joints.[41] This test is performed with the child supine, hip flexed to 90 degrees. The knee is passively extended until resistance is felt. The angle is measured from the lateral aspect of the leg to the vertical. In contrast the popliteal angle is the measurement of the angle made by the leg and thigh.

A variety of methods to examine *muscle strength* are also available; their use depends on the age and ability of the child. For infants and children younger than 3 or 4 years, evaluation of strength is most often accomplished through observation of movement and function such as squatting, stair climbing, or reaching up on tiptoes. A child must be able to follow the directions in the testing procedure to ensure accurate results using either manual muscle testing (MMT) or dynamometry.[42] Handheld dynamometry has been found to be a reliable and sensitive method of assessing strength in various populations of children.[43,44] Gajdosik determined that handheld dynamometry could be used reliably with typical developing children between the ages of 2 and 5 years as long as they could follow the directions and understand the command to push as well as agree to participate in the process.[45] Children in the 2-year age range were more likely than the 3- and 4-year-olds to refuse to participate in the testing sessions. Strength may also be reliably tested using isokinetic machines if the child is tall enough to reach the components.[46] The method of strength testing will depend upon measurement devices available to the physical therapist, the cognitive status of the child, and the child's ability to follow directions.

POINT TO REMEMBER

Strength Testing

The method of strength testing will depend upon the measurement devices available to the physical therapist, the cognitive status of the child, the child's age, and child's ability to follow directions.

During the initial examination, a *postural screen* may be appropriate. The physical therapist examines skeletal alignment in a variety of positions, depending on the age of the child. Skeletal alignment should include spinal and lower extremity alignment and limb length. An example of the basic components of a physical therapy musculoskeletal examination can be found in Appendix B.

A frequent reason for referral to outpatient physical therapy is a concern by parents on the way their child walks. Frequently it is due to the presence of an in-toed gait pattern. Physical therapists working in a pediatric setting must be aware of the rotational or torsional and skeletal alignment changes of bones and joints that occur with normal growth and development. Often a parent's concerns can be eased through education on the normal development of gait in children. However, these normal developmental processes may be altered secondary to abnormal muscle pull or weight-bearing forces that may be present in a child with a neurologic diagnosis. Therefore, a physical therapist also needs to be able to identify these abnormal deforming forces and potential for development of excessive rotational deformities that will impact function as the child grows.

Staheli et al. has developed a rotational profile to assess lower extremity alignment and assist in determining which component of the lower extremity contributes to the rotational variation.[47] The rotational profile consists of six measurements, including:

1. foot-progression angle,
2. medial rotation of the hip,
3. lateral rotation of the hip,
4. thigh-foot angle,
5. angle of the transmalleolar axis, and
6. configuration of the foot.

Normal values have been established for the first five measurements and can be used to determine whether the variation falls within the wide range of normal or if intervention is indicated (refer to Appendix C).

Lower extremity angular alignment also changes over the course of normal growth and development. An infant who presents with a varus position of the lower extremities will gradually progress to a valgus position by 2.5 to 3 years of age and then to a relatively straight lower extremity position by early school age. Lower extremity angular alignment continues to gradually change over time until skeletal maturity, when girls exhibit a slightly valgus posture and boys often exhibit a straight or varus position of the lower extremities.

POINT TO REMEMBER

Common Referral

A frequent reason for referral to outpatient physical therapy is a concern by parents on the way their child walks.

The examination of *gait* in a child is similar to that in an adult, and can be performed through systematic clinical observation or with more objective measures, ranging from video analysis to use of an instrumented gait laboratory. There are several observational gait analysis scales, such as the Physician Rating Scale or Rancho Los Amigos Gait Observation Rating Scale, that can be used clinically to assist with consistency among physi-

cal therapists and to document change over time. Many facilities often develop their own check-off gait observation lists that can be easily modified for use with a wide range of children. Whatever the scale or tool that is used for gait examination, the age of the child must be considered and knowledge of the characteristics of early walking must be incorporated into the examination.

A variety of evaluation tools are available to determine a child's *developmental level or functional abilities.* Information on the child's mobility, functional skills, and gross motor abilities can often be gained by observation and augmented through interview questions. Useful information can often be obtained by asking the parents to report a typical day for their child. While talking with the parents, the physical therapist should be observing the child's posture, play, spontaneous movements, and activities and note any asymmetries or difficulty with age-appropriate skills.

The Bayley Scales of Infant Development, Bruininks-Oseretsky Test of Motor Proficiency, Second Edition (BOT II), Peabody Developmental Motor Scale, PEDI, and the GMFM are all functionally based tests. All have moderate to good reliability ($r \geq 0.50$), and most have established construct or concurrent validity. They can be used as discriminative tools, if focus is directed toward specific items within the test, and can also serve the purpose of evaluation and monitoring progress. Caution is warranted, however, in that these tests are typically designed for specific age groups and populations, thus they are not widely applicable to all children.[48]

When comparing the various tests used to assess *balance*, there was one that surpassed all others. The Berg Balance Scale (BBS) is thought to be the gold standard in functionally measuring balance.[49,50] The BBS was designed to test elderly patients' level of balance and consists of 14 balance items deemed safe for elderly patients to perform. The BBS takes approximately 15 to 20 minutes to complete and is scored during administration. The independent items are scored on a five-point ordinal scale, with zero indicating inability to perform the task and four representing independence in completing the task. A higher score is indicative of improved or better balance. Although typically thought of as a standard test for measuring balance in the elderly population, recent research demonstrated the application of the BBS with the pediatric population.[49,51] The BBS highlights function, targeting a variety of skills such as sit to stand, pivot transfer, standing unsupported, reaching forward while standing, and picking up an object from the floor. As Berg states, ". . . the scale may well apply to any population . . . regardless of age."[49] Studies have shown that the BBS possesses high inter-rater reliability and test-retest reliability in assessing balance in children with varying degrees of motor impairment ($r = 0.997$ and $r = 0.998$, respectively).[49,51] Scores on the BBS also correlate highly with those from the GMFM, a highly validated test that measures balance at a functional level in children with cerebral palsy.[49]

The Pediatric Quality of Life Inventory (PEDS-QL) is a generic quality-of-life measurement used with children ages 8 to 12 years. This inventory tool has been shown to have test-retest reliability, sensitivity to changes in quality of life, and differences between healthy children and children with health concerns.[52,53] This inventory has been validated with children who have cancer, diabetes, rheumatoid arthritis, and orthopedic conditions.[54] The PEDS-QL has a child's version and a parent's version. The child's version asks the child to rate his own quality of life in the past month in areas of health and activities; his general feelings; how he gets along with others; and school performance. A five-point scale is utilized which ranges from 0 = never a problem, to 4 = almost always a problem. The items are reverse-scored (0 = 100; 4 = 0) so that the higher the total score, the better the quality of life. The parental version asks questions in the same categories but seeks the parent's perception of how they feel their child does in these same situations.

Measurements of quality of life are beginning to be utilized for children with disabilities.[55] This is an important factor to consider when examining the effects of rehabilitation services on a child and correlating that change or influence with a meaningful change to the child's quality of life.

When all of the necessary examination information is obtained, an evaluation and diagnosis are made to facilitate the development of a plan of care.

Evaluation

The physical therapist should review the examination findings, including any tests scores and their meaning such as age equivalency, with the parent. A diagnosis is needed to receive payment in the outpatient setting and should be listed on the plan of care. The diagnosis can include the child's medical diagnosis, if known, but should definitely include a rehabilitation diagnosis that reflects the examination findings.

Part of any physical therapy examination could include information gained from diagnostic imaging either by report or direct observation of the image. Chapter 4 presented an overview of a basic way to read an imaging film, and pointed out the use of this information in understanding the extent of a pathology. The information gained from this type of test can aid in the selection and prescription of certain interventions and provide information on the patient's response, or lack of response, to intervention provided. Information gleaned from radiology reports or imaging can also aid with patient and family education and provide additional information on the patient's condition and prognosis for functional recovery.

In the outpatient setting, the plan of care is developed in coordination with the parent. The parent and the child, if applicable, have identified their goals or concerns that they would like physical therapy to address. The physical therapist may need to guide the parent to goals that can realistically be accomplished within an episode of care. The frequency of services will be determined by the goals identified and the effectiveness of the interventions to reach those goals. Parent input and participation is vital in this process. Some children and parents will be able to carry out specific exercises at home on a regular basis and will only need to attend outpatient sessions for updates to this program. Other parents may need to attend more frequent outpatient physical therapy sessions to insure compliance and understanding of the home exercise program and the activities that promote the attainment of the identified goals.

The duration or episode of care to accomplish the goals and the criteria for discharge should be determined at the onset of physical therapy. If increased ROM to improve gait is a goal, the child may initially only need to attend physical therapy as frequently as the serial casts need to be changed. The frequency may increase as the ROM is obtained and the intervention shifts toward functional training. An increased frequency level may be needed if the child is initially using specialized equipment such as a body weight support device for gait training. Other children may benefit from services once a week with a parent who is able to follow through on a program several times a week at home.

Some third party payers will require that the plan of care be sent to them or the child's pediatrician or primary care physician for review and authorization for a specified number of physical therapy visits. These reviewers often request that scores from an objective measure or standardized test be included on the plan of care for measurement of functional change over time. Scores could include developmental ages or functional scores from standardized assessments or timed scores such as the Timed-Up-and-Go (TUG) or timed walk tests.

POINT TO REMEMBER

Frequency and Duration

The frequency and duration of services provided will be determined by goals identified and the effectiveness of the interventions to reach those goals.

INTERVENTION

Just as in the inpatient setting, the interventions will be determined by the goals on the plan of care and the expected outcomes, and should focus on improving function for the child in his home and community setting. Intervention may also be focused on training of the parent or caregiver if a change in status, such as growth or weight gain, has effected how the child accomplishes ADLs and transfers in the home. The *Guide to Physical Therapist Practice* describes the interventions that will be utilized to improve the child's functional status.[38] The key points that have a different emphasis in the outpatient setting are emphasized below.

Coordination and communication differ significantly in an outpatient setting compared to an inpatient facility. The multidisciplinary team that may be involved in the child's care is no longer under one roof, and regular meetings between team members rarely occur in this setting. The physical therapist may need to request information from other medical professionals to learn the child's full medical status and plan. An organized intentional effort will be required to communicate the physical therapy examination findings, plan of care, and progress of the child to other medical professionals participating in the care of the child. The physical therapist may need to refer the child for other services or consult with equipment vendors, orthotists, or other providers to further define and augment the plan of care. Coordination of additional services and consultations requires time as well as effective communication skills. It is important to remember in this setting that HIPAA regulations must be adhered to when communicating patient information with other professionals or organizations.

In the inpatient setting, *instruction* often occurs initially with other members of the interdisciplinary team to insure carryover of the plan of care. In the outpatient setting, instruction is focused on the child and the parent. The physical therapist must communicate with the parent to determine the parent's current level of understanding of the child's diagnosis and care, how the parent best learns, and what activities or stress that are currently in the parent's life that may limit a physical therapy program at home. A study by Rone-Adams et al. concluded that parental stress is one factor that interferes with compliance of home programs.[56] Client instruction focuses on activities for carryover at home that can be incorporated into the child's day or trials of functional skills practiced during the outpatient visit. Feedback from the parent at subsequent therapy visits will help to determine the compliance and the effectiveness of training and carryover of new skills in the home setting.

POINT TO REMEMBER

Home Exercise Programs

Home exercise programs should focus on activities that can be incorporated into the child's routines and activities of the day.

Most procedural interventions that are utilized in other settings can also be incorporated into the outpatient therapy session. A high percentage of children attending outpatient physical therapy will at some point require an adaptive or assistive device; a topic that is presented later in this section.

Therapeutic exercise and strengthening have long been used by physical therapists for orthopedic conditions. Reviews of the literature show that strengthening and resistive exercise programs can yield positive improvements in impairments and function for children with neurologic diagnoses.[57,58] Children with cerebral palsy exhibit significant weakness in their muscles compared to their able-bodied peers, whereas children who have sustained a TBI have lost strength due to inactivity and possible loss of refined movements. Strengthening programs, as well as increased activity levels, will benefit children of all ages with a neurologic diagnosis.

Flexibility exercises, endurance and conditioning programs may also be appropriate for many children with a wide range of diagnoses including neurologic conditions, musculoskeletal injuries, rheumatologic conditions, and obesity, as well as those children recovering from a transplant procedure or oncologic medical treatment. The physical therapist will need to design a program based on the child's age, present level of conditioning, and resources available.

Specific conditioning or training programs such as treadmill training with and without body weight support systems are beginning to demonstrate positive outcomes for young children and adolescents of varying diagnoses.[59–62] Treadmill training programs incorporate practice of a specific task while also addressing strengthening and balance impairments. Constraint-induced movement therapy is another type of specific training that has begun to demonstrate effectiveness in children with neurologic diagnoses with asymmetrical upper extremity limitations.[63–65] Many of the studies vary in their intensity and severity of constraint, so it is difficult at this time to recommend a specific protocol.

Functional training will be determined by the goals developed in the plan of care with the parent or caregiver. Functional training typically involves transfer training, mobility training, or training in the use of a new adaptive or assistive device to promote increased independence for the child.

The physical therapist working in the outpatient setting must be frequently communicating with the parent to determine if *adaptive devices* would ease the burden of care in the home or facilitate functional independence for the child. Progress as well as growth may necessitate a change in either an orthotic or assistive device. The physical therapist in the outpatient setting is frequently relied upon to provide significant input in determining the type of orthotic device that is most beneficial for the child. Progression in use of assistive devices is often determined by the physical therapist. Equally important is an understanding of a child's ambulation potential and the ability to identify an alternative method of mobility when appropriate.

For ease in ordering assistive and adaptive devices an effective working relationship should be established with local vendors for durable medical equipment. Most third party payers now require that the child have tried a device prior to ordering and that several styles of the same device are trialed. For example, if the physical therapist is helping the family order a bath seat for home, the child should be trialed in several styles of seats prior to submission of the final order. The physical therapist may be requested to write a *letter of medical necessity* to explain the device, benefits for the child, how it will increase function or ease of burden of care at home, and what other devices were tried that were not optimal for the child. Sample letters of medical necessity can be found in Appendix D. Anything that supports use of the particular device should be added to the letter as well as functional levels or safety concerns that would justify why the device is needed are always beneficial.

The vast array of wheelchairs, both power and manual, and especially the options to safely access and drive a power wheelchair make it almost impossible to remain fully knowledgeable of all of the options available to a child and his family. For this reason, not all outpatient centers are able to prescribe sophisticated power wheelchairs, seating systems, and driving array options for children. Specially trained personnel who work in a multidisciplinary team are needed for these unique and expensive equipment options. The team usually consists of a physician, physical therapist, occupational therapist, rehabilitation engineer, and possibly a case manager or social worker. The Rehabilitation Engineering and Assistive Technology Society of North America (RESNA) offers credentialing examinations both for providers to assess and train a patient in the use of equipment and for vendors who sell and service assistive technology devices.

The outpatient physical therapist plays an important role in instructing both the child and family members in the safe use of assistive devices. When the family receives the device, the physical therapist should insure that they are able to competently and safely use it. If the device is delivered to the home and the physical therapist cannot make a home visit, arrangements should be made so that a representative from the vendor delivering the equipment or a home health physical therapist can instruct the family in safe and proper use of the device.

POINT TO REMEMBER

Vendors

A good working relationship with your local medical equipment vendors may make it easier to order and utilize assistive and adaptive devices.

OUTCOMES

Expected outcomes are based on the successful achievement of the goals established at the onset of the episode of care. Children who have sustained a musculoskeletal injury often can be expected to return to their baseline level of function in a short period of time. Defining the expected outcomes for children with neurologic diagnoses can be more difficult but can help assist in defining the episode of care. For some children the Gross Motor Classification System not only provides a classification for children with cerebral palsy but can also provide an evidence-based prognosis regarding the child's expected gross motor progress.[66] A prognosis for expected outcomes will assist the physical therapist and family with planning the intervention strategy and monitoring the child's progress over time.

■ CASE STUDY ■

Inpatient Rehabilitation
Maria
Medical Diagnosis: Traumatic Brain Injury
Setting: Inpatient Rehabilitation

EXAMINATION

History

Maria is a 7-year-old girl who sustained a TBI injury 4 weeks ago as a result of a car versus pedestrian accident. Maria sustained a subdural hematoma requiring surgical evacuation, intracranial hemorrhages, and multiple contusions. She spent 4 weeks in the intensive care unit of a pediatric acute care hospital and was just admitted to the inpatient rehabilitation unit. Prior to her accident she attended second grade and enjoyed swimming and dancing. Maria lives with her parents and two younger siblings in a two-story home 30 miles from the hospital.

Her mother reports that her development has been typical. Maria has no significant past medical history and has been a very healthy and active little girl. Currently she is taking oral baclofen, is fed by gastrostomy tube (g-tube) and is wearing bilateral short leg serial casts. Her parents were unable to define specific goals for rehabilitation other than "we want her to learn to do as much as she can" and "we want her to be able to do what she could before the accident."

Current Condition/Chief Complaint

Maria is dependent for all mobility and ADLs. She is difficult to position due to periods of dystonic posturing in trunk and extremity extension.

Systems Review

Cardiovascular/Pulmonary
Heart rate	92 bpm
Blood pressure	124/74
Respiration rate	14 bpm
Edema	Absent
Integumentary	Unremarkable

Tests and Measures

Assistive and Adaptive Devices: Maria is wearing bilateral short leg serial casts. The first set of casts were applied 1 week ago. She currently does not possess any durable medical equipment, but has been out of bed in a reclining manual wheelchair with head support for 30 minutes at a time.

Circulation: Capillary refill time in her toes <3 seconds.

Cognition: Maria has definite awake and sleep periods. She responds to family members' voices, especially her younger siblings, and is beginning to visually track a light and other bright objects. She consistently blinks her eyes at her mother's request and attempts to reach toward family members. Maria also becomes agitated at times.

Environmental/Home/Work Barriers: Maria lives in a two-story house with four steps to enter; there is a railing on the left. Her bedroom is currently on the second floor. There is a full bathroom on the first and second floors. Maria's school is one story with a ramp at the curbside near the building entrance. She moves from her classroom only for special classes such as music, art and for lunch.

Joint Integrity and Mobility: ROM of extremities is within functional range except for ankles bilaterally. Short leg casts were removed for the examination; ankle dorsiflexion ROM: $-10°$ with knees flexed and $-20°$ with knees extended. Cervical motion is within functional limits. Trunk mobility is also within functional limits, but can be difficult to achieve due to dystonia.

Motor Function: Maria demonstrates significant impairments in motor control, especially the ability to initiate movement and to move through her available ROM. She is unable to hold her head erect in any position or to support her trunk in a sitting position. Maria needs total assistance for all mobility and ADLs with a total raw score of 19 on the WeeFIM.

Muscle Performance: Significant dystonia is present that interferes with positioning and comfort; score of 19 on BAD scale. Voluntary movement includes head turning in the supine position in response to a family member calling her name. Maria also attempts to reach for her mother, but attempts at voluntary movement are often accompanied by increased dystonic postures.

Sensory Integrity: Maria withdraws in response to painful stimuli.

EVALUATION

Impairments: Maria presents with impairments in her cognitive function and expressive and receptive communication, limited passive ROM at her ankles, dystonia, lack of head and trunk control, and poor control of voluntary movements.

Functional Limitations: Her present clinical presentation shows significant functional limitations in bed mobility, all transitional skills, ambulation, and gross motor skills.

DIAGNOSIS

Diagnostic Pattern: Impaired Motor Function and Sensory Integrity Associated with a Nonprogressive Disorder of the Central Nervous System Acquired in Childhood

Rationale: Maria is most limited by her dystonia and lack of motor control and motor function secondary to a recent injury to her central nervous system.

PROGNOSIS
Plan of Care

Short term:
1. Maria will demonstrate 25 degrees of increased ankle dorsiflexion ROM to ultimately assist with standing and transfer activities.
2. Maria will sit in a manual wheelchair with seat angle at 90 degrees for 45 minutes without dystonic extensor postures while listening or interacting with her family.

Long term:
3. Maria will perform bed mobility and transition to sitting over edge of bed with moderate assistance.
4. Maria will sit in a chair with arm supports with good head and trunk control for 30 minutes during daily activities such as eating.
5. Maria will perform a stand-pivot transfer from bed to wheelchair with moderate assistance.

Expected range of visits for this episode of care given this Guide Practice Pattern is 10 to 60 visits. (Note: The course of treatment and range of visits is anticipated for 80% of the patients/clients who are classified into this pattern, during a single episode of care.)[38]

INTERVENTIONS

Coordination/Communication/Documentation: Review plan of care at multidisciplinary meeting. Contact the school's special education program to coordinate with any physical education or related services being offered. Discuss with physicians the significant dystonia exhibited by Maria and the difficulty with positioning, movement, etc., with recommendation to enhance baclofen with other medications for dystonia. Discuss possibility of botulinum toxin A injections to plantarflexor muscle group to augment effects of serial casting.

Patient/Client Related Instruction: Receive input as to methods for best interaction, levels of commands to be used, and how to confirm Maria's responses to requests. Provide education to other team members in transfer and bed mobility techniques to be initiated with Maria for carryover throughout the entire day. Instruct mother and other relevant family members in proper lifting and body mechanics to assist with transfers. Provide team members and parents with written information regarding transfer and bed mobility techniques to be used with Maria.

Procedural Interventions

Prescription, Application, and Fabrication of Devices and Equipment: Application of weekly serial casts to improve ankle dorsiflexion to minimum of 0 to 10 degrees with knee extended. After serial casting is completed, reassess need for orthotic device such as an ankle-foot orthosis (AFO) to maintain newly acquired ankle ROM.

Discuss with family and team members at weekly meetings the need for durable medical equipment in the home after discharge. Begin ordering process for large equipment such as a manual wheelchair.

Therapeutic Exercise: ROM exercises to extremities and trunk. Facilitation of active movements, especially head control, through activities or visual or auditory stimuli that are enticing and interesting to Maria.

Functional Training: Self Care/Home: Practice with bed mobility and transfers. Practice in upright weight-bearing positions with use of body-support gait-training device. Sessions focus on active movement with correct musculoskeletal alignment, symmetry of head and trunk, and decreased need for assistance and/or cues.

Determining Frequency and Duration

Maria will be receiving occupational therapy, physical therapy and speech therapy on a daily basis. She will initially be seen twice a day for 30-minute visits by physical therapy; the length of sessions will increase as her tolerance to intervention increases and as she improves in her functional skills. She is expected to remain in inpatient rehabilitation for 2 months unless she does not exhibit any changes in function. Within 2 months, the team will have better knowledge of her expected long-term outcomes to plan for her discharge home and possible return to her second grade classroom. Prior to discharge, a home visit will need to be made and equipment ordered to assist with her care at home and facilitate her independence. Extensive communication with school personnel will be needed prior to discharge to determine both her needs at school and the best placement for her if cognitive impairments persist.

OUTCOMES

After discharge from the inpatient rehabilitation hospital, Maria is expected to require outpatient physical therapy services to continue to advance her functional skills. At time of discharge from the hospital, it is expected that Maria will be assisting with transfers and sitting erect in a chair with arm rests or in a wheelchair, and that she will be mobile in her home with an assistive device. Her function will be reassessed weekly and at discharge using the WeeFIM instrument.

Reflection Questions

1. What other assessment tools might you use in addition to the WeeFIM to complete your examination?
2. Maria scored a 19 on the BAD scale. How do you think this level of dystonia will interfere with her care or movement? Give examples.
3. At the time of admission to the rehabilitation unit, Maria is unable to communicate. How will you monitor how she is tolerating sitting out of bed in a wheelchair or her tolerance to your physical therapy interventions?
4. When you begin the ordering process for Maria's wheelchair, what components do you think she will require?
5. Assuming that Maria transfers her physical therapy care to an outpatient facility closer to home after discharge from your inpatient unit, what will be important to communicate to her new outpatient physical therapist?

SUMMARY

The physical therapist is an integral part of the rehabilitation team serving a child in either the inpatient or outpatient setting. Many pediatric rehabilitation hospitals were started more than 100 years ago to care for children with impairments as a result of polio or other congenital orthopedic conditions. Today facilities provide comprehensive multi- or interdisciplinary services aimed at the restoration of function for children and adolescents who have congenital conditions, have sustained injuries, have illnesses, or have undergone surgery. In addition, today's inpatient and outpatient facilities are influenced by many federal and state laws and regulations as well as external accrediting agencies such as CARF to protect the patients' rights and to promote quality and patient satisfaction. Major differences between inpatient and outpatient service provision are seen in the frequency and type of services available and in the health and availability of the patient.

The role of the physical therapist and the communication needed may change depending upon the setting, but the physical therapist is a key member to help identify the activity limitations of the child. The parents also serve as vital members of the team, and the physical therapist must communicate with the parent to develop appropriate goals, establish an appropriate plan of care, and efficiently provide interventions that will optimize the child's functional skills and ease the parent's burden of care. The progress that is often accomplished by a child in the rehabilitation or outpatient setting can be very rewarding for all members involved and reinforces the successful teamwork and communication that fostered the child's progress toward functional independence.

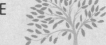

PARENT PERSPECTIVE

Matt and P. T.

My son, Matt, is a happy, healthy, normal teenager. He owes it to lots of prayer and to a terrific physical therapist.

Matt spent his grade school years participating in every sport: baseball, basketball, and his favorite—football. Over the years he developed knee and leg pain. In the summer of his eighth grade year, Matt's pain was so severe that he had to quit every sport. Any movement, touch, or activity would produce acute pain. We took Matt to several physicians and specialists. We did vitamin therapy and chiropractic. He had x-rays and MRIs. He was prescribed various braces and crutches. Still the pain got worse. Matt developed depression, was estranged from his peers, and was incredibly discouraged with the medical community. It appeared to us that each doctor listened with half an ear, prescribed tests, and mostly gave us the feeling that because the tests showed nothing, that Matt was somehow creating this problem. One even suggested it was Mom's fault because of her back pain. Each doctor treated Matt's feeling and his knees in a very rough manner. Our family is very close, and we all suffered with and for Matt.

Because we tried everything, we decided to also try outpatient physical therapy. Immediately, many things were different. First, our physical therapist listened. She listened to Matt . . . and to me. She even listened to Matt's siblings. She recommended that we see a rheumatologist. Matt was diagnosed with reflex neurovascular dystrophy (RND). We were told that there was a cure, it was relatively easy, but we would have to wait 2 to 3 months to be admitted for a 2-week inpatient stay at the local rehabilitation hospital.

That's it . . . go home . . . see you next month. We were happy to finally have a diagnosis, but extremely discouraged to have to wait because Matt's pain was amazing. During this time, Matt was missing out on football, was vomiting in school every day from the pain, and was so depressed. Each member of our family suffered with Matt.

Here is where outpatient physical therapy is so great. Our physical therapist (who made us feel every day that she cared about Matt and for each one of us) understood that, for us, 2 to 3 months was too long to wait. She knew that Matt and I would do everything it took to get back to normal. She was able to secure the protocol from the rehabilitation hospital, and we planned to take 2 weeks off from school to do daily physical therapy. Everyone was excited because we felt progress was going to begin. Note: I had tried in vain to get the rehabilitation hospital to allow Matt to come on an outpatient basis, but they refused because they only treated one child with RND at a time!

The protocol was to find out what hurt, and to do it again and again. Stairs, walking, touching the skin, running . . . all produced acute pain for years. Well, let's say that our physical therapist worked a miracle with her support, listening, and caring! By the end of the first week, Matt was running on a treadmill. By the end of the second week, he was pain free!! All because this physical therapist saw a boy . . . who was physically in pain . . . who was emotionally in pain . . . who had a family who would do anything to take that pain away. She saw us, and she heard us. Forever we will be grateful for her and her ideal way of caring for each individual person wherever they are in their journey.

We are now 9 months later. Matt is trying out for his high school golf team. He is currently a yellow belt in Tae Kwon Do. He is also taking Latin and the Honors Sciences with hopes of a career in physical therapy.

REVIEW QUESTIONS

1. You are treating a 12-year-old child in your outpatient clinic. The child informs you that he receives physical therapy at his school. In order to promote consistency with interventions and coordination of services, you wish to contact the physical therapist at the school to discuss the treatment and programming for this child. Which of the following would be the most appropriate course of action?
   a. The child's parent or guardian must sign consents for release of information before you contact the school's physical therapist.
   b. You may contact the school's physical therapist at any time, as long as you obtain written consent from the child's parent or guardian before the child is discharged from your services.
   c. You may contact the school's physical therapist at any time without the written consent from the par-

ent or guardian as communication and coordination of services is within the scope of practice of a physical therapist.
   d. The school's physical therapist must sign consents for release of information before you obtain written consent from the parent or guardian of the child.
2. Your patient presents with marked increase in muscle tone of his left upper extremity. You are performing passive ROM during your examination. The increase in muscle tone is noted through most of the ROM, but the affected part can be easily moved. What Ashworth grade would you assign?
   a. 1
   b. 2
   c. 3
   d. 4
3. You are working in an outpatient physical therapy clinic. Outpatient services are typically billed:
   a. in accordance with the appropriate DRG.
   b. as a fee for service related to the service performed and the time the physical therapist spent with the patient.
   c. as a fee for service related to the actual time the physical therapist spent with the patient.
   d. according to a predetermined rate regardless of the individual services provided or adaptive equipment provided to the patient.
4. Pain assessment should be performed during the initial examination and should include questions about pain during activity or movement and waking from sleep secondary to pain, along with identification of what alleviates the pain and what medications or other interventions have been tried that address the pain. A common way of rating pain is by using a Visual Analog Scale from 0 to 10. What is the minimum age of the patient for which this would be a valid test?
   a. 4 years
   b. 8 years
   c. 14 years
   d. 18 years
5. You are asked to evaluate a 14-year-old boy who is status post (s/p) TBI secondary to a motor vehicle accident 2 months ago. He was transferred from the hospital to the inpatient rehabilitation unit 2 days ago and has been evaluated by occupational therapy yesterday. In an interdisciplinary setting, much of your initial history can be gathered:
   a. from an interview with the child and his parents.
   b. from the child's attending physician and primary care nurse.
   c. from the child's medical record rather than asking the parent or caregivers the same questions repeatedly.
   d. after the physical therapy examination so as to not bias your test and measurement findings.

6. As a physical therapist on a CARF-accredited inpatient rehabilitation unit you are aware of the need for an outcome measurement that can be used with your patients. Which of the following statements is true regarding the outcomes required?
   a. A standardized assessment tool that assists with goal development and a system that monitors outcomes will be required in most inpatient rehabilitation facilities that are CARF accredited.
   b. CARF does not require the use of a standardized assessment tool for inpatient rehabilitation as long as there is documented evidence that the patient and family participated in the initial development of the plan of care.
   c. CARF requires that a standardized assessment tool be used only at the time of admission to an inpatient rehabilitation unit.
   d. The use of a standardized assessment tool for inpatient rehabilitation is not necessary as long as the outcomes are monitored and compiled into an annual outcomes report that is shared with CARF.

7. CMS criteria for admission to an inpatient rehabilitation hospital include a patient who is medically stable and:
   a. able to tolerate a minimum of 1 hour of rehabilitation therapy a day for at least 3 days per week.
   b. able to tolerate a minimum of 2 hours of rehabilitation therapy a day for at least 7 days per week.
   c. able to tolerate a minimum of 3 hours of rehabilitation therapy a day for at least 5 days per week.
   d. able to tolerate a minimum of 5 hours of rehabilitation therapy a day for at least 7 days per week.

8. Functional training begins at the time of admission to an inpatient rehabilitation unit and may include such activities as bed mobility and transfers. In order to facilitate functioning in a patient, which of the following is the most important?
   a. Functional training should be carried out by all team members.
   b. Training should be done at a minimum of twice a day while in the hospital.
   c. Functional training should only be carried out by qualified professionals who have been educated in the importance of this type of intervention.
   d. Functional training goals should be developed only by the physical therapist after the examination has been completed.

9. Kevin is a 14-year-old boy who has been receiving rehabilitative services through the inpatient rehabilitation hospital in your local community. Kevin is medically stable and has achieved his goals in occupational and speech therapy. He lives at home (two-story house) with both parents who are able to care for his present needs. Kevin continues to receive only physical therapy services in which he continues to make progress on stair negotiation (not independent) and balance skills (minimal impairment). He has not had a recent fall, and his parents are able to provide the necessary level of supervision and support that make him a minimum falls risk. The insurance company has asked for an update on Kevin's current functional status to determine his need for additional inpatient rehabilitation. Which of the following would be the most appropriate course of action, given this information?
   a. Document Kevin's progress in physical therapy and request authorization for additional inpatient physical therapy to maximize his functional potential before discharge.
   b. Document Kevin's progress in physical therapy and coordinate outpatient therapy services with a plan to discharge to home.
   c. Document Kevin's progress in physical therapy and plan discharge to home.

10. You are employed as a physical therapist by the local inpatient rehabilitation hospital. The director of the program informs you of the two standardized tests that are used for outcome measurements for the inpatient rehabilitation program. Both are functional assessments with strong validity and reliability properties. The director informs you that they are the only tests that need to be done for an initial evaluation in physical therapy. Given this information, which of the following statements is true?
   a. Standardized functional assessments are not meant to replace the physical therapy evaluation that may include additional items such as developmental assessments, balance tests, and measurements of impairments.
   b. Standardized functional assessments should have strong reliability properties as they are completed upon admission and discharge, but the validity is not important.
   c. Standardized functional assessments can be used in place of a physical therapy evaluation in CARF-accredited rehabilitation hospitals.

APPENDIX A

Orthotic Devices

Orthotic devices are listed by body part. A brief description of the orthotic's common application in the pediatric population is provided.

ORTHOTIC DEVICES FOR THE NECK AND TRUNK

Cervical collars: Used to support or immobilize the cervical spine. Often used after trauma, until the cervical spine has been radiographically examined and cleared of any injury or malalignment.

Thoracolumbosacral orthosis (TLSO): Often used in the management of spinal scoliosis or when immobilization of the spine is warranted. A one- or two-piece custom molded TLSO provides support to the trunk. A bivalved (or two piece) TLSO is easier to put on.

Abdominal binder: Used to support the abdominal contents. May be used after a kidney transplant, when the new kidney is placed in the lower anterior abdomen, or with placement of pharmaceutical pumps.

ORTHOTIC DEVICES FOR THE LOWER EXTREMITY

Hip abduction wedge or pillow: Maintains the hip joint in abduction.

Standing, walking, and sitting hip (SWASH) orthosis: Assists in maintaining the hip joint in alignment during these activities.

Reciprocating gait orthosis (RGO): hip knee ankle foot orthosis (HKAFO) with a mechanical assist for reciprocal lower extremity movements. Often used with children who have spina bifida or spinal cord injuries to make ambulation more energy efficient.

Knee ankle foot orthosis (KAFO): Used for support of the knee, ankle, and foot during standing or ambulation. Quadriceps muscle strength and knee joint stability are major factors in determining the need for a KAFO versus an AFO.

Knee immobilizers: Immobilize the knee joint, typically in extension, for medical reasons or if the quadriceps muscle is too weak to hold the knee in extension.

AFO: Commonly used to maintain proper alignment of the ankle and foot during weight-bearing activities. The upright aspect can influence knee control or positioning during ambulation. The ankle joint can either be fixed or allow for a certain degree of plantar and/or dorsiflexion of the talocrual joint. AFOs are also used for muscle tone reduction in the lower extremity.

Foot orthotic (FO): Used to provide support to the subtalar joint, especially with inversion and eversion, in addition to the midfoot articulation, with supination and pronation of the foot. Provides support to the arches of the foot. Can also be used for muscle tone reduction.

Components of a Musculoskeletal Examination

Joint or Body Segment	Normal Findings	Interventions for Abnormal Findings
Head	–Fontenelles: closed by 18 months –Head circumference: refer to head circumference charts –Symmetry of cranium	–If closed early, refer to MD. –Refer to MD if large head circumference for age compared with weight and height, if cranium asymmetrical, child irritable; may indicate early closure of cranial sutures. –Asymmetry or plagiocephaly: could be due to head preference to one side or torticollis. –Position to encourage head symmetry; may require cranial band for severe cases.
Neck	–Symmetrical ROM and position	–If asymmetrical in infant, look for torticollis, palpate muscle tightness. –If asymmetrical in preschool and school-age child, check for other signs of neurologic involvement such as ataxia, headache—refer immediately to MD; may be early symptoms of posterior fossa tumor. –If asymmetrical in older child or adolescent, is there a history of injury?
Trunk	–Trunk symmetry (scoliosis screen) –A/P curvature of the spine, not present in infants. Cervical and lumbar lordosis develops as child gains head control and prone skills. –Symmetrical excursion during breathing with minimal use of accessory muscles	–Asymmetrical positioning: check for scoliosis. Scoliosis secondary to asymmetrical muscle pull with neurological diagnosis: consider positioning, seating system, etc. Idiopathic scoliosis: refer to MD. –Kyphosis, positioning to increase trunk extension.
Shoulder	–Full ROM present at birth except shoulder abduction limited to 130 degrees. –Actively moves UEs from birth with movements and reaching becoming more refined during first year. –Symmetry of landmarks such as nipple line, scapula, and muscle bulk.	–Full shoulder abduction ROM present by 3 months. –Lack of active movement or symmetrical movement may be early signs of neurological disorder. –Holds UE in shoulder extension with IR and minimal active movement at shoulder, elbow, and/or wrist may indicate brachial plexus injury. –Congenital elevation of scapula indicative of Sprengel's deformity. Associated with other musculoskeletal anomalies; requires orthopedic workup. –Asymmetrical muscle bulk may indicate absence or hypoplasia of muscles such as Poland's syndrome or absence of the pectoralis major muscle. –Scapular winging-WB and NWB. Indicative of weakness. If asymmetrical and accompanied by shoulder retraction, may be early sign of neurologic involvement. Intervention focuses on achieving full scapular mobility and increasing stability of surrounding muscles. –Pain or lack of active movement at the shoulder in the school age or adolescent requires full musculoskeletal examination of the shoulder.
Elbow and Forearm	–Newborn: Flexion contracture 25 to 30 degrees. –Normal elbow motion and alignment throughout childhood and adolescence.	–Full elbow extension present by 3 to 6 months. –Limited forearm supination and prominent radial head indicate radial head dislocation. May be congenital or result of trauma.
Wrist and Hand	–Full ROM present at birth. –2 to 3 months: reach and grasp for toys, brings hands to mouth. –Raking grasp present at 6 to 8 months. –Refined pincer grasp present by 12 months. –Handedness not apparent until 4 to 5 years of age.	–Child should not show strong preference for one hand before age 4 years.

(continued)

Joint or Body Segment	Normal Findings	Interventions for Abnormal Findings
Hip and Femur	–Newborn: hip flexion contracture 30 to 50 degrees. –Hip abduction and ER posture. –Hip IR/ER: 35 to 90 degrees/50 degrees to 90 degrees* –Femoral anteversion 40° to 60°. –Femoral antetorsion 35 to 40 degrees. Lateral bowing of femur. *External rotation is greater than internal at birth but exact numbers are variable. –Toddler (1 to 2 years old): Hip flexion contracture 10 to 20 degrees at 1 year of age, reduces to < 5 degrees by 2 years and resolved by 3 years of age. –Hip IR/ER: external rotation decreases and internal rotation increases from birth values but slightly greater ratio of ER to IR. By 3 years of age, IR slightly greater than ER. –Femoral anteversion decreases significantly from birth to 2 years. –School-age: –Hip IR/ER ratio: IR slightly > ER. –Femoral antetorsion: Near 20 to 25 degrees by 4 years and <20 degrees by age 5 years. –Adolescent: –Hip IR/ER ratio: Ratio near equal in 14-year-olds, then begin trend of ER slightly > IR. –Femoral anteversion: adult values of 5 to 16 degrees by 16 years of age. –Femoral antetorsion: by 16 years, approaches adult values of 5 to 16 degrees.	–Hip flexion contracture decreases to 10 to 20 degrees by 1 year and 0 to 5 degrees by 3 years. –Asymmetrical hip abduction ROM: look for hip dysplasia (DDH). Barlow and Ortolani tests used 0 to 2 months. Asymmetrical thigh and gluteal folds, asymmetrical hip ROM and positive Galeazzi's sign (femoral shortening with hip flexed) in children >2 months; Refer to orthopedist. –Decreased spontaneous or active movement of the hip may be indicative of synovitis or osteomyelitis. –Onset of limp in 4- to 10-year-old may indicate Legg-Calve-Perthes disease. PT exam findings include limited hip IR and abduction on affected side without history of trauma, limp, Trendelenburg sign may be present; refer to orthopedist. –Onset of limp or pain in knee or groin in young adolescent may indicate slipped capital femoral epiphysis (SCFE). PT exam findings of minimal hip IR, leg held in ER and slight abduction may be consistent with SCFE.
Knee and Tibia	–Newborn: knee flexion contracture 20 to 30 degrees. –Tibial varum 15 degrees. –External tibial torsion 0 to 5 degrees, gradual increase through childhood. –Toddler (1 to 2 years old): knee flexion contracture resolved. –Tibial varum <5 degrees –External tibial torsion near 5 degrees –Mid-childhood to adult: tibial varum 0 to 2 degrees. Mean of 22 to 25 degrees external tibial torsion with a range of 0 to 40 degrees.	–Knee flexion contracture may persist or develop with abnormal muscle pull or development as seen with cerebral palsy or myelomeningocele. –Excessive tibial varum with severe bowing of proximal portion of tibia may indicate Blount's disease. Tibial varum of Blount's disease progresses with time; physiological tibiofemoral angle improves with time. –Complaint of in-toeing: age related, reference rotational profile. Not correctable by type of shoes worn, shoe inserts, or cable twisters. Internal tibial torsion is indicative of abnormal or imbalanced muscle pull.
Leg (tibiofemoral angle)	–Newborn: genu varum 15 to 17 degrees. –18 months: nearly straight –2 to 4 years: gradually progresses to genu valgum with peak of 15 degrees near 3.5 years. –7 years: adult values of 5 to 8 degrees. genu valgum (girls slightly greater valgum than boys).	–Natural course of genu varum as an infant, progressing to genu valgum as a preschool-age child with decrease to mild genu valgum by 7 years of age. Natural course includes broad ranges of normal. If excessive or asymmetrical, may require surgical correction through stapling or osteotomy.
Foot and Ankle	–Newborn: ankle dorsiflexion 40 to 80 degrees, Ankle plantarflexion neutral to 20 degrees. –Ankle dorsiflexion decreases to 45 to 50 degrees by 3 months. –Nonweight bearing: calcaneal varus of 10 degrees and forefoot varus of 5 to 10 degrees. –In weight-bearing position, calcaneal valgus of 5 to 10 degrees with no apparent longitudinal arch.	–Multiple congenital foot anomalies and deformations are possible. May be due to intrauterine positioning or failure of development of the foot. Examples include clubfoot deformity (talipes equinovarus) and metatarsus adductus. Less severe forms respond to serial casting; severe forms of equinovarus will require surgical correction. –Positional deformations of the foot often associated with DDH. –Toe walking: may be idiopathic or neurological in origin. Check for spasticity of plantarflexors or ankle clonus;

Joint or Body Segment	Normal Findings	Interventions for Abnormal Findings
	–Toddler: ankle dorsiflexion 0 to 45 to 50 degrees. Ankle plantarflexion 0 to 20 to 30 degrees. –Forefoot' varus neutral. –Stands in calcaneal valgus posture, pronation normal aspect of development. Longitudinal arch may be present in sitting but not in stance. –Gait, developing heel strike. –4 to 7 years of age: adult gait pattern established. Longitudinal arch present by age 4 years in stance. Stance in 0 to 2 degrees calcaneal varus.	check ankle dorsiflexion ROM needed for normal gait pattern. Limited ankle dorsiflexion may respond to serial casting and/or use of orthotic devices. –In-toeing may result from multiple causes. Shoe inserts and orthopedic shoes will not correct in-toeing gait.

Note: MD, medical doctor; ROM, range of motion; UE, upper extremity; IR, internal rotation; WB, weight bearing; NWB, non-weight bearing; ER, external rotation; DDH, development dysplasia of the hip; SCFE, slipped capital femoral epiphysis.

Rotational Profile

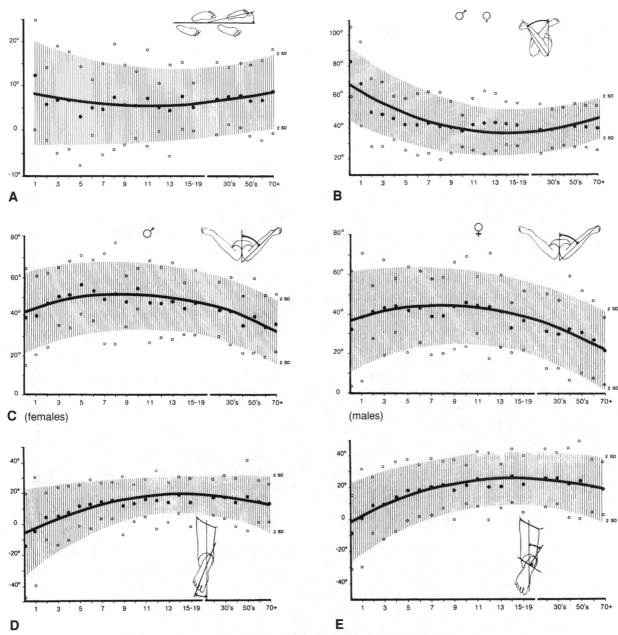

A

B

C (females)

(males)

D

E

From Tecklin J. *Pediatric Physical Therapy*, 3rd ed. Baltimore: Lippincott Williams & Wilkins; 1999.

Sample Letters of Medical Necessity for Durable Medical Equipment

LETTER OF MEDICAL NECESSITY SAMPLE 1

Name:

DOB:

DOE:

Diagnosis: medulloblastoma, status post cerebral vascular accident

Recommended Equipment: Snug Seat Bronco Gait Trainer. The Bronco Gait Trainer is a durable gait trainer that can be utilized in both the indoor and outdoor settings. The base of support is wider and includes larger wheels that accommodate uneven surfaces without tipping. The trunk support and pommel are fully adjustable. Seth will require the padded armrest attachment.

Medical Justification: Seth is a nine-year-old boy with a complex medical history including resection of medulloblastoma at age five years with right CVA and resulting left hemiplegia, seizure disorder. Seth presents with a dense left hemiplegia with his left upper extremity in a strong and tight flexed posture. Functionally, Seth is nonambulatory and is unable to utilize his left arm or hand for stability to utilize a walker.

Upright positions and movement offer Seth an increased activity level and the ability to interact with his family and peers. In addition, the upright standing posture and walking activity promote improved bowel function and reduce his episodes of constipation, enhance muscle activity to promote bone growth and bone density as well as improved respiratory and pulmonary function.

Seth was evaluated in the physical therapy department of Children's Hospital to assess the appropriateness of the Bronco Gait Trainer for home use. Home use of a gait trainer will allow Seth to increase his activity level and participate in activities with his family and peers. Examples of activities include walking in his neighborhood or local park with his family, walking outside in his yard, and participating in community age-appropriate programs with his peers.

Seth was evaluated using the Bronco Gait Trainer both inside and outside on uneven surfaces. Due to his inability to utilize his left upper extremity, he will require the padded armrest attachment to support his left arm for safety when in the upright position. Seth was able to independently propel the Bronco, including turning corners and moving around stationary objects, inside in tight rooms. He was able to maintain his arms on the armrests; the armrests eliminated any possibility of Seth getting his nonfunctional left arm caught in a doorway or on other nearby objects. Seth also independently ambulated outside over the grass and up and down hills utilizing the Bronco Gait Trainer. The Bronco was very stable on uneven surfaces and did not tip as other gait trainers did on this occasion.

The Snug Seat Bronco Gait Trainer best meets Seth's needs due to the support it provides and the independence it offers Seth. The gait trainers offered by both _____ and _____ do not offer Seth the safe independent mobility that the Bronco offers Seth. Both of these models have narrower bases of support and small wheels that make mobility on uneven surfaces impossible and unsafe with the gait trainers tipping over.

In summary, it is recommended that Seth receive a Snug Seat Bronco Gait Trainer for home use. With the Bronco Gait Trainer, Seth was able to safely and independently ambulate with good support and proper alignment of his head and trunk. Seth was very cautious when asked to trial the Bronco but became very ecstatic when he realized that he was able to independently explore over a variety of terrains with the Bronco. He was very upset when he realized that this was a trial and he could not take the Bronco home. Other gait trainers have been tried but do not provide safe ambulation for Seth.

Thank you for your attention to this matter. Questions may be referred to myself at ......

LETTER OF MEDICAL NECESSITY SAMPLE 2

Name:

DOB:

Date:

Diagnosis: Cerebral Palsy, spastic triplegia

Equipment Recommended: (Insert brand name and style) Power Wheelchair with swing and solid back and seat system. Additional components include batteries and battery ch adjustable desk-length flip-back removable armrests, footrest platform, removable head

Medical Justification: Deshae is an 11-year-old boy with a diagnosis of cerebral palsy, s ambulates but falls frequently in both the community and classroom settings. He transfe sitting to standing and can walk distances of 50 to 75 feet but exhibits frequent losses of b by holding onto walls and objects with his functional hand. He is unable to use a walker device for ambulation due to the significant spasticity and dystonia of his involved left arm. Deshae falls easily when bumped and when he needs to change direction or turn. In addition, he exhibits very poor upper extremity protective reactions when he falls. He has had two falls during the past year that have resulted in cuts to his head; one fall required seven stitches on the posterior aspect of his head from a fall when walking on a level surface. Deshae scores a 24 out of a possible 56 points on the Berg Balance Scale, which clearly indicates his significant balance deficits that impact his ambulation safety.

Deshae requires a power wheelchair for safe mobility outside of his house including his community and school settings. He has trialed several power wheelchairs, including the _____ that is being requested and the _____. He was able to transfer in and out of the _____ independently due to the lower seat height compared to a _____. Deshae was able to independently drive the chair with use of a carrot type joystick; his driving was safe and accurate. Deshae is unable to operate a one-arm drive chair as this method is very slow and fatiguing when trialed.

He will require flip-back desk-length armrests to allow him to pull the chair up to desks and counters of varying heights either in school or out in the community. A removable headrest is needed for safe transportation in a school bus or van and when using other wheelchair-accessible vehicles. The lap belt is also needed for safety; Deshae is able to independently fasten and unfasten the lap belt.

A _____ power wheelchair with the above mentioned attachments will allow Deshae to safely participate in activities that require mobility outside of the home with his peers at school and in the community and with his siblings at home. This wheelchair will also be used as his mobility in middle school, where he must change classes and travel distances much greater than 150 feet between classes. Prognosis for use of the wheelchair is excellent as Deshae was trialed in the wheelchair and was able to drive the wheelchair safely and complete a transfer in and out of the wheelchair independently. This power wheelchair will further add to Deshae's developing independence.

Please refer any questions regarding this letter to _____. Thank you for your attention to this matter.

REFERENCES

1. Technology-Related Assistance for Individuals with Disabilities Act of 1988. Public Law 100-407.
2. Americans with Disabilities Act of 1990. Public Law 101-336.
3. Patient Self-Determination Act of 1990. Public Law 101-508.
4. Health Insurance Portability and Accountability Act of 1996. Public Law 104-191.
5. Commission on Accreditation of Rehabilitation Facilities. CARF Standards 2006. Available at www.carf.org. Last accessed February 27, 2007.
6. Child Abuse Prevention and Treatment Act of 1974. Public Law 93-247.
7. Centers for Medicare and Medicaid Services. U.S. Department of Health and Human Services. 2004. Available at www.cms.gov. Last accessed July 27, 2006.
8. Teasdale G, Bennett B. Assessment of coma and impaired consciousness: a practical scale. *Lancet*.1974;2:81–84.
9. Simpson D, Cockington R, Hanieh A, et al. Head injuries in infants and young children: the value of the Paediatric Coma Scale. Review of the literature and report on a study. *Childs Nerv Syst*. 1991;7:183–190.
10. Hagen C, Makmus D, Durham P, et al. Levels of cognitive functioning. In: *Rehabilitation of the Head-Injured Adult: Comprehensive Physical Management*. Downey, CA: Professional Staff of Rancho Los Amigos Hospital; 1979;87–90.
11. Ewing-Cobbs L, Levin H, Fletcher J, et al. The Children's Orientation and Amnesia Test: relationship to severity of acute head injury and to recovery of memory. *Neurosurgery*. 1990;27:683–691.
12. Greco C, Aner M, LeBel A. Acute pain management in infants and children. In: Warfield CA, Bajwa ZH, eds. *Principles and Practice of Pain Medicine*. New York: McGraw-Hill; 2004;541–552.
13. Bieri D, Reeve R, Champion P, et al. The Faces Pain Scale for the self-assessment of the severity of pain experienced by children: development, initial validation, and preliminary investigation for ratio scale properties. *Pain*. 1990;41:139–150.
14. McGrath PA, Seifert CE, Speechly KN, et al. A new analog scale for assessing children's pain: an initial validation study. *Pain*. 1996;64:435–443.
15. Beyer J, Knott C. Construct validity estimation for the African-American and Hispanic versions of the Oucher scale. *J Ped Nurs*. 1998;13:20–31.
16. Ashworth B. Preliminary trial of carisoprodol in multiple sclerosis. *Practitioner*. 1964;192:540–542.
17. Bohannon R, Smith M. Interrater reliability of a modified Ashworth scale of muscle spasticity. *Phys Ther*. 1987;67:206–207.
18. Sanger T, Delgado M, Gaebler-Spira D, et al. Classification and definition of disorders causing hypertonia in childhood. *Pediatrics*. 2003;111:89–97.
19. Hass B, Bergstrom E, Jamous A, et al. The inter-rater reliability of the original and of the modified Ashworth scale for the assessment of spasticity in patients with spinal cord injury. *Spinal Cord*. 1996;34:560–564.
20. Sloan R, Sinclair E, Thompson J, et al. Inter-rater reliability of the modified Ashworth scale for spasticity in hemiplegic patients. *Int J Rehabil Res*. 1992;15:158–161.
21. Clopton N, Dutton J, Featherston T, et al. Interrater and intrarater reliability of the modified Ashworth scale in children with hypertonia. *Ped Phys Ther*. 2005;17:268–274.
22. Boyd R, Graham H. Objective measurement of clinical findings in the use of botulinum toxin type A for the management of children with cerebral palsy. *Eur J Neurol*. 1999;6:S23–S35.
23. Mackay A, Walt S, Lobb G. Intraobserver reliability of the modified Tardieu scale in the upper limb of children with hemiplegia. *Dev Med Child Neurol*. 2004;46:267–272.
24. Burke R, Fahn S, Marsden C, et al. Validity and reliability of a rating scale for the primary torsion dystonias. *Neurology*. 1985;35:73–77.
25. Barry M, VanSwearingen J, Albright A. Reliability and responsiveness of the Barry-Albright dystonia scale. *Dev Med Child Neurol*. 1999;41:404–411.
26. Damiano D, Quinlivan J, Owen B, et al. What does the Ashworth scale really measure and are instrumented measures more valid and precise? *Dev Med Child Neurol*. 2002;44:112–118.
27. Pandya S, Florence J, King W, et al. Reliability of goniometric measurements in patients with Duchenne muscular dystrophy. *Phys Ther*. 1985;65:1339–1342.
28. Stuberg W, Metcalf W. Reliability of quantitative muscle testing in healthy children and in children with Duchenne muscular dystrophy using a hand-held dynamometer. *Phys Ther*. 1988;68:977–982.
29. Focus on Therapeutic Outcomes, Inc. P.O. Box 11444, Knoxville, TN. Available at www.fotoinc.com. Assessed August 1, 2007.
30. Haley S, Coster W, Ludlow L, et al. Pediatric evaluation of disability index: development, standardization and administration manual. Boston: New England Medical Center Hospitals; 1992.
31. Uniform Data System for Medical Rehabilitation. WeeFIM II System. Buffalo, NY; 2003.
32. Uniform Data System for Medical Rehabilitation. The WeeFIM System Clinical Guide, Version 6.0. Buffalo, NY; 2006.
33. Roberts S, Wells R, Brown I, et al. The FRESNO: a pediatric functional outcome measurement system. *J Rehabil Outcomes Meas*. 1999;3:11–19.
34. Nichols D, Case-Smith J. Reliability and validity of the pediatric evaluation of disability inventory. *Pediatr Phys Ther*. 1996;8:15–24.
35. Tokcan G, Haley S, Gill-Body K, Dumas H. Item-specific functional recovery in children and youth with acquired brain injury. *Pediatr Phys Ther*. 2003;15:16–22.
36. Ottenbacher K, Msall M, Lyon N, et al. Interrater agreement and stability of the functional independence measure for children (WeeFIM): use in children with developmental disabilities. *Arch Phys Med Rehabil*. 1997;78:1309–1315.
37. Thomas-Stonell N, Johnson P, Rumney P, et al. An evaluation of the responsiveness of a comprehensive set of outcome measures for children and adolescents with traumatic brain injuries. *Pediatr Rehabil*. 2006;9:14-23.
38. American Physical Therapy Association. *Guide to Physical Therapist Practice*, 2nd ed. 2001; S151–S176.
39. Michaud L, Rivara F, Grady M, et al. Predictors of survival and severity of disability after severe brain injury in children. *Neurosurgery*. 1992;31:254–264.
40. Dumas H, Haley S, Ludlow L, et al. Recovery of ambulation during inpatient rehabilitation: physical therapist prognosis for children and adolescents with traumatic brain injury. *Phys Ther*. 2004;84:232–242.
41. Bleck E. *Orthopedic Management in Cerebral Palsy*. Philadelphia: Lippincott; 1987.
42. Kendall F, McCreary E. *Muscles: Testing and Function*. Baltimore: Williams & Wilkins; 1993.
43. Effgen S, Brown D. Long-term stability of hand-held dynamometric measurements in children who have myelomeningocele. *Phys Ther*. 1992;72:458–465.
44. Stuberg W, Koehler A, Wichita M, et al. Comparison of femoral torsion assessment using goniometry and computerized tomography. *Pediatr Phys Ther*. 1989;1:115–118.

45. Gajdosik C. Ability of very young children to produce reliable isometric force measurements. *Pediatr Phys Ther.* 2005;17:251–257.

46. Merlini L, Dell'Accio D, Granata C. Reliability of dynamic strength knee muscle testing in children. *J Sports Phys Ther.* 1995;22:73–76.

47. Staheli LT, Corbett M, Wyss C, et al. Lower-extremity rotational problems in children. *J Bone Joint Surg.* 1985;67A:39–47.

48. Wescott S, Lowes L, Richardson P. Evaluation of postural stability in children: current theories and assessment tools. *Phys Ther.* 1997;77:629–646.

49. Kembhavi G, Darrah J, Magill-Evans J, Loomis J. Using the Berg balance scale to distinguish balance abilities in children with cerebral palsy. *Pediatr Phys Ther.* 2002;14:92–99.

50. Riddle DL, Stratford PW. Interpreting validity indexes for diagnostic tests; an illustration using the Berg balance test. *Phys Ther.* 1999;10:939–948.

51. Franjoine M, Gunther J, Taylor M. Pediatric balance scale: a modified version of the Berg balance scale for the school-age child with mild to moderate impairment. *Pediatr Phys Ther.* 2003;15:114–128.

52. Varni J, Burwinkle T, Seid M, Skarr D. The Peds-QL as a pediatric population health measure: feasibility, reliability, and validity. *Ambul Pediatr.* 2003;3:329–341.

53. Varni J, Seid M, Knight T, Szer I. The Peds-QL 4.0 Generic Core Scales: sensitivity, responsiveness, and impact on clinical decision making. *J Behav Med.* 2002;25:175–193.

54. Varni J, Seid M, Kurtin P. PedsQL 4.0: reliability and validity of the Pediatric Quality of Life Inventory version 4.0 generic core scales in healthy and patient populations. *Med Care.* 2001;39:800–812.

55. Bjornson K, McLaughlin J. The measurement of health related quality of life in children with cerebral palsy. *Eur J Neurol.* 2001;5:183–193.

56. Rone-Adams S, Stern D, Walker V. Stress and compliance with a home exercise program among caregivers of children with disabilities. *Pediatr Phys Ther.* 2004;16:140–148.

57. Darrah J, Fan J, Chen L, et al. Review of the effects of progressive resisted muscle strengthening in children with cerebral palsy: a clinical consensus exercise. *Pediatr Phys Ther.* 1997;9:12–17.

58. Dodd K, Taylor N, Damiano D. A systematic review of the effectiveness of strengthening for people with cerebral palsy. *Arch Phys Med Rehabil.* 2002;83:1157–1164.

59. Schindl M, Forstner C, Kern H, et al. Treadmill training with partial body weight support in nonambulatory patients with cerebral palsy. *Arch Phys Med Rehabil.* 2000;81:301–306.

60. Ulrich D, Ulrich B, Angulo-Kinzler R, et al. Treadmill training of infants with Down syndrome: evidence-based developmental outcomes. *Pediatrics.* 2001;108:e84.

61. Bodkin A, Baxter R, Heriza C. Treadmill training for an infant born preterm with a grade III intraventricular hemorrhage. *Phys Ther.* 2003;83:1107–1118.

62. Day J, Fox E, Lowe J, et al. Locomotor training with partial body weight support on a treadmill in a nonambulatory child with spastic tetraplegic cerebral palsy: a case report. *Pediatr Phys Ther.* 2004;16:106–113.

63. Charles JR, Wolf SL, Schneider JA, et al. Efficacy of a child-friendly form of constraint-induced movement therapy in hemiplegic cerebral palsy: a randomized control trial. *Dev Med Child Neurol.* 2006;48:635–642.

64. Naylor C, Bower E. Modified constraint-induced movement therapy for young children with hemiplegic cerebral palsy: a pilot study. *Dev Med Child Neurol.* 2005;47:365–369.

65. Taub E, Ramey SL, DeLuca S, et al. Efficacy of constraint-induced movement therapy for children with cerebral palsy with asymmetric motor impairment. *Pediatrics.* 2004;113:305–312.

66. Rosenbaum PL, Walter SD, Hanna SE, et al. Prognosis for gross motor function in cerebral palsy, creation of motor development curves. *JAMA.* 2004;288:1357–1363.

ADDITIONAL RESOURCES

National Dissemination Center for Children with Disabilities (NICHCY)

NICHCY compiles disability-related resources in each state and creates State Resource Sheets. This site will help you locate organizations and agencies within your state that address disability-related issues, including:

- state agencies serving children and youth with disabilities;
- state chapters of disability organizations and parent groups;
- parent training and information projects; and
- much more, including the official state web site, governors and U.S. senators, and other useful associations and organizations.

Available at http://www.nichcy.org/states.htm. Accessed July 28, 2006.

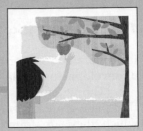

CHAPTER 6

Providing Services in an Early Intervention Program

Mark Drnach and Nikki Kiger

LEARNING OBJECTIVES

1. Understand the basic structure and function of early intervention services under the Individuals with Disabilities Education Act (IDEA), Part C.
2. Understand the process of classifying and applying eligibility criteria for early intervention services.
3. Explain the difference between an evaluation and assessment in an early intervention program.
4. Demonstrate the appropriate use of physical therapy in an early intervention program.
5. Explain the role of the physical therapist in Individualized Family Service Plan (IFSP) development.
6. Differentiate between discipline-specific interventions and interventions that will assist a family and child in their daily routines.

A physical therapist who works with children in a variety of settings should appreciate that the services provided through an early intervention system are unique in their focus on the family as well as the child, and that those services are provided in the most natural environment for the child, namely the home. Service providers (who include physical therapists) are often utilized to provide education and strategies to aid the family in daily routines, to coordinate services, and to provide support to a family as they learn how to live and manage the day with their new infant.

Early intervention services are based on early childhood development and the role of the family in that process. General principles for best practice include a family-focused service delivery in which the parents are both recipients and providers themselves, a relationship between parents and providers in which they are both equally respected, and a team that shares the same goals and values while working collaboratively.[1]

Early intervention services are mandated by federal law under Part C of the Individuals with Disabilities Education Act (IDEA) (PL 108–446).[2] States that participate in this program have the latitude to comply with the federal law in accordance with what the state determines is appropriate, within the federal guidelines. Therefore, early intervention services can vary from state to state. The information provided in this chapter is a general outline with regard to the implementation of early intervention services under IDEA.

One thing that remains constant from state to state is the emphasis on a *family-centered approach*. The family and early intervention service (EIS) providers work closely to construct a living environment that benefits the family and child by influencing the child's development during the years that provide the most chance for remodeling the nervous system. A family-centered approach is reflected in the chosen services and interventions that are based on the concerns and priorities of the family and not primarily on the diagnosis or level of developmental delay of the child.

Throughout this chapter, the Part C sections of the IDEA law are abbreviated by the section of the law in which they are found and denoted by Section 631 through Section 644. The Code of Federal Regulations (CFR) is the codification of the general and permanent rules published in the Federal Register that pertain to early intervention programs and is referenced as 34CFR303 along with the appropriate subpart.

HAVING AN INFANT WITH A DISABILITY

Having an infant with a developmental delay or a disability can be difficult for a family. Every parent has the expectation that his or her child will grow and develop into an independent and fully functioning adult. When those perceptions are challenged by new information, parents can be left with feelings of loss, bewilderment, fear, incompetence, or anger. What does the future hold for their child? How will these "special needs" influence the parent's ability to parent, allow the family to function as a family, or influence the child's ultimate ability to participate in the family and society? What can the parent do to ensure the best possible outcome? For many years professionals have associated the lack of acceptance of the disability or skill acquisition of the child with the grieving process associated with loss.[3] Although there are many similarities with this association, there is a significant difference in that the child with a disability is in the parent's life for many years. With every new milestone or social event, such as beginning preschool, making friends, graduating from middle school, or learning to drive a car, there is another reminder of the lack of ability in their child.[3] Being the parent of a child with special needs is a lifelong process, as with any parenting, but with fewer role models or appropriate road maps to follow. A natural behavior, when confronted with this new information, is for families to seek out competent and knowledgeable people who can help them answer questions about their child. Unfortunately, the answers or information are not always clear or definitive. What is known is that families need information and support. Interventions that are family centered, family oriented, or family focused, have developed and acknowledge the child with a disability and the demands associated with the diagnosis, and have introduced appropriate and sustainable strategies and activities to promote family and child development. Over a lifetime, the family and the child will require skills to face recurrent and unpredictable situations. Early intervention services are some of the first resources and support systems in this process.

THE PRACTICE ENVIRONMENT: THE FEDERAL GOVERNMENT

Since 1968, the federal government has provided essential guidelines for the implementation of early intervention services for infants and toddlers with disabilities and their families. This has been completed through a series of laws, regulations, supports, and incentives that collectively have shaped the nature and extent of the current practice.[4] Federal leadership is provided to all states, but individual states are able to modify their state practices under federal guidelines listed in the IDEA. In the Individuals with Disabilities Education Improvement Act (IDEIA) of 2004, Congress stressed the importance of enhancing the development of infants and toddlers with disabilities, decreasing the likelihood of a developmental delay, and being aware of the rapid changes in brain development that occur during the child's first 3 years of life [Sec. 631(a)(1)].[2] In addition, Congress stated that all states must strive to decrease the educational costs to society through the implementation of early intervention services, to maximize the potential for individuals with disabilities to live independently in the community, to enhance families' capacities to meet the needs of their children with disabilities, and to meet the needs of minority children, such as native Americans, homeless children, and children in foster care [Sec. 631(a)].

Federal guidelines expect states to bring about a comprehensive, multidisciplinary, statewide system in order to provide early intervention services for children under the age of 3 and their families. The federal government works to provide coordination of payment for services through multiple sources, to enhance state quality of early intervention services, and to encourage states to expand opportunities for children who would be at risk for delay if services were not rendered.[5] Federal requirements for states must include at a minimum the following:

1. a rigorous definition of the term developmental delay
2. a guarantee that early intervention services are based upon current, scientifically based research
3. a guarantee that a timely, comprehensive, multidisciplinary evaluation of the child is completed
4. the implementation of an Individualized Family Service Plan (IFSP)
5. the incorporation of a child find system
6. the implementation of a public awareness program focusing on the identification of children from birth to 3 years old who have a disability
7. a directory of services, resources, and experts available in the early intervention program
8. the development of policies and provision of training for service providers to assure that practitioners maintain the appropriate level of quality care
9. the identification of a *lead agency* to supervise services and coordinate resources for families

10. the arrangement of contract agreements for service providers with timely reimbursement for services provided
11. a guarantee that services are primarily provided in a natural environment (Sec. 635)
12. the establishment of a State Interagency Coordinating Council (Sec. 641)

In 2001, approximately 2% of the population of infants and toddlers were served under Part C, with 2-year-olds making up the largest percentage of children served.[6]

POINTS TO REMEMBER

Goals of Early Intervention

Enhance the development of infants and toddlers with disabilities.
Maximize the child's potential to be independent.
Decrease the likelihood of a developmental delay.
Decrease future educational costs.
Help families acquire or develop the tools necessary to meet the needs of their child.

INDIVIDUALS WITH DISABILITIES EDUCATION ACT, PART C

Child Find

Child Find is the process in which an early intervention system identifies children who are eligible for IDEA, Part C services. Public awareness activities, events, screenings, and evaluations are performed in order to locate and refer appropriate children to the early intervention program as soon as possible. Each state differs in its method for child find, but IDEA requires each state to have a comprehensive child find system [Sec. 635(a)(5)]. In order to make sure numerous children do not "slip through the cracks," the lead agencies in each state are responsible for planning and implementing a comprehensive plan to locate children in need (34CFR303 Subpart C). A comprehensive child find process must first target the appropriate population, children from birth to 35 months, and then work to provide awareness to the public on early identification of children who may have a developmental delay. Physical therapists can be involved in the child find process by participating in developmental screenings and public education sessions, and by educating other health care providers or individuals who work with children about early intervention services and eligibility requirements.

When a child is identified, referral guidelines are followed to assure appropriate and timely delivery of services. The primary referral sources should notify the appropriate lead agency in order for a formal evaluation

and assessment to be done in accordance with IDEA (34CFR303 Subpart C). The primary referral source may be a health care provider, but can also include any adult who has identified a concern regarding a child. This may include parents, day care center staff, social services, or a friend of the family. Referrals should be made within a timely manner after identification of a child with a possible delay to assure that the lead agency begins the process of eligibility determination as soon as possible.

After the referral is made, the early intervention program appoints a *service coordinator* for the child. The service coordinator is responsible for taking the initial information from the family in order to determine which evaluations are appropriate for this particular child and family. He is also responsible for coordinating meetings, making contact with the family, and notifying appropriate EIS providers to facilitate the process of eligibility determination as soon as possible. Federal law requires that the multidisciplinary team complete the evaluations and assessments and hold an eligibility and IFSP meeting, if appropriate, within 45 days (34CFR303 Subpart C). State legislation has the power to set the exact timeline for completion as long as it does not exceed the federal guideline.

POINT TO REMEMBER

The Next Step

After a referral is made to the early intervention program, the program appoints a service coordinator for that child and family.

Determining Eligibility

Eligibility meetings are held prior to the implementation of the IFSP in order to determine if the child qualifies for services based on state guidelines and the evaluations of the multidisciplinary team. The meeting may consist of the service coordinator, parents, licensed health care providers involved in the evaluation process, and any other individual the family may want to include. The meeting typically begins with a review of the evaluation findings with the family, identifying the child's strengths and family concerns. It is not necessary to have every team member complete an evaluation before the eligibility meeting. If an EIS provider has enough information to formulate a clear opinion about the child's developmental skills from the initial packet of information gathered by the service coordinator and the other relevant evaluations (e.g., physician's report, standardized test information), the EIS provider can attend the eligibility meeting without having formally met the child or family.

BOX 6-1
A Sample List of Established Conditions from the West Virginia Birth To Three Early Intervention System

Autistic Disorder
Cerebral Palsy
Congenital Rubella Disease
Down Syndrome
Hearing Impairment
Intraventricular Hemorrhage (Grade III or IV)
Muscular Dystrophy
Neural Tube Defect (Including Spina Bifida)
Pervasive Developmental Disorder
Spinal Cord Injury
Vision Impairment

Established Condition Categories. West Virginia Birth to Three Principles of Practice. Evaluation and Assessment Handout Materials. West Virginia Birth To Three Program. 2004:8.

BOX 6-2
Example of At-Risk Categories. West Virginia Birth To Three Early Intervention System

Birth weight of ≤1,500 grams

Born at 32 weeks' gestation or less

Technology dependent (includes ventilator)

Child-specific trauma (child abuse or acute injury)

Family stressors (may include: a single parent with no other adult in the house, lack of social support, physical or social isolation, primary caregiver with four or more preschool children, primary caregiver with another child who has a diagnosed disability)

Family barriers to accessing support (may include: primary caregiver younger than 18 years, primary caregiver with an educational level less than a high school degree, a family income level which qualifies for federal assistance, no health insurance coverage, no permanent residence, multiple changes in residence)

Serious parental concern

An example of At Risk Categories. West Virginia Birth to Three Principles of Practice. Evaluation and Assessment Handout Materials. West Virginia Birth To Three System. 2004:9.

After the evaluations are reviewed, the team must determine if the child is eligible for the state's early intervention services under the state's guidelines for eligibility. Under federal guidelines, the child can be eligible for Part C services through one or more of three ways. First, a child can be qualified if she has a substantial delay as diagnosed by the multidisciplinary team [Sec. 632(5)(A)(i)]. She may present with atypical or delayed development in one or more of the following areas: cognitive, physical, communication, social, or emotional development, or in self help skills. The decision from the multidisciplinary team that the child is delayed could be based on a numeric value, such as a 25% delay based on a standardized test, or based on the EIS provider's clinical decision, depending on the individual state interpretation of the federal law.[4] Some states may allow the child to qualify for services by an informed clinical opinion without the completion of a standardized test (34CFR303 Subpart C). The second area of qualification is a diagnosis of an established condition in which there is a high probability of a developmental delay [Sec. 632(5)(A)(ii)]. If the child has a diagnosed condition, such as Down syndrome, which has published evidence of its association with a developmental delay, then the child is eligible for early intervention services. A list of established conditions is provided on a state-to-state basis. If a child has a condition that is not designated on the official list and the EIS provider wishes to add the condition, he must obtain the medical diagnosis from the child's physician and provide published information to support a probable risk for developmental delay. (See Box 6-1 for a sample list of established conditions.)

The third method to deem a child eligible for early intervention services, if a state so chooses, is to determine that the infant or toddler is at a significant risk for developmental delay if early intervention services are not provided [Sec. 632(5)(B)]. Each state defines the "at risk" classification. West Virginia, for example, requires that a family must have four risk factors to be considered "at risk." (Box 6-2 provides a partial listing of criteria used in West Virginia.) In addition, the following have been added as eligibility criteria under the most recent reauthorization of Federal law:

"Appropriate early intervention services are available to all infants and toddlers with disabilities in the States and their families, including Indian infants and toddlers with disabilities and their families residing on a reservation geographically located within the State, infants and toddlers with disabilities who are homeless children and their families, and infants and toddlers with disabilities who are wards of the State" [Sec. 634(1)].

According to the Office of Special Education Programs, younger infants and toddlers are more likely to have either a medical diagnosis or be considered "at risk" than are older toddlers who are more likely to be eligible because of a developmental delay.[6]

Determining eligibility is an important component of the law and early intervention services, which emphasize the importance of identifying appropriate children for whom this federal entitlement is available. Eligibility determination requires some form of evaluation.

Eligibility Criteria

1. An infant or toddler age birth to 35 months who has been diagnosed by a multidisciplinary team as having a substantial developmental delay
2. An infant or toddler age birth to 35 months who has been diagnosed with an established physical or mental condition that has a high probability of resulting in a developmental delay
3. An infant or toddler age birth to 35 months who is at significant risk of a developmental delay if early intervention services are not provided (state specific)

The Evaluation and Assessment

The terms "evaluation" and "assessment" are frequently used interchangeably, yet under IDEA they possess two distinct meanings. An *evaluation* consists of procedures used to determine initial and continued eligibility for early intervention. The evaluation must be comprehensive, multidisciplinary, and timely. The *assessment* is defined as the ongoing procedures to identify (i) the child's unique strengths and needs; (ii) the services appropriate to meet those needs; (iii) the resources, priorities, and concerns of the family; and (iv) the support services needed to enhance the family's capacity to meet their child's developmental needs (34CFR303 Subpart C).

The evaluation and assessment process should be guided by the family's needs and concerns for their child. The role of the physical therapist is to ask appropriate questions to gain insight on how the family goes about their day and where problems arise concerning the child. The physical therapist can evaluate the child based on parent interview, observation, and formal or informal testing. Asking the parent or primary caregiver questions such as "What is the most difficult part of your day?" "In what ways do you expect early intervention services to help your child accomplish his everyday routines?" or "Do you have any difficulty taking your child on community outings with your family?" can facilitate the process of clarifying family concerns and priorities. This clarification is vital to the family-centered process of early intervention.

Evaluation and Assessment

Evaluation is defined as process used to determine initial and continued eligibility for early intervention.

Assessment is defined as the ongoing process of the child's and family's response to the services.

Although standardized testing is not mandated in the federal law, several states require the use of a standardized test to diagnose a developmental delay. The Peabody Developmental Motor Scales (PDMS) and the Hawaii Early Learning Profile (HELP) are two examples of tests that may be used in an early intervention program. The PDMS-2 is a standardized, norm-referenced, discriminative test, composed of six subtests that measure interrelated motor abilities that develop early in life.[7] The test assesses the gross and fine motor skills of children from birth to 6 years by using a three-point rating scale (i.e., 2,1,0). Reliability (inter-rater and test-retest) and validity of the PDMS-2 has been empirically determined with a normative sample of 2,003 children from 46 states.[7] The six subtests that form the basis for testing are reflexes, stationary skills, locomotion skills, object manipulation, grasping, and visual-motor integration. The primary uses for the PDMS-2 in early intervention is to estimate the child's motor performance in respect to his peers, to assess both qualitative and quantitative aspects of individual skills for goal development, and to evaluate the child's progress over multiple administrations.[7]

The HELP is a widely used, curriculum-based assessment that provides a comprehensive look at the child's skills in all areas of development from birth to 3 years of age.[8] The assessment tool is criterion referenced, allowing the tester to measure the mastery of skills in the child over time.[9] The tool is divided into sections addressing cognitive, expressive, and receptive language and gross and fine motor, social-emotional, and self-help skills. It also has a small section devoted to the child's sensory system and how she interacts with the environment. The EIS provider can address all areas within the testing tool should it be necessary to complete a comprehensive examination of the child to determine eligibility or for further evaluation. The HELP places the child in a developmental age range as well as provides the family with information as to when skills should emerge and develop.[9] If the state requires eligibility for early intervention services to be based on a percentage of developmental delay, the tester should note that the HELP does not result in a standard score. The test is scored with a plus and minus system, then an average of the child's functioning is made based on a clinical judgment. It does, however, give credit for emerging skills and can be helpful with the intervention planning.

The evaluation by a physical therapist could cover all of the domains of development either by standardized testing or observation and parental reporting. The physical therapist should observe the child's developmental skills as she moves about the house and interacts with her toys and favorite objects. Identification and discussion of the primary concerns of the family provide the physical therapist with the goals of the family and help to establish the priorities of intervention. In addition to the gestational, birth, and developmental histories, an identification of current medications, immunizations, and nutritional intake is appropriate to include in the examination process. Studies have shown that a child's cognitive and behavioral development can be compromised if her nutritional status is abnormal.[10] Dietary guidelines for infant nutrition can be misconstrued. (Refer to Chapter 2 for additional information on nutrition for infants and children.) Asking about the child's birth weight, current weight, and any concerns with feeding will provide the physical therapist with basic information in this area. The need for additional consultation may be warranted. Appendix A contains one example of an evaluation form that could be used by a physical therapist in an early intervention program. After the child has been evaluated and determined to be eligible for early intervention services, the next step in the process is the formulation of an IFSP.

POINTS TO REMEMBER

The Evaluation

Family involvement is necessary and vital in the process. The evaluation should include the family's concerns and the priorities placed on those concerns. It should capture the child's daily functioning in family routines and should include a dietary aspect.

The Individualized Family Service Plan

After eligibility has been determined, a meeting is held with the multidisciplinary team to develop the IFSP. If the family so desires, the IFSP meeting can take place immediately following determination of eligibility. The *IFSP* is a plan written in "family-friendly" language that addresses the family's primary concerns, priorities, and resources, and identifies how the team can work together to improve the family's situation [Sec. 636(a)(2)]. The IFSP must include the following elements:

A statement of the child's present level of functioning based on objective criteria;

A statement of the family's resources, concerns, and priorities;

A statement of the measurable results or outcomes expected, including preliteracy and language skills;

A statement of the specific early intervention services based on peer-reviewed research, to the extent practicable, necessary to meet the unique needs of the child and family;

A statement of the natural environment in which the early intervention services will be provided;

Identification of the dates of service, including the intensity, frequency, and duration;

Identification of the service coordinator from the profession most immediately relevant to the child's or family's needs; and

Identification of the steps to be taken to support the transition of the child to preschool or other appropriate services [Sec. 636(d)].

The IFSP includes the major outcomes the family wishes for the child to achieve within a specific time frame, and identifies which team member(s) will be providing the services in order to help the family reach their goals (see Appendix B for an example of an IFSP outcome page). If parental consent is not given with respect to a specific early intervention service, then only the services for which consent has been obtained will be provided [Sec. 636(e)]. Individual state policy will determine the minimum length of time before IFSP goals are updated and rewritten, but for a child who has been evaluated for the first time and determined to be eligible, a meeting to develop the initial IFSP must be conducted within the 45-day time period (34CFR303 Subpart C).

The service coordinator, parents, and at least one professional who completed an evaluation of the child should be present during the IFSP process. The other involved professionals should attempt to attend in person. If this is not possible, making phone contact (real-time electronics), sending another qualified representative, or providing written communication are also accepted forms of participation in most states. The family may include whomever they wish as well. The service coordinator organizes the meeting in the location and at the time convenient for the family (34CFR303 Subpart C).

The IFSP meeting begins with the service coordinator providing education to the family on their rights and the role of early intervention. The family's primary concerns for their child are then discussed with the team. The team addresses the child's current level of development and assists the family in formulating appropriate ideas to incorporate into their daily routine in order for the identified goals or outcomes to be reached. It is important for the team to address the family's concerns and priorities and not to unduly influence the family to identify outcomes that are more meaningful to a specific professional.

After outcomes have been created, the team works together to develop *strategies* that can be taught to the family in order for them to implement the activities on a daily basis. The service coordinator writes down strategies needed to meet the major outcomes established on the IFSP, as well as who in the child's life, and which professionals, are responsible for making this happen. The IFSP also addresses what adaptive equipment may be needed to reach the outcomes developed, if necessary.

Also included in the IFSP is the identification of where the services will take place. The physical therapist is mandated to provide services in the child's natural environment, whether that is at her home, the day care facility, or the park. One purpose of early intervention is to help the child better interact with her environment, whether through activities that help to strengthen her muscles so that she can be more independent in her movements, or by adapting the environment so that she can function as well as possible. If the sessions are consistently held in an area that is not in the child's home, documentation in the IFSP should support why this alternate location is most beneficial for the child to achieve the identified goals. In 2000, 71.8% of infants and toddlers served under IDEA Part C were served primarily in the home.[6]

It is the responsibility of the team to decide the frequency and duration of the services. These decisions should be made after the goals and outcomes have been identified and the appropriate team member has been selected to assist in this process. A discussion on how frequently the intervention should be applied and for what duration of time should follow, taking into consideration the parent's schedule and the type of intervention under consideration. The intervention should have an influence on an activity or routine that has been identified as problematic and that is a priority for the family. This discussion could begin with the family or parent first identifying how often she could fit a service provider into her schedule. Determining frequency of services can be challenging. The team should remember that the IFSP is a flexible document, and the frequency of services can be updated or changed as needed. The initial agreement on frequency of services does not have to stay in place for the next 3 to 6 months. Any team member can initiate the process of changing the IFSP to better meet the needs of the family and child. The team can meet to review the child's IFSP as many times as necessary throughout the year, depending on the achievement of goals or the need to change the type or intensity of services. When a new need arises (such as the child having difficulty with textures when feeding), the team would meet to determine who is qualified on the team to address the parent's new concerns. If a current EIS provider working with the child and family is competent in feeding issues, the team may hold off on calling in another professional until the basic interventions and strategies have been tried. An annual IFSP meeting with a minimum of a 6-month review of the child's progress is mandatory [Sec. 636(b)].

Finally, the service coordinator talks with the family about transitioning out of the early intervention program [Sec. 636(d)(8)]. This *transition plan* is included in the IFSP in order to assure a seamless transition into the school system or other appropriate setting. Although the transition process can officially appear in the IFSP when the

child is 26 months old, the service coordinator and other service providers should begin talking about transitioning long before this mandated timeline. This allows the family to mentally prepare for the transition before they see it in the IFSP.

The parent does have the right to disagree with the type, location, intensity, frequency, or duration of services presented by the team. The parent also has the right to refuse certain services as well (34CFR303 Subpart C). If this is the case, the IFSP should list the services declined by the parent before the parent and providers sign the document. Refusal of one type of service does not influence the availability of additional services. The parent can also request another IFSP meeting or mediation, or can request a *due process hearing* (the right to be heard) in order to work out any disagreements there may be before services begin. Box 6-3 outlines some of the options that parents have available to them when a team cannot work out disagreements.

BOX 6-3
Grievance Procedure

Steps involved in a grievance process include:

Mediation–The parent has a right to access mediation services in order to address disputes related to the identification, evaluation, or provision of appropriate early intervention services under Part C of the IDEA. A written request by the parents must be made to the appropriate state-appointed individual in order for the mediation process to begin.

Due Process Hearings—The parent may submit a written request to the appropriate state-appointed individual in order to begin the process. Mediation to resolve the issue will first be offered to the parent. If the parent declines, an impartial hearings officer will be assigned to the case in order to listen to both parties. The hearing proceedings along with a written decision will be made within 30 days from the parent's complaint. If either party is unhappy with the decision, they have a right to bring a civil action in state and federal court.

State Complaint—A written complaint must be filed by either party to the director of the early intervention program in the state in which they practice. The complaint must state that there has been a violation of required services under Part C of the IDEA and who or what agency is responsible for this violation. The complaint must be made within 1 year of the supposed violation. A decision from the state must be made within 60 days of the received complaint, and the state will declare corrective actions to be made in order to achieve compliance with the law. Information retrieved from the Overview of General Parents Rights from the West Virginia Birth to Three System.[22]

After the IFSP has been developed, services are initiated that provide a family with strategies and activities to help their child develop. These are listed in the IFSP and can include service coordination; physical, occupational, and speech therapies; child development; medical services for diagnostic reasons; vision and audiology checks; and dietary services.

Services and Outcomes

Empowering the family by giving them strategies to help their child progress and show them how to take an active role in their child's unique development is one of the best things that the EIS provider can give to a family. As mentioned previously, there are various professional services available to children who are eligible for early intervention services. The role of the team is to continually assess the child's needs and family's concerns as they both develop and change over the course of the first 3 years of life and to ensure that an appropriate amount of services is being provided to meet the family's and child's current needs.

Establishing outcomes for children in an early intervention program differs from the typical goal setting in other pediatric settings. The entire team, including the parents, using easily understood language, establishes the outcomes. In addition, the outcomes are written so they are attainable within a specific time period, typically within 6 months. (Appendix B is one example of an outcome page in an IFSP.) The outcome should reflect the child's and parent's needs, while being functional in nature. This may be as basic as "Jack will walk." The family must then state why they want Jack to walk. They may say, "We want Jack to walk so we don't have to carry him all over town." The outcome could then be "Jack will be able to walk with his family on community outings." The team also documents what the child is doing currently in the process of achieving that goal, such as "Jack creeps all over his home as his main means of movement." The agreement of the measurement or activity that would indicate that the outcome has been reached is also identified. For example, the team could write, "Jack will walk in his home and community as his primary means of mobility."

After the outcome for the child has been described, the team brainstorms on ways to help the family achieve this outcome. The strategies can be from all disciplines and people involved with the family's or child's care, working together to develop the most comprehensive plan of action for the child and family. For example, the team may agree to work on various techniques to encourage walking along with strengthening exercises to provide the child with the ability to walk independently (Box 6-4). These activities and strategies should be

BOX 6-4
Strategy Examples

Strategies for Jack to meet his goal include:

• Start with playtime at the couch (standing).
• Begin to place toys out of reach so Jack has to step to the right and left in order to get to the toys on the couch.
• Work on moving from the couch to the coffee table by placing his toys on both surfaces or in different places.
• Have Jack walk in the home with a push toy. The toy can be weighted down to provide stability.
• Walk with Jack in the home with two hands held; move to one hand held and assistance at the opposite shoulder; move to one hand held.
• If the parent is alone, have Jack stand with his back to the couch and encourage one to two steps to the parent, increasing the distance with each successful step. If two family members are present, encourage Jack to walk from one family member to the other.

incorporated into typical activities of children such as playing, climbing, bathing, or dressing. The IFSP also lists which individuals with the special skills and knowledge are needed to help make this happen and identifies who is responsible for this aspect of the plan. These individuals could be the parents, extended family, church family, day care workers, or even friends of the family. Another area of the IFSP addresses any adaptations, equipment, or accommodations that can be utilized to make this happen.

In addition to outcomes for the child, the family should have a set of outcomes to enable them to provide appropriate care for the child. Family outcomes should be a focus throughout the early intervention experience. The service coordinator assists the family in knowing their rights and responsibilities and how to advocate appropriately for their child. The coordinator is also responsible for linking the family to available services in their community to provide any needed support. All EIS providers can help the family understand their child's abilities and needs as well as teach them how to help their child participate in community and home activities. The family environment is considered one of the most influential factors in the early development of a child. The emotional, physical, and community aspects of the family can have an impact on their child's development.[11] Because most families feel alone when they first find out their child has a developmental delay or disability, an available and strong support system can be invaluable. The positive benefit received from a support system seems to come more from how the family perceives the quality of support versus the quantity of support. The type of support that is considered quality support differs from family to family based on the community they live in and their cultural beliefs.[11] Although the avenues of support provided to families differ, the key point to remember is to help link the family to a support system best suited for that individual family.

POINTS TO REMEMBER

Outcomes of Early Intervention

The outcomes established by the team should be meaningful to the family, functional in context, and measurable. The team, including the family, decides which services are needed, where they will be delivered, who will deliver the services, and how frequently the services are needed at this time. The outcomes of early intervention services should address the child's development as well as the family's ability to promote that development throughout the child's lifetime.

INTERVENTIONS

The IFSP identifies the priorities and anticipated outcomes of early intervention services. The outcomes, stated in the family's words, help the physical therapist to develop intervention strategies that will assist the family and child with activities that are carried out in the environments most natural for them. The interventions focus on the utilization of objects and toys that the family owns or are found in the child's environment. It is important for the physical therapist to use items that the family has readily available. If the physical therapist enters the home with balls and bolsters, uses them, and then takes them away at the end of the session, he may not have helped the family understand or deal with their child in everyday activities or routines. Equipment or adaptive devices in the home used to promote participation in daily activities would be more appropriate.

The categories of interventions used by a physical therapist within an early intervention program are the same as in other settings, and are outlined in the *Guide to Physical Therapist Practice.*[12] One of the main interventions is the *coordination, communication, and documentation* of information regarding the child and family. These three areas may include the following: coordinating eligibility and transition planning, documenting and communicating developmental skills and family routines (i.e., IFSP development), communicating

and collaborating with other agencies (i.e., day care program), and collecting data and analyzing outcomes with communication to the appropriate persons. *Patient/client- or child/caregiver-related instruction* is the most important intervention provided to a family. Family education is vital in creating an environment in which a child will grow and develop over many years. It is the main emphasis of early intervention services, and one that the physical therapist should utilize at each visit. The physical therapist's role is to provide interventions in a way that teaches the family what to do with their child when the physical therapist is not present. The 167 hours that the family experiences over the week are just as important as the 1 hour of service that the physical therapist, or any other EIS provider, delivers.

Activity-based instruction is primarily used in the early intervention environment. This type of intervention was first developed in the special education environment.[13,14] Activity-based instruction observes what the child's interests are and works on functional skills that are applicable to her versus what a developmental book states that a child should be doing at a certain age. For example, by the age of 24 months a child should be able to step up a step in the house. What if the child, during a visit, does not want to step up a step? The physical therapist could look at the components of stepping and promote those components in a more functional and meaningful way for that individual child for this particular visit. Instead of stepping up a step, the physical therapist could work on alternate ways to have the child develop lower extremity strength, coordination, and one-legged stance. The child and physical therapist could build a tower out of large blocks and then push them over to make it more fun and appropriate for that child. From this one activity, the physical therapist can work on lower extremity strengthening by encouraging multiple squats to build one-legged stance by encouraging the child to step over the blocks, and lower extremity coordination by asking the child to run toward the blocks to knock them over. It is important to remember that, if the child is not willing to participate in an activity, it may not be that she is uncooperative; she may not like the activity. The service delivery in early intervention should be child driven. Through experience, the physical therapist will learn to quickly adapt a play activity to allow the child to feel as though she is in charge, but still address the desired goal (Fig. 6-1).

In addition to activity-based instruction, the physical therapist should ensure that the outcomes set forth by the family are seamlessly woven into their day. For example, if the parent wants the child to go up and down the steps on her own, the physical therapist could teach the parents to encourage their child to step up the steps when going upstairs instead of carrying her up the steps

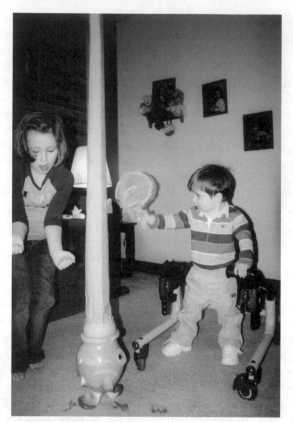

Figure 6-1 ■ Jacob participates in an activity with his sister while exhibiting independence with the use of his walker. The intervention session is child driven, so the child feels as though he is in charge.

throughout the day. The parents do not have to set aside time each day to practice going up and down the steps 10 times. The parents could just take a few extra minutes before the child's nap or bath time and allow the child to walk up the steps during these functional and appropriate activities.

Because teamwork among EIS providers is highly encouraged, it is important to maintain communication between all the members of the team and set aside time to discuss the interventions and how each team member can reinforce the interventions during his or her session with the family. For example, if a child has hypotonia and tongue protrusion that is impairing the child's speech due to decreased oral motor control, the physical therapist can incorporate a strengthening activity that would address both proximal and oral motor weakness. The physical therapist could engage the child in a game of tug of war or in pushing a large object across the room to help strengthen the base of the tongue to get tongue retraction, while working on shoulder girdle and lower extremity strengthening. This simple play activity could also incorporate improvement of grip strength that the occupational therapist is working on to open packages or draw with a crayon. The physical therapist should work to

encompass as many of the goals from each EIS provider while participating in one play activity, thus eliminating the need for three individual exercises focusing on each individual area.

A child, depending on her individual needs, may require extra assistance from external support devices (such as therapeutic taping to promote lower extremity alignment, a walker, or a standing frame) to develop skills while maintaining some level of independence. If a child always requires assistance to ambulate in her home, a walker might be a logical choice to give the child independence while relieving the parent of constant supervision to assist the child. *Assistive technology* is another intervention that may be used in certain situations. Public Law 100-407 defines assistive technology as any item, piece of equipment, or product system whether acquired commercially off the shelf, modified, or customized that is used to increase, maintain, or improve functional capabilities of individuals with disabilities (Figs. 6-2 and 6-3).[15]

The reasons for the implementation of assistive technology in early intervention are to promote participation of the child in various environments, increase the child's functional independence, improve the

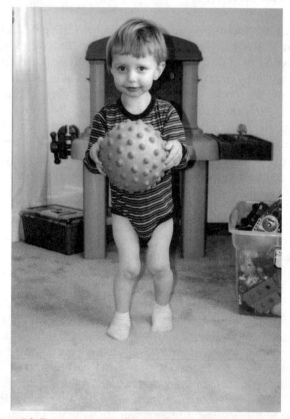

Figure 6-2 ■ Logan possesses ligament laxity with internal rotation and a crouched gait pattern, causing genu valgum and ankle hyperpronation bilaterally.

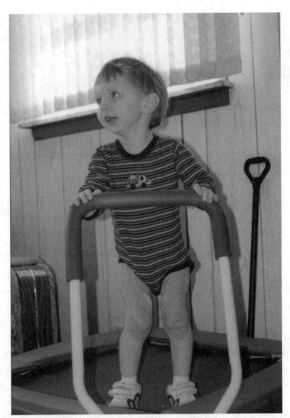

Figure 6-3 ■ Using kinesiotape to provide structural alignment and muscle facilitation of the quadriceps. Bilateral AFOs are also worn to provide stability at the ankle but are not pictured here.

child's alignment and postural control, minimize the effects of atypical system impairments, and prevent secondary impairments that could arise if assistive technology was not used.[15] The physical therapist should work closely with the family to develop a plan of care for their child using assistive equipment if necessary.

POINT TO REMEMBER

Intervention

Interventions provided in an early intervention system may include:

- Communication, documentation, and coordination;
- Child and caregiver education;
- Functional training; and
- Manual therapy techniques, including handling and positioning.

Remember: Families should be taught strategies to help with daily routines and to promote their child's development within a natural environment.

SERVICE DELIVERY

Early intervention programs strive to provide services in a natural environment for children in hopes to provide the best chance to generalize the child's goals to her everyday surroundings. *Natural environments* for children in the early intervention program are defined as "the home, community, and early childhood settings where children learn to develop everyday abilities and skills. Natural learning environments include the places, settings, and activities where children from birth to three years of age would typically have learning opportunities and experiences."[16]

Part C of the IDEA requires services to be provided in a natural setting to the maximum extent appropriate for the needs of the child [Sec. 635(16)]. There are instances in which the clinic environment is the only available setting for the delivery of the interventions. The argument for this situation is that this arrangement does not clearly reflect the philosophy of early intervention in promoting child development in the natural environment. If a physical therapist works in a clinic using suspended equipment, ball pits, etc., and then sends the child home with the parent, the intervention, on the surface, has no correlation with the everyday routines of the family. The clinic and other environments are acceptable when (i) all other options for natural environments have been attempted without success, (ii) the IFSP team can justify why services cannot be provided in a natural setting in order to meet the child's outcomes, (iii) justification states that the EIS provider is not working in a clinical setting for convenience (there should also be documentation on how the interventions are to be incorporated into the family's daily routine in their natural environment), and (iv) the need exists for the team to bring the family out of the natural environment to network or provide other family supports as identified in the IFSP.[17]

Intervention in the community setting could occur at the child's day care facility, where the physical therapist educates the day care staff on how to facilitate different movements or activities with the child. It could occur at the playground, where the child has difficulties climbing the jungle gym like the other children. Parents must analyze their day and decide in which environments they need most help to maximize their child's function. If the team decides that the child will consistently be seen in a different setting than the home, this must be documented in the child's IFSP.[18]

POINT TO REMEMBER

Service Delivery

Services should be delivered to the maximum extent appropriate to the needs of the child in the child's natural environments, including the home and community setting in which children without disabilities participate.

Researchers Dunst and Bruder[16] conducted family interviews to identify the benefits of home therapy. Families stated that the greatest benefit of therapy in a natural environment was improving child-learning opportunities, inclusion, and fostering parent–child play episodes. When asked what the parents felt were the benefits of early intervention, they listed improving child development and functioning, better child quality of life, and increased confidence working with their child.[16] Recent research shows that these two areas of practice are highly intertwined.[16,19]

When discussing frequency of services in the natural environment, the physical therapist could begin by looking at the child's current level of functioning. What are the child's limitations in function, and what is impairing the child from acquiring additional skills? Does she have the potential to improve her function? What interventions can be used to render change in the child and her family? By answering these questions, the physical therapist can clarify which specific areas to address in order to help the child progress toward her goals and obtain a better understanding of the frequency of visits needed to make this happen.[20] Because early intervention is a team approach in which the physical therapist educates the parents in techniques to facilitate acquisition of goals, the frequency of services need not be two to three times per week as seen in the outpatient setting. The parent takes over as the interventionist when the EIS provider leaves the home. Going one time a week to the natural environment in order to reassess the child's changes and develop strategies for continued improvement may be sufficient depending on the individual family and child situation.

Another aspect to consider in the delivery of services is the family's personal situation and schedule. It is important to listen to what the family is saying, verbally and nonverbally. The parents may both work and then spend time with other children at sporting events or educational activities and have limited time for several EIS providers to come into their home each week. The family may desire to have the EIS provider come to the home two times a month versus one time per week. Actively listening to the concerns of the family and understanding the current needs is important in this process. Giving the parent the lead in setting the frequency of services will allow her to identify her availability at this point in time. Conversely, the family may feel that their child is in need of frequent service provision by whomever the team recommends. Reinforcing the purpose of early interventions services, as compared to outpatient rehabilitation services or other traditional medical services, may be necessary. Parental and team education on the intent of IDEA Part C is key to making the team, including the parents, understand the intent of early intervention services. When conflicts arise that cannot be resolved through one-on-one discussions, a team meeting should be called with the service coordinator in order to discuss resolutions to the conflict.

POINTS TO REMEMBER

Determining Frequency of Services

When making decisions on frequency of services, the following factors should be considered:

What is the availability of the parent or primary caregiver?

What is impairing the child?

What types of interventions are available and are they effective?

Who are people involved in providing this help?

Are the people involved in the child's life willing and able to help?

The physical therapist should also be cognizant of the family's nonverbal and verbal language from session to session. Some families who are unsure of what to do or who feel as though there are too many suggestions that do not easily fit within their daily routine may just give up and wait for the physical therapist or other EIS provider to return to work with their child. Working on a few strategies reinforced by all EIS providers who come into the home, and progressing or adding more strategies only after the old ones have been evaluated for effectiveness or incorporated into a daily activity, may be more manageable for a family and may foster more compliance, acceptance, and understanding. The physical therapist should also be cognizant that the family or other EIS providers may not easily understand medical terminology. Parent-friendly language is emphasized to promote understanding. For example, instead of using common physical therapy terms such as prone and supine, the physical therapist could talk to the parent about the child being on his stomach or back.

Other factors that can influence service delivery are family culture and practices. Language barriers and the potential for misunderstandings should be a concern in the home of a family with limited English-speaking skills, or with an EIS provider with limited skills in the language of the family. A translator should be made available and accompany the EIS provider if he is unable to communicate verbally with the family.[21] Nonverbal communication is also important to consider when interacting with the child and family. Physical touch is an integral part of physical therapy, yet in some cultures this is not an accepted method of interaction. For example, in some families of Chinese descent, the head is considered sacred and an inadvertent touch on the child's head can be viewed as offensive, even if it was an endearing mode of communication by the service provider.[22] In addition, sensitivity to the parent's beliefs about their child with a disability and the cause of the disability should be understood. Some cultures consider that having a child with a disability is a special calling, whereas other cultures believe the disability results from the child's or parent's wrongdoings in this or a previous life.[23] Being aware of

BOX 6-5
Examples of Cultural Differences

1. Some families may not view teenage pregnancy as a negative issue.
2. Some families may view the grandmother as the primary decision maker for a child rather than the mother.
3. Parenting styles and behaviors may be acceptable in one culture, but not in another. One example is not correcting boys if they are too aggressive.
4. Some families place a child's respect for elders above the child's educational success.
5. Participation in religious ceremonies and rituals are more important in some families than in others.

the family's cultural beliefs before entering the home is important in order to avoid inadvertent offensive comments or actions on the part of the service provider. Box 6-5 presents some additional cultural differences.

ANNUAL SUMMARY

The child in the early intervention program is evaluated at least annually to determine if she continues to qualify for services. The yearly review date must be set before the 1-year anniversary of the child entering the early intervention system. The summary should include the child's progress within the last year along with support for the continuation or the discontinuation of early intervention services. Each team member may write his own synopsis of the child's current level of functioning and recommendations. If the child is eligible for another year of services, then the IFSP process may continue with the development of new goals and identification of the appropriate service provider.

To assure that the family has received the proper guidance and training within a family-centered context, some states have currently implemented a survey for the family to complete after their early intervention experience. Appendix C contains a survey developed by the National Center for Special Education Accountability Monitoring, for families receiving early intervention services.

POINTS TO REMEMBER

Annual Summary

An annual summary is done to evaluate the child's progress and continued eligibility for early intervention services. It does not have to be a separate process from the scheduled visits to the child's home, but rather a review of the information acquired over the last 12 months.

REIMBURSEMENT

Early intervention under Part C of IDEA is a federal grant program administered by the Office of Special Education Programs (OSEP) that assists states in operating a comprehensive statewide program of early intervention services. Grant monies are allocated by the federal government to a particular state based on a census formula of a state's 0- to 2-year-old population. State Medicaid monies and federal grant monies are the primary sources of revenue for early intervention services, as well as the family's health insurance when allowed by the state. Services are provided at no cost to the family except where federal or state law allows, including the establishment of a *sliding scale fee schedule* (fees that are based on the family's income level) [Sec. 632(4)(B)]. Services provided that cannot be charged to a family include the following:

Implementing the child find requirements,
Evaluation and assessment,
Service coordination, and
Administrative and coordinative activities related to (i) the development, review, and evaluation of IFSPs; and (ii) implementation of the procedures.

If a state has in effect a state law requiring the provision of a free appropriate public education to children with disabilities from birth, the state may not charge parents for any services (e.g., physical or occupational therapy) required under that law that are provided to eligible children and their families (34CFR303 Subpart F).

There are various methods for reimbursement to EIS providers used by early intervention programs. In addition to the annual salary or hourly rate provided to an employee of a company that provides early intervention services, many physical therapists in private practice can also bill for services rendered if they are participating in the state's early intervention program. Four common methods outlined below are fee for service, capitated, partially capitated, and cost based. The type of method used is determined by the payer.

The first type of reimbursement is the *fee-for-service* method. The EIS provider is compensated for each unit of service provided to the child. The level of reimbursement is decided by the state and could be different depending on the EIS provider's profession. With a fee-for-service method, research shows that families have a higher rate of satisfaction, although processing claims can be problematic in the tracking of units and in the budgeting, which can be more difficult because revenue is based on the amount of services delivered, which may be hard to predict.[24]

Capitated reimbursement methods pay the EIS provider in advance a fixed dollar amount for each child enrolled in the early intervention program. Research shows that capitated payment methods can lead to a better coordination of care along with the inclusion of preventative methods to manage the visit frequency. Because individual units of service do not have to be tracked with this system, budgeting is easier.[24]

Cost-based reimbursement methods look at the number of children cared for per year and then bases future annual payments on the historical numbers of children served. Cost-based methods, as in capitated services, also make budgeting easier because reimbursement is predictable, producing less inconvenience because individual services do not have to be billed.[24]

The final and least used approach for reimbursement is the *partially capitated reimbursement* method. This method of repayment looks to combine the fee-for-service and capitated systems. The payer who reimburses the EIS provider on a fee-for-service basis up to a certain number of visits and no more (For more information see Chapter 14).[24]

TRANSITIONING

Transitioning a child from early intervention services into Part B (preschool) services is generally the responsibility of the child's service coordinator. He is responsible for beginning the process when the child reaches 26 months of age. Many families are not thinking of this transition yet, as they are primarily focused on their child's progress within the early intervention program. It is therefore important to include the entire team in the child's transitioning to assure as smooth a transition as possible. The IDEA includes the following with regard to transitioning:

> . . . to ensure a smooth transition for toddlers receiving early intervention services under this part to preschool, school, other appropriate services, or exiting the program, including a description of how (i) the families of such toddlers and children will be included in the transition plans . . . (ii)(II) in the case of a child who may be eligible for preschool services, with approval of the family of the child, convene a conference among the lead agency, the family and the local education agency, not less than 90 days (and at the discretion of all such parties, not more than 9 months) before the child is eligible for preschool services, to discuss any such services that the child may receive [Sec. 637(a)(9)(A)].

The family may meet with the service coordinator and discuss options for future placement of their child in order for services to continue without disruption. Options vary from state to state, but educational services that provide special needs preschool classes are the primary choice for the majority of families. The families can choose to meet with the teachers at the school and discuss the needs of their child before the child turns 3 years old in order to facilitate and complete the transition. States have a right to stop early intervention services when the child turns 3 years of age. Federal law allows

for early intervention services to continue until the age of 5 years if the state is willing to provide these services. The family must decide along with the team what they feel is best for the child. If given the option, some families may prefer that their child be placed in the educational system and receive related services in the school, whereas other families may prefer to continue home-based services. The majority of children in an early intervention program are eligible for IDEA Part B services when they turn 3 years old.[6]

> **POINTS TO REMEMBER**

Transitioning

Transitioning should begin when the child reaches 26 months of age but no less than 90 days before he is eligible for preschool. Early intervention services can be extended to age 5 years if allowed by the state.

PARENT PERSPECTIVE

EARLY INTERVENTION SERVICES

When you become a new parent, you experience feelings of love, joy, excitement, anticipation, and a whole lot of nerves! When you become a new parent to a child with special needs, the nerves multiply exponentially. You enter a new world full of unknowns that cannot be answered by going to the local bookstore and looking in a section full of books for new parents. However, when you start receiving early intervention services, the service providers become your resource guide and start answering some of those unknowns.

One of the biggest challenges of caring for children with special needs is the ability to access and find resources. Early intervention service providers not only supplied the resources, they brought them right to my doorstep. After having to travel to pediatricians, neurologists, neurosurgeons, cardiologists, and pulmonologists, it was a nice reprieve not having to travel for services. Every week, I had a physical therapist, speech therapist, occupational therapist, or child development specialist visit my children and me at our home. This enabled the service providers to see and understand my children in their environment. It also allowed me the opportunity to witness the service providers working with my children and to learn first hand about specific techniques that I could use to further my children's development during my daily interactions with them. They also supplied me with information, support, and the comfort of knowing I was not alone in my determination to do what was best for my children.

Through early intervention services, my children received the help and support that was desperately needed. The service providers gave me the assistance and guidance to build my confidence and strength, and to overcome the fear of the unknowns of the future.

—*Shannon L, mother of twins Reed and Nico, who have cerebral palsy, and their triplet sister Alessa*

CASE STUDY

An Evaluation to Determine Eligibility for Early Intervention Services

Child's Name: Jiada R.
Date of Birth: 02-12-05
Chronological Age: 14 months
Date of Examination: 04-23-06
Parent's Name: Rachel D.
Address: 107 Grant Avenue. Anywhere, MX
Referral Source: Mother
Family's Concerns: Jiada is 14 months old and does not walk.
Primary Physician: Dr. Wright

MEDICAL HISTORY

Jiada is the second child of Rachel D. She was born at 39 weeks gestation and weighed 7 pounds 3 ounces. Mom reports that Jiada passed her hearing screen at birth and had chicken pox when she was 2 weeks old. The chicken pox resolved without any complications.

CURRENT HEALTH STATUS

Immunizations are up to date. Jiada is presently taking Albuterol for her chest congestion, which she has had for 2 weeks. She currently weighs 22 pounds.

DEVELOPMENTAL HISTORY

History report is unremarkable, with the exception of independent walking. Mom has been using a commercial walker since Jiada was 9 months old to promote this activity and also to give Mom some time to perform housework while Jiada is occupied. Jiada is in the walker for approximately 2 hours every other day by Mom's report.

OBSERVATIONS

Jiada's vision and hearing do not appear to be impaired. She does say "ba ba" and "da da" but is not specific. She is cruising along furniture. Jiada will pull to stance using a half kneel, leading with her right leg. Jiada will attempt to maintain her balance in stance, lifting her toes and moving over her ankles. She took three steps independently during the examination, demonstrating a typical gait pattern of a new walker. (Legs spread apart, knees straight, legs turned out, arms held high). Jiada will throw a toy, by report, and demonstrated the ability to crawl up steps. With her hands Jiada will hold two objects or toys when presented to her. She will hold onto a cracker or cookie and bite it. She is developing the use of her fingers to grasp. She points and will search and uncover a hidden toy. Jiada laughs and will look at you when you say her name. She will hand you a toy. Jiada finger feeds and uses a sippy cup. Jiada is dressed by her mother and will cooperate by pulling off her socks.

Today, Jiada sat on my lap while I read a book to her. She appeared interested and reached out for the pages. After the story (approximately 2 minutes in length), Jiada played with the book, turning and pulling at the pages.

RESULTS

Jiada demonstrates age-appropriate developmental skills today. She also walks like a new walker.

RECOMMENDATIONS

Today, Mom and I discussed:

1. Giving Jiada more opportunities to walk, holding onto her hand;
2. Limiting the use of the commercial walker to once or twice a week, if needed;
3. Spending time every day (2 to 5 minutes) reading to Jiada;
4. Following through with the eligibility meeting that is scheduled for next week; and
5. Providing information and education to Mom on the general development of children from 1 to 3 years.

Reflection Questions

1. The parent's concern was that Jiada does not walk; yet during the examination she took three steps independently. What questions could the physical therapist ask to clarify Mom's concern?
2. Why do you think the physical therapist recommended reading to Jiada daily? What is the role of the physical therapist regarding preliteracy skills?
3. According to this information, Jiada does not present with a developmental delay. Why do you think the physical therapist recommended that Mom follow through with the eligibility meeting that is scheduled for next week? What other factors may make Jiada or her family eligible for early intervention services?

SUMMARY

Raising a child is a daunting undertaking. Raising a child with a disability can add additional obstacles and joys to that process as the child and parents grow in their respective roles. Early intervention services under IDEA, Part C, is a joint attempt by the federal government and state governments to enhance the development of infants and toddlers with disabilities within a state, to improve the educational results of such children, and to maximize the potential for individuals with disabilities to live independently in society. The focus on the family's role and the recognition of its influence makes the delivery of these services significantly different from that practiced in other health care and educational environments. A physical therapist who is knowledgeable in child development and the delivery of family-centered services is an appropriate and valuable professional to engage in a state's child find activities and evaluations to determine eligibility, and to assist with the development and implementation of the IFSP. Physical therapy interventions provided to enhance the family's ability to care for their child and to promote her development are naturally done in those environments in which the family and child live and participate on a daily or routine basis. Periodic reporting and a focus on the future, through a formal transitioning process, provide the physical therapist with the opportunity to evaluate and report on the effectiveness of the services provided and to plan for the child's future when she becomes eligible for the public education system.

REVIEW QUESTIONS

1. You are a physical therapist working in a rural area of the state. You are aware that early intervention services are available for eligible children and their families. Which of the following federal legislations established this entitlement?
   a. The IDEA
   b. The Rehabilitation Act
   c. The Americans with Disabilities Act
   d. The No Child Left Behind Act

2. Which of the following is the process in early intervention of increasing public awareness, screening young children, and being involved in other community activities that identify children who are eligible for Part C services?
   a. Multidisciplinary evaluations
   b. Eligibility determination
   c. Child find
   d. IFSP teaming

3. Under IDEA Part C, the federal government defines the procedure used to determine initial and continued eligibility for a child as which of the following terms?
   a. Assessment
   b. Evaluation
   c. Eligibility
   d. IFSP

4. The federal government requires that all necessary evaluations are completed and, if appropriate, an IFSP developed within how many days?
   a. 30
   b. 45
   c. 60
   d. 90

5. Chaz is a 27-month-old child who has cerebral palsy and spastic hemiplegia. He is receiving early intervention services as well as attending a day care program while his parents are working. On the weekends, he and his parents attend functions at their local church. Under IDEA, early intervention services for Chaz are to be provided in his natural environment. This would be defined for Chaz as which of the following?
   a. In the physical therapy department where other children with cerebral palsy receive services
   b. In his home
   c. In his home or day care setting
   d. In his home, day care setting, or local church

6. Which of the following would be considered the greatest resource for a child in an early intervention program?
   a. The professional resources available through the state program
   b. The child's family
   c. The federal and state resources available through IDEA
   d. The skills of the members of the IFSP team

7. The federal requirements for early intervention services include which of the following?
   a. The need for services to be based on scientifically based research, to the extent practicable
   b. The provision of any medical services necessary for the treatment of a condition that results in a developmental delay in the child
   c. The provision of any assistive technology desired by the family
   d. The inclusion of a child development specialist on the eligibility team

8. Curt is the 15-month-old son of Bryan and Lydia. One of the goals of the early intervention program is to enable Curt to walk independently around the house so that his mother does not have to carry him so often. Of the following strategies, which would be most reflective of an early intervention strategy to promote increased walking skills?
   a. Instruct Lydia to encourage Curt to crawl up and down stairs at least three times a day to encourage strengthening of Curt's hip muscles.
   b. Instruct Lydia and Bryan to encourage Curt to ride a tricycle or riding toy daily to promote increased strength in his legs.
   c. Instruct Lydia to encourage Curt to crawl up the steps when going to bed or to take a nap, crawl onto the couch to have a story read to him, and to walk in between rooms when the family is moving from one room to another (e.g., when it is time for dinner).
   d. Instruct Bryan to carry Curt whenever necessary, and have Lydia make Curt walk wherever she wants him to go.

9. Jack is 35 months old and is receiving early intervention services to address his developmental delay. His parents would like to continue receiving the same services for Jack until he begins kindergarten. What options do Jack's parents have?
   a. The parents have no options. Early intervention services are only available for Jack until he turns 3 years old.
   b. They will have to pay privately for needed early intervention services that must discontinue when Jack turns 3 years old.
   c. They will continue to receive services under the current IFSP if the service duration is documented "until Jack enters kindergarten."

d. If the state allows, Jack can continue receiving early intervention services until he is 5 years old.

10. Kara is a 16-month-old girl with Down syndrome. When she turns 3 years old, her mother would like her to attend the local preschool along with her older sister Helena. Transitioning from early intervention services to Part B services should begin by what age?

a. No more than 9 months before she is eligible for preschool services but no less than 90 days before she is eligible for preschool

b. When the child turns 18 months old, but before she turns 30 months

c. No more than 90 days before she is eligible for preschool services in her state

d. When the child turns 30 months old, but before she turns 36 months old

An Evaluation: Early Intervention Physical Therapy Evaluation

PHYSICAL THERAPY

General Information:
Child's name: _____   ___ male ___ female
Exam date:_____
Parent's names: _____
Address: _____ Phone: _____
Date of Referral: _____

Date of Birth: _____ Chronological Age: _____
Medical diagnosis: _____
Precautions: _____
Medications: _____
Pediatrician: _____
Other health care services/agencies: _____
_____
Medical and Birth History: _____
_____
_____
_____
                                                              _____
Other EI services: _____
_____
Parent's concerns and priorities: _____
_____
_____
_____

Systems Review:

Child's current height: _____ weight: _____

Communication: ___ verbal ___ non verbal ___ vocal ___ sign
Device: _____

Vision: _____ WFL: Impaired: _____
Hearing:_____WFL: Impaired _____

Emotion/behavior during exam: ___cooperative ___ uncooperative ___ passive ___other:_____
Motor control: ___ impaired ___not impaired
Motor learning: ___ impaired ___not impaired

Sensation to touch :   ____ impaired____ not impaired
Oral motor skills: ____ impaired____ not impaired

Additional comments: _____
_____

Caregiver availability and capability:
                    _____ Lives with mom who is primary caregiver
                    _____ Other:
                    _____ Also attends daycare center. Staff: _____

Tests and Measurements:

Range of Motion and Muscle Tone
        _____ Range of motion and muscle tone are WNL throughout the trunk and extremities
        _____ Range of motion and muscle tone are WNL throughout the trunk and extremities with the following
                exceptions: _____

Functional Strength
        _____ Able to touch the back of the head
        _____ Able to touch the middle of the back
        _____ Able to pronate/supinate the forearm
        _____ Able to oppose fingers to thumb
        _____ Able to rise from a chair
        _____ Able to step up a six-inch step

Rises from the floor:
        _____ using half kneel
        _____ via squat
        _____ via modified plantargrade
        _____ requiring: _____ assist
        _____ Other: _____

Neuromotor development

Reflexes: Primitive reflexes ___ appear integrated ___ are present
Comments:_____

Reactions: _____ Righting _____
                      Protective extension _____

Equilibrium: ___prone ___ supine ___ quadruped ___ sitting ___kneeling ___ standing
Balance:___ not impaired ___impaired
Sitting: _____

Standing: _____

Walking: _____

During ADLs: _____

Coordination: UE: ___ not impaired ___ impaired
                  LE: ___ not impaired ___ impaired

Mobility:

Transfers: ___ independent ___ dependent

Description with level of assistance needed: _____

Ambulation: ___ independent ___ assist ___ non-ambulatory

Gait pattern: _____

Assistive device: _____

Level of assistance needed: _____

Stair negotiation: _____

Child is independent in the developmental sequence to _____

Self Care (mark the level of assistance needed to complete the task)

___ undressing ___ dressing ___ eating ___ toileting ___ bathing ___ other

comments: _____

_____

Assistive technology or adaptive equipment presently used:

_____

_____

_____

The following information was obtained by ___ report ___ observation

Accessibility of the natural environment: _____

_____

Child's primary position during play/activities: _____

_____

Analysis of child's motor skills while playing: _____

_____

Analysis of child's participation in activities: _____

_____

List of family's leisure activities: _____

_____

DEVELOPMENTAL SKILLS CHECKLIST

Developmental Checklist:
(Numbers in parentheses indicates the average age in months at which a child typically demonstrates this skill)

Gross Motor
Prone suspension: head at body (2); head above body (3)
Bears weight through legs (4)
Rolling: prone to supine (5); supine to prone (6)
Sitting (6)
Assumes hand and knee (7)
Crawling (8)
Sits on floor for 10 minutes (8)
Pull to Stand (10)
Standing (10)
Walking (12)
Throws ball (13)
Squats (15)
Crawls up steps (15)
Begins to jump (18)
Climbs into adult chair (18)
Carries large toy 2 hands (19)
Walks backwards (24)
Runs (24)
Stairs: step to step (24); alternates up (36)

Fine Motor
Grasp reflex (1)
Hold rattle for 10 sec (2)
Reaches for object (3)
Hands to mouth (4)
Ulnar grasp (4); Palmar grasp (5); Radial grasp (6)
Picks up spoon (5)
Rakes and bangs (6)
Manipulates (7)
Plays with paper (7)
Hold two objects (8)
Developing precision grasps (8)
Hands used for separate functions (9)
Holds, bites and chews cracker (9)
Points (10-11)
Uncovers toy (10)
Holds with one hand and manipulates with another (12)
Unwraps toy (14)

Holds 3 items (14)
Finer motor development (15-24)
Attemps to fold paper (24)
Turns pages of book separately (24)
Imitates vertical and horiz. line, and circle (27)
Hold crayon with thumb and index (30)
Copies a circle (36)
Cuts across paper with scissors (36)

Cognitive
Watches caregiver (1)
Follows object 180 (2-3)
Smiles (2)
Watches hand (4)
Localizes sound (4)
Laughs (5)
Discriminates strangers (6)
Resists removal of toy (6)
Mouths toy (6)
Bangs and shakes (7)
Understands no (8-10)
Responds to name (9)
Looks when asks "Where is the ball?" (13)
Plays peek a boo (11-14)
Ask for objects by pointing (15)
Looks at pictures and turn pages (18)
Points to one named body part (18); 4 body parts (24)
Follows two directions (18); three directions (21)
Refers to self by name (24)
Understands size difference (27)
Know full name (30)
Knows if they are a boy or girl (36)
Joins in song (36)

Language
Coos (2-3)
Produces single vowel sounds (2)
Squeals (5)
"ba", "ka", "na" (8)
Shakes head no (9)
Ma Ma and Da Da (8-10)
2 words (12)
Speaks in 2 word sentences (21)
Asks for food when hungry (21)
Uses pronouns (24)
Uses plurals (3)

Self Help

Holds bottle (6)
Holds, bites, and chews (9)
Finger feeds (12)
Takes off hat or shoe (12)
Cooperates with dressing (12)
Pulls off socks (14)
Vocalizes or gestures wants (15)
Imitates housework (16)
Uses spoon (18)
Empties dish when done (18)
Uses toilet (18)
Puts toys away where they belong (21)
Attempts to put shoes on (22); Put on pants (24)
Take off clothes (24); Undresses completely (36)
Spoon feed (24)
Dry hands (30)
Dress with supervision (33)
Unbuttons (36)

Emotional/Social

Crying decreases dramatically (3)
Stranger anxiety (6-8; 15)
Expresses protest (6)
Responds to verbal request (10)
Gives toy to adult upon request (12)
Wants to be near adults (14)
Imitates grown up activities (16)
Parallel play (18); Enjoys roll play (24); Associative play begins (33)

Impairments:

_____ impaired range of motion	_____ impaired respiratory function
_____ impaired motor learning	_____ impaired muscle strength
_____ impaired balance	_____ impaired motor control
_____ impaired coordination	_____ impaired mobility
_____ impaired endurance	

Functional limitations: _____
_____
_____
_____
_____

Other services, equpiment or assistive device recommendations: _____ none

_____
_____
_____
_____

SUMMARY: _____
_____
_____
_____
_____
_____
_____
_____

_____   _____
Physical Therapist signature   Date

_____   _____
Parent's signature   Date

APPENDIX B

An IFSP Example

WV Birth to Three
Office of Maternal, Child and Family Health
Bureau for Public Health
Department of Health and Human Resources

Child's name: _____
Child's date of birth: _____
Date: _____

Family and Child Centered Outcomes

Outcomes are statements of changes families would like to see happen for themselves and their children

Outcome # what do we want to happen in the next six months?	What is happening now related to this outcome?

How will we, as a family, work toward achieving this outcome within our daily activities and routines?	Special skills and knowledge needed that can help make this happen.
	How will other team members support the family in achieving this outcome?
People in the child's life who can make this happen.	Special accommodations/adaptations/equipment that can help make this happen:

We will know this outcome has been met when:

WV Birth to Three. Office of Maternal, Child and Family Health. Bureau for Public Health. Department of Health and Human Resources. 2007. With permission.

Family Survey—Early Intervention. National Center for Special Education Accountability Monitoring

Family Survey - Early Intervention

This is a survey for families receiving Early Intervention services. Your responses will help guide efforts to improve services and results for children and families. For each statement below, please select one of the following response choices: very strongly disagree, strongly disagree, disagree, agree, strongly agree, very strongly agree. You may skip any item that you feel does not apply to your family

Use pencil only

Fill in circle completely:
Incorrect:

Response columns: Very Strongly Disagree | Strongly Disagree | Disagree | Agree | Strongly Agree | Very Strongly Agree

Family-centered services

	Very Strongly Disagree	Strongly Disagree	Disagree	Agree	Strongly Agree	Very Strongly Agree
1. I was offered help I needed, such as child care or transportation, to participate in the individualized Family Service Plan (IFSP) meeting(s).	O	O	O	O	O	O
2. I was asked whether I wanted help in dealing with stressful situations.	O	O	O	O	O	O
3. I was given choices concerning my family's services and supports.	O	O	O	O	O	O
4. My family's daily routines were considered when planning for my child's services	O	O	O	O	O	O
5. I have felt part of the team when meeting to discuss my child.	O	O	O	O	O	O
6. The services on our IFSP have been provided in a timely way	O	O	O	O	O	O

My family was given information about:

	Very Strongly Disagree	Strongly Disagree	Disagree	Agree	Strongly Agree	Very Strongly Agree
7. Modifications of routines, activities, and the physical setting that would help my child.	O	O	O	O	O	O
8. The rights of parents regarding Early Intervention services.	O	O	O	O	O	O
9. Community programs that are open to all children.	O	O	O	O	O	O
10. Organizations that offer support for parents of children with disabilities.	O	O	O	O	O	O
11. How to participate in different programs and services in the community.	O	O	O	O	O	O
12. Opportunities for my child to play with other children.	O	O	O	O	O	O
13. How to advocate for my child and my family.	O	O	O	O	O	O
14. Who to call lif I am not satisfied with the services my child receives.	O	O	O	O	O	O

Someone from the Early Intervention Program:

	Very Strongly Disagree	Strongly Disagree	Disagree	Agree	Strongly Agree	Very Strongly Agree
15. Helped me get services like child care, transportation, respite care, or food stamps.	O	O	O	O	O	O
16. Helped me get in touch with other parents for help and support.	O	O	O	O	O	O
17. Asked whether the services my family was receiving were meeting our needs.	O	O	O	O	O	O
18. Went out into the community with me and my child to help us get involved in the community activities and services.	O	O	O	O	O	O

The Early Intervention service provider(s) that worked with my child:

	Very Strongly Disagree	Strongly Disagree	Disagree	Agree	Strongly Agree	Very Strongly Agree
19. Are dependable.	O	O	O	O	O	O
20. Are easy for me to talk to about my child and my family.	O	O	O	O	O	O
21. Are good at working with my family.	O	O	O	O	O	O
22. My service coordinator is available to speak with me on a regular basis.	O	O	O	O	O	O
23. My service coordinator is knowledgeable and professional.	O	O	O	O	O	O
24. Written information I receive is written in an understandable way.	O	O	O	O	O	O
25. I was given information to help me prepare for my child's transition.	O	O	O	O	O	O

Please turn page over

National Center for Special Education Accountability Monitoring (NCSEAM) LSUHSC/SAHP/HDC. New Orleans, LA. 2007. Web address: www.acountabilitydata.org. Accessed August 25, 2007.

Impact of Early Intervention Services on Your Family

	Very Strongly Disagree	Strongly Disagree	Disagree	Agree	Strongly Agree	Very Strongly Agree
Over the past year, Early Intervention services have helped me and/or my family:	○	○	○	○	○	○
26. Participate in typical activities for children and families in my community.	○	○	○	○	○	○
27. Know about services in the community.	○	○	○	○	○	○
28. Improve my family's quality of life.	○	○	○	○	○	○
29. Know where to go for support to meet my child's needs.	○	○	○	○	○	○
30. Know where to go for support to meet my family's needs.	○	○	○	○	○	○
31. Get the services that my child and family need.						
32. Feel more confident in my skills as a parent.	○	○	○	○	○	○
33. Keep up friendships for my child and family.	○	○	○	○	○	○
34. Make changes in family routines that will benefit my child with special needs.	○	○	○	○	○	○
35. Be more effective in managing my child's behavior.	○	○	○	○	○	○
36. Do activities that are good for my child even in times of stress.	○	○	○	○	○	○
37. Feel that I can get the services and supports that my child and family need.	○	○	○	○	○	○
38. Understand how the Early Intervention system works.	○	○	○	○	○	○
39. Be able to evaluate how much progress my child is making.	○	○	○	○	○	○
40. Feel that my child will be accepted and welcomed in the community.	○	○	○	○	○	○
41. Feel that my family will be accepted and welcomed in the community.	○	○	○	○	○	○
42. Communicate more effectively with the people who work with my child and family.	○	○	○	○	○	○
43. Understand the roles of the people who work with my child and family.	○	○	○	○	○	○
44. Know about my child's and family's rights concerning Early Intervention services.	○	○	○	○	○	○
45. Do things with and for my child that are good for my child's development.	○	○	○	○	○	○
46. Understand my child's special needs.	○	○	○	○	○	○
47. Feel that my efforts are helping my child.	○	○	○	○	○	○

---

48. State of Residence

49. Child's Age at Time of Survey Completion

1. ○   Birth to 1 year
2. ○   1-2 years
3. ○   2-3 years
4. ○   Over 3 years

50. Child's Age When First Referred to Early Intervention

1. ○   Birth to 1 year
2. ○   1-2 years
3. ○   2-3 years

51. Child's Race / Ethnicity

1. ○   White
2. ○   Black or African-American
3. ○   Hispanic or Latino
4. ○   Asian or Pacific Islander
5. ○   American Indian or Alaskan Native
6. ○   Multi-racial

For Office Use Only

--Thank you for your participation--

REFERENCES

1. Carpenter B. Early intervention and identification: finding the family. *Children & Society*. 1997;11:173–182.
2. Individuals with Disabilities Education Improvement Act of 2004. Public Law 108–446. 20 USC 1400.
3. Simpson J. Parenting a Child with Cerebral Palsy (or Parent's Rights). United Cerebral Palsy. 2007;1–6. Available at http://www.ucp.org/ucp_channeldoc.cfm/1/11/51/51-51/775. Accessed August 25, 2007.
4. Baily D. The federal role in early intervention: prospects for the future. *Top Early Child Spec*. 2000;20:2.
5. Butler J. Individuals with Disabilities Education Improvement Act of 2004 compared to Individuals with Disabilities Education Act (IDEA) of 1997 (Draft). The Council of Parents Attorneys and Advocates, Inc.; 2004.
6. Office of Special Education Programs. 25th Annual Report to Congress on the Implementation of the Individuals with Disabilities Education Act. Infants and Toddlers Served Under IDEA, Part C. Washington, DC: U.S. Department of Education; 2003.
7. Folio MR, Fewell RR. *Peabody Developmental Motor Scales*, 2nd ed. Austin, TX: PROED Inc.; 2000.
8. Furuno, O'Reilly K, Hosaka C, et al. Hawaii Early Learning Profile (Inside HELP). Palo Alto, CA.: VORT Corporation; 1994.
9. Goff HE. Hawaii Early Learning Profile (HELP) 2002. Available at http://www.kaimh.org/slides/help/index.htm. Accessed December 2006.
10. Worobey J, Pisuk J, Decker K. Diet and behavior in at-risk children: evaluation of an early intervention program. *Public Health Nurs*. 2004;21:122–127.
11. Early Childhood Outcomes Center. Family and child outcomes for early intervention and early childhood special education. Office of Special Education Program 2005. Available at http://www.fpg.unc.edu/~eco/pdfs/eco_outcomes_4-13-05.pdf. Accessed December 2006.
12. American Physical Therapy Association. *Guide to Physical Therapist Practice*, 2nd ed. Rev. Alexandria VA: American Physical Therapy Association; 2003:98–101.
13. Bricker D, Pretti-Frontczak K, McComas N. *An Activity-based Approach to Early Intervention*, 2nd ed. Baltimore: Brookes; 1998.
14. Pretti-Frontczak KL, Barr DM, Macy M, Carter A. Research and resources related to activity based intervention, embedded learning opportunities, and routines-based instruction. *Top Early Child Spec Ed*. 2003;23:29–39.
15. Technology-Related Assistance for Individuals with Disabilities Act: Public Law 100-407. 1994; reauthorized 1998.
16. Dunst CJ, Bruder MB. Valued outcomes of service coordination, early intervention, and natural environments. *Except Child*. 2002;68:361–375.
17. Chiarello LA, Shelden M, Rapport M, et al. *Early Intervention Services: Natural Learning Environments*. Alexandria, VA: American Physical Therapy Association; 2001.
18. Vanderhoff M. *Maximizing Your Role in Early Intervention*. Alexandria, VA: American Physical Therapy Association; 2004.
19. Scarborough AA, Spiker D, Mallik S, et al. A national look at children and families entering early intervention. *Except Child*. 2004;70:469–483.
20. O'Neil M, Palisano R. Attitudes towards family-centered care and clinical decision making in early intervention among physical therapists. *Pediatr Phys Ther*. 2000;12:173–182.
21. Lattanzi J, Purnell L. *Developing Cultural Competence in Physical Therapy Practice*. Philadelphia, PA: F.A. Davis Company; 2006.
22. Geissler EM. *Mosby's Pocket Guide: Cultural Assessment*. 2nd ed. St. Louis, MO: Mosby; 1998.
23. Zhang C, Bennett T. Multicultural views of disability: implications for early intervention professionals. *Infant Toddler Intervention*. 2001;11:143–154.
24. McCall CH. Early Intervention Program Reimbursement Methodology. State Controller Division of Management Audit and State Financial Services. State of New York: Department of Health; June 1998.

Additional Online Resources

The Regional Resource and Federal Centers (RRFC) Network is made up of the six Regional Resource Centers for Special Education (RRC) and the Federal Resource Center (FRC). The purpose is to assist state education agencies in the systemic improvement of education programs, practices, and policies that affect children and youth with disabilities. These centers offer consultation, information services, technical assistance, training, and product development. Web site: http://www.rrfcnetwork.org/

The National Early Childhood Technical Assistance Center (NECTAC) supports the implementation of the early childhood provisions of IDEA. Our mission is to strengthen service systems to ensure that children with disabilities (birth through age 5) and their families receive and benefit from high quality, culturally appropriate, and family-centered supports and services. Web site: http://www.nectac.org/default.asp. For individual state regulations and policies, the reader is referred to the NECTAC Web site at http://www.nectac.org/partc/statepolicies.asp.

National Dissemination Center for Children with Disabilities. Information on children with disabilities, IDEA, and No Child Left Behind as it relates to children with disabilities and research-based information on effective educational practices. Web site: http://www.nichcy.org/

Access to the Code of Federal Regulations can be found at http://www.access.gpo.gov/nara/cfr/waisidx_06/34cfr303_06.html.

Families and providers can link themselves to their state's Part C Coordinator and Early Intervention Program's Web page by visiting http://nectac.org/contact/Ptccoord.asp#.html.

CHAPTER 7

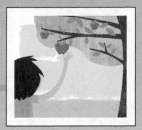

Providing Services in the Educational Environment: Regular Education

Mark Drnach and Joel Clark

LEARNING OBJECTIVES

1. Understand the purpose of Section 504 of the Rehabilitation Act of 1973 as it relates to primary and secondary regular education.
2. Apply the influences of Section 504 to the patient/client management process of a student enrolled in regular education.
3. Understand the general role and responsibilities of the physical therapist in the regular education system.
4. Explain the role of the physical therapist in providing screenings for students in regular education.
5. Articulate the appropriate use of the physical therapist with a select group of high school athletes.

The goal of physical therapy within the regular education setting is to promote the life of the student within the academic community. The role of a student is not limited to learning textbook knowledge. A student is continually participating and adapting to his environment, learning lifelong skills to function as an adult in society. To restrict a student from fully participating in this enriching community would be to deny him the full opportunity for social, psychological, emotional, and intellectual development. Physical therapists must strive to incorporate services into this environment that promote participation and inclusion within the academic community for all children, providing an opportunity for success in academic and extracurricular endeavors.

This chapter will explore the role and practice of physical therapy with children enrolled in the regular education environment, with an emphasis on the Rehabilitation Act of 1973, Section 504.[1] It will review the major aspects of this section of the law and how it can influence the delivery of physical therapy in the school setting. This chapter will also address the general role of a physical therapist in promoting health and fitness in the school-aged child as well as a general understanding of some basic issues of the student athlete.

Throughout this chapter, the Rehabilitation Act of 1973 (PL 93-112), Section 504, which addresses the civil rights of individuals with disabilities, is referred to as Section 504. The Code of Federal Regulations (CFR) is the codification of the general and permanent rules published in the Federal Register that pertain to Section 504 and is referenced as 34CFR104.

THE STUDENT WITH A DISABILITY

In 1973, the federal government of the United States passed the *Rehabilitation Act of 1973* (PL 93-112).[1] This law prohibits discrimination against an individual based on his or her disability in any program that receives federal funds. Generally applied to the issue of discrimination in the workplace and in the employment and training of adults with disabilities, this important piece of civil rights legislation also addressed the failure of the public schools to appropriately educate students with disabilities. It identified and established the need for rehabilitation services (including physical therapy) for the student with a disability in order to meet his educational needs as adequately as the needs of the nondisabled student. This civil rights law provided the framework for the delivery of educational services to children with disabilities that would provide them with the equal opportunity to succeed in the educational environment (emphasis on opportunity, not guaranteeing identical outcomes or level of achievement). Any student with a disability, whether he receives regular education or special education services, is protected under this law, because all public, and some private schools receive federal funding. Section 504 of this law states that no otherwise qualified individual with a disability in the United States, as defined in section 706(8) of this title, shall, solely by reason of her or his disability, be excluded from the participation in, be denied the benefits of, or be subjected to discrimination under any program or activity receiving federal financial assistance [34CFR104.4(a)].

Approximately 4 million students with disabilities are enrolled in public elementary and secondary schools in the United States.[2] A large majority of students with disabilities are spending a significant part of their school day attending classes with nondisabled students.[3,4] Students not requiring specialized instruction (special education services) may still be eligible to receive rehabilitation or *related services* (services that assist a student with a disability to benefit from special education, including physical therapy services) in order to access the general curriculum and school activities. Other students with disabilities may not require modifications or accommodations. Identification of students with impairments or disabilities that are not easily seen (such as a coordination disorder, cardiac disease, or asthma, to name a few) is necessary to ensure an appropriate public education. These hidden disabilities often cannot be readily known without the administration of appropriate diagnostic tests.

THE PRACTICE ENVIRONMENT

The Macroenvironment

The provision of physical therapy services within the educational setting has been firmly established for the past several decades. For years, individual states have required that children receive a formal education. Public education is typically mandated by 6 to 8 years of age, depending on the state. In some states, children can be eligible to voluntarily attend school as early as 4 years of age. These state-led initiatives were precipitated by the earlier forms of education that were completely voluntary.[5] These earlier private and voluntary schools began in Boston, Massachusetts, in the 1600s and continued to gain popularity over time.[6] It was not until the mid 1800s that mandatory education of all children became law in several states, beginning with Massachusetts, which created a system of "common-schools," based on the belief that every child was entitled to the same content in education. This concept of education continued to spread, and by 1918 all states had laws requiring education of children at the elementary school level.[7]

It is important to note that the education of children in the United States is primarily the responsibility of the state and local communities, with some financial assistance provided by the federal government. This federal involvement would ultimately bring about fundamental changes in society, allowing for equal opportunity in education for all children regardless of race, gender, or physical or mental capability.

The Federal Government

For most of our nation's history, schools were allowed to exclude and often did exclude certain children, especially those with disabilities. In the era of the Civil Rights Movement and the passage of significant civil rights legislation, the federal government, in 1965, passed the *Elementary and Secondary Education Act* (PL 89-10). This legislation provided a plan for addressing the inequality of educational opportunity for economically underprivileged children and became the statutory basis upon which early special education legislation was later drafted. In 1972, President Nixon signed into law the *Educational Amendments to the Civil Rights Act* of 1964, which included the landmark *Title IX,* which prohibits sex discrimination in any educational program or activity within an institution that receives any type of federal financial assistance. Under this law, boys and girls are expected to receive fair and equal treatment in all areas of public schooling: recruitment, admissions, educational programs and activities, course offerings, financial aid, scholarships, and athletics. Subsequent legislation included PL 94-142, the Education for All Handicapped Children Act of 1975, which mandated a free appropriate public education (FAPE) for all children with disabilities, and became the core of federal funding for special education. (This law, subsequently amended, is now known as the Individuals with Disabilities Education Act [IDEA]; see Chapter 8.) The Rehabilitation Act of 1973 is not considered educational law; rather, it addresses the civil rights of an individual. This law has been amended and reauthorized a number of times since its inception. In 1978, PL 95-602 expanded the scope of Section 504 to include agencies of the executive branch of the federal government. PL 98-221 was passed in 1983 authorizing demonstration projects for the transition of individuals with disabilities from school to work, and the Rehabilitation Act Amendments of 1986 (PL 99-506) provided programs in supported employment services for individuals with disabilities. A subsequent and more current law that protects the civil rights of a person with a disability is the 1990 Americans with Disabilities Act (ADA; see Chapter 10).[8]

POINT TO REMEMBER

The Rehabilitation Act

The Rehabilitation Act addresses the civil rights of an individual. It prohibits the discrimination of an individual based on his or her disability in programs and activities that receive federal financial assistance. It is a civil rights law, not an educational law like the IDEA.

Most federal laws passed by the U.S. Congress establish minimum standards that the states have to follow in order to receive federal funds. Some flexibility with state laws and regulations are allowed but they cannot be more restrictive than the federal law if the state wishes to receive federal monies. Most education regulations come from state and local governments with the exception of special education, which is strictly regulated under the IDEA.

POINT TO REMEMBER

Title IX

The Educational Amendment of the Civil Rights Act, Title IX, requires that boys and girls receive fair and equal treatment in all areas of public education. This legislation is a major influence on female participation in school sports.

PARENT PERSPECTIVE

DAUGHTERS IN SCHOOL SPORTS

Regarding daughters in sports. When I grew up in the 1960s and early 1970s, there were virtually no sports for girls. Going to a catholic school certainly did not help the situation as we didn't even have gym class. My choices were to either be a cheerleader or majorette. Since I took dance lessons since I was 4 years old, I chose to be a high school majorette.

When we had our first daughter in 1979, our second in 1980, and our third in 1983, we thought we would be spending endless hours in dancing schools and watching dance recitals. But thanks to Title IX, things certainly changed for our daughters. They are all athletic, and as a result we were the cheerleaders for our daughters as they played softball, basketball, soccer, gymnastics, volleyball, and rugby. Had it not been for Title IX, they would not have had the opportunity to experience sports and reap the benefits of good competition and team spirit.

—*Sharon D., mother of three daughters.*

The State Government

It is important to understand the specific state regulations that affect the delivery of educational services and the utilization of rehabilitative or related services for students. A physical therapist should contact the state's department of education and obtain a copy of the policies and procedures, as well as the rules and regulations for the provision of educational services in the state.

Although Section 504 of the Rehabilitation Act does not provide direct funding to schools, it does carry the threat of losing funding if the school does not comply. The majority of funding comes from the state level, but the federal government does contribute to the revenues received for educating a student. During the 2002–2003 school year, the median school district in the United States received $8,891.00 per student in revenues from local, state, and federal sources.[9] On average, about 8% of those revenues came from the federal government, 50% from the state government, and 42% from local taxes.[9] Each child, by law, is entitled to a FAPE. Educational costs paid by parents of a student with a disability are to be no different than those paid by parents of a student without a disability. (Examples include such things as fees for class pictures, special field trips, or class social functions.) This is a basic tenet of FAPE. See Box 7-1 for additional information regarding FAPE.

BOX 7-1
Free Appropriate Public Education

An appropriate public education will include:

1. educational services designed to meet the individual educational needs of students with disabilities as adequately as the needs of nondisabled students;
2. the education of each student with a disability with nondisabled students, to the maximum extent appropriate to the needs of the student with a disability;
3. nondiscriminatory evaluation and placement procedures established to guard against misclassification or inappropriate placement of students, and a periodic re-evaluation of students who have been provided special education or related services; and
4. the establishment of due process procedures that (i) enable parents and guardians to receive required notices, review their child's records, and challenge identification, evaluation, and placement decisions; (ii) provide for an impartial hearing with the opportunity for participation by parents and representation by counsel; and (iii) include a review procedure.

FAPE for Students with Disabilities: Requirements under Section 504 of the Rehabilitation Act of 1973. U.S. Department of Education. Office of Civil Rights. July 1999.

Additional funding may be obtained through the states medicaid program. The Medicare Catastrophic Coverage Act (PL 100-360) prohibits Medicaid from denying payment for services that are covered by the state's Medicaid plan to children with disabilities solely because such services are included in the student's Individualized Education Program (IEP) or the child's Individualized Family Service Plan (IFSP).[10] This legislation, often used to provide funding for related services in early intervention and special education, generally does not include Section 504 services.

The role of the local board of education is to provide guidance to the schools in the district and to oversee the running of the educational services. The board functions as an elected board of directors, working with the chief educational officer, the superintendent of the schools, in developing and implementing policies and procedures for the district. The local board of education is responsible for all legal matters, financial reports and budgets, and the hiring of all employees upon the recommendation of the superintendent. The board of education, upon the recommendation of the superintendent, authorizes the hiring or contracting of a physical therapist for the district. The board is also responsible, along with the local school district administration, for establishing policies and procedures for implementing Section 504 and the designation of a *Section 504 Coordinator*, who is the person responsible for assisting the school in meeting the requirements of Section 504 of the Rehabilitation Act by providing resources and helping the school make the necessary accommodations for qualified students.

At least annually, the local school district has a duty to conduct a *child find* activity during which the school district must make efforts to identify and locate every qualified student with a disability who resides in their jurisdiction, and to notify the parents of a student with a disability of the district's obligations to provide a FAPE (34CFR104.32).

POINT TO REMEMBER

Board of Education

The local board of education authorizes the hiring of all school employees and contracted services, such as physical therapy.

THE REHABILITATION ACT, SECTION 504

To be eligible for services under Section 504, a student must qualify as an individual with a disability. As defined in the law, an individual with a disability means any person who:

1. has a mental or physical impairment which substantially limits one or more major life activities;
2. has a record of such an impairment; or
3. is regarded as having such an impairment [34CFR 104.3(j)(1)].

Impairment may include any disability, chronic illness, or disorder that substantially limits the student's ability to learn in the educational setting and substantially limits one or more major life activities. Major life activities can include, but are not limited to, self-care, manual tasks, walking, seeing, speaking, sitting, learning, breathing, interacting with others, and working.

Anyone can refer a student for an evaluation under Section 504, but the school must also have a reason to believe that the student is in need of services due to a disability. The school district does not have to evaluate a student based solely on the recommendation of the referral source (parent, physician, physical therapist, etc.). The deciding factor is whether the school staff suspects that the student has an impairment that substantially limits a major life activity and is in need of services in order to access an education.

According to federal regulations, placement decisions are to be made by a group of persons, the *Section 504 Committee*, who are knowledgeable about the child, the meaning of the evaluation data, placement options, *least restrictive environment* requirements, and comparable facilities [34CFR104.35(c)(3)]. (Least restrictive environment is defined in the IDEA as: To the extent appropriate, the education of students with disabilities with students who are not disabled, in a regular classroom [34CFR300.550].) Unlike special education, the federal requirements under Section 504 do not require the parents to be a member of the committee. Best practice guidelines and local policies may dictate otherwise. In addition, a school district has the option of attempting to address any identified impairments through traditional school-based interventions (those interventions that would be used on a student without an impairment or disability) prior to conducting an evaluation. If such interventions are successful, a district is not obligated to evaluate a student for additional modification or accommodations.

POINT TO REMEMBER

Disability Defined

As defined in the law, an individual with a disability means any person who:

1. has a mental or physical impairment which substantially limits one or more major life activities;
2. has a record of such an impairment; or
3. is regarded as having such an impairment.

The Evaluation

Parental consent is required prior to beginning an evaluation. Under Section 504, no formalized testing is required to determine the student's eligibility, but the Section 504 Committee should consider a variety of information from more than one source. These sources could include health records, grades from previous years, information from the parents, physical therapy reports, attendance records, etc. Decisions on placement should be made based on information about the specific student and the identified accommodations or modifications that will be needed. According to the law, the tests and other evaluation materials that are used must be validated for the specific purpose of their use and administered by trained personnel. The test results should also reflect the student's aptitude or achievement rather than a measurement of the student's impairment, except where those areas are the factors that the test purports to measure. Re-evaluations are required periodically or if any significant changes in placement are anticipated (34CFR104.35).

Having information on any established medical diagnosis that the student has may aid in the understanding of the prognosis and in the selection of appropriate intervention strategies. Parental involvement is essential in this process as the educational record seldom contains the necessary information often found in a medical record to aid in this process. Knowing the pathology will help in understanding the possible impairments to movement and function that may be seen or expected in the student (see the physical therapy evaluation in the Appendix of Chapter 8). Some key issues to also consider are the medications taken by the student, either at school or at home. This information will aid in understanding the factors that may influence the student's motor learning or motor control. Measurements of the student's height and weight will also come in handy if future dimensions for assistive technology or accommodations are needed.

There are two main factors in determining eligibility that could be addressed in a physical therapy evaluation. First, what is the physical impairment? Second, how does this impairment substantially limit the student's ability to participate in a major life activity?

Physical therapists have several tests and measurements that examine and quantify impairments such as range of motion, muscle strength, or endurance, as well as capture functional skills such as walking or stair negotiation.

Standardized tests can also be used to obtain comprehensive information on a student's motor development. The Peabody Developmental Motor Scales, Second Edition (PDMS 2) is a norm referenced standardized test used to evaluate a child's (1 month to 6 years) level of motor skill.[11] It is composed of six subtests that evaluate a range of gross and fine motor skills. These subtests include reflexes, stationary abilities, locomotion, object manipulation, grasping, and visual-motor integration. The scores for each subtest are combined to provide a total motor quotient, which is then compared with norm-referenced data. The PDMS-2's psychometric properties include a test–retest reliability of 0.94, inter-rater reliabil-

ity of 0.99, construct validity in the range of 0.63 to 0.83, and a content validity in the range of 0.35 to 0.69.[11]

Another standardized test is the Bruininks-Oseretsky Test of Motor Performance, Second Edition (BOT-2).[12] The BOT-2 is a norm-referenced, standardized test that evaluates the child's (4.5 to 14.5 years) motor skills. The BOT-2 is composed of eight subtests including fine motor precision, fine motor integration, manual dexterity, bilateral coordination, balance, running speed and agility, upper-limb coordination, and strength. The subtest scores are combined to provide an overall comprehensive measure of motor proficiency. The BOT-2 has a test–retest reliability of 0.87 and an inter-rater reliability of 0.63 to 0.97.[12]

In addition to the administration of tests and measurements, there should be observation of the student performing basic motor skills needed to function in the educational environment. Mobility within the environment, positioning during educational activities, manipulation of tools used in the learning process, and participation in group and leisure activities are all important aspects of a student's school day. Consultation with the student's teachers and school staff regarding the unique tasks assigned to the particular student during this time in his educational process (current lesson plans) is important to help identify the educational impact of the student's disability and plan for the education of the student in the least restrictive environment possible.

If the student is determined to be eligible, the Section 504 Committee will create an accommodation plan, or a *Section 504 Plan*, for the student. Section 504 does not require a student to be enrolled in special education in order to receive related services.

POINT TO REMEMBER

Testing for Eligibility

Under Section 504, no formalized testing is mandated to determine a student's eligibility.

The Section 504 Plan

There is no legal requirement stating what should be included in the Section 504 Plan like there is for an IFSP in early intervention or an IEP in special education. Basically the plan should address the identified impairment or disability, how it impacts a major life activity, and how this impact relates to the student's education. The plan should also clearly spell out the necessary accommodations or modifications needed that would allow the student to access his educational program in the classroom or in the least restrictive environment identified.

If for some reason the parents do not agree with the Section 504 Plan, the local school district is required to provide an impartial hearing with regard to the identification, evaluation, or placement of a student. The physical therapist should be familiar with a district's policy and procedures that address due process. Parents who have a complaint regarding Section 504 should contact the Office for Civil Rights, which has the authority to enforce Section 504 and will assist in mediation.

The Section 504 Plan does not reduce the academic expectations of the student, but provides the necessary modifications to enable the student with a disability or impairment to participate and have an equal chance to compete in the classroom. A physical therapist could assist in the modifications necessary to achieve this goal.

POINT TO REMEMBER

The 504 Plan

Unlike the IEP or IFSP, there are no federal mandates requiring that a Section 504 Plan be in writing or that specific content be included. Other possible names for a Section 504 Plan are an Individual Accommodation Plan (IAP), a Modified Education Plan (MEP), or a service agreement.

Physical Therapy and Section 504

Typically the education of a student in the regular education system is the primary responsibility of the classroom teacher who is part of a multidisciplinary team. This team can include allied health professionals in physical and occupational therapy, speech language pathology, and nursing. Other support personnel may include dieticians, psychologists, social workers, and academic counselors. It must be remembered that the provision of physical therapy services is only one part of a larger plan to enhance the ability of the student to learn. Services should be limited to those that are most beneficial and appropriate for the student at this particular time in his educational process. Duplication of services should be avoided.

Students who are receiving services, modifications, or accommodations under a Section 504 Plan may appear to be less disabled than students enrolled in special education. Physical therapists are called to understand their role as a team member in the regular education environment and to provide appropriate interventions that meet the intent of the law in providing an FAPE for all children in the least restrictive environment available. A collaborative effort from all persons involved can assure that the most appropriate level and type of intervention is being incorporated into the student's daily educational routines and activities in order to optimize his ability to access and utilize his educational environment, comparable to his nondisabled peers. Collaboration and consultation with the school administration, teacher, and classroom staff are important aspects of service delivery in the educational setting. Unlike an IFSP or IEP, the identification and recording of the frequency and duration of intervention

in the Section 504 Plan is not mandatory under the Rehabilitation Act, but may be a policy or procedure required by the state. Also, the State's Practice Act for Physical Therapy will also dictate the need for a physician's referral and the supervisory guidelines for the utilization of a physical therapist assistant.

A physical therapist can be a key member of the team when working with students who have impairments that affect their ability to access or utilize materials in the educational environment, yet are not eligible for services under the IDEA. An important intervention is communication, coordination, and education of the members of the team and classroom staff in identifying impairments and promoting an understanding of how the impairment affects the student. The physical therapist can provide information and impart knowledge regarding movement and disabilities with function in the classroom, educating everyone involved on the nature and extent of which the impairment can be alleviated through the use of modifications or accommodations. It is said that attitudes about a disability are more disabling than the disability itself. Understanding the impairments of a student with a coordination disorder or attention deficit disorder, for example, is the first step in the process of enablement.

Documentation of accessibility and the dimensions of desks, chairs, and other items will provide the basic information needed for modifications to the environment or the use of assistive technology, if needed. Under the ADA, the federal government mandated structural modification and/or construction allowing for environmental access for individuals with disabilities.[8] It is within the scope of practice of a physical therapist to examine and assist in the creation of an accessible environment for the student with a disability enrolled in regular education. Are the doorways large enough to accommodate a wheelchair? Is the ramp used to access the school at the appropriate slope to allow for self-propulsion? Are the thresholds small enough to allow a student using crutches or a walker to safely walk over them? Is the lighting sufficient and properly directed to allow the student to see the educational materials? (Some of the key aspects of accessibility can also be found in Chapter 10.) These criteria are based on adult design and may not be applicable to young children. The Federal Access Board provides advisory guidelines on specifications for accessible building elements for children 12 years old or younger. Student and teacher instruction on the use of assistive technology in the classroom or environmental modifications in the school would also be appropriate.

Procedural interventions could include functional training in the school to allow for better participation in the classroom, physical education (PE) class, and extracurricular activities, such as field trips or outings into the community. Teaching a student compensatory movement strategies may also be necessary in order for

BOX 7-2
Examples of Adaptive Equipment That Can be Utilized in School

- pencil grips
- adaptive scissors
- adaptive seating
- inclined boards/writing surface
- magnification devices
- computer touch screens
- adaptive equipment for eating
- standing and mobility devices
- bowling ramps
- beeper balls
- playground equipment
- adaptive toilet
- electronic communication devices

him to function efficiently. Interventions provided should be developmentally appropriate as well as educationally relevant. Environmental modifications have been greatly enhanced with the growth of the assistive technology field. On the low-tech end of the spectrum, a student may only need a built-up pencil grip to assist with writing activities. At the other end of the spectrum, a host of highly specialized and computerized equipment is available to help promote function (Box 7-2). The prescription or application of splints, assistive devices, or orthotics may be necessary to provide the student with increased stability and/or mobility or to provide better energy conservation (and therefore endurance) throughout the school day. With the realization that most students are provided services in a financially finite program, the physical therapist should explore creative and least costly modifications whenever appropriate. Some of the easiest solutions to everyday problems are created through cooperation and communication with the classroom staff, student, and parents.

PE has been, and in some areas remains, a significant contribution to the physical activity of a student with a disability. The goal of PE is to provide the student with activities that promote movement and interaction with peers to aid in physical development and a sense of fitness and wellness. The physical therapist can provide guidance in activity modification or staff education regarding a student's abilities. In many school districts, adaptive PE has been restricted due to the decreasing budget for overall PE. For this reason, the physical therapist should work closely with the PE teacher to provide appropriate activities for the student. It should be remembered that PE is part of the education law and an aspect of FAPE, the desired outcome of all interventions.

Physical Therapy Interventions

Physical therapy interventions may include:

- communication, coordination, and documentation;
- direct client/student-related instruction;
- functional training in the school;
- environmental modifications; and
- the teaching of compensatory strategies.

Outcomes

The desired outcome of public education is to provide a student with the necessary skills to enable him to participate in society at whatever level is the optimal and most appropriate for him. Parents and professionals should always keep in mind the ultimate reason for developing plans, interventions, and education for the child, with or without a disability: the goal of independent functioning as an adult. Five criteria can be used to assess whether a student is developing skills to function independently, in addition to his academic goals.

1. The degree of independence in the communication of wants, needs, and interests, and the ability to make decisions for oneself. This is much larger than the ability to communicate to another person, but to communicate thoughts, feelings, opinions, and desires. This ability forms the basis of relationships, autonomy, and feelings of self-worth.

2. The degree of socially acceptable behavior. The student must behave in socially acceptable ways in a variety of social situations, especially during school or work hours. Consistent behavioral outbursts that are verbally or physically aggressive are detrimental to the student's ability to learn or work with others in an educational or employment situation. They can also be detrimental to relationships and to the feeling of self-control.

3. The degree of independence in personal care and hygiene. The ability of a student to maintain his appearance and to manage his own personal needs provide a level of independence and autonomy.

4. The degree of independence with self-feeding and drinking. Not only is this necessary for nutritional reasons, but mealtime is a highly social aspect of a student's day. The ability to manage this motor task efficiently will allow time for him to socialize and to build relationships.

5. The degree of independence in mobility and accessing the environment. With the ever-increasing ability of assistive technologies to provide a means of mobility, and with federal laws that mandate accessibility, more and more students are finding this type of independence a possibility. The more a student moves about

his environment and can access public transportation or drive, the more people he comes in contact with, and the more opportunities he has for social interaction. The more social interactions he has, the more opportunities for relationship development. Relationships can lead to opportunities for more community involvement, friendships, and ultimately independence from his family.

P O I N T   T O   R E M E M B E R

Outcomes

Suggestions for student outcome areas in addition to academic performance:

- Communication
- Behavior
- Personal care and hygiene
- Self-feeding and drinking
- Mobility

An annual summary that addresses these outcomes provides a method for assessment of functional gains and the identification of the benefits received from the accommodations and modifications made during the prior school year. A re-evaluation of the impairments and limitations of the major life activities identified could also be done at this time to assure compliance and continued eligibility. The law requires periodic (defined under the IDEA as at least every 3 years) re-evaluation of the education program. A re-evaluation should also occur if any changes in placement are being considered or if the student is changing schools, which may require a re-evaluation of accessibility.

TRANSITIONING

The term *transition services* means a coordinated set of activities for a student, designed within an outcome-oriented process, that promotes movement from school to postschool activities, including postsecondary education, vocational training, integrated employment (including supported employment), continuing and adult education, adult services, independent living, or community participation. The coordinated set of activities is based on the individual student's needs, taking into account the student's preferences and interests, and includes instruction, community experiences, the development of employment and other postschool adult living objectives, and, when appropriate, acquisition of daily living skills and functional vocational evaluation.[13]

Unlike the IDEA, no written transition plan is mandated under Section 504, but the process is required. Preparation and transitioning from one program to

another, and from one stage of life to the next, is a continual process that both parents and students experience throughout their lifetime. Moving from one program to another, or approaching a developmental milestone such as obtaining a job or graduating from high school, can be a difficult and stressful experience. Adequate preparation for transitioning will provide the parents and student with resources, information, and time to make an informed decision regarding their individual needs and preferences for the future. Box 7-3 provides some examples of lifelong transitioning. The future plans and aspirations of any student should always be considered as part of his educational program, including any plan or interventions provided by the physical therapist. Early education and planning by the parents and student will allow them to better understand the student's potential and to identify and discuss the possible choices he will have available to him as he matures into a young adult.

BOX 7-3
Lifelong Transition Planning

Infant (0 to 1 year): Begin financial planning for the future. Encourage movement, exploration, basic communication, and learning.

Toddler (1 to 3 years): Encourage language development, outdoor play, mobility, and exploration of the toddler's larger environment. Read to your child and encourage pre-literacy skills. Celebrate accomplishments. Lay the foundation for a positive self-image. Promote independence. Plan for the type of school in which your child will be enrolled.

Young Child (preschool; 4 to 6 years): Encourage independence in self-help skills. Involve your child in chores around the house. Give the child responsibilities and feedback on performance. Teach basic life skills, meal preparation. Teach your child how to handle emergency situations. Teach your child about his abilities and his disability. Involve your child in social activities. Encourage cooperative play. Seek inclusion in the educational environment as much as possible.

The Child (elementary; 7 to 12 years): Plan for high school and what he will do after he graduates from high school. Encourage a sleepover with a friend or relative. Encourage independence in his ADLs.

The Adolescent (high school; 13 to 18 years): Teach your adolescent instrumental ADLs (IADLs): shopping, managing money, budgeting expenses, earning income. Have him volunteer in community or religious programs. Teach him how to use public transportation and basic public services. Encourage steps towards personal independence. Plan for a career, activities beyond high school. Support his rational decisions and allow him to make independent choices. Let your adolescent experience appropriate consequence of his decisions and help him work through the outcomes.

THE STUDENT WITHOUT A DISABILITY

All students, with or without a disability, have the right to an appropriate public education, including the right to participate in PE and extracurricular activities. The physical therapist can also provide a valuable service to students without disabilities through general screenings and examinations of the musculoskeletal and cardiopulmonary systems, nutritional screenings, preparticipation screenings for sports, and education on prevention of injury and sport-specific training.

Screenings and Examinations of the Student

Postural evaluation and screening are common aspects of the physical therapist's role in the educational setting. Many times the physical therapist is evaluating the posture of a student before the official examination has even begun. This process can begin with observation of the student as he walks within the school hallway or is seated in a classroom. To examine posture on an objectified basis, several key anatomic landmarks must be identified in relation to the body's position in the frontal plane. A plum line should pass through the external auditory meatus, the lateral aspect of the acromioclavicular joint, the greater trochanter of the femur, just anterior to the midline of the lateral femoral condyle (excessive anterior displacement of the plum line in relation to the knee signifies genu recurvatum), and finally through the lateral malleolus. An anterior and posterior perspective should also be taken when examining posture.

A common component of a postural screen is the examination of the spine. Visual examination should include observation of the normal alignment and spinal curves. The human spinal column is composed of naturally occurring curves, which add to its structural stability. When the spine curves laterally, the normal processes of articulation, mobility, and support can be compromised. These lateral curves, occurring primarily in the frontal plan, are termed scoliosis.[12] Screening for scoliosis is a common practice in many of our public schools for grades five through eight. To date no standard procedure for the screening of scoliosis has been universally adopted. Box 7-4 includes some commonly asked questions when performing a scoliosis screening. The physical therapist should remember that curves <20 degrees may be difficult to identify without the use of radiographs. In addition, female adolescents, who are tall for their age, may have a predisposition to this problem.[14]

In addition to posture, an examination of a student's fitness level can be done. This type of examination has traditionally been overlooked or summarily included in a general PE course. The use of standardized tests and measures to assess fitness levels provides reliability and validity that were previously underutilized. As part of the initial evaluation, vital signs should be examined to

---

BOX 7-4
Screening for Scoliosis

Standing Position
Is one shoulder higher than the other, or is there more muscle fullness on one side of the neck?
Is one scapula higher or more prominent than the other?
Is there more distance between the arm and the body on one side than the other?
Is there a deeper crease on one side of the waist compared to the other?
Does the spine itself appear to curve?
Is one hip higher than the other?
Does the person have a kyphosis?
Does the person have a lordosis?

Bending Forward
Is there a hump in the rib area?
Is there a hump in the lumbar region?

Leg Length Discrepancy
Is there a leg length discrepancy?

---

determine general health values as compared to established normative values.[15] Upon completion of vital sign evaluation, a number of options are available to the physical therapist. A program with established criteria has been published by The President's Challenge for Kids, which provides useful information for daily activity and monitoring of caloric expenditure.[16] In relation to fitness evaluations, data have been collected and normalized for ages 6 through 17 plus years. The areas of evaluation include curl-ups, shuttle run, V-sit and reach, sit and reach, 1-mile run-walk, pull-ups, right angle push-ups, and flexed arm hang.[17] Testing of a student in any of these activities results in determining the level of fitness for that particular activity in relation to national percentiles for age-adjusted values, providing the physical therapist with an accurate and repeatable testing pattern for evaluating a student fitness level in respect to normative data. (The normalized data did not take into account physical or mental disability and the subsequent impact on individual scores. An adjustment and baseline value in each of these areas for children with disabilities has not been established to date.)

Another area that can be reviewed by the physical therapist is nutrition. Food insufficiency has been sited as a significant contributing factor to decreased cognitive, academic, and psychosocial development.[18] Research has shown that the peak of human brain glucose utilization occurs between 4 and 7 years of age in conjunction with synaptogenesis.[19] At a point in time when students are maturing both physically and mentally, proper nutrition is essential. Restrictive diets, physical disabilities, distorted body images, eating disorders, and obesity all play a role in limiting the intake of proper nutrition.

The United States Department of Agriculture (USDA) has established a food guide pyramid for both children and adults. This guide was established to provide a recommended allowance of nutrients derived from a person's daily diet. Research has shown that only 1% of youth in America are meeting the required allowances put forth by the USDA.[20] Physical therapists should recognize the importance of adequate nutrition in the healing process of injured tissues as well as the maintenance of homeostasis. Although direct dietetic counseling is not within the scope of practice, it is the responsibility of health care professionals to identify risk factors in students and make a proper referral when appropriate. There are a number of ways in which this can be accomplished. Commonly used within a variety of settings is a food journal or dietary intake log. This involves the student recording the quantity and type of food and beverage consumed over the course of approximately 1 week's time. Although this can provide valuable insight into the typical dietary patterns of a student, there are a number of drawbacks readily identifiable. First, a young child should not be held responsible for constant recording and monitoring of food intake. The reliability of this action could be questioned. Second, a student typically has the majority of his daily intake provided by a parental figure, which would transfer the responsibility and subsequent need for education of that individual. A more reliable option for the physical therapist within an educational setting is the utilization of a nutritional screening. Currently, there are no clinically validated nutrition screenings for application to students within the educational setting. The position statement of the American Dietetic Association is that all children and adolescents, regardless of age; gender; socioeconomic status; racial, ethnic, or linguistic diversity; or health status should have access to food and nutrition programs that ensure the availability of a safe and adequate food supply that promotes optimal physical, cognitive, and social growth and development.[21] According to the current policy, nutritional considerations should be made upon the diagnosis of the individual and not the fact that he or she has a disability. For this reason, it is recommended that the physical therapist be familiar with the common medical diagnoses seen in children and the related nutritional deficiencies that may occur. Box 7-5 presents some commonly asked questions of the student or parents related to a nutritional screening that may be beneficial when determining if a referral to a registered dietician is appropriate. In addition, clinical signs and symptoms of an eating disorder may require a referral to a qualified professional. These may include reports of a recent dramatic weight loss, an obsession with weight, calorie counting, or excessive exercising. Additional clinical signs may include hair loss, dizziness, frequent reports of a sore throat, low

> **BOX 7-5**
> Nutrition
>
> *Questions for a nutritional screen*
>
> Does the student have an illness or disability that affects the kind or amount of food they can eat?
>
> Does the student eat two or fewer meals a day?
>
> Does the student eat few fruits, vegetables, or dairy products?
>
> Does the student have oral dysfunction that makes eating difficult?
>
> Is proper assistance provided for the student if eating independently is impaired?
>
> Has the student had an abnormal change in body weight in the past 6 months not associated with a growth spurt?
>
> Does the student participate in physical activity on a regular daily basis?
>
> Does the student's body mass index score fall within an acceptable range for his age?
>
> Do the student's height and weight correlate with accepted growth charts for his age?
>
> Adapted from American Academy of Family Physicians[22]

blood pressure, or a loss of a menstrual cycle. Early detection through the use of screening allows the physical therapist to provide earlier intervention.

These general screenings and evaluations can be beneficial to all students, especially those involved in school sports.

POINT TO REMEMBER

Physical Therapy for All Students

Additional services may include:
- Postural screenings
- General fitness evaluations
- Nutritional screenings

The Student Athlete

Organized sport participation plays an intricate role in the growth and development of many school-aged children. The international level of participation in sports has reportedly ranged from 64% to 79% for school-aged children.[23,24] A national trend has emerged in recent years of recruiting children at younger ages to begin training for competition. The resultant effect is a population of children who are presenting with high stress and overuse injuries at a point in their development that previously did not exist. To fully appreciate this change in philosophy, the physical therapist must take into consideration the developmental pattern of a prepubescent and pubescent child. A number of issues have been identified physiologically in relation to pediatric athletes. These issues typically center on possible injury to the apophyseal growth center, fibrocartilaginous insult, musculotendinous injury, or the decreased resistance of bone to external stresses with physical maturity.[25-27] The extent to which a child has matured physically will greatly impact the long-term effects of his injury and, consequently, his recovery.

POINT TO REMEMBER

The Pediatric Athlete

Physical immaturity in pediatric athletes exposes them to an increased risk of injury when participating in sports.

In a study that analyzed the prevalence of sports-related injury in pediatric athletes, 28% of injuries were located in the wrist and/or hand, 22% in the head or face, and 18% in the ankle or foot.[28] There were four sports related to the majority of injuries seen in an emergency department. These sports included basketball (19.5%), football (17.1%), baseball/softball (14.9%), and soccer (14.2%).[28] Of particular interest was a study conducted by Powell and Barber-Foss, which analyzed the incidence of sports-related injuries between boys and girls. Among the sports previously mentioned (with the exception of football), girls had a higher incidence of injury than their male counterparts in all sports. The author noted that female basketball and soccer players had a higher number of anterior cruciate ligament (ACL) surgeries than did female or male players in any other sport.[29]

The following section will examine four common sports and the physical demand that they place on the pediatric athlete. Common orthopedic injuries will also be discussed in relation to each sport to provide the reader with an appreciation of how a physical therapist can be utilized.

THE PREPARTICIPATION SPORT EXAMINATION

The preparticipation sport examination (PPSE) has been an area traditionally provided by the physician. Although some aspects of the traditional examination should still be referred to a physician for clearance before participating in sports, the scope of physical therapy practice includes many aspects of the PPSE. It is recommended that the physical therapist performing a PPSE be familiar with orthopedic sports medicine diagnoses and have further continuing education in this field before performing a school-wide annual examination. Unfamiliarity with correct examination techniques has been cited as a major concern for allied health professionals in performing a PPSE.[30] The following is a brief overview of the format and reasoning behind the examination.

The examination begins with a thorough description of the student's past medical history. It is here that underlying pathology and areas of concern can be identified for further inspection. The physical therapist should be aware of cardiac, congenital, neurologic, visual, or genitourinary pathologies that warrant referral to a physician before clearance for participation in sports. The next step involves a general upper and lower quarter screening. The student is assessed for musculoskeletal, neuromuscular, and integumentary impairments through a range-of-motion examination, manual muscle testing, observation, and examination of functional and sports-related movements. The author recommends including several additional special tests as part of the PPSE, although they are not required in a traditional upper and lower quarter screen. These tests include the anterior apprehension test of the shoulder, Lachman's test for ACL instability in the knee, the talar tilt test and anterior drawer test of the ankle, drop arm test, and Patrick's test. These six tests provide a quick method for determining joint stability in the four most commonly injured joints associated with athletes. Box 7-6 lists the procedure for these tests and the positive test result.

Of critical importance when performing the PPSE is an evaluation of functional core strength. This evaluation can be done in conjunction with the upper and lower quarter screenings as a transition between the two. This evaluation should include an endurance test as well as a test of functional strength. Core strength of the athlete has been identified as the vital component in athletic performance.[32] In order for the athlete to be able to perform at a competitive level both effectively and safely, the extremities must have a strong platform. Allowing a student athlete to compete with proximal muscle weakness can place that athlete at an increased risk for injury.

Two issues of increasing concern with high school and middle school athletes are eating disorders and the use of steroids. Both of these issues can be touched upon during the PPSE. The first is typically associated with female athletes but can include male athletes. People who are close to the individual most often identify the eating disorder. This identification may first come from a friend or coach who spends a significant amount of time with the athlete. Although direct intervention of eating disorders such as anorexia nervosa and bulimia nervosa are outside the scope of practice for the physical therapist, a team-oriented approach is strongly recommended. Referral to a physician, registered dietician, or psychological therapist and inclusion of the team coach are necessary in providing support and help for the athlete with an eating disorder. A second concern for athletes is the abuse of anabolic steroids. A growing trend has been identified of increased usage at all levels of organized sports. Although abuse in an athlete may be harder to identify due to natural growth changes, diligent observation and the use of an annual PPSE can aid in identifying these individuals. Education

BOX 7-6
Common Special Tests Used During the PPSE[31]

Lachman's Test for ACL instability of the knee: With patient supine and with 30 degrees of knee flexion, the examiner anteriorly translates the tibia on the femur while stabilizing the distal femur. Excessive movement of the tibia and laxity at the end range of motion indicate anterior cruciate ligament laxity (when compared with the contralateral ACL).

Anterior Apprehension Test of the shoulder: Passive abduction and external rotation of the shoulder elicits a feeling of apprehension or alarm that the shoulder may dislocate (positive). The positive test indicates anterior glenohumeral instability.

Talar Tilt Test of the ankle: With the ankle in the anatomic position, an inversion force is applied to the calcaneus. Excessive range of motion is indicative of calcaneofibular ligament laxity.

Anterior Drawer Test of the ankle: After proximal stabilization of the tibia/fibula, examiner anteriorly translates the talus in the ankle mortise (ankle positioned in 20 degrees plantar flexion). Excessive translation as compared with the contralateral ankle is positive for anterior talofibular ligament laxity.

Drop Arm Test of the shoulder: With patient seated, perform passive abduction of the upper extremity to 90 degrees. Patient is unable to return the arm to his side slowly or without pain (positive). A positive test indicates a tear or mechanical insult to the rotator cuff; most commonly the supraspinatus.

Patrick's Test (FABER): With patient supine, perform passive flexion, abduction, and external rotation of the hip. The patient is unable to allow the knee of the involved leg to approximate the table or at least become parallel with the contralateral leg (positive). A positive test warrants further examination. Limitations that result in a positive test without pain are typically due to muscular tightness of the adductor group. Limitations from pain, which result in a positive test, are referred from three common locations: inguinal pain (hip joint pathology), lateral thigh pain (trochanteric bursitis), posterior buttock pain (sacroiliac or appropriate pathology).

of the athletic population is the best source for prevention at this time. The National Strength and Conditioning Association has developed an action plan for coaches to identify and respond to the problem of anabolic steroid abuse among athletes that may be useful to the physical therapist.[33] The long-term side effects of usage greatly outweigh any short-term gains the athlete may experience. As a health care professional, the physical therapist must take a proactive role in the prevention of steroid abuse. Referral to a physician, counselor, and/or the school administration is appropriate upon identification of an

involved student athlete. Common signs of steroid abuse may include an increased problem with acne, abnormally rapid increase in muscle mass, increased secretion of skin oils, excessive development of the male's breasts or *gynecomastia*, and altered patterns of hair growth.

The goals of the PPSE are to identify the strengths and weaknesses of a student who wishes to participate in school sports and to provide education and training to lessen the risk of injury and allow the student to safely participate in this school activity.

POINT TO REMEMBER

Preparticipation Sports Examination

PPSE should include musculoskeletal, neuromuscular, cardiovascular/pulmonary, and integumentary systems. A thorough history during the PPSE can elicit information that requires referral or further examination before clearance to participate in sports. Elements of a PPSE include: a history, system review, upper and lower quarter screenings, special stress tests, and an evaluation of core muscle strength.

PREVENTION

The saying that an "ounce of prevention is worth a pound of cure" is an understatement when considering the detrimental effects of many sports injuries. External protective devices have historically been the primary prevention measure in sports. The physical therapist should look to the manufacturer guidelines if the fitting and provision of protective equipment falls within her job description. Beyond external devices to prevent injury, there are a number of internal factors that must be considered. As previously mentioned, core strength is a vital component of any movement-based activity. Weakness of the core musculature (i.e., rectus abdominus, transverse abdominus, external oblique, internal oblique, and the superficial and deep erector spinae) is often hidden by compensatory strategies. It is recommended that any deficiency in strength that is identified during the PPSE be addressed before the athlete is allowed to participate in the sport. Failure to strengthen the body's core has been cited as one of the primary predisposing factors for lumbar spine injury in the high school athlete.[34] In addition to core stabilization, numerous sports injuries are related to the distal joints of the body. At a time when the young athlete is continuing to develop physically, it is important for the physical therapist to recognize faulty biomechanical patterns. Female high school athletes display an increased susceptibility to ACL tears due to the biomechanical stresses placed on the knee while jumping.[35] This susceptibility is one example of how the developing athlete may be at an increased risk for injury during sports activities. To minimize the risk of injury, it is recommended that athletes be included in both in-season and off-season strength and conditioning programs.

TRAINING

Unfortunately, in today's public school system, funding is typically not available to provide for strength and conditioning coaches for high school athletes. The responsibility is left to the coach to create and implement a program for the athletes. The level of training a coach may have in the area of strength and conditioning varies widely. As specialists in the area of movement, physical therapists could provide useful information for both coaches and athletes. This information could include the formation of in-season and off-season training programs specific to the nature of the sport involved. All programs should emphasize the areas of flexibility, endurance, speed, agility, strength, and power.

Static stretching to promote flexibility has traditionally been included within most sport programs' warm-up drills before practice and before competition. Conflicting research has been published as to the efficacy of static stretching to prevent injury. The use of static stretching has been shown to improve range of motion when performed after warming up (after increased localized blood flow to the muscle has occurred).[36] At this time, it is recommended that static stretching be included in the warm-up and cool-down periods of physical activity in both practice and competition. The purpose is to maintain or (if needed) increase the functional length of the muscle. Stretching before participation should also involve dynamic movements of the expected muscles involved in the activity. An example of this approach would be to perform high knee jogging and heel kicks while jogging to promote increased blood flow and stretch to the anterior and posterior aspects of the lower extremity. Sports that have an increased risk for injury due to decreased range of motion for any given joint (i.e., baseball pitchers lacking shoulder internal rotation) should implement stretching protocols to minimize these adverse effects.

Endurance training of the adolescent athlete should focus on cardiovascular performance. The exercise prescription should be set at the level of 65% to 90% of the age-adjusted maximal heart rate (HR) for high school athletes.[37] The Karvonen method of determining the age-adjusted maximal HR is commonly used among clinicians (Box 7-7). Debate still remains over the clinical

BOX 7-7
Exercise Intensity: The Karvonen Method

220 – Age of athlete = x
x – Resting HR = y
$y \times$ Chosen percentile (70% to 90%) = z
z + Resting HR = Maximal age-adjusted HR for exercise

Traditional Method
220 – Age = x
$x \times$ Chosen percentile (70% to 90%) = Maximal age-adjusted HR for exercise

validity of the traditional method for calculating target HR workload.[38] The duration of exercise should be approximately 50% of competition play per day to maintain adequate cardiovascular response during the off-season. Endurance training should not be limited to the traditional forms of aerobic exercise of running, swimming, and biking. Training methods of circuit, interval, and low-intensity–high-repetition workouts have all been shown to maintain elevated HR levels, which is a critical aspect of endurance training.[39]

Muscular endurance in the athlete can be defined as the ability of the muscle to perform repeated movements without premature fatigue. This aspect of training varies widely on the basis of sport involvement. For example, football players typically use short bursts of fast-twitch muscle fiber activity to execute plays on the field. In contrast, a cross-country runner may only recruit his fast-twitch fibers in explosive moves at the beginning or end of a race. The prescription of muscular endurance training should be based upon the necessity of the athlete to perform such movements.

The common misconception that speed is based solely on the genetic predisposition of fast-twitch muscle fibers has been proven false in current research.[40] Training to improve speed can focus on factors such as form, reciprocal arm swing speed, unilateral force production in each leg, and methodology of the training program. Current research has shown that training programs that include resisted sprinting and over-speed drills have significant increases as compared to traditional sprint drills.[41] Techniques that focus on the factors affecting speed include seated/standing resisted reciprocal arm swing, core stabilization to decrease excessive trunk rotation, single leg squats, single leg bounding, resisted sprints (chutes and weighted vests), and over-speed sprints (with tubing).

Speed training should be performed with the specific sport requirement taken into consideration. The maximum distance a football player will sprint at any given time is 100 yards. A softball player will sprint 60 to

240 feet (first base versus a home run) after a hit. Speed training of the athlete is a vital component of all sports programs. Proper development of a speed-training program should include a variety of drills and techniques. The physical ability of the athlete must be taken into consideration. Subsequent speed program modifications may be necessary. Appropriate rest periods of three to five times the duration of the drill should be allowed for recuperation from anaerobic work.

Agility training falls closely in line with that of speed training. Agility should be considered a skill that is trainable and not an inherent aspect of a person's physical abilities. The skill of agility incorporates speed, accuracy, form, and adaptability. To create training programs that are beneficial to agility, one must look at the sport involved. Traditionally, sports such as soccer, football, and hockey have utilized footwork drills. These include running through a series of cones, practicing quick decisive turns, and hopping/jumping forms. Sports that revolve around upper extremity movement such as tennis, volleyball, and field hockey focus their training on hand–eye coordination drills and reaction time. Although all sports incorporate both upper and lower extremity agility, prescription of training techniques to increase agility should be as sport specific as possible. If an athlete is experiencing difficulty in this area, a building block approach should be used to increase his skill level. Training should first focus on the form of the student. Does he have the correct biomechanical and kinesiologic movement patterns for proper performance? After form has been corrected, accuracy of that form should be emphasized. After accuracy has been achieved, speed should be encouraged to perform the movement at increasing levels until competition play has been achieved. Following form, accuracy, and speed, the adaptability of the movement pattern should be emphasized. As most sports take place in an open and changing environment, a variety of competition-equivalent training drills should be performed.

Strength training has become increasingly popular in the recreational setting following an overflow from the sport population. This increase has created numerous opportunities and sources of information concerning technique and philosophy. Exercise prescription for the adolescent athlete should be based upon established principles and a sound scientific foundation. High school male athletes have a notorious reputation for displaying their machismo in the weight room by trying to "out do" their peers. This attitude leads to an environment that is more hazardous than beneficial. Long-term damage and overuse injuries are more likely when strict guidelines are not established for strength training. Basic lifting exercises that promote whole-body development should be initiated before isolated movements are prescribed. Following this idea, the training program should emphasize balance between all major muscle groups, not just those

BOX 7-8
Guidelines for Intervention on Strengthening

For strength: set resistance ≥85% of 1 RM
For power and speed: perform submaximal effort with emphasis on velocity of movement
For muscle hypertrophy and endurance: move resistance at submaximal effort to fatigue

that are aesthetically pleasing. Beginning at a level of 60% to 75% of the athlete's one repetition max (1 RM) will allow for safe evaluation of lifting technique and progression of resistive exercise. Submaximal prediction equations are valid when establishing baseline data for exercise prescription.[42] Some sources have cited the benefits of lifting at 90% to 100% of the athlete's 1 RM.[43] Although strength benefits are gained at this intensity, it must be remembered that the athlete is still developing physically. Caution and proper safety guidelines should be followed when performing maximal intensity lifts. Research suggests that a 1-day-per-week strength-training program is sufficient to maintain strength during the competitive season.[44] A general guideline for exercise intensity should be based upon the desired outcome of the program (Box 7-8).

Olympic lifts are an excellent method of strength training that promotes total body strength within the context of explosive movement that is characteristic of many sports. A key principle of Olympic lifts is the idea of triple extension. Extension movements take place at the ankle, knee, and hip simultaneously; thus recreating the motion of jumping or running while applying additional resistance. In addition, these lifting movements are ground based and multiplanar. Both of these factors simulate sport-based movement patterns.[45] The rationale for using Olympic lifts with athletes include improved rate of force development (RFD), power output, acceleration, dynamic flexibility, torso strength, and economy of time.[46]

There is a negative connotation with the prescription of Olympic lifts in today's society. As with other forms of strength training, Olympic lifts are to be properly instructed and monitored for proper technique and execution. Failure to do so can place the athlete at an increased risk. Instruction in the Olympic lifting technique should begin with an unweighted bar until the athlete is able to safely and efficiently perform the lift. Upon accomplishment of the technique, progression of resistance can take place under the proper supervision. Although these lifts are safe to perform, it cannot be stressed enough that inadequate preparation and training can lead to injury.

Power is a product of strength (force) and speed (velocity). There is an inverse relationship between the two factors. As speed is increased, the force production of the muscle (strength) is decreased. Likewise, the most powerful force-producing moments are those that eliminate speed altogether (isometric). Power training has traditionally been accomplished through the prescription of *plyometric exercises*. Any exercise that utilizes the stretch-shortening cycle of a muscle should be considered plyometric. Plyometric exercises incorporate an eccentric muscle contraction immediately followed by a concentric contraction of the same muscle. Traditionally, these exercises have included box jumps and leaping and bounding drills. A quick screening performed by the physical therapist to ascertain whether the athlete is physically able to complete plyometric exercises is called the *rebound test*. The athlete is placed on a box (typically 12 inches in height) and asked to step off and immediately jump as high as he can when contacting the ground. The height jumped after rebounding can be recorded with either a vertical jump stick or by placing tape on a wall where the athlete was able to touch. If the athlete is able to rebound to the height of the box jumped from, then he can be cleared for plyometric training. This test can also be used to determine the starting box height for advanced plyometric exercises by increasing the initial box height until the athlete can no longer rebound to a given height. Another method of assessing an athlete's ability to perform plyometric training is based upon strength. The ability to perform a parallel squat with a load equal to body weight on the back and perform a chest press with one third of body weight are the minimum requirements for lower and upper extremity plyometric training.[47]

When creating a plyometric program, the nature of the sport involved should be taken into consideration. Historically, plyometric training has been restricted to the training of contact sports, primarily football. Inclusion of other sports, such as cheerleading, in a plyometric program can be beneficial. The nature of cheerleading includes plyometric movements performed numerous times within a single performance. For this reason, the creation of a program should not be limited to only one sport or type of athlete. Rather, the physical therapist should look to include this aspect of a training program into a variety of settings in order to fully maximize the benefit of that program. Plyometric training simulates real-world activities to a greater degree than does traditional resistance training.

POINT TO REMEMBER

Training

Flexibility—range-of-motion interventions with a warm-up and cool-down period
Endurance—cardiovascular performance at approximately 65% to 90% of age-adjusted maximum HR over a sport-specific time period
Speed—a variety of timed drills and exercises
Agility—a factor of biomechanics (form), accuracy, speed, and adaptability
Strength—percentage of 1 RM
Power—a product of strength and speed. Plyometric exercises are an example.

COMMON HIGH SCHOOL SPORTS

Soccer

Soccer has been gaining national recognition at all age levels over the past several decades. In the United States approximately 3 million children participate in a high school or a youth soccer association.[48] Soccer can be thought of as an endurance-oriented sport that requires intermittent bursts of explosive power. Although it may seem that this type of movement would place the athlete most at risk for overuse injuries, traumatic injuries secondary to external forces and acceleration/deceleration injuries are more common. The movement patterns required during soccer are frequently changing and therefore minimizing the risk of overuse repetitive injuries. Traumatic injuries secondary to external forces, which are more common, typically include ACL tears and inversion ankle sprains. These two injuries occur most often when the athlete has his foot planted firmly in the ground and an external force is applied, causing lower extremity rotation or range of motion beyond normal physiologic barriers. The acceleration/deceleration injuries occur predominantly in the dominant kicking leg. These injuries tend to manifest as either hamstring muscle strains or adductor muscle (groin) strains. The physical therapy rehabilitation plan for either of these traumatic injuries will be determined by the extent of injury and the decision by the athlete and parents to undergo orthopedic correctional surgery, if applicable. As with all athletic injuries, the rehabilitation plan's goal is to ultimately return the athlete to competitive play (Box 7-9). This area of rehabilitation is best achieved after normal physiologic movement and strength are restored to the affected extremity. Progression for return to play is then only limited by the level of internal motivation of the athlete and any psychological barriers that may be present regarding future re-injury.

Baseball and Softball

Fast-pitch softball and baseball are two sports with similar presentation of injuries. According to the mechanism of injury (MOI), injuries in these two sports would fall predominantly under the overuse and acceleration/deceleration categories. Players of both sports experience traumatic injuries ranging from contusions to fractures that are

BOX 7-9
Sport Injuries: Implication for the Physical Therapist

Soccer[49]

Common injuries: ankle sprains, shin splints, compartment syndrome, ACL injuries, myositis ossificans, thigh/groin strains
Prevention: warm-up (10 minutes of cardiovascular exercise), stretching, strengthening, power, speed, agility, endurance, prophylactic devices
Sport-specific return guideline: The athlete should be able to complete the following: single-leg hop test, shuttle run, starting, stopping, cutting, jumping, running, kicking, passing, and running through cones while controlling a ball. Progression should be 50% to 75% to 100% of competition level. Practice sessions progress from one quarter, one half, three quarters, and then full practices. After three full practices without pain or soreness, the athlete can return to competition.

Baseball/Softball[52]

Common injuries: rotator cuff tears, impingement, glenohumeral instability
Prevention: warm-up (10 minutes of cardiovascular exercise), stretching, strengthening, power, speed, agility, endurance, prophylactic devices
Sport-specific return guideline: Throwing begins with 25 to 30 throws in a session, progressing to 70 throws per session. Distance is gradually increased from 20 feet up to 120 feet. Athlete should be sprinting base paths, using proper sliding technique, and practicing proper throwing biomechanics. Progression should be 50% to 75% to 100% of competition level. Practice sessions progress from one quarter, one half, three quarters, and then full

practices. After three full practices without pain or soreness, the athlete can return to competition.

Basketball[55]

Common injuries: Lateral ankle sprains, patellar tendonitis (jumper's knee), finger fractures, meniscal injuries
Prevention: warm-up (10 minutes of cardiovascular exercise), stretching, strengthening, power, speed, agility, endurance, prophylactic devices
Sport-specific return guideline: The athlete should be able to complete the following: line drills, box jumps, agility drills, vertical jumping, lay-ups, jump shots, set shots, and rebounding. Progression should be 50% to 75% to 100% of competition level. Practice sessions progress from one quarter, one half, three quarters, and then full practices. After three full practices without pain or soreness, the athlete can return to competition.

Football[56]

Common injuries: Heat exhaustion, brachial plexus injuries, concussions, posterior shoulder instability
Prevention: warm-up (10 minutes of cardiovascular exercise), stretching, strengthening, power, speed, agility, endurance, prophylactic devices
Sport-specific return guideline: The athlete should be able to complete position-specific running drills in all planes. Clearance by a physician postconcussion is required. Progression should be 50% to 75% to 100% of competition level. Practice sessions progress from one quarter, one half, three quarters, and then full practices. After three full practices without pain or soreness, the athlete can return to competition.

---

attributed to on-field collisions and the variations in playing surfaces.[50] The prevalence of overuse and acceleration/deceleration injuries can be attributed to the biomechanics of throwing. For a detailed description and analysis of throwing biomechanics, the reader is referred to other literature.[51] The biomechanical difference in the pitching motion between fast-pitch softball and baseball should not be understated. A repeated high-velocity overhand throw, as performed with baseball pitching, places excessive forces on the anterior shoulder and medial elbow. The result of the repeated activity can be seen in many postgame events when a pitcher has multiple ice bags surrounding his shoulder and elbow to minimize the inflammatory response created by this repetitive trauma. Fast-pitch softball also requires high-velocity movement around the shoulder and elbow, but in an underhand delivery. This minimizes the excessive forces placed on the anterior shoulder and medial elbow. Postgame icing is also present in this sport, but typically due to the volume of pitches made, not the mechanics. The injuries sustained secondary to traumatic external forces and acceleration/deceleration forces

are treated in accordance with their severity. Sprains, strains, and contusions are allowed appropriate healing time while minimizing the detrimental effects of the initial inflammatory response. Overuse injuries require the physical therapist to address not only the immediate symptoms, but also the underlying pathology. Without proper correction of the biomechanical forces underlying the athlete's complaint, ongoing treatment will be required. Observation of the athlete performing his or her sport-specific skill will provide the physical therapist with valuable information as to the cause of the injury (Box 7-9).

Basketball

Basketball injuries for both male and female athletes are predominantly the result of traumatic external forces. Two major pathologies associated with this sport are ACL tears and lateral ankle sprains. ACL tears, as previously mentioned, have a high incidence in female basketball players. Likewise, lateral ankle sprains have a high incidence and recurrence rate for both male and female athletes.[53] Both of these injuries are typically caused by the environment within which the sport is played. An athlete with an ACL tear will likely describe his injury as occurring after having planted his foot and rotating to make the next move. An athlete with a lateral ankle sprain will typically describe having stepped on or landed on someone's foot and feeling his ankle "roll" (inversion). Although research suggests the involvement of hormonal changes and biomechanical factors in ligamentous laxity, the physical therapist must remember the nature of the injury.[54] Traumatic external forces cannot be eliminated from competitive sport. Therefore, preseason and in-season training necessitate the need to focus on strengthening of the musculature surrounding highly susceptible joints and the flexibility of those muscles to avoid injury. As with all injuries involving ligamentous insult, rehabilitation should focus on minimizing the immediate detrimental effects of inflammation. Following this, full functional range of motion should be achieved and strengthened within that range. When these three objectives have been met, the functional sport performance of the athlete should be addressed. Return to play guidelines will vary between each athlete (Box 7-9). It is recommended that the athlete be allowed to progress up to competitive play status instead of allowing a full return to play immediately after rehabilitation goals have been met.

Football

The sport of football has had a history of highly publicized injuries secondary to traumatic external forces. All areas of the body are susceptible to injury, and the incidence of injury to each area can be largely attributed to the various positions played. One major injury area that has not been previously discussed involves the central nervous system. Cranial, cervical, thoracic, and lumbar injuries have been the focus of on-field and off-field management. The physical therapist should be familiar with signs of a spinal cord injury (SCI) and the necessary precautionary measures needed during on-field play. Rehabilitation protocols can vary widely with the severity of the injury (Box 7-9). More common is the occurrence of a concussion. Signs and symptoms of concussion can include headache, dizziness, confusion, tinnitus, nausea, vomiting, and/or vision changes. Later developing signs can include memory disturbances, poor concentration, irritability, sleep disturbances, fatigue, and personality changes.[58] General guidelines are available that establish return-to-play criteria postconcussion. The American Academy of Neurology (AAN) has established a simplified format to follow when assessing the athlete.[59] AAN guidelines for return to play are located in Box 7-10. In addition, the Sport Concussion Assessment Tool (SCAT) was one of the outcomes of the 2nd International Conference on Concussion in Sports.[60] This tool was developed for use by physicians, physical therapists, health professionals, coaches, and other people involved with athletes. The SCAT can be found in the Appendix.

POINTS TO REMEMBER

General Return to Sport Guidelines[59]

1. No persistent swelling in the injured area.
2. Time constraints for tissue healing have been observed.
3. Pain free full ROM of the injured joint is possible.
4. Injured area has 90% of pre-injury strength.
5. Proprioception of the involved joint is not impaired.
6. Flexibility of the injured area is equal to contralateral non-injured area.
7. Joint stability maintained by muscle control and/or brace or tape.
8. Cardiovascular fitness is able to meet demands of the sport.
9. Sport specific skills have been regained.
10. No biomechanical dysfunction is evident.

BOX 7-10
AAN Guidelines for Return to Play After a Concussion[57]

Grade 1

Symptoms: Momentary confusion, but no loss of consciousness. Mental status abnormalities last <15 minutes.

Management: The athlete must be removed from the game and be examined immediately and at 5-minute intervals for signs of disorientation. The athlete may return to the game only if confusion and other symptoms clear within 15 minutes. Any athlete who incurs a second Grade 1 concussion the same day should be removed from play until symptom-free for 1 week.

Grade 2

Symptoms: Brief confusion, but no loss of consciousness. Mental status abnormalities last >15 minutes but <60 minutes.

Management: The athlete must be removed from the game and not allowed to return. A medical examination is necessary. If symptoms persist, a more extensive diagnostic evaluation is required. Get a magnetic resonance imaging (MRI) of the brain if symptoms persist for >1 week. The athlete may resume playing only after 1 week without symptoms. Any athlete who incurs a Grade 2 concussion subsequent to a Grade 1 concussion on the same day should be removed from play until symptom-free for 2 weeks.

Grade 3

Symptoms: Loss of consciousness, either seconds (brief) or minutes (prolonged). Mental status abnormalities last >60 minutes.

Management: If the athlete is unconscious or if abnormal neurologic signs are present at the time of initial evaluation, the athlete should be transported to the nearest emergency room. No sports for at least 1 week after brief loss of consciousness (seconds) and 2 weeks after prolonged loss of consciousness (minutes). If subsequent brain scan shows brain swelling, contusion, or other intracranial pathology, the athlete should be removed from sports for the season and must discuss the findings with the doctor. Returning to contact sports is discouraged.

CASE STUDY

Sam Oliver—Regular Education and a Section 504 Plan

History

Sam Oliver is a 9-year-old boy who is enrolled in the local elementary school (fourth grade, regular education). He has a medical diagnosis of cerebral palsy spastic left hemiplegia. He is right hand dominant. Presently he is neither taking medications nor receiving any type of physical therapy. He has no history of past surgeries. He did wear an articulating ankle foot orthoses (AFO) to aid with ambulation efficiency, but discontinued wearing the brace 2 years ago. He reports that he could not run in the brace.

Sam is independent with ambulation in school. He is able to transition from his desk and work tables independently. He can negotiate the stairs in the school as well as the steps onto the school bus. He presents with a typical gait pattern of a child with his medical diagnosis, with noted gait deviations. He can run and jump but with noted decrease in distance and form.

Presently Sam is having difficulty managing his books and other supplies. He also takes longer than other students in walking to class when it is located on the other side of the school building. The students are given 2 minutes to change classes. He enjoys PE class but is not successful with the gross motor tasks this year, which include more sport-specific activities such as basketball, baseball, and dodgeball.

After review of additional information, the Section 504 team agreed that Sam is eligible for a Section 504 Plan to address his mobility in school and his participation in PE.

EXAMINATION

The following information was obtained during the physical therapy examination. Sam's left lower extremity demonstrates 15 degrees of passive ankle dorsiflexion and 5 degrees of active dorsiflexion with the knee fully extended. There is limitation in the left hamstring range (popliteal angle of 130 degrees on the left, 160 on the right) and hip joint rotation (20 degrees of external rotation in the left hip and 45 degrees on the right, measured in prone). Sam presents with an apparent leg length difference of 1 cm on the left, with a noted pelvic obliquity; left iliac crest higher than the right upon visual examination.

Ankle eversion muscle strength was 5/5 on the right and 1/5 on the left. Sam was able to perform 20 toe raises in stance without upper extremity assist. One-legged stance on the right was >30 seconds; on the left, it was 5 seconds.

Sam's left forearm demonstrates full passive supination and 90 degrees of active supination. Active wrist extension with finger extension is difficult. He demonstrated limitations in active shoulder flexion (160 degrees) and external rotation (60 degrees) on the left. Right shoulder range of motion is within functional limits. Sam is independent in activities of daily living (ADLs) by his mother's report. He does have some difficulty with fasteners at times, and requires more time to complete the task.

Sam can walk 50 feet in 30 seconds. Running is slow with posturing of his left arm in flexion and his left foot internally rotated. He can broad jump 20 inches. He is impaired in his ability to perform coordinated activities such as jumping jacks or skipping, although he attempts with noted effort. He does ride a two-wheeled bike by report. He ascends and descends stairs reciprocally. He can throw a ball overhand accurately with his right, but has difficulty catching with his left. He does maintain eye contact with the ball when thrown to him but has difficulty with eye–hand coordination on the left, to catch, as well as finger opposition to close the glove over the ball. Sam reports that he enjoys riding a bike and playing basketball with his dad.

DIAGNOSIS

Impaired motor function association with a nonprogressive disorder of the central nervous system acquired in infancy.

IDENTIFIED GOALS

1. Sam will be able to manage his books and school items from class to class.
2. Sam will be able to transition from class to class in a reasonable amount of time.
3. Sam will consistently participate in and be successful with his PE activities.

ACCOMMODATIONS AND/OR MODIFICATIONS

Management of his classroom items: Sam will be provided with an organizer with a shoulder strap to carry his books and notebooks from class to class. He will be seated in the row next to the door to provide a clear pathway for him to walk. Additional textbooks will be provided in the classroom so that Sam does not have to carry more than two books at one time from class to class. If the classrooms are more than 50 feet apart, Sam will be allowed an additional 1 to 2 minutes to arrive to class. If appropriate, Sam should be allowed to leave class 1 to 2 minutes early, so that he is on time for the beginning of the next class.

Sam will be provided with activities to practice at home 2 months prior to the activities for his PE class. No modifications will be made at present to the activities in class (by request of Sam and his mother).

PHYSICAL THERAPY INTERVENTIONS

Communication and coordination: Physical therapist will consult with the PE teacher regarding what to expect of Sam and what his medical diagnosis may impair him from doing. The PE teacher will work with the physical therapist in planning for home activities that would prepare Sam to more successfully participate in the basketball, baseball, and dodgeball activities planned for the class this school year. The physical therapist will consult with the classroom teacher regarding the type of organizer that Sam will use and how he will carry/manage his educational materials from class to class. Strategies will be explored and the most efficient one will be adopted.

Client-related instruction: The physical therapist will design a home exercise program for Sam to address the discrete tasks associated with the activities of baseball, basketball, and dodgeball.

Therapeutic exercise: Sam will be provided with exercises to address his impairments in range of motion, muscle strength, and power of his left hemibody. These will be incorporated into his home exercise program.

Functional training: Sam will be provided with interventions to address his stride length and cadence. His ability to participate in the general tasks of baseball (batting, running, throwing, catching), basketball (dribbling, running, jumping, shooting), and dodgeball (throwing, dodging, running, catching) will be addressed. In addition, bilateral use of his upper extremities for carrying textbooks and his organizer will also be addressed.

Service delivery and frequency: Consultation will be provided to the classroom teacher three times throughout the school year to evaluate the effectiveness of the accommodations suggested. Consultation with the PE teacher will occur six times throughout the school year, to plan for future activities and to evaluate the effectiveness of the home program on Sam's performance in PE. Consultation with the family will occur six times throughout the school year to update the home exercise program as needed.

OUTCOMES

By the end of the second quarter, Sam was arriving to his classes prior to the start of class, consistently. The organizer and extra textbooks made the transition between classes more efficient. His family was independent in carrying out the home exercise program, and Sam was participating in PE class with more success. He even made several baskets during basketball games in class! An unexpected outcome was the interest Sam's father developed for coaching basketball. He and Sam participated in a recreational basketball league in the community this year.

Reflection Questions

1. If accommodations were not provided, how do you think Sam's inability to consistently arrive to class on time would have affected his overall school experience?
2. What are some of the discrete movements associated with playing basketball? How would a diagnosis of cerebral palsy, spastic hemiplegic, affect Sam's ability to perform these movements?
3. If the Section 504 Committee did not identify physical therapy as an appropriate related service for this student, what other disciplines or school personnel may have been identified to address Sam's mobility in school and his participation in PE classes? What is the benefit of a physical therapist over the other choices?

SUMMARY

The Rehabilitation Act, Section 504, is a civil rights legislation that is often eclipsed by the IDEA with regard to education of children with disabilities. Children with disabilities who do not qualify for special education under the IDEA are still entitled to a FAPE. Physical therapists working in the school setting are poised to be advocates for all children, aiding in the identification, evaluation, and planning for eligible students, making recommendations on appropriate modifications and accommodations to their educational programs and their school environment.

The role of the physical therapist in the educational setting extends beyond the students with disabilities into the general education, fitness, and wellness of all school-aged children. This role can include:

1. Screening of students for posture, fitness, nutrition, and preparticipation sports examinations.
2. Education of athletes, coaches, and staff encompassing substance abuse, eating disorders, and training programs.
3. Creation of safe and effective sport-specific training programs to prevent injury.

REVIEW QUESTIONS

1. You are working as a physical therapist at your local elementary school. A teacher informs you that one of the students in her afternoon math class is frequently late to class. She knows that this student has asthma and wonders if she has to tolerate the student's tardiness. Which of the following response statements would be correct?
   a. Yes, she does have to allow for additional time for class changes because the student has a disability.
   b. No, she does not have to allow or provide any accommodations for this student as having asthma does not make the student eligible for any additional services.
   c. She should talk to the student's other teachers and discuss the possibility that this student may be defined as being disabled under Section 504 of the Rehabilitation Act. If he qualifies, he may require accommodations to his schedule.
   d. Asthma is not associated with any cognitive impairment or significant impairments in the student's ability to manage his time appropriately. She should talk to the superintendent and student's parents about his tardiness.
2. Which of the following students would least likely qualify as an "individual with a disability" under Section 504 of the Rehabilitation Act given only the information below?
   a. A student has a mental impairment that limits his ability to read and perform computer tasks.
   b. A student has a complete SCI at T12 and is independent in wheeled mobility.
   c. A student has cystic fibrosis.
   d. A student has a history of multiple fractures of his upper and lower extremities.
3. You have been asked to evaluate a student in the ninth grade to determine if she is eligible for accommodations under Section 504. She is 15 years old and has a diagnosis of spina bifida at the S2 level. Which

of the following statements are true regarding evaluations under Section 504?

a. The evaluation must be norm referenced to her same-age peers.

b. The evaluation must be criterion referenced and relevant to her functioning in the school environment.

c. No formalized test is required under Section 504 to determine the student's eligibility.

d. The evaluation must be designed to provide information to make a decision based exclusively on the results of the test.

4. After the student has been determined to be eligible for accommodations, a plan is developed to address the accommodations or modifications that will be considered. Which of the following statements is true regarding a Section 504 Plan?

a. The Section 504 Plan is less structured than an IEP.

b. The Section 504 Plan is the same as an IEP, and must include adjustments to the student's academic performance standards in accordance with the outcomes of the evaluation.

c. The Section 504 Plan is similar to an IFSP and should cover all areas of a student's development.

d. The Section 504 Plan must include the frequency and duration of any related services that will be provided to the student.

5. By law, the Section 504 Plan should be reviewed how often?

a. Every 6 months

b. At the end of each school year

c. Every 2 years

d. Periodically, at least every 3 years

6. It is close to the end of the school year, and the parent of a child to whom you are providing services is not satisfied with the modifications and accommodations as outlined in her son's Section 504 Plan. She does not feel that the school made an effort to implement the recommendations in a timely manner, and several of the recommendations have not been addressed. She has met with the school administration but does not feel that the meetings were productive. She wishes to file a complaint. Which of the following agencies would be ultimately responsible for enforcing Section 504?

a. U.S. Department of Education

b. Local Board of Education

c. Office for Civil Rights

d. Office of the Superintendent

7. As a physical therapist, you are asked to participate in the school's health fair to screen for scoliosis. Which of the following grades would be most appropriate to screen for scoliosis?

a. First through fifth grade

b. Fifth through eighth grade

c. Eighth through tenth grade

d. Ninth through twelfth grade

8. As a physical therapist, you are asked to participate in the school's health fair to evaluate students' general fitness. Which of the following groups of activities would best reflect a student's fitness level?

a. Number of sit-ups/curl-ups; time to perform a shuttle run; distance measured in a sit and reach

b. Upper and lower quarter screens

c. Throwing, beginning with 25 to 30 throws in a set and progressing to 70 throws. Distance to the target is gradually increased from 20 feet up to 120 feet.

d. Calculation of 1 RM

9. Which of the following is considered the most important component in athletic performance, allowing the athlete to be able to perform effectively and safely?

a. Flexibility

b. Endurance

c. Core muscle strength

d. Power

10. You are the physical therapist for the high school football team. Part of your responsibility is to decide if and when an athlete can return to play following an injury. According to the AAN guidelines on return-to-play criteria postconcussion, which of the following grades is associated with a loss of consciousness?

a. Grade 1

b. Grade 2

c. Grade 3

d. All of the above

Sport Concussion Assessment Tool (SCAT)

FIFA   OOOOO   IIHF

The SCAT Card
(Sport Concussion Assessment Tool)
Medical Evaluation

Name: _____   Date _____

Sport/Team: _____   Mouth guard? Y N

1) SIGNS

Was there loss of consciousness or unresponsiveness?   Y   N
Was there seizure or convulsive activity?   Y   N
Was there a balance problem / unsteadiness?   Y   N

2) MEMORY
Modified Maddocks questions (check correct)

At what venue are we? __; Which half is it? __; Who scored last?__

What team did we play last? __; Did we win last game? __?

3) SYMPTOM SCORE
Total number of positive symptoms (from reverse side of the card) = _____

4) COGNITIVE ASSESSMENT

5 word recall	(Examples)	Immediate	Delayed (after concentration tasks)
Word 1 _____	cat	____	____
Word 2 _____	pen	____	____
Word 3 _____	shoe	____	____
Word 4 _____	book	____	____
Word 5 _____	car	____	____

Months in reverse order:
Jun-May-Apr-Mar-Feb-Jan-Dec-Nov-Oct-Sep-Aug-Jul   (circle incorrect)

or

Digits backwards (check correct)

5-2-8	3-9-1	_____
6-2-9-4	4-3-7-1	_____
8-3-2-7-9	1-4-9-3-6	_____
7-3-9-1-4-2	5-1-8-4-6-8	_____

Ask delayed 5-word recall now

5) NEUROLOGIC SCREENING

	Pass	Fail
Speech	____	____
Eye Motion and Pupils	____	____
Pronator Drift	____	____
Gait Assessment	____	____

Any neurologic screening abnormality necessitates formal neurologic or hospital assessment

6) RETURN TO PLAY
Athletes should not be returned to play the same day of injury. When returning athletes to play, they should follow a stepwise symptom-limited program, with stages of progression. For example:
1. rest until asymptomatic (physical and mental rest)
2. light aerobic exercise (e.g. stationary cycle)
3. sport-specific exercise
4. non-contact training drills (start light resistance training)
5. full contact training after medical clearance
6. return to competition (game play)

There should be approximately 24 hours (or longer) for each stage and the athlete should return to stage 1 if symptoms recur. Resistance training should only be added in the later stages. Medical clearance should be given before return to play.

Instructions:
This side of the card is for the use of medical doctors, physiotherapists or athletic therapists. In order to maximize the information gathered from the card, it is strongly suggested that all athletes participating in contact sports complete a baseline evaluation prior to the beginning of their competitive season. This card is a suggested guide only for sports concussion and is not meant to assess more severe forms of brain injury. **Please give a COPY of this card to the athlete for their information and to guide follow-up assessment.**

Signs:
Assess for each of these items and circle Y (yes) or N (no).

Memory: If needed, questions can be modified to make them specific to the sport (e.g. "period" versus "half")

Cognitive Assessment:
Select any 5 words (an example is given). Avoid choosing related words such as "dark" and "moon" which can be recalled by means of word association. Read each word at a rate of one word per second. The athlete should not be informed of the delayed testing of memory (to be done after the reverse months and/or digits). Choose a different set of words each time you perform a follow-up exam with the same candidate.
Ask the athlete to recite the months of the year in reverse order, starting with a random month. Do not start with December or January. Circle any months not recited in the correct sequence.
For digits backwards, if correct, go to the next string length. If incorrect, read trial 2. Stop after incorrect on both trials.

Neurologic Screening:
Trained medical personnel must administer this examination. These individuals might include medical doctors, physiotherapists or athletic therapists. Speech should be assessed for fluency and lack of slurring. Eye motion should reveal no diplopia in any of the 4 planes of movement (vertical, horizontal and both diagonal planes). The pronator drift is performed by asking the patient to hold both arms in front of them, palms up, with eyes closed. A positive test is pronating the forearm, dropping the arm, or drift away from midline. For gait assessment, ask the patient to walk away from you, turn and walk back.

Return to Play:
A structured, graded exertion protocol should be developed; individualized on the basis of sport, age and the concussion history of the athlete. Exercise or training should be commenced only after the athlete is clearly asymptomatic with physical and cognitive rest. Final decision for clearance to return to competition should ideally be made by a medical doctor.

For more information see the "Summary and Agreement Statement of the Second International Symposium on Concussion in Sport" in the April, 2005 Clinical Journal of Sport Medicine (vol 15), British Journal of Sports Medicine (vol 39), Neurosurgery (vol 59) and the Physician and Sportsmedicine (vol 33). ©2005 Concussion in Sport Group

This tool represents a standardized method of evaluating people after concussion in sport. This Tool has been produced as part of the Summary and Agreement Statement of the Second International Symposium on Concussion in Sport, Prague 2004

Sports concussion is defined as a complex pathophysiological process affecting the brain, induced by traumatic biomechanical forces. Several common features that incorporate clinical, pathological and biomechanical injury constructs that may be utilized in defining the nature of a concussive head injury include:

1. Concussion may be caused either by a direct blow to the head, face, neck or elsewhere on the body with an 'impulsive' force transmitted to the head.
2. Concussion typically results in the rapid onset of short-lived impairment of neurological function that resolves spontaneously.
3. Concussion may result in neuropathological changes but the acute clinical symptoms largely reflect a functional disturbance rather than structural injury.
4. Concussion results in a graded set of clinical syndromes that may or may not involve loss of consciousness. Resolution of the clinical and cognitive symptoms typically follows a sequential course.
5. Concussion is typically associated with grossly normal structural neuroimaging studies.

Post Concussion Symptoms

Ask the athlete to score themselves based on how they feel now. It is recognized that a low score may be normal for some athletes, but clinical judgment should be exercised to determine if a change in symptoms has occurred following the suspected concussion event.

It should be recognized that the reporting of symptoms may not be entirely reliable. This may be due to the effects of a concussion or because the athlete's passionate desire to return to competition outweighs their natural inclination to give an honest response.

If possible, ask someone who knows the athlete well about changes in affect, personality, behavior, etc.

Remember, concussion should be suspected in the presence of ANY ONE or more of the following:
- Symptoms (such as headache), or
- Signs (such as loss of consciousness), or
- Memory problems

Any athlete with a suspected concussion should be monitored for deterioration (i.e., should not be left alone) and should not drive a motor vehicle.

For more information see the "Summary and Agreement Statement of the Second International Symposium on Concussion in Sport" in the April, 2005 edition of the Clinical Journal of Sport Medicine (vol 15), British Journal of Sports Medicine (vol 39), Neurosurgery (vol 59) and the Physician and Sportsmedicine (vol 33). This tool may be copied for distribution to teams, groups and organizations. ©2005 Concussion in Sport Group

The SCAT Card
(Sport Concussion Assessment Tool)
Athlete Information

What is a concussion? A concussion is a disturbance in the function of the brain caused by a direct or indirect force to the head. It results in a variety of symptoms (like those listed below) and may, or may not, involve memory problems or loss of consciousness.

How do you feel? You should score yourself on the following symptoms, based on how you feel now.

Post Concussion Symptom Scale	None		Moderate			Severe	
Headache	0	1	2	3	4	5	6
"Pressure in head"	0	1	2	3	4	5	6
Neck Pain	0	1	2	3	4	5	6
Balance problems or dizzy	0	1	2	3	4	5	6
Nausea or vomiting	0	1	2	3	4	5	6
Vision problems	0	1	2	3	4	5	6
Hearing problems / ringing	0	1	2	3	4	5	6
"Don't feel right"	0	1	2	3	4	5	6
Feeling "dinged" or "dazed"	0	1	2	3	4	5	6
Confusion	0	1	2	3	4	5	6
Feeling slowed down	0	1	2	3	4	5	6
Feeling like "in a fog"	0	1	2	3	4	5	6
Drowsiness	0	1	2	3	4	5	6
Fatigue or low energy	0	1	2	3	4	5	6
More emotional than usual	0	1	2	3	4	5	6
Irritability	0	1	2	3	4	5	6
Difficulty concentrating	0	1	2	3	4	5	6
Difficulty remembering	0	1	2	3	4	5	6
(follow up symptoms only)							
Sadness	0	1	2	3	4	5	6
Nervous or Anxious	0	1	2	3	4	5	6
Trouble falling asleep	0	1	2	3	4	5	6
Sleeping more than usual	0	1	2	3	4	5	6
Sensitivity to light	0	1	2	3	4	5	6
Sensitivity to noise	0	1	2	3	4	5	6
Other: _____	0	1	2	3	4	5	6

What should I do?
Any athlete suspected of having a concussion should be removed from play, and then seek medical evaluation.

Signs to watch for:
Problems could arise over the first 24-48 hours. You should not be left alone and must go to a hospital at once if you:
- Have a headache that gets worse
- Are very drowsy or can't be awakened (woken up)
- Can't recognize people or places
- Have repeated vomiting
- Behave unusually or seem confused; are very irritable
- Have seizures (arms and legs jerk uncontrollably)
- Have weak or numb arms or legs
- Are unsteady on your feet; have slurred speech

Remember, it is better to be safe. Consult your doctor after a suspected concussion.

What can I expect?
Concussion typically results in the rapid onset of short-lived impairment that resolves spontaneously over time. You can expect that you will be told to rest until you are fully recovered (that means resting your body and your mind). Then, your doctor will likely advise that you go through a gradual increase in exercise over several days (or longer) before returning to sport.

McCrory P, Johnston K, Meeuwisse W, Aubry M, et al. Summary and Agreement Statement of the 2nd International Conference on Concussion in Sport, Prague 2004. Clin J Sport Med 2005;15:48–55. and Br J Sports Med 2005;39:196–204. With permission.

REFERENCES

1. Section 504 of the Rehabilitation Act of 1973, 29 USC §794.
2. The Civil Rights of Students with Hidden Disabilities, under Section 504 of the Rehabilitation Act of 1973. Washington, DC: U.S. Department of Education. Office for Civil Rights. Available at: http://www.ed.gov/about/offices/list/ocr/docs/hq5269.html. Accessed August 24, 2007.
3. Office of Special Education Programs. 26th Annual Report to Congress on the Implementation of the Individuals with Disabilities Education Act. Washington, DC: U.S. Department of Education; 2004.
4. Kaye HS. Education of Children with Disabilities. Disabilities Statistics Abstract Number 19. 1997. Washington, DC: U.S. Department of Education, National Institute on Disability and Rehabilitation Research.
5. Kauerz K, McMaken J. Access to Kindergarten: Age Issues in State Statutes. ECS StateNote. February 2005. Available at: http://www.ecs.org/clearinghouse/58/27/5827.doc. Accessed March 15, 2006.
6. Johnson JA, Collins HW, Dupuis VL, et al. *Foundations of American Education.* Boston: Allyn & Bacon, Inc.; 1969.
7. Education in the United States. Wikipedia, The Free Encyclopedia. Availiable at: http://en.wikipedia.org/w/index.php?title=Education_in_the_United_States&oldid=45838654. Accessed March 28, 2006.
8. Americans with Disabilities Act of 1990, 42 USC §12101.
9. Hill J, Johnson F. Revenues and Expenditures for Public Elementary and Secondary Education: School Year 2002-2003. Education Statistics Quarterly. Washington, DC: U.S. Department of Education, National Center for Educational Statistics; 2005. Available at: http://nces.ed.gov/programs/quarterly/vol_7/1_2/4_14.asp. Accessed March 2006.
10. Medicare Catastrophic Coverage Act of 1988 (Public Law 100-360) Title IV; Section 411.
11. Folio M, Fewell R. *Peabody Developmental Motor Scales. Examiner's Manual,* 2nd ed. Austin, TX: Pro-Ed; 2000.
12. Bruininks RH. *Bruininks-Oseretsky Test of Motor Proficiency Examiner's Manual.* Circle Pines, MN: American Guidance Service; 1978.
13. Rehabilitation Act Amendments of 1998. Section 7 (37).
14. Drnach M, Paleg G. *Back to Basics. The Latest on Bracing and Exercise to Treat Scoliosis.* Physical Therapy Products 2001;12:51–53.
15. Beers MH, Berkow R, et al. *Merck Manual,* 17th ed. Whitehouse Station, NJ: Merck Research Laboratories; 1999:2429.
16. The President's Council on Physical Fitness and Sports. The President's Challenge. Available at: http://www.presidentchallenge.org/educators/program_details.aspx. Accessed March 29, 2006.
17. The President's Council on Physical Fitness and Sports. The President's Challenge. Curl-ups for boys. Available at: http://www.presidentschallenge.org/pdf/normative_data.xls. Accessed March 29, 2006.
18. Alaimo K, Olson CM, Frongillo EA Jr. Food insufficiency and American school-aged children's cognitive, academic, and psychosocial development. *Pediatrics.* 2001;108:44–53.
19. Dowling JE. *The Great Brain Debate: Nature of Nurture?* Joseph Henry Press [serial online]. 2004;doc 14.
20. Munoz KA, Krebs-Smith SM, Ballard-Barbash R, et al. Food intakes of U.S. children and adolescents compared with recommendations. *Pediatrics.* 1997;100:323–329.
21. American Dietetic Association Position Paper. Child and adolescent food and nutrition programs. Position Paper 2006;106:1467–1475. Available at: http://www.eatright.org/cps/rde/xchg/ada/hs.xsl/advocacy_1730_ENU_HTML.htm. Accessed March 18, 2006.
22. Hark L, Deen D. Taking a nutrition history: a practical approach for family physicians. *Am Fam Physician.* 1999:59. Available at: http://www.aafp.org/afp/990315ap/1521.html. Accessed March 18, 2006.
23. Sharma P, Luscombe KL, Maffulli N. Sports injuries in children. *Trauma.* 2003;5:245–259.
24. Pratt M, Macera C, Blanton C. Levels of physical activity and inactivity in children and adults in the United States: current evidence and research issues. *Med Sci Sports Exerc.* 1999;31:S526–S533.
25. Patel DR, Nelson TL. Sports injuries in children. *Med Clin North Am.* 2000;844:983–1007.
26. Maffulli N, Bruns W. Injuries in young athletes. *Eur J Pediatr.* 2000;159:59–63.
27. Micheli LJ. Sports injuries in children and adolescents. Questions and controversies. *Clin Sports Med.* 1995;14:727–745.
28. Taylor BL, Attia MW. Sports-related injuries in children. *Acad Emerg Med.* 2000;7:1376–1382.
29. Powell JW, Barber-Foss KD. Sex-related injury patterns among selected high school sports. *Am J Sports Med.* 2000;28:385–391.
30. Koester MC, Amundson CL. Pre-participation screening of high school athletes. *Phys Sportsmed.* 2003;31:35–38.
31. Magee DJ. *Orthopedic Physical Assessment,* 2nd ed. Philadelphia: W.B. Saunders Co.; 1992.
32. Allen H. Training the trunk for improved athletic performance. *Strength Cond J.* 2000;22:50–61.
33. Performance Enhancing Substance Abuse Committee. Combating anabolic steroid abuse. National Strength and Conditioning Association. 2001. Available at: http://www.nsca-lift.org/Publications/combating.pdf. Accessed March 22, 2006.
34. Ladeira CE, Hess LW, Galin BM, et al. Validation of an abdominal muscle strength test with dynamometry. *J Strength Cond Res.* 2005;19:925–930.
35. Ford K, Myer G, Hewett T. Valgus knee motion during landing in high school female and male basketball players. *Med Sci Sports Exerc.* 2003;35:1745–1750.
36. de Weijer VC, Gorniak GC, Shamus E. The effect of static stretch and warm-up exercise on hamstring length over the course of 24 hours. *J Orthop Sports Phys Ther.* 2003;33:727–733.
37. Roitman JL, Herridge M, Kelsey M, et al. *ACSM'S Resource Manual for Guidelines for Exercise Testing and Prescription,* 4th ed. Philadelphia: Lippincott Williams & Wilkins; 2001:452.
38. Robergs RA, Landwehr R. The surprising history of the "HRmax = 220-age" equation. *J Exerc Physiol.* 2002;5:1–10.
39. Pierce K, Rozenek R, Stone MH. Effects of high volume weight training on lactate, heart rate, and perceived exertion. *J Strength Cond Res.* 1993;7:211–215.
40. Roozen M. Progressive drills to improve agility skills. Presented at the National Strength and Conditioning Association's Sport Specific Training Conference; January 7–8, 2005; Louisville, KY.
41. Coleman G. Speed enhancement for the baseball player. Presented at the National Strength and Conditioning Association's Sport Specific Training Conference; January 7–8, 2005; Louisville, KY.
42. Whisenant MJ, Panton LB, East WB, et al. Validation of submaximal prediction equations for the 1 repetition maximum bench press test on a group of collegiate football players. *J Strength Cond Res.* 2003;17:221–227.
43. Benedict T. Manipulating resistance training program variables to optimize maximum strength in men: a review. *J Strength Cond Res.* 1999;13:289–304.
44. DeRenne C, Hetzler RK, Buxton BP, et al. Effects of training frequency on strength maintenance in pubescent baseball players. *J Strength Cond Res.* 1996;10:8–14.

45. Ragan TJ. Maximizing the transference of Olympic lifts to athletics – increasing acceleratory power. Presented at the National Strength and Conditioning Association's Sport Specific Training Conference; January 7–8, 2005; Louisville, KY.

46. Phillips J. The Olympic lifts and their application to baseball/softball. Presented at the National Strength and Conditioning Association's Sport Specific Training Conference. January 7–8, 2005; Louisville, KY.

47. Voight ML, Draovitch P, Tippett SR. Plyometrics. In: Albert MS. *Eccentric Muscle Training in Sports and Orthopedics.* New York: Churchill Livingstone; 1995:67–98.

48. American Academy of Pediatrics. Committee on Sports Medicine and Fitness. Injuries in Youth Soccer: A subject review. *Pediatrics.* 2000;105:659–661.

49. Gasse S. Soccer. In: Shamus E, Shamus J. *Sports Injury: Prevention & Rehabilitation.* New York: McGraw-Hill; 2001.

50. Meyers MC, Brown BR, Bloom JA. Fast pitch softball injuries. *Sports Med.* 2001;31:61–73.

51. Zachazewski JE, Magee DJ, Quillen WS. *Athletic Injuries and Rehabilitation.* Philadelphia: W. B. Saunders Co.; 1996:332–352.

52. Mohr KJ, Brewster CE. Baseball. In: Shamus E, Shamus J. *Sports Injury: Prevention & Rehabilitation.* New York: McGraw-Hill; 2001.

53. Hertel J. Functional instability following lateral ankle sprain. *Sports Med.* 2000;29:361–371.

54. Hewett TE. Neuromuscular and hormonal factors associated with knee injuries in female athletes. *Sports Med.* 2000;29:313–327.

55. Shamus E, Kelleher W, Foran B. Basketball. In: Shamus E, Shamus J. *Sports Injury: Prevention & Rehabilitation.* New York: McGraw-Hill; 2001.

56. Vermillion RP. Football. In: Shamus E, Shamus J. *Sports Injury: Prevention & Rehabilitation.* New York: McGraw-Hill; 2001.

57. American Academy of Neurology. Practice parameter: the management of concussion in sports. *Neurology.* 1997;48:581–585.

58. Harmon KG. Assessment and management of concussion in sports. *Am Acad Fam Physicians.* 1999;60:1–8. Available at: http://www.aafp.org/afp/990901ap/887.html. Accessed March 22, 2006.

59. Shamus E, Shamus J. *Sports Injury: Prevention & Rehabilitation.* New York: McGraw-Hill; 2001:365.

60. McCrory P, Johnston K, Meeuwisse W, Aubry M, et al. Summary and Agreement Statement of the 2nd International Conference on Concussion in Sport, Prague 2004. *Clin J Sport Med.* 2005;15:48–55.

Recommended Web sites

1. American College of Sports Medicine (ACSM) provides guidelines for exercise prescription for a healthy population as well as those with physical limitations. http://www.acsm.org

2. National Strength and Conditioning Association (NSCA) provides information on performance enhancement through strength training. http://www.nsca-lift.org

3. The President's Challenge Web site provides standardized testing parameters for school-aged children in physical fitness. http://www.presidentschallenge.org

4. The National Council on Disability (NCD) is an independent federal agency making recommendations to the President and Congress to enhance the quality of life for all Americans with disabilities and their families. http://www.ncd.gov

5. The American Alliance for Health, Physical Education, Recreation and Dance (AAHPERD) is the largest organization of professionals supporting and assisting those involved in physical education, leisure, fitness, dance, health promotion, education, and all specialties related to achieving a healthy lifestyle. http://www.aahperd.org

6. American Sports Medicine Institute (ASMI) Web site contains information relating to sport injury and sport-specific conditioning programs. http://www.asmi.org

7. The National Association for Sport and Physical Education (NASPE) seeks to enhance knowledge and professional practice in sport and physical activity through scientific study and dissemination of research-based and experiential knowledge. http://www.aahperd.org/naspe/template.cfm

8. The Secretary for Health and Human Services and the Secretary of Education created a report to the President on promoting better health for young people through physical activity and sports. The appendices can be accessed at: http://www.ed.gov/offices/OSDFS/physedapndc.pdf

9. The President's Council on Physical Fitness and Sports provides information and resources related to health, physical activity, fitness, and sports. http://www.fitness.gov/

10. The Active and Healthy Schools Program is an evidence-based program for elementary and middle schools that improves the health of students by increasing their activity levels and improving their eating habits. http://www.active-andhealthyschools.com/

Additional Online Resources

Access 34CFR104-Nondiscrimination on the basis of handicap in programs or activities receiving federal financial assistance. Available at http://www.access.gpo.gov/nara/cfr/waisidx_06/34cfr104_06.html. Accessed August 24, 2007.

A listing of individual states' Departments of Education can be accessed through the U.S. Department of Education, Education Resource Organizations Directory at http://wdcrob-colp01.ed.gov/Programs/EROD/org_list.cfm?category_ID=SEA.

The Office for Civil Rights enforces Section 504 and can be accessed at http://www.hhs.gov/ocr/discrimdisab.html.

Specifications of accessibility are listed in the ADA and can be accessed at http://www.ada.gov/stdspdf.htm.

Federal Access Board guidelines on specifications for accessible building elements for children aged 12 years and younger are available at http://www.access-board.gov.ada-aba/final.htm

CHAPTER **8**

Providing Services in the Public Schools: Special Education

Mark Drnach

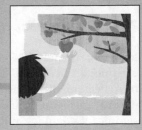

LEARNING OBJECTIVES

1. Comprehend the role and responsibility of the physical therapist in the special education environment.
2. Understand the basics of the Individuals with Disabilities Education Act (IDEA) and the service delivery model for physical therapy in the special education environment.
3. Recognize the physical therapist's role in the Individualized Education Program (IEP) process and the promotion of intellectual development and functional independence in the student enrolled in special education.
4. Understand the patient/client management process as it relates to a student in special education.
5. Understand the role and responsibility of the physical therapist as a member of the IEP team and in the IEP plan.
6. Understand how to compile and critique information used in decision making regarding the need and frequency for the related service of physical therapy.
7. Recognize the role of the physical therapist in transitioning a student from special education into an appropriate postgraduation situation.

This chapter will explore the role and practice of physical therapy in the special education environment. It will present some of the external and internal influences on this system and suggest a framework for making decisions and assessing outcomes of students in special education who receive physical therapy under the IDEA Part B.[1,2] This part of the law provides federal funds to states to assist them in providing a public education to children with disabilities within the state. Physical therapists working in this environment should have an understanding of the federal law and the appropriate utilization of physical therapy services to aid in the education of the student with a disability. Physical therapists have provided services to children with disabilities throughout the history of the profession, and today can contribute specific evaluations and intervention strategies that may help a student with a disability benefit from her educational experience.[3]

Throughout this chapter, the IDEA law (PL 108-446) is abbreviated by the section of the law in which the information is found (Section 611 through Section 619). The Code of Federal Regulations (CFR) is the codification of the general and permanent rules published in the Federal Register that pertain to special education programs and is referenced as 34CFR300.

THE CHILD WITH A DISABILITY

Approximately 5 million children participate in federally supported programs for students with disabilities. This, according to the U.S. Department of Education, accounts for approximately 12% of the students enrolled in American public schools.[4,5] Of these students, approximately half have been identified as having a specific learning disability. Students who have impairment in speech or language, significant cognitive impairment (mental retardation), or emotional problems make up the next largest group of students. The smallest groups of students are those who have an orthopedic impairment, hearing or visual impairment, or multiple disabilities.[5,6]

A large majority of students with disabilities (96%) are being educated in regular school buildings, and almost half spend most of the school day in classrooms with students who are not disabled.[6] These students are more likely to have a speech or language impairment. Those students with orthopedic, hearing, visual, or emotional impairments typically spend less than half of the school day in classrooms with students who do not have a disability. Those least likely to spend time with their nondisabled peers are students with significant cognitive impairments or multiple disabilities.[5,6]

Approximately 51% of students with disabilities graduate from secondary school, receiving a standard diploma along with their nondisabled peers.[6] Approximately 13% graduate and receive a certificate of completion or a modified diploma. The likelihood of graduating is related to the nature of the disability. Most students with visual or hearing impairments graduate with an ordinary diploma. Approximately 65% of students with orthopedic impairments, significant cognitive impairment, learning disabilities, or multiple disabilities graduate with a modified diploma or certificate. Students with emotional problems have the lowest graduation rate of any of the categories and the highest dropout rate.[5,6]

Children with disabilities may require special educational instruction, which is defined in each student's Individualized Education Program (IEP). The IEP is the legal document that describes the educational program for an individual student enrolled in special education. The student in special education is expected to participate and progress in her education and to participate in school activities, as much as possible, with her peers in regular education. The ability to travel to and from school, move or be transported through the school building, be positioned at a desk or table in the classroom, and participate in educational activities is expected. The ability to manipulate tools in order to learn or to assess learning is necessary, whether it is the use of a no. 2 pencil with a built-up grip or a head pointer to activate a touch screen on a computer.

Physical therapists, teachers, physicians, and parents may have misconceptions about eligibility requirements and the role of physical therapy in the educational setting. The provision of physical therapy and other services depends in part on an understanding of the laws that influence the delivery of services to students with disabilities.[7]

POINT TO REMEMBER

Students with Disabilities

Most students with a disability spend most of the school day in classrooms with students who are not disabled. Students with emotional problems are at the highest risk of dropping out of school.

THE PRACTICE ENVIRONMENT

The Federal Government

The practice of physical therapy in the public educational environment was clearly defined with the passage of Public Law 94-142: The Education for All Handicapped Children Act of 1975 (PL 94-142).[8] This law provided for a "free and appropriate public education" (FAPE) for all children with disabilities, beginning whenever the individual state provides public education to children who are not disabled (age 5 or 6 years, depending on the state). Contained in PL 94-142 are several provisions commonly encountered in the special education classroom today, including the IEP, education in the least restrictive environment (LRE; to the extent appropriate, the education of students with disabilities with students who are not disabled, in a regular classroom), and the right to related services (services that assist a student with a disability to benefit from special education), which includes physical therapy services.

As with many other federal laws, periodic reauthorization is required to assure continued appropriations and to provide for an opportunity to re-evaluate the components of the current law for necessary updates, clarifications, or deletions. PL 94-142 was reauthorized with amendments in 1986 as the *Education of the Handicapped Act Amendments*, or PL 99-457, which contained a significant update, extending educational services to children age 3 to 5 years.[9] In 1991, PL 99-457 and PL 94-142 were reauthorized and amended into the *Individuals with Disabilities Education Act, PL 102-119*. With this reauthorization, Congress added autism and traumatic brain injury to the eligibility category, required transition services for students with disabilities who were 16 years of age, and added assistive technology and rehabilitation counseling as related services. Subsequent reauthorization in 1997 as PL 105-17 added related services such as physical therapy to transition services, funding to students with disabilities who are placed in private schools to meet the requirements of special education, greater emphasis on integrating students with disabilities and students without disabilities as they progress through the general curriculum, and a greater emphasis on program accountability for student outcomes.[1]

Clarification of the goals and objectives of special education were highlighted by Congress, which stated "disability is a natural part of the human experience and in no way diminishes the right of individuals to participate in or contribute to society. Improving educational results for children with disabilities is an essential element of our national policy of ensuring equality of opportunity, full participation, independent living, and economic self sufficiency for individuals with disabilities" [PL 105-17, Sec 601 (c)]. Again in 2004 the IDEA was reauthorized as the Individuals with Disabilities Education Improvement Act (PL 108-446) and established a 60-day (or state-established) timeline from the receipt of the parental consent for an evaluation to determine eligibility to the actual determination of eligibility for special education services.[2] This current version of the law also clarified the frequency of re-evaluations, which cannot occur more than once a year, unless agreed upon by the parent and local education agency (LEA). It also states that a re-evaluation must occur at least once every 3 years unless the parents and LEA agree that it is unnecessary. PL 108-446 also clarified that members of the IEP team may be excused from the meeting upon consent of both parties [Sec 614 (d)(1)(C)] and that IEPs may be amended in writing without reconvening the IEP team [Sec 614 (d)(3)(D)].[2]

The IDEA does not require special education programs to maximize the educational opportunities of children with disabilities; it only requires that children receive some educational benefit from the special educational program. That benefit should revolve around the students learning skills necessary to access opportunities that will allow them to participate in society after graduation.

With the passage of the *No Child Left Behind Act of 2001* (NCLB), Congress reauthorized the *Elementary and Secondary Education Act* (ESEA), the principal federal law affecting education from kindergarten through high school.[10] This law represents an overhaul of federal efforts to support elementary and secondary education in the United States. It is built on four pillars: accountability for states, school districts, and schools regarding the test results of their students; an emphasis on doing what works best in education based on scientific research; expanded parental options, particularly for those parents of students attending consistently low performing schools; and expanded local control and flexibility for the state and local educational agencies in the use of federal education monies. The NCLB addresses accountability by requiring a statewide system of accountability for all public school students, including students with disabilities. The system is based on state standards in reading and math, with annual testing of all children from third through eight grades.

The federal government plays a significant role in promoting the education of children with disabilities, but the education of all children in the United States is primarily the responsibility of the state and local communities that also pass laws and regulations that affect the provision of services in the educational environment.

The State Government

Each state has a Physical Therapy Practice Act, which is the state law intended to protect the public from imposters or fraudulent billing practices. These laws do not prohibit school personnel from using interventions associated with physical therapy, such as passive range of motion, positioning, or therapeutic exercise, as long as the person providing them does not represent himself or herself as a physical therapist or as providing physical therapy. In the educational setting, it is important that the student, parent, school district personnel, and any third party payer are not misled by the application of an intervention that is physical therapy (provided by a physical therapist or physical therapist assistant) from an intervention provided to a student by classroom personnel as part of the educational program. Physical therapists in the educational setting may delegate selected interventions to appropriately trained and supervised personnel. Current states' Practice Acts do not specify that only a physical therapist may use certain interventions or procedures.[11] It is the responsibility of the physical therapist to perform the appropriate evaluations and supervision in accordance with the law.

In addition, Practice Acts may also provide for the direct access (access to physical therapy evaluation and treatment without the referral of a physician) to physical therapy services without a referral from a physician. Not all states allow for direct access, nor is all direct access created equal. Some states put limits on the amount of time a physical therapist can provide services before a referral to continue to treat is needed. It is important to understand that, when physical therapy services are listed on the IEP, a contract to provide those services has been made under the IDEA law. If the need for a referral from a physician is a requirement of the state Practice Act, it is the responsibility of the physical therapist delivering services to obtain that referral, and to act accordingly.

Many states that allow for direct access also require a certain number of continuing education credits for renewal of the physical therapist's license to practice. Each state may vary on the number of credits and what constitutes an approved credit. In addition, as with licensing, there are rules and regulations governing educational certification and recertification. It is the responsibility of the physical therapist to assure that he maintains a current license to practice within the state and that he obtains the continuing education credits necessary for licensure in the state.

Each Practice Act may also contain the supervisory relationship between the physical therapist and physical therapist assistant with regard to supervision (typically 1:2 in most states) and what constitutes supervision. Does it mean in direct line of sight, in the same physical location, or that the physical therapist is available via telecommunication? It is important to remember that the physical therapist assistant is required to work under the direction and supervision of the physical therapist and it is the responsibility of the physical therapist to delegate and supervise the physical therapist assistant appropriately.

In addition to Practice Acts, a state is also responsible for the administration of the state's Medicaid program. Medicaid is a joint federal and state program under the Social Security Act (Title XIX) that provides reimbursement for certain services to eligible populations, namely the poor. Medicaid programs are administered by the individual state; therefore, regulations may vary from state to state. Medicaid is required to pay for the IDEA-related services that are medically necessary and already provided by the state's Medicaid program, for Medicaid-eligible students. The services that are covered and listed on the IEP are subject to the state's Medicaid requirements for coverage, which may include the need for a physician prescription for the services, prior authorization, and appropriate and specific documentation of services rendered. Even if the state's Physical Therapy Practice Act does not require a referral for the provision of services by a physical therapist, the state Medicaid program may require a referral from a physician for payment to the school district. Proper documentation and submission of additional paperwork for those students eligible for Medicaid would be required. The LEA that is responsible for the education of the student and is reimbursed by the Medicaid program for the appropriate services rendered will most likely require this information.

A state's board of education will also have specific policies that address issues of employment or retention of qualified personnel, as well as those relating to the provision of services. Many boards of education accept physical therapy licensure alone as an adequate level of professional skills and knowledge to work in the school system, whereas some may require a teaching certificate or additional certification for employees of the school.

Local boards of education (school districts) also establish specific procedures relating to the IDEA. For example, in accordance with federal law, a local school district may have specific procedures to follow to establish or modify an IEP. Depending on the nature of the change, some districts may require only parental notification and agreement, whereas others might require a face-to-face meeting. If a family decides to send their child to a private school, or choose home schooling, the school district may not be obligated to pay for the special education or related services unless the child is placed in a private school as a means to obtain a special education that is not available in the public school.

INDIVIDUALS WITH DISABILITIES EDUCATION ACT

Determining Eligibility

Child Find is a required state system to identify, locate, and evaluate all children with disabilities who reside in the state and are in need of special education and related services (34CFR300.125). A parent, professional, or the school district's system of Child Find can request that the school perform an evaluation of a student to see if she is eligible for special education. A student is eligible for special education if he or she is between the ages of 3 and 21 years, if she has a diagnosis of 1 of the 13 categories of disabilities specified in the IDEA, and if it is determined that the disability adversely effects her educational performance. Box 8-1 lists the categories of disabilities as identified in the IDEA. If the parents disagree with the results of the eligibility evaluation, they have the right to

BOX 8-1
Categories of Disabilities Specified by IDEA

Autism
Deaf-blindness
Deafness
Hearing impairment
Mental retardation
Multiple disabilities
Orthopedic impairment (that adversely affects a child's educational performance)
Other health impairment (e.g., having limited strength, vitality, or alertness)
Serious emotional disturbance
Specific learning disability
Speech or language impairment
Traumatic brain injury
Visual impairment, including blindness
Developmental delay for children 3 to 9 years old (at the state's discretion)
34CFR §300.7

an *Independent Educational Evaluation* (IEE) for which the school system is obligated to pay.

After the eligibility evaluations are complete, a group of qualified professionals and the parents sit down together and determine if the student is eligible for special education. Again, the parents have the right to challenge the eligibility decision if they are in disagreement. If a student is then enrolled in special education and has a disability that adversely affects her ability to learn, the student can receive physical therapy as a necessary related service in order for her to benefit from the educational program. In a study by Borkowski and Wessman,[12] the authors found that determining the need for physical therapy services in the public school setting is done in a variety of ways, from the use of checklists to priority lists, which assist in determining the eligibility for physical therapy services. Nationally, there is no formula or automatic requirement based on disability that adds physical therapy as a related service to the IEP. Special education and the related services needed to meet the educational goals of the student are to be designed and provided on an individual basis and not on a system needs or capacity basis. No established criteria can supplant the IEP process in determining the unique educational needs of the student.

Related Services

Related services are defined as those services necessary in special education for a student to benefit from special education. These services include, but are not limited to, audiology services, medical services for diagnostic purposes, occupational therapy, physical therapy, rehabilitation counseling, and speech–language pathology services (34CFR300.24). If a student does not need special education, she does not need a related service for special education. Understanding the role of a related service in special education is important in facilitating a collaborative approach toward achieving IEP goals.[13] Many professionals are educated and trained to function independently within their profession rather than collaboratively with an educational team. Understanding the interrelatedness of the service providers, the educational relevance of the intervention, and the skills of each person involved with the student helps to foster a more collaborative and, hopefully, more efficient system of service delivery. The physical therapy evaluation can significantly add to the understanding of the student's functional ability in the classroom.

The Evaluation

The physical therapy evaluation can be helpful in identifying any orthopedic impairments or developmental delays in the student as well as impairments in movement or manipulation that may impair a student's ability to learn in the classroom. The evaluation can be helpful in

both identifying a disability and gathering information in order for the physical therapist to participate effectively in the creation of the IEP. It is not undertaken to establish physical therapy or discipline-specific goals, as is the case in other settings. The physical therapy evaluation is only one part of a comprehensive student evaluation that should identify those impairments or functional limitations that may affect the student from participating and benefiting from the educational experience.

The evaluation can begin with an examination of the student's transportation to school, if appropriate, and how she enters the building and begins the school day. It can also include an examination of her mobility or transport to and from classrooms, and the accessibility of the emergency evacuation routes that will be used during the school year. Positioning and manipulation during the educational activities, mobility to and from the lunch room, positioning during lunchtime, and the skills used for eating lunch and snacks are also appropriate areas to examine. The student's functioning during leisure or group activities, classroom outings, and school field trips could also be included in the examination. (See the Physical Therapy Evaluation Form in the Appendix.)

The physical therapist is mandated to provide services in the LRE. Physical therapy in the school should not be something that occurs only in a special therapy room with special therapy equipment for a blocked period of time. Rather, the physical therapist should identify and examine school environments and classroom activities that could be used throughout the day by members of the IEP team or classroom aides. Specific strategies should be explored that decrease or eliminate the barriers to the student's education.

It should be noted that the identification of impairments, by itself, cannot adequately specify the functional outcomes for an individual child. In a study by Mancini et al.[14] on predicting school participation in children with disabilities, functional information was better than the severity of the impairment in identifying participation outcomes in children with disabilities. It is the purpose of the evaluation to ultimately describe a student's ability to function in the school environment and participate in her educational program, taking into consideration the multiple factors that can influence that ability.

The IDEA does not mandate specific information in the physical therapy evaluation, or any standardized testing instrument. Each student's program should be designed to address the unique individual needs of that student in order for that student to have an appropriate public education. According to the IDEA, any standardized tests that are given to a student are administered by trained and knowledgeable personnel in accordance with the instructions provided by the producer of the test. If a standardized test is not conducted under standard conditions, a description of the extent to which the conditions varied from the standard must be included in the evaluation report (34CFR300.532). The School Function Assessment (SFA) and the Pediatric Evaluation of Disability Inventory (PEDI) are two examples of standardized tests that could apply to the school setting.

The SFA is a criterion-referenced standardized test used to assess a student's ability (kindergarten through sixth grade) to participate and function in the educational setting.[15] The SFA is composed of three parts: Part I, Participation, which examines the student's level of participation in a variety of school settings (e.g., the classroom, during lunch, on the playground); Part II, Task Supports, which examines the supports that the student needs to effectively participate in the educational program (e.g., type of assistance needed from adults, modifications to the environment); and Part III, Activity Performance, which examines the student's performance of functional activities (e.g., moving around the classroom, following rules, using materials). The SFA has good test–retest reliability (intra-class correlation coefficient [ICC] = 0.80 to 0.98).[15] Its content validity indicates that the SFA is comprehensive and relevant for elementary students with disabilities.[16] Correlations were also found between the Gross Motor Function Measure-66 and the physical task dimension and cognitive components of the SFA.[17]

The PEDI is a norm-referenced standardized test used to evaluate a child's (6 months to 7.5 years) functional performance and capabilities in the domains of self-care, mobility, and social function.[18] It can be used to detect functional deficits or developmental delays, to monitor progress in pediatric rehabilitation programs, and to evaluate outcomes of pediatric rehabilitation programs or therapeutic programs in an educational setting. The PEDI is composed of three parts: Part I, Functional Skills Scales, which examine the child's level of functioning in self-care, mobility, and social functions; Part II, Caregivers Assistance Scales, which examine the amount of help a child needs to carry out functional activities; and Part III, the Modifications section, which is a frequency count of the type and extent of environmental modifications needed for completion of a functional activity. Due to the way the test items are constructed, it is more likely to identify subtle differences in functional performance between children with limited or slowly emerging competencies. Scores on the PEDI can indicate the child's standing in relation to age expectations for functional skills and performance (normative standard score) and indicate the child's performance along a continuum (scaled scores). Reliability has been shown to increase when the PEDI is administered by both the parent and the physical therapist as their perception of the child differ on some PEDI test items.[19] Studies by the authors of the PEDI and others have shown that it is a reliable and valid instrument for the evaluation of young children with disabilities.[18–20] After the evaluation is complete, the physical therapists can more actively participate in the IEP process.

POINTS TO REMEMBER

Purpose of Student Evaluation

The physical therapist may be asked to evaluate a student to:

1. determine if she is eligible for special education, or
2. gather information about a student who is eligible, in order to develop an IEP.

The Individualized Education Program

When a student has been determined to be eligible for special education, an IEP must be developed within 30 days [34CFR300.343(b)(2)]. The IEP is a legal document, developed by a team of professionals and parents to address the educational needs of the student. Adherence to the goals identified in the IEP and the agreed-upon frequency of service delivery are required unless formally changed by the team and appropriately signed. A physical therapist working in the school system is obliged to adhere to the established IEP whether or not he took part in the construction of the program.

The IEP consists of two parts: *the team* and *the plan*. The physical therapist, as a member of the IEP team, is a valuable resource in identifying and implementing the appropriate interventions to address any identified limitations of the student or classroom in the educational process. Using the disablement model, the physical therapist identifies any impairments or functional limitations of the student that would have an affect on her ability to learn and function in the educational environment.[21] Decisions regarding the need for related services, as well as the frequency and duration of the intervention, are decided upon by the IEP team and become part of the IEP document. The physical therapist should participate in the development of the student's educational goals and identify how the services of a physical therapist could facilitate the achievement of those goals. It is the IEP that guides the delivery of the special education program and related services for the student with a disability. Without a doubt, constructing, designing, and implementing an effective IEP require open communication and teamwork.

The IDEA requires certain information to be included in each student's IEP. States and local school systems often include additional information in order to document that they have met certain requirements of federal or state law. The flexibility that states and school systems have to design their own IEP forms is one reason why IEP forms may look different from school system to school system or from state to state.

It is the school's responsibility to contact the parent and schedule an IEP meeting early enough to allow them the opportunity to attend. An agreeable time and location are determined with the parents. The parents should be

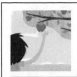

BOX 8-2
An Example of an Annual Goal

Student annual goal: Luke will sit in a classroom chair, and on the floor, in order to participate in a variety of educational activities during the school day so that he can more fully participate in the educational program with his peers.
Student annual goal: Grace will negotiate the stairs in the school independently while carrying her book bag so that she can safely access resources within the school.

informed of who will be attending the IEP meeting and are allowed to invite people who would have special knowledge or expertise about their child. Physical therapists are not mandated to attend the IEP meeting but should do so in order to more effectively assist in the design of the special education program and the utilization of physical therapy services in that process. It is not appropriate to establish goals for the IEP before the team has a chance to meet and develop the educational program. Also, the physical therapist cannot know how his services can aid in the implementation of an individualized special education program before the program is developed.

The next step in this process is the actual IEP meeting. The information gained from the physical therapy evaluation should be brought to the meeting to add to the discussion in the development of an IEP. Although the law does not explicitly require that an IEP team consist of the related service provider, if the student has a possible need for a related service it would be appropriate for that provider to be a part of the team and attend the IEP meeting. The related service provider should be included when his or her particular related service will be discussed, or at the request of the student's parents or the school.

Annual goals are established by consensus and are discipline free. (See Box 8-2 for an example.) The goals are the student's goals and are developed by all members of the IEP team, which include the student, if appropriate. Goals should be measurable and clearly reflect the student's educational program and her ability to participate in this process [34CFR300.347(a)(2)]. Randall and McEwen,[22] in their article "Writing Patient-Centered Functional Goals" identified steps that can aid in this process. Applying these steps in the educational environment, the IEP team would first determine the desired outcomes as they relate to the education of the student. Next, the team would identify the environments or times in the school day in which specific activities related to the outcomes occur. Finally, the team establishes measurable goals that relate to the identified educational outcomes.

At the IEP meeting, the actual IEP plan is written and signed by all the members present. If the parents do not agree with the IEP, they should discuss their concerns

with the other members. A solution to the disagreement should be devised. Possible disagreement is another reason to have all the members at the meeting, including the related service personnel. If the IEP team cannot work out a solution, the parents are entitled to mediation. Parents can also file a complaint with the state department of education, and may request a due process hearing. Open communication, active listening, efficient planning, and adherence to a student-focused process can help avoid this path.

By law, the IEP must include certain information about the student and her educational program [Sec 614(d)(1)(A)]. This information includes a statement on the student's current performance in school and how her disability affects her involvement in the educational process, annual goals that are measurable and reasonable to achieve within the school year, and the identification of the special education and related services needed to assist the student in meeting her goals.

The IEP must identify the participation of the student with students who are nondisabled and explain the extent (if any) to which the student will not participate with students who are nondisabled in the regular class and in other school activities. The IEP must also identify what modifications in the administration of tests for the state or district that the student will need. The physical therapist can aid in the identification and modifications needed to take the test, assuring that the tests will accurately reflect the student's knowledge and that the scores on the test will not be limited by the student's ability to physically complete the test.

The IEP must also identify the parameters of service provision: when services will begin (date), how often they will be provided (frequency), where they will be provided (location), and how long they will last (duration). It is important that the physical therapist assist in this process with the team to assure efficient and effective delivery of the interventions needed to help the student work toward and achieve her annual goals.

POINTS TO REMEMBER

The IEP

An IEP is a legal document and consists of two parts:

1. the team, and
2. the plan.

The IEP must state the starting date of services to be provided, as well as their frequency, location, and duration.

The IEP must also identify how the student's progress will be measured and how parents will be informed of that progress. The Education for All Handicapped Children Act of 1975 (PL 94-142) formalized the participation of the parent by requiring their involvement in program planning. Parents of minors have the right and obligation to grant permission to evaluate, consent to the release of information, and provide information about the student in a broader context than the confines of the school building, and they have the right to all educational records about their child. They have a lifelong commitment to the education, growth, and social development of their child that extends well beyond the age of 21. Members of the IEP team must learn to actively listen to parents in order to help in the process of developing a truly individualized educational program for their son or daughter. Parents can be powerful advocates for their child, as well as a wealth of information on the child's functional strengths and needs.

The special education teacher and school must make sure that the student's IEP is being carried out as it was written. Parents are provided a copy of the IEP. Each of the student's teachers and service providers also have access to the IEP and should know their responsibilities toward the achievement of the student's goals.

Writing goals that focus on function not only helps the physical therapist conform to public laws and reimbursement systems, but also can motivate the student to work toward the desired outcome. According to **Kettenbach**,[23] appropriate goals should contain the following components: an Audience, an identified Behavior, the Conditions under which the behavior will be observed, and the Degree to which the behavior will be observed (ABCD). In the educational setting, the goal should also reflect the educational relevance, which would extend **Kettenbach**'s acronym to ABCDE. The *audience* would most often be the student, but could also be the parent, teacher, or classroom staff (the student will; the teacher will...). The *behavior* is something that can be described or measured accurately. They are generally action verbs, describing what the student or teacher is to do (demonstrate the ability to sit, independently manipulate...). The *condition* is the circumstance in which the behavior is done (in the classroom, during physical education, while walking in the hall...). The *degree* is the minimal number of times, or the determination of success or mastery of an objective, and is used to identify when the goal is achieved (for 35 minutes, 3 days a week; for 5/5 trials). The *educational relevance* is the relationship of this goal to the student's education (in order to participate in group discussions, in order to complete the in class assignment, in order to interact in the school environment, in order to progress in the general curriculum).[24] Writing the educational relevance at times may seem redundant, but it helps the IEP team understand the reason for the goal and can also identify inappropriate goals for the educational environment. This structure clarifies for the IEP team for whom the goal was developed: the student, classroom teacher, classroom aide, transportation personnel, etc. It identifies the behavior that is expected and under what conditions it would be seen. It

also provides the criteria for objective attainment, noting the degree to which the behavior must be performed in order for the goal to be considered met.

POINTS TO REMEMBER

Constructing Goals

When constructing goals, remember:
A: audience
B: behavior
C: condition
D: degree
E: educational relevance

Goals must be identified and agreed upon by the IEP team. The educational system was never intended to provide for all of the student's needs. The special education program should address those needs that will enable the student to participate in her educational program. Goals should be identified and written that reflect the student's ability to function in the educational environment. They also assist the physical therapist in the identification and selection of appropriate interventions.

PARENT PERSPECTIVE

THE IEP MEETING

As parents of a child with a disability, we experienced fear and intimidation in our first IEP meeting. Thinking we knew a little about special education, we soon realized we knew nothing about the laws or our rights. We had to read, study, and go to support groups to learn how to help our child and to work and understand the special education system. Today we would never think of going to an IEP meeting without an advocate or documentation to support our child's needs. After the meeting, we continued to monitor the implementation of the IEP and our son's progress. Being this involved can lead to an attitude of "us against them," which only creates no-win situations. Open and honest communication, mutual understanding, and respect are so important to assuring an appropriate education, which is guaranteed by law, for our son or for any child.
—*Charlie and Mary B., parents*

INTERVENTIONS

The interventions that physical therapists use in the school system are not typically listed on the IEP, but they are instrumental when making decisions on implementation, how often the intervention will be provided, whether specialized training or education is required, and in what specific school setting the intervention will be provided. It is the purpose of the therapy in this environment that is different from other environments such as the hospital or outpatient setting. The purpose is to optimize the student's ability to participate in her IEP to achieve the identified goals. Physical therapists have a variety of interventions that can be used in the educational setting. The Guide to Physical Therapist Practice identifies those interventions that include, but are not limited to, the following:[25]

Coordination and communication. Effective communication with the student, teachers, parents, classroom staff, administrators, physicians, and the IEP team is frequently utilized and an important intervention that physical therapists are asked to use in the school environment. It is the responsibility of the physical therapists to successfully educate others on the role of physical therapy in the special education program and to work with the IEP team in developing a truly individualized and educationally relevant program for the student. Physical therapists are the movement specialists and are called upon to optimize the student's ability to function in the classroom. As in all practice environments, it is important to remember the audience when communicating information. Other members of the team may not be as well versed in the use of medical and professional jargon that a physical therapist uses daily in his professional documentation. Teachers, classroom staff, school nurses, neurologists, and speech language pathologists most likely speak at different levels regarding health care. It is necessary to modify what is communicated in order to promote understanding on the part of the recipient and all members of the IEP team. Nonverbal communication is also a form of communication that is especially noted when disagreements arise. It is important to remember the perception and the responsibility of the parent who is trying to do what she feels is in the best interest of her child. Looks of impatience, confrontation, or disinterest are not effective means of fostering a collaborative team approach in special education. Active listening, the use of open ended probing questions, identification of the student's strengths as well as weaknesses, and honest discussions about the student's future add to the likelihood of a successful outcome and are a few aspects of a collaborative team approach.

Client-related instruction. Instruction on the various interventions that a physical therapist recommends is vital for successful implementation. The positions that the student assumes during the many activities that she participates throughout the day influence her ability to effectively participate in those activities. How does she sit in a classroom chair, wheelchair, on the floor, or on the school bus? How is she positioned during educational activities, leisure activities, recess, or physical education? Assuring optimal positioning of the student during educational or leisure activities to promote function is one of the most important duties of the physical therapist in the educational setting.

Therapeutic exercise. Therapeutic exercises are the most common procedural interventions provided by a physical therapist.[25] The ability to stretch, strengthen, increase endurance, promote the proper use of body mechanics, and facilitate task-specific skills are just a few of the many therapeutic exercises that a physical therapist can use in the school.

Functional training. Functional training is the natural progression of therapeutic exercise, which should be aimed at impairments and functional limitations of the student. Functional training in the educational setting can include the ability to move about the school building while carrying books or backpacks. It can include the ability to open a locker, carry a tray, hold a pen, turn a page, or participate in group activities and community field trips. Functional training can also include job coaching or simulated work environments and tasks.[25] It is the ultimate goal of the intervention to increase the student's ability to function in the classroom and, ultimately, in society.

Prescription, application, and use of assistive technology. Often, when working to compensate for skills that are absent or movement that is nonfunctional, interventions can be augmented by the use of external devices or equipment referred to as assistive technology. The use of these devices can help to compensate for the student's lack of motor development or skill by providing support or environmental modification when indicated.

The following questions are important to consider when deciding a student's needs: What type of assistive technology will provide the maximum amount of function for the student in the school environment? How will an external device aid, as well as limit, the student's ability to move and learn? How frequently will the assistive technology be used, and for what duration of time?[26] In determining the answers to these questions, the physical therapist first identifies the factors that impair the student from acquiring a particular motor skill. In the patient management process, as identified in the Guide to Physical Therapist Practice, six steps can be identified in the determination and utilization of assistive technology for the student.[25] These include the examination, the evaluation, and the diagnosis of what is impairing the student's motor or educational development; the provision of an appropriate level of intervention by appropriate personnel; and the monitoring and identification of the outcomes of the intervention. The first step should include such information as medical diagnosis; the student's age and weight; identification of the accessibility and barriers in the environment; the mode of transportation that the student will use to move about the school; classroom support/aides; financial abilities and limitations; cognitive and motivational level of the student; and, most importantly, what the IEP team hopes to gain from the assistive technology. In addition, it is important to clarify for the team the expected duration of the use of the technology. Will it be for the school year or over several years? When will the technology be used during the school day, and who would be involved in teaching the student, classroom staff, and family to use the device? Acquiring the technology will include identification of specific components of the device for the student; securing payment, delivery, and assembly; and proper training in the fitting, use, and care of the device. Periodic reassessments and follow-up on the use of the assistive technology is vital to assure that the maximum benefit is derived from its utilization.

Any type of technology that is introduced into a student's life has both positive and negative aspects. The IEP team should be aware of the effect the technology will have on the student in terms of peer acceptance and restrictions. Supported standing devices are appropriate in providing necessary support, allowing the student to be positioned more upright, have eye-level contact with peers and staff, and participate in a natural activity such as standing, but the device may also limit the student from moving around her environment, which limits her opportunities to interact with others, impairing to some extent her ability to initiate interactions in her immediate environment. The complete educational plan should be taken into consideration whenever assistive technology is considered. Everyone involved should be aware of the responsibility and time that are associated with the use of assistive technology. Problems may arise if there are negative attitudes toward the use of the technology, or if there is insufficient staff training and support in the utilization of the technology in the classroom.[27]

The interventions selected will influence, and be influenced by, the service delivery model needed to implement the interventions.

POINTS TO REMEMBER

Interventions

When choosing interventions, the physical therapist should keep in mind:

1. Coordination, Communication, and Documentation
2. Client-Related Instruction
3. Procedural Interventions

Common interventions used in the school setting may include:

1. Therapeutic exercise
2. Functional training in the school
3. Application of assistive technology

MODELS OF SERVICE DELIVERY

Physical therapists can be challenged to understand their role in special education as compared to their more common role in the health care system. Before 1975, physical therapists primarily followed a medical model of providing care that focused on direct hands-on intervention.

With the passage and implementation of PL 94-142, the practice of physical therapy in the educational environment became clearer, with an increased responsibility on the part of the physical therapist in understanding the law and the types of service delivery models that are available to meet the intent of the law in providing an appropriate education for all children.[7]

After the IEP team determines annual goals and objectives, the physical therapists can assist with delineating what interventions would be appropriate to use in order to work toward those goals. Taking into consideration the student's present level of functioning, the identified goals, the type of intervention that applies, and the availability and capability of other members of the team, the IEP team should determine the most appropriate model of service delivery. Various authors use different terminology to describe different levels or types of service delivery, but basically they are describing either a direct or indirect service provision or a combination of the two. *Direct* service provision, for which the skills and interventions for this particular student are available only by the professional, requires the provision of the intervention by the physical therapist directly to the student in the classroom (where the skill learned in isolation may be generalized to aid in education) or in the community.[28] *Indirect* service provision may be appropriate when the skills and interventions for this particular student are available by consultation and education of the classroom staff and parent by the physical therapist. With indirect service, the recipient of the physical therapy intervention shifts more toward the teacher, classroom staff, school environment, or parent, rather than directly to the student. A collaborative effort by all persons involved can assure that the most appropriate interventions are being incorporated into the student's daily routines and activities, in order to optimize her ability to benefit from the IEP. This integrated model of service delivery is the preferred model of service provision today.[29] An *integrated approach* requires consultation with the IEP team. Many authors expound the importance of consultation with the members of the IEP team, and agree that this is one of the most important forms of service delivery in the educational setting.[30] Collaboration with team members requires an understanding of each team member's role, the routines and activities in the classroom, and a shared responsibility for the implementation of the IEP.[28,31] Frequent communication with the classroom staff and parents, individual flexibility on the part of the physical therapist and classroom staff (so that the physical therapist can be in the classroom during appropriate activities or routines), the functionality of the interventions, and the individual responsibility of each member toward achieving the student's IEP goals are important factors in achieving a successful program.[28,29]

The model of service delivery is influenced by the needs of the student, the type of intervention needed, and the capability of other providers, including the classroom staff. In many cases direct, indirect, or an integrated approach to the provision of services will be determined by the needs of the student and the classroom. A continuum of service delivery models may be necessary and appropriate to meet the individual needs of a student.[31] The type of service delivery model may also influence the frequency of intervention.

FREQUENCY OF INTERVENTION

Making decisions on the frequency of physical therapy services is a key point in the formation of an IEP. Many times members of the IEP team may not agree upon the recommended frequency of a related service, typically feeling that a higher frequency of intervention would produce a better outcome. Education, communication, and documentation are vital in this process to ensure that all members of the team have an understanding and agree upon the level of related services provided (for additional information see Chapter 1).

In a study by Kaminnker et al.,[32] 626 physical therapists who were members of the American Physical Therapy Association (APTA) Pediatric Section and who identified themselves as school-based physical therapists were surveyed. The survey presented four case studies and evaluated the clinical choices of the respondents with regard to several factors, including frequency and intensity of services. The study examined the thought process used in clinical decision making. The most important characteristics of the student, which influenced the physical therapists' decisions, were the student's present level of functioning, the student and family goals, and the identified functional limitations of the student. A study done by Effgen[33] surveyed 686 members of the APTA Pediatric Section, in which 325 worked in the school setting, and found that the most important factor when considering the termination of physical therapy services was when the student met his or her functional goals.

The evaluation of function plays an important role in this process, as does the selection of interventions used to address the functional limitations. Can the impairment that constrains function be changed through intervention? Is the student performing optimally, and can intervention improve her function by making it more efficient? If the impairment cannot be changed by a physical therapy intervention, could a compensatory strategy or the use of assistive technology improve the student's function?[34] These questions are important to ask in the process of determining the frequency of services. In addition, the student's age, health, diagnosis and prognosis, motivational level, and cognitive status are also used in deciding if an intervention would be appropriate and beneficial. The school environment, the availability and capability of classroom staff, the student's schedule, and compliance with the program are additional factors to consider and highlight the importance of a team approach in the construction and implementation of a student's IEP. At times, the student's behavior may impact the effectiveness of the intervention or the ability to provide a service.

POINT TO REMEMBER

Frequency and Duration

Frequency and duration of intervention are dependent on the individual situation of each student.

Behavioral Issues

Many behaviors can arise when students have to comply with an educational or any structured program. Students with and without disabilities can be noncompliant and/or aggressive, and they can present a danger to themselves or to other students. The IDEA does allow the removal of a student for up to 10 days at a time for any violation of the school rules. This applies to students with or without a disability as long as the identified behavior is not a manifestation or part of the student's disability. There is nothing in the IDEA that restricts schools from disciplining students with disabilities.

A student's behavior at times can become disruptive and/or offensive. If no formal behavioral modification program is part of the IEP, ignoring the behavior would be recommended, as long as there is no potential harm to the student or other students, and the behavior does not violate the school's code of conduct. Collaboration with the IEP team will help in identifying the triggers, frequency, and possible strategies used to address the behavior. Positive reinforcement for appropriate behaviors is recommended to foster the development of these characteristics. Receiving praise is not only instantly gratifying, but also increases the likelihood of the behavior being repeated. An effective way of developing a positive supportive environment is to recognize and reinforce positive behaviors instead of focusing on correcting and redirecting negative behaviors.[35] Negative reinforcement can be just as powerful as positive reinforcement. Becoming visibly upset, or demonstrating nonverbal displeasure with a student's actions may be reinforcing to the student, encouraging her to behave in the same manner. Controlling and understanding verbal and nonverbal skills is an essential aspect of communication.

If the student's behaviors impair her ability to participate and progress through the curriculum, a behavioral consultation and the development of a behavioral aspect of the IEP may be necessary. The school's psychologist can help facilitate this process. A Functional Behavior Assessment (FBA) is one example of a formal assessment taken to identify problem behaviors and the events that cause them to occur.[36] This assessment is taken to better understand the context in which the behavior is seen and to guide the development of effective, relevant, and efficient interventions to address the behavior.[36] For those students who have an established behavioral modification program incorporated into their IEP, it is imperative that the physical therapist follows the established program to address the behavior. Failure to address the behavioral issues in a consistent manner can jeopardize the entire process. Kevin Dwyer, the Assistant Executive Director of the National Association for School Psychologists, has outlined several principles to increase positive behavior and reduce the need to suspend or expel a student from school[37] (see Box 8-3). These principles include the estab-

---

BOX 8-3
Principles to Increase Positive Behavior

1. Schools have the responsibility to maintain a safe environment conducive to learning. This responsibility includes the establishment and enforcement of a code of conduct.
2. Schools have a responsibility to assure that all students, including those receiving special education, and their families are familiar with the code of conduct and the consequences for violations of the code.
3. Students who have disabilities that may cause them to be unable to follow the code of conduct should have their expectations addressed in their IEP.
4. Behavioral goals, like specific discipline goals, should be incorporated into the IEP and not be separate "behavioral plans."
5. Parents should be involved with the team in finding effective strategies to address a change in the student's behavior. Behavioral goals, like other annual goals and objectives, should be measurable.
6. Any behaviors that impair a student's ability to learn should be addressed. Any new behaviors that develop that may lead to a suspension should cause the school to initiate an IEP meeting before the behavior or repeated suspensions becomes a problem.
7. Weapons or drug violations require an IEP meeting within 10 days.
8. The IEP team, assisted by the appropriate professionals, determines if the student's behavior is related to his disability. Review of the student's behaviors and the interventions tried should be comprehensive and focus on multiple factors, not solely behavioral goals.
9. When dangerous behavior is a result of a disability, a re-evaluation of the student's placement and the identification of the necessary related services would be appropriate and identification of related services to assure that the behavior will be addressed and to prevent its reoccurrence. When dangerous behavior is not a result of a disability, the student may be subject to the regular process for violations of the code of conduct, provided that the intervention does not violate FAPE.

Adapted from: Dwyer K. Disciplining Students with Disabilities. Behavioral Interventions 1998; 26:18–21.

---

lishment of a School Code of Conduct with clear communication on the consequences of violating that code. A student with a disability who is unable to follow that code should have her expectations addressed in her IEP. It is expected that the physical therapist, or any school personnel, would be familiar and comply with the school's Code of Conduct.

ANNUAL SUMMARY/OUTCOMES

The IDEA emphasizes the importance of teaching and learning, with a specific focus on the utilization of the IEP as the primary tool for enhancing a student's involvement and progress in the general school curriculum. At least every 3 years, the student undergoes a complete re-evaluation. This evaluation is often called a triennial. Its purpose is to find out if the student continues to be a child with a disability, as defined by IDEA, and to identify the student's current educational needs. The student's IEP is reviewed by the IEP team at least once a year, or more often at the request of the parents or appropriate school personnel. The student's progress toward the annual goals are measured, as stated in the IEP, and reported to her parents. Progress reports must be given to parents at least as often as parents are informed of their nondisabled children's progress.

One method of tracking the goals and objectives for which physical therapy is utilized can be listed on the documentation form (see the Appendix). A monthly summary of the student's performance toward the established IEP goals is also helpful in assessing the rate of goal attainment and the progress of the student (Fig. 8-1). This summary can help the physical therapist and teacher keep up to date on the student's performance, or encourage identification and timely problem solving for goals that are not progressing as expected (or for goal attainment that has progressed more quickly than expected). This information could facilitate early planning, re-evaluations, scheduling of meetings, and updating of the IEP. The tracking of goals also makes annual summaries of the student's progress more expedient. Based on the IEP and the appropriate goals that were addressed by the physical therapist, an annual assessment of the number of goals achieved would reflect one outcome measurement in this process (Fig. 8-2). This interpretation makes several assumptions regarding the appropriateness of the goals established, the criteria set for mastery of the goal, and the system of measuring goals. This process can be used to demonstrate, at one level, the appropriate utilization and effectiveness of physical therapy in a student's educational program.

REIMBURSEMENT

In addition to the annual salary or hourly rate provided to an employee of a company that provides physical

Physical Therapy Documentation Form

Student:_____   School year:_____

Frequency of services as noted on the IEP: _____

IEP GOAL	DATE	COMMENT
Monthly Summary:		

_____
Physical Therapist

Figure 8-1. ■ Physical therapy documentation form.

therapy services to a school, many physical therapists in private practice can also sign a contract with the local school district to provide physical therapy services to one or more schools. Fees are determined by the individual physical therapist and are usually based on an hourly rate (see Chapter 14).

States are allocated federal grant monies to assist them in providing special education and related services to children with disabilities in accordance with the IDEA Part B (34CFR300.701). The grant is based on the number of students with disabilities in the state who are receiving special education and related services. In addition, school districts are given the ability to bill third party payers for services, including physical therapy or other related services, mandated by a student's IEP, with the approval of the parents. In doing so, the state must insure that there is no delay in the implementation of a student's IEP (34CFR300.301). Any insurance funding that requires copayments, decreases the lifetime benefit, or results in a loss or decrease in service benefit cannot be accessed without a parent's permission. Parents are not required to provide the school with their insurance information, and refusal by the parents cannot impair or jeopardize the student's right to an appropriate education.

In 1988, the *Medicare Catastrophic Coverage Act* (PL 100-360)[38] was signed into law by President Reagan. This law allows states to obtain funds through public health insurance programs, namely Medicaid, to pay for health-related services in special education as long as there is no cost to the family. A family does not have to enroll in Medicaid in order to receive a related service.

County School District
Example of a Physical Therapy End-of-Year Report

Student: Alek Smith
Number of IEP goals: five
Number achieved: four
Goal achievement rate: 80%
PT service frequency on IEP: 60 minutes per week; direct.

Annual Summary:

During this school year Alek has made significant progress in his prewalking skills, sitting skills, and moving skills. In October, we initiated bench sitting with the seat tilted forward. This activity was done to encourage a more upright posture of his trunk and to encourage him to move his trunk during seated activities. By December, he was able to move from bench sitting to stance with one hand assist. In January, we initiated standing against the wall while holding onto a standard walker. By the end of the month, Alek demonstrated the ability to maintain a grasp on the walker for 10 seconds, with both hands, independently! He received new braces in January, and we initiated walking forward with his walker by the end of the month. In February, Alek received a new wheelchair and made progress in his sitting posture and use of a standard walker during assisted walking exercises. By March, Alek demonstrated the ability to stand for 5 seconds independently and to walk with one hand held for 10 feet in the classroom. On March 12, he took one step on the right independently. By the end of April, Alek was able to walk 50 feet down the hall with one hand held, far enough to walk to the physical education class with his classroom peers. In May, Alek was demonstrating the ability to knee walk 3 to 5 feet, move from lying on his back into a full kneel independently, and move from a full kneel to stance with one hand assist. He can stand at the table in the art room for 5 to 10 minutes. His walking with one hand held has improved in speed, accuracy of foot placement, posture, and control.

Figure 8-2. ■ Examples of a physical therapy year-end report for an individual student **(A)** and an annual physical therapy program report **(B)**.

EXTENDED SCHOOL YEAR

The term extended school year (ESY) means special education and related services that are provided to a child with a disability beyond the normal school year (34CFR300.309). The need for ESY services is based on the individual student's needs and the progress made toward the identified goals in her IEP. The ESY services should be structured and provided in relation to the established special educational program for the student, to facilitate the attainment or maintenance of the student's goals or performance. No one person can decide if a student is eligible for ESY services or if she should receive them. The IEP team makes that decision based on the student's performance and need. Decisions regarding goal attainment, regression, and recoupment should be supported by documented evidence of these occurrences. It is necessary, to the extent possible, that the physical therapist, as well as other members of the IEP team, incorporate reliable and valid tests and measurements to aid in this decision-making process.

TRANSITIONING

Transitioning refers to the process that prepares students with disabilities to move from school to postschool activities. These postschool activities can include postsecondary education, vocational training, integrated employment (including supported employment), continuing and adult education, adult services, independent living, or community participation (34CFR300.29). The ultimate goal of special education is to enable the student to become a productive and contributing member of society. "Improving

During the school year, the classroom reports that Alek has demonstrated an increased use of his left hand. He is more socially interactive and has improved in his listening and following directions skills. Alek is making requests regarding his wants and needs more consistently, and he is compliant with physical activities during gym class.

Recommendations:

After consultation with Alek's teacher, the classroom staff, his parents, and other IEP team members, goals were developed and discussed at the IEP meeting. The IEP goals address Alek's functional skills in the classroom, as well as his mobility and walking skills. The need for direct physical therapy services was determined to be 30 minutes every other week, with indirect services provided to the teacher, parent, and classroom staff for 60 minutes once a month.

_____
Physical Therapist

Figure 8-2. ■ **(A)** (*Continued*).

educational results for children with disabilities is an essential element of our national policy of ensuring equality of opportunity, full participation, independent living, and economic self sufficiency for individuals with disabilities" [PL 105-17, Sec 601(c)].

Transition plans to vocational programs, employment, and services beyond public education must be included in each student's IEP. These plans can begin at any time, but must be identified in the student's IEP no later than the first IEP to be in effect when the student is 16 years old [Sec 614(d)(1)(A)(VIII)]. Early discussions with the student and parents to identify the student's interests and preferences after graduation are paramount to achieving the optimal outcome for the student. Identifying appropriate opportunities that are available for the student in the community, the degree of her participation, the level of independence she can achieve, and the

amount and type of employment that is appropriate is one goal of a transition plan. Some of the transition services that are available include formal assessment of career skills or interests, job readiness or prevocational training, and specific job skills training.[5] The physical therapist can assist in this process by clarifying the student's level of motor functioning and use of assistive technology to aid in activities of daily living (ADLs), community participation, vocational training, integrated employment, or postsecondary education, to name a few of the options. Physical access of the identified sites and the training needs of the personnel with whom the student will come in contact are other transition services that can be provided by the physical therapist. Ultimately, upon graduation from high school, the student's ability to participate as a member of society reflects the influence and outcome of special education.

Example of an Annual Physical Therapy Program Report
School Year

Administrator:

During this school year, I provided physical therapy services to 9 students at Central High School. Their end of the year reports are attached.

From the data collected, the overall goal attainment rate for this group of students was 78%. This reflects all of the goals identified on their IEPs that were addressed with physical therapy as a related service. If you eliminate the one outlier from the group, who had a 50% goal attainment rate for this year, the group rate increases to 83%.

It has been great working with you again. You have a great program. Keep up the good work.

Professionally:

_____
Physical Therapist

Figure 8-2. ■ (B) (*Continued*).

CASE STUDY

John

STUDENT EVALUATION

John is a 17-year-old boy who presents with cerebral palsy, spastic quadriplegia. His hearing and vision are intact by professional report. He is nonverbal, nonambulatory, and frequently demonstrates self-abusive behaviors that require the use of a protective helmet. John presents with impairments in his cognitive and communicative functions. His active and passive ranges of motion are limited due to spasticity. He has a fixed lateral curvature, with rotation, of the spine (nonprogressive adolescent neurogenic scoliosis, left thoracic with rotation to the left; 55 degrees by radiographic measurement). Impairments in muscle performance and motor control are evident, most noted by John's inability to perform transitional skills higher than rolling and in the use of his hands. He demonstrates the ability to hold a built-up-handled spoon with a gross grasp, and performs a voluntary release.

John presents with functional limitations in his ability to effectively and efficiently communicate his wants or needs to another person, transition from supine or prone into a sitting position, transition from sitting in his wheelchair into stance (which requires the assist of one), stand, or walk. John is dependent with all his ADLs and instrumental ADLs.

John is enrolled in the special education program at the local high school. He utilizes a prone stander and his wheelchair as his primary positioning and mobility devices. John will gaze and reach during his educational activities to make choices and answer one-step requests. He is presently transitioning to a day program at the local behavioral health center. His parents plan on John living at home with them after he graduates and desire that he assist with ADLs as much as possible. They are also interested in him using a gait trainer for exercise ambulation. Presently John requires the assistance of another person to perform the necessary mobility functions to utilize the community and school environments.

DIAGNOSIS

Impaired Motor Function and Sensory Integrity Associated with a Nonprogressive Disorder of the Central Nervous System Congenital in Origin (Pattern 5C)

Secondary diagnosis: Impaired Joint Mobility, Motor Function, Muscle Performance, and Range of Motion Associated with Spinal Disorders (Pattern 4F)

ANNUAL GOAL

John will successfully participate in his educational activities with the minimal amount of assistance necessary.

INTERVENTIONS

1. *Coordination and communication.* Because of John's self-abusive behavior, which frequently interrupted his educational program, consultation with a behavioral specialist and the implementation of his recommendations into John's daily activities was coordinated among all team members (including the family at home) and classroom staff. Consistency with the type and administration of the behavioral modification techniques was imperative in the evaluation of their effectiveness.
2. *Client-related instruction.* Instruction was provided on the proper use of John's supportive stander, gait trainer, and wheelchair, in order to optimize his upper extremity function during educational activities, speech therapy, and his self-feeding program. The proper and timely use of these assistive devices was important to assure that John had the appropriate support and the necessary freedom of movement to participate in a variety of school activities. Instruction to his classroom staff on transfers to and from his wheelchair, gait trainer, toilet, a classroom chair, and the mat on the floor, and into and out of his stander, was necessary to promote consistency and safety.
3. *Procedural interventions.* Therapeutic exercises were incorporated into John's daily routine and adaptive physical education program to strengthen and promote motor control of his trunk and lower extremities, which aided in the development of his transition and assisted ambulation skills. These exercises included moving into and out of quadruped, sit-to-stand exercises, and stepping activities with proper foot placement, while in his gait trainer.

Functional training in the school included the maintenance of optimal positions in both supported sitting and stance throughout the school day. Proper positioning was necessary to promote upper extremity function in order for John to participate in his educational and related service programs and activities. These included such activities as reaching forward, grasping and releasing appropriate objects, touch switch activation, and eye–hand and hand-to-mouth coordination activities. The use of a gait trainer was also incorporated into his school day when a change of classrooms occurred, which was scheduled to happen twice a day.

Application of supportive and assistive devices involved adjustments and adaptations to the equipment that John used in the classroom and lunchroom and during his adaptive physical education. The proper use and fit of his gait trainer was monitored, and the appropriate adjustments were made as he progressed in this area.

OUTCOMES

Number of IEP goals that the physical therapist was involved in: 5

Number achieved: 4

Goal attainment: 80%

Frequency of physical therapy as listed on the IEP: Weekly for 30 minutes, direct, and 30 minutes indirect, monthly

During this school year, John has demonstrated consistent attainment of his goals. He continues to consistently demonstrate the ability to transition out of bed with moderate assistance. He will assist in repositioning himself in his wheelchair with verbal cues and physical cues, holding his hands on the armrest. If this is done, John will scoot his pelvis backwards into the seat. His goal was to do this 50% of the time. He has demonstrated the ability to do this 100% of the time, upon request. John uses his gait trainer 3 to 5 days a week. He will consistently move his feet for 100 to 300 feet, independently. John appeared to enjoy this activity of exercise ambulation as noted by decreasing his self-abusive behaviors, making noises associated with pleasure, and on occasion, smiling during this activity. John will maintain a quadruped position when placed for >1 minute. He will move from quadruped to prone with controlled movements. John will assist transferring from lying on the floor to stance. He requires moderate assistance to transition from prone to quadruped and moderate to maximum assistance to move from quadruped to full kneel position. John requires maximum assistance to transition from full kneel to stance. This is unchanged from the beginning of the school year.

Reflection Questions

1. How could John's self-abusive behavior impair his ability to use assistive technology in school? What activities could it impair the most?
2. What specific interventions could be used during John's functional training at school? Discuss which interventions could be delegated to support staff. What qualifications or characteristics of the support staff would be necessary for the successful delegation and implementation of the selected interventions?
3. Discuss the educational relevance of ambulation. What justification can be made for the purchase of a gait trainer for this student?

SUMMARY

Millions of children with disabilities participate in special education programs under the guidance of the federal law currently known as the IDEA. This federal program's primary purpose is to improve the education of children with disabilities in order to ensure that they have an equal opportunity to succeed as individuals in society as do children without disabilities. Physical therapists play an important role in this process as related service providers, assisting with the identification and remediation of impairments to movement, function, and learning.

The practice of physical therapy in the educational environment is structured around the IEP, which includes a team, a plan, and the identification of annual goals for the student in special education. Interventions commonly used by a physical therapist in this environment include the communication and coordination of services and information, as well as functional training in the school environment. These and other appropriate interventions are provided directly to the student through a hands-on application, indirectly to the student through the education and support of the parents and classroom staff, or a combination of the two, with an emphasis on collaboration and integration. Physical therapy can also be provided throughout an ESY and during the transition process, if necessary.

With an understanding of the special education practice environment, along with a collaborative participation in the special education program, the physical therapist can truly make an impact on the student and effectively promote "equality of opportunity, full participation, independent living, and economic self sufficiency for individuals with disabilities" [PL 105-17, Sec 601(c)].

REVIEW QUESTIONS

1. You are working at a local school as a physical therapist. You are evaluating the integration of students with disabilities into the school environment. Which of the following groups of students is least likely to spend time with their nondisabled peers in an educational setting?
   a. Students with a diagnosis of a learning disability
   b. Students who have multiple disabilities
   c. Students who have an emotional problem
   d. Students who have impairment in speech or language

2. One difference between the provision of physical therapy services in a traditional medical model versus that in an educational model is that in an educational model of service delivery the physical therapist
   a. does not require the input or direction of the physician.
   b. is acting solely as a health care provider.
   c. is a member of the IEP team.
   d. provides services directed solely by a physician's prescription.

3. Which of the following laws introduced the concept of an FAPE for all children with disabilities?
   a. PL 94-142: Education for All Handicapped Children Act of 1975
   b. PL 99-457: Education of the Handicapped Act Amendments of 1986
   c. PL 102-119: IDEA of 1991
   d. PL 108-446: IDEA of 2004

4. In the school setting, information on the need for a physician's prescription to provide physical therapy services as well as guidelines on the utilization of the physical therapist assistance are determined by which of the following?
   a. The local educational agencies policies and procedures
   b. The state Practice Act for Physical Therapy
   c. The IDEA
   d. The APTA's policies and procedures

5. Your friend has a child with a disability and is sending the student to a private religious school in the local area for his education. According to the IDEA, is this student entitled to receive related services in his special education program?
   a. Yes. All students are entitled to an FAPE.
   b. Yes. All students enrolled in special education are entitled to receive related services to optimize their ability to learn.
   c. No. The IDEA is a federal law applicable to public education and does not apply to private education.
   d. It depends. If the student was placed in a private school in order to obtain special education not available in the local public school, then the local school district may be held accountable for payment for these services.

6. After a student has been determined to be eligible for special education, a physical therapist may be asked to do an evaluation. At this point in the process, the physical therapy evaluation most likely would be done to accomplish which of the following?
   a. To evaluate and gather information in order to more effectively participate in the IEP team meeting
   b. To determine if the student has any of the identified disabilities specified by the IDEA
   c. To establish specific therapy goals in order for the student to benefit from the special educational experience
   d. To determine the frequency of physical therapy services needed by the student

7. Which of the following statements regarding the evaluation process (after eligibility has been determined) is *incorrect*?
   a. If appropriate, the PEDI can be done to gather data on the student to be used throughout the school year, as a means to monitor progress.

b. The evaluation can identify specific orthopedic impairments present in the student that may impair his ability to learn.

c. The evaluation can establish specific physical therapy discipline goals to be added to the IEP.

d. The evaluation can identify functional limitations that impair a student's ability to participate in educational activities.

8. You are participating in the development of goals on a student's IEP. In this process you identify the audience, behavior, condition, and degree. You should also be able to identify the "E" component of this objective. What does the "E" stand for?

a. Extent to which this goal should be mastered

b. Environment in which this goal will be demonstrated

c. Educational relevance of this goal

d. Educational needs of the classroom staff

9. It is the beginning of the school year, and you are a member of Jason's IEP team. You are working with him to improve his ability to stand up from his classroom desk and transfer into his wheelchair. You decide that he needs one on one instruction in order to learn the steps involved in this process. You decide to take him out of the classroom and teach him these skills in a more quiet and controlled environment. Which of the following statements correctly applies to this situation?

a. Procedural interventions should always take place in the classroom, and removing Jason from this environment is inappropriate.

b. It is not appropriate to teach Jason skills in a controlled environment. They should always be taught in the natural environment.

c. Physical therapy services that address impairments to movement activities should be provided outside the classroom so as not to disrupt the other students.

d. At times it is appropriate to pull a student from the classroom to address specific impairments or functional limitations to his participation in classroom activities.

10. According to the IDEA, a student's plan to transition into a vocational program after he graduates from high school must be included in the student's IEP

a. by the time he completes the eighth grade.

b. by the time he is 16 years old.

c. at least 2 years before graduation from high school.

d. by the time he is 18 years old.

APPENDIX

Evaluation, Documentation, and Outcome Forms

The clinical evaluation form provided is one example of the type of information gathered on students in special education. The form is self-explanatory. The following comments are presented to clarify the process:

Prescription for physical therapy: If needed, the physician's prescription for physical therapy should be obtained and filed in the student's educational record. Although there is no law stating how often the prescription needs to be renewed, best practice is to have a new prescription written annually.

Medical diagnosis: A student in special education may have one or more medical diagnoses that provide information on the possible impairments and prognosis for functional independence.

Medications: Medications play an important role in the general health of a student. They may also affect the interventions provided by the physical therapist. It is important that the physical therapist is aware of the medications that the student is taking, and understands their possible affect on the student's performance.

Student's height and weight: These are important objective measurements to obtain when considering equipment specifications, lifting requirement, and general growth of the student.

Range of motion: The range-of-motion chart contains two columns for comparison in measurements taken over time.

Muscle performance: Standard manual muscle testing may not be appropriate for students for a number of different reasons. As the testing is subjective, it is difficult to determine the results of a break test in a student who is very young or has a cognitive impairment that could jeopardize the test results. For these reasons, assessing the student's functional strength may provide more helpful information. Through observation, the physical therapist can determine how much functional strength or active range of motion a student has to perform daily classroom and personal care activities.

Educational concerns: Note your discussions with the teacher regarding the student's physical limitations and her educational goals. This is an important aspect of the evaluation, and is instrumental in determining interventions and the need for a related service.

Goals: Note that there are no discipline-specific goals identified on this evaluation form. Goals for the student are created at the IEP meeting with input from all team members.

Information for the Physical Therapist at School

Student's name: _____

Parent's name: _____

My name is _____ , and I am the physical therapist at your child's school. In order to assure efficiency in the provision of service to your child, please complete the questions below and return this letter to the school.

The physical therapy examination for your child is scheduled on _____

If you have any questions, you can reach me by calling _____

Thank you.

1.   What is your child's medical diagnosis? _____

2.   Has he/she had any surgeries in the past?   ____ Yes ____ No
      If yes, what was done then?

      _____

3.   Are you planning for any surgeries or purchase of special equipment in the next 9 months?
      ____ Yes ____ No   *If yes, please explain.*

      _____

4.   What equipment does your child use or have at home? How often is the equipment used?
      (Please list.)

      _____

5.   Does your child receive therapy services at another facility, in addition to what he/she is receiving
      in the school?   ____ Yes ____ No

      If yes, please describe.

      _____

Identification of services does not authorize contact. If contact with an agency or person is required, prior authorization will be requested.

Physical Therapy Evaluation Form

General Information:

Student's name: _____   Exam date: _____

School: _____   Classroom: _____

D.O.B. _____ Age: _____   ____ Male ___ Female

Medical diagnosis: _____

Precautions: _____

Medications: _____

Service provision by: ___ IEP   ___ Service Agreement

Secondary insurance*:   ___ N/A   ___ MA   ___ other: _____

   *Secondary funding sources may require additional documentation for reimbursement.

Significant Medical History

   ___ See Parent/Guardian Report, attached

   ___ Other

_____

_____

_____

Previous therapy services: _____

Systems Review:

Communication: ___ vocal ___ nonverbal ___ verbal ___ sign language

       Device: _____

Vision: ___ WFL ___ Impaired

Hearing: ___ WFL ___ Impaired

Cognitive level by report: _____

Emotion/behavior during exam: ___ cooperative ___ uncooperative ___ passive ___ other:

Student's height: _____ weight: _____

Is the student continent of bowel? ___ yes ___ no   of bladder?   ___ yes ___ no

Heart rate: _____ Respiratory rate/pattern _____

Circulation: ___ impaired   ___ not impaired

Edema: ___ not present ___ present   Describe: _____

Hand dominance: ___ right ___ left ___ not established

Motor function:

     Motor control: ___ impaired ___ not impaired

     Motor learning: ___ impaired ___ not impaired

     Sensation to touch: ___ impaired ___ not impaired

     Oral motor skills: ___ impaired ___ not impaired

Additional comments:

Tests and Measures:

___ Standardized Test: _____

   Outcome: _____

___ Additional tests or measures: _____

_____

Range of Motion

___ Range of motion and strength are WFL throughout the trunk and extremities

___ Range of motion and strength are WFL throughout the trunk and extremities
   with the following exceptions: _____

___ Range of motion and strength are present as follows

Goniometric Measurements: ___ **Passive**   ___ **Active**

	Dates	ROM __/__		ROM __/__			Dates	ROM __/__		ROM __/__	
Upper Extremities		L	R	L	R	**Lower Extremities**		L	R	L	R
Shoulder Flex	0-180					Hip Flex	0-182				
Ext	0-60					Ext	0-30				
Abd	0-180					Abd	0-45				
Horz. Add.	0-135					Add	0-135				
Int. Rot.	0-70					I.R.	0-45				
Ext. Rot.	0-90					E.R.	0-90				
Elbow Flex.	0-150					Knee Flex.	0-135				
Ext.	0-150					Ext.	0-150				
Wrist Flex	0-80					Ankle Dorsi.	0-20				
Ext.	0-70					Plant.	0-50				
Rad. Dev.	0-20					Inver.	0-35				
Uln. Dev.	0-30					Ever.	0-15				
Forearm Pro.	0-80					Trunk					
Sup	0-80					Neck					
Fingers						Toes					

Comments:

_____

_____

_____

Muscle Performance
Muscle Tone:
____ is WNL throughout trunk and extremities with active and passive movements.
____ is hypotonic in _____.
____ is hypertonic in _____.

Functional Strength
____ able to touch the back of head
____ able to touch the middle of back
____ able to pronate/supinate forearm
____ able to oppose fingers to thumb
____ able to rise from a chair
____ able to step up a 7-inch step

Rises from the Floor:
____ using half kneel
____ via squat
____ via modified plantargrade
____ requiring: _____ assist
____ Other: _____

Student is independent in the developmental sequence to _____

Neuromotor Development
Reflexes: Primitive reflexes   ____ appear integrated   ____ are present

DTR's are (0 +1 +2 +3 +4) in _____

Reactions:
Righting _____
Protective extension _____

Equilibrium: ___ prone ___ supine ___ quadruped ___ sitting ___ kneeling ___ standing

Balance:
Sitting: _____
Standing: _____
Walking: _____
During ADLs: _____

Coordination:
UE: _____
LE: _____

Mobility:

Transfers: ___ independent ___ pivot ___ dependent
Description with level of assistance needed: _____

Wheelchair mobility: ___ N/A ___ independent ___ assist ___ dependent
Description with level of assistance needed: _____

Ambulation   ___ independent ___ assisted ___ nonambulatory
Gait pattern: _____
Device: _____
Level of assistance needed: _____
Stair negotiation: _____

Self-care in School (mark the level of assistance needed to complete the task)
 ___ undressing ___ dressing ___ eating ___ toileting ___ grooming ___ other
Comments: _____
_____

Orthotics: _____

Equipment: _____

The following information was obtained by ___ report ___ observation

Analysis of the school environment: _____
_____

Student's position during educational activities: _____
_____

Analysis of student's motor skills for education: _____
_____

Analysis of student's participation in school activities: _____
_____

Analysis of student's leisure activities: _____
_____

Educational Concerns: _____

_____

_____

_____

Impairments:

    ___ impaired range of motion   ___ impaired respiratory function

    ___ impaired motor learning   ___ impaired muscle strength

    ___ impaired balance   ___ impaired motor control

    ___ impaired coordination   ___ impaired mobility

    ___ impaired endurance

Functional Limitations: _____

_____

_____

_____

_____

Summary/current level of functioning: _____

_____

_____

_____

_____

Other services, equipment, or assistive device recommendations or considerations: _____

_____

_____

_____

Signature, title, and date

This form should be kept in the student's file.

REFERENCES

1. Individuals with Disabilities Education Act Amendments of 1997. Public Law 105-17.
2. Individuals with Disabilities Education Improvement Act of 2004. Public Law 108-446.
3. American Physical Therapy Association. Physical Therapy for Individuals with Disabilities: Practice in Educational Environments. HOD 06-95-14-03 (Program 32).
4. Kaye S. Education of Children with Disabilities. Disability Statistics Abstract. U.S. Washington, DC: Department of Education, National Institute on Disability and Rehabilitation Research; 1997;19.
5. Office of Special Education Programs. 25th Annual Report to Congress on the Implementation of the Individuals with Disabilities Education Act. Washington, DC: U.S. Department of Education; 2003.
6. Office of Special Education Programs. 26th Annual Report to Congress on the Implementation of the Individuals with Disabilities Education Act. Washington, DC: U.S. Department of Education; 2004.
7. Rapport MK. Laws that shape therapy services in educational environments. In: McEwen IR, ed. *Occupational and Physical Therapy in the Educational Environments*. New York: The Hawthorne Press Inc.; 1995:5–32.
8. The Education of All Handicapped Children Act of 1975. Public Law 94-142.
9. The Education of All Handicapped Children Act. Amendments of 1986. Public Law 99-457.
10. No Child Left Behind Act of 2001. Public Law 107-110.
11. Rainforth B. Analysis of physical therapy practice acts: implications for role release in educational environments. *Pediatr Phys Ther*. 1997;9:54–61.
12. Borkowski MA, Wessman HC. Determination of eligibility for physical therapy in the public school setting. *Pediatr Phys Ther*. 1994;6:61–67.
13. Giangreco MF. Related service decision-making: a foundational component of effective education for students with disabilities. *Phys Occup Ther Pediatr*. 1995;15:47–68.
14. Mancini M, Coster W, Trombly C, et al. Predicting elementary school participation in children with disabilities. *Arch Phys Med Rehabil*. 2000;81:339–347.
15. Coster W, Deeney T, Haltiwanger J, Haley S. *School Function Assessment Materials*. San Antonio, TX: The Psychological Corporation; 1998.
16. Coster W, Deeney T, Haltiwanger J, Haley S. *Technical Report: School Function Assessment*. San Antonio, TX: The Psychological Corporation; 2000.
17. Footer C, Babayan X, Fuentes J, et al. Comparison of the Gross Motor Function Measure (GMFM) and the School Function Assessment (SFA) in evaluating school function for children with cerebral palsy. *Pediatr Phys Ther*. 2004;16:72.
18. Haley S, Coster W, Ludlow L, et al. *Pediatric Evaluation and Disability Inventory (PEDI): Development, Standardization and Administration Manual*. Version 1.0. Boston, MA: New England Medical Center Hospitals, Inc., and PEDI Research Group; 1992.
19. Nichols D, Case-Smith J. Reliability and validity of the Pediatric Evaluation of Disability Inventory. *Pediatr Phys Ther*. 1996;8:15–24.
20. Ketekaar M, Vermeer A. Functional motor abilities of children with cerebral palsy: a systematic literature review of assessment measures. *Clin Rehabil*. 1998;12:369–380.
21. Jette A. Physical disablement concepts for physical therapy research and practice. *Phys Ther J*. 1994;74:230–386.
22. Randall E, McEwen I. Writing patient-centered functional goals. *Phys Ther*. 2000;80:1197–1203.
23. Kettenbach G. *Writing SOAP Notes*. Second Edition. Philadelphia: FA Davis Company; 1995:83–88.
24. Dole R, Arvidson K, Byrne E, et al. Consensus among experts in pediatric occupational and physical therapy on elements of individualized education programs. *Pediatr Phys Ther*. 2003;15:159–166.
25. American Physical Therapy Association. *Guide to Physical Therapist Practice*. 2nd ed. *Physical Therapy Journal*. 2001;81: 39–50.
26. Drnach M. Expanding their world. Choosing and using pediatric mobility equipment. *Physical Therapy Products*. 2001;12:33–36.
27. Copley J, Ziviani J. Barriers to the use of assistive technology for children with multiple disabilities. *Occup Ther Int*. 2004;11:229–243.
28. Cross A, Traub E, Hutter-Pishgahi L., et al. Elements of successful inclusion for children with significant disabilities. *Topics in Early Childhood Special Education*. 2004;3: 169–183.
29. Nolan K, Mannato L, Wilding G. Integrated models of pediatric physical and occupational therapy: regional practice and related outcomes. *Pediatr Phys Ther*. 2004;16:121–128.
30. Bundy A. Assessment and intervention in school-based practice: answering questions and minimizing discrepancies. In: McEwen IR, ed. *Occupational and Physical Therapy in Educational Environments*. New York: The Hawthorne Press Inc.; 1995:69–88.
31. Sekerak D, Kirkpatrick D, Nelson K, et al. Physical therapy in preschool classrooms: successful integration of therapy into classroom routines. *Pediatr Phys Ther*. 2003;15:93–104.
32. Kaminner M, Chiarello L, O'Neil M, et al. Decision making for physical therapy service delivery in schools: a nationwide survey of pediatric physical therapist. *Phys Ther J*. 2004;84:919–933.
33. Effgen S. Factors affecting the termination of physical therapy services for children in school settings. *Pediatr Phys Ther*. 2000;12:121–126.
34. Shumway-Cook A, Woollacott M. *Motor Control: Theory and Practical Application*. Baltimore, MD: Lippincott Williams & Wilkins; 2001.
35. Mitchem K. Be proactive: including students with challenging behavior in your classroom. *Intervention in School and Clinic*. 2005;40:188–191.
36. Sugai G, Horner R, Dunlap G, Hieneman L, et al. Applying positive behavioral support and functional assessment in schools. Technical Assistance Guide 1. Washington DC. OSEP Center on Positive Behavioral Interventions and Support. 1999.
37. Dwyer K. Disciplining students with disabilities. In: National Association of School Psychologist. *Behavioral Interventions: Creating a safe environment in school*. Bethesda MD: National Association of School Psychologist, 1998; 26:18–21.
38. Medicare Catastrophic Coverage Act of 1988. Public Law 100-360.

Other Resources

McEwen I. *Providing Physical Therapy Services Under Parts B & C of the IDEA* Arlington, VA. Section on Pediatrics, American Physical Therapy Association; 2000.

U.S. Department of Health and Human Services (for information on Disabilities and Health Policy Issues). Web site: www.aspe.hhs.gov

U.S. Department of Education (for information on current legislation and regulations relating to public education and access to the Office of Special Education Programs [OSEP]). Web site: www.ed.gov

The Council for Exceptional Children (CEC) is the largest international professional organization dedicated to improving educational outcomes for individuals with exceptionalities, students with disabilities, and/or the gifted. Also a source for references on the IDEA. Web site: www.cec.sped.org

The Division for Early Childhood (DEC), a division of the Council for Exceptional Children, is especially for individuals who work with or on behalf of children with special needs, birth through age 8 years, and their families. Web site: www.dec-sped.org

The Family Education Network is a source of educational content, resources, and shopping for parents, home schoolers, teachers, and kids. Web site:www.fen.com

AbilityHub's purpose is to help people find information on adaptive equipment and alternative methods available for accessing computers. Web site: www.abilityhub.com

The 34CFR300 can be accessed at http://www.access.gpo.gov/nara/cfr/waisidx_02/34cfr300_02.html.

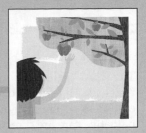

CHAPTER 9

Pediatric Hospice

Christine Constantine and Mark Drnach

LEARNING OBJECTIVES

1. Define and delineate the differences between hospice care and palliative care.
2. Describe the role of physical therapy in hospice care.
3. Understand the general issues around dying in children.
4. Identify the role of the interdisciplinary hospice team in addressing clinical, psychosocial, spiritual, and emotional needs of the child and family.
5. Recognize the individuality of each child and his or her family experience, and understand the importance of supporting their wishes, decisions, and beliefs.

There is growing empirical evidence that the health care system is failing children and families when they are confronted by a life-threatening illness. Too many children undergo painful procedures and suffer from the symptoms of advancing disease without adequate relief, despite the fact that modern medicine has the means to relieve their pain and improve most symptoms. Families of gravely ill children can feel abandoned and overwhelmed, often suffering emotional and sometimes financial consequences for years. Social supports for children and families before and after death are woefully inadequate, and health care professionals themselves are often left without emotional support for the difficult work they do. In their training, health care professionals have received either minimal training to deal with the dying patient or virtually no opportunities to practice the skills necessary for communicating effectively with dying children and their families. Many times, practicing health care professionals also lack guidance on how best to manage the conflicting goals and values that can arise in difficult cases. Such conflicts are made all the more challenging by the broad cultural and religious diversity represented in the United States population. Although there is an ongoing national effort to improve palliative care among adult patients, very little has been done so far in the United States on behalf of children and their families.[1]

This chapter presents hospice care and the general issues that patients and families may encounter. Palliative care is emphasized, which focuses on care (not cure) of the patient. This chapter will also include the role for the physical therapist as an integral part of an interdisciplinary team providing hospice care.

WHAT IS HOSPICE?

Hospice is a philosophy of care that is available to anyone with a terminal prognosis, measured in months not years. The focus of medical intervention shifts from treatment to cure, to providing care and alleviating pain. The management of the disease itself begins to fade, and the dominating focus turns to the management of symptoms. Along with the expertise to control pain and associated symptoms, the hospice team provides emotional, psychosocial, and spiritual support to the patient and family. Hospice believes that each patient has a right to die with dignity and without pain.

Palliative care is a main component of hospice care. The word "palliate" comes from the Latin word, palliure, "to cloak." It is defined as making (the symptoms of a disease) less severe without removing the course. Goals of palliative care are directed toward physical comfort, emotional support, and quality of life. Although all hospices provide palliative care, not all palliative care reflects hospice care. Palliative care expands the definition of hospice, and confusion is not uncommon. Table 9-1 presents a list of questions, compiled by Caring Connections, comparing palliative care and hospice care.[2] Although a child has a terminal illness with a short prognosis, palliative care is about living until you die. Dying happens with the last breath, on the last day.

POINT TO REMEMBER

Hospice

Hospice is a philosophy of care that is available to patients in the end stage of their terminal illness. The focus of intervention is on palliative care and alleviating pain, not on curing the patient of the disease.

THE PRACTICE ENVIRONMENT

The term hospice dates back to medieval times and refers to a place where weary travelers could find rest and temporary shelter on their journey. The modern terminology reflects a concept of care for a terminally ill patient and his or her family. Up until the early part of the 20th century, death, like birth, happened at home. It was seen as a natural part of life. However, with the advances in medicine and the growth of hospitals, dying began to occur more in the hospitals and was often seen as a failure of modern medicine to cure a patient or prolong life. Dr. Cicely Saunders, a British physician, opened St. Christopher's Hospice in London in 1967 and is largely responsible for the modern movement of hospice, to bring more dignity to dying.[3] The inpatient care setting was the concentration of care in England. The first hospice in the United States was established in 1974 in Branford, Connecticut: the Connecticut Hospice. This program was funded by the National Cancer Institute and provided hospice services in the home. The basic concept and philosophy of care formulated by Dr. Saunders were maintained, but the primary setting for the delivery of care shifted from an inpatient care setting to the patient's home. Although initially designed to meet the needs of adults, it soon became apparent, as more children were served in adult hospice programs, that there was a need to have a hospice program for children. In 1979, the first pediatric hospice programs were opened in the United States in the state of Virginia.

Most hospice programs in the United States developed from grassroots organizations, mainly from home health care organizations. In 1982, the U.S. Congress included a provision to create a *Medicare hospice benefit* in

TABLE 9-1 Palliative versus Hospice Care		
Question	**Palliative Care**	**Hospice Care**
Who can receive this care?	Anyone with a serious illness, regardless of life expectancy.	Someone with an illness with a life expectancy measured in months, not years.
Can I continue to receive treatments to cure my illness?	You may receive palliative care and curative care at the same time.	Treatments and medicines aimed at relieving symptoms are provided by the hospice.
Does Medicare pay?	Some treatments and medications may be covered.	Medicare pays all charges related to hospice.
Does Medicaid pay?	Some treatments and medications may be covered.	In 47 states, Medicaid pays all care related to hospice.
Does private insurance pay?	Some treatments and medications may be covered.	Most insurance plans have a hospice benefit.
What organization provides these services?	Hospitals, hospices, nursing facilities, health care clinics.	Hospice organizations, hospital-based hospice programs, other health care organizations.
Who provides these services?	It varies. However, usually there is a team including doctors, nurses, social workers, and chaplains, similar to the hospice team.	A team including a doctor, nurse, social worker, chaplain, volunteer, home health aide, and others.
How long can I receive care?	This will depend upon your care needs and the coverage you have through Medicare, Medicaid, or private insurance.	As long as you meet the hospice's criteria of an illness with a life expectancy of months, not years.
Where are services provided?	In home, assisted living facility, nursing facility, hospital.	Usually, wherever the patient resides, in home, assisted living facility, nursing facility, or hospital; some hospices have facilities where people can live.
Do they offer expert end-of-life care?	This varies; be sure to ask.	Yes, staff are experts in end-of-life care.

the Tax Equity and Fiscal Responsibility Act of 1982 (PL 97-248).[4] This Medicare benefit provides hospice care coverage for terminally ill Medicare beneficiaries who elect to receive care from a participating hospice. The regulations established eligibility requirements and reimbursement standards and procedures, defined covered services, and delineated the conditions a hospice must meet in order to be approved for participation in the Medicare program. By 1986, the Medicare hospice benefit was made permanent by Congress, and states were given the option of including hospice in their Medicaid programs. The hospice coverage in Medicaid is patterned after the Medicare benefit but does not have to match Medicare payment, and capitated payment programs may apply depending on the individual state system. A Medicare-certified hospice agency provides services such as nursing care; counseling; physician services; spiritual care; physical, occupational, and speech therapy; durable medical equipment (DME); and short-term inpatient and respite care.

POINTS TO REMEMBER

The Hospice Benefit

In 1982, the U.S. Congress created a hospice benefit for Medicare beneficiaries. Medicaid programs, which are administered by state governments, may include a hospice benefit for eligible children.

According to the National Hospice and Palliative Care Organization (NHPCO), >1 million patients sought hospice care in 2004, a 10% increase from the previous year.[5] Additionally, the number of hospice programs continues to grow. In 1974, there was one hospice program in the United States. Today, there are >3,600 programs serving the terminally ill. Although cancer diagnoses accounted for 46% of hospice admissions in 2004, other conditions, such as end-stage heart or kidney disease, dementia, debility, and lung disease, were prevalent diagnoses in the adult hospice patients. Children, in contrast, die from different factors. According to the American Academy of Pediatrics, approximately 53,000 children in the United States die each year because of trauma, lethal congenital conditions, extreme prematurity, genetic disorders, or an acquired illness.[6]

As hospice continues to grow, it is becoming an option for more and more adults with terminal illness (Box 9-1), but the philosophy of hospice care can be at odds with the provision of mainstream health care in the United States, especially as it applies to children. In a culture that strives to cure and uses leading edge technology to prolong life, death can still represent failure, and although death is inevitable, society expects that children will outlive their parents. It is an emotional and social challenge to

BOX **9-1**
What Americans Want

A nationwide Gallup survey conducted for the NHPCO found the following:

1. Nine of 10 adults would prefer to be cared for at home rather than in a hospital or nursing home if diagnosed with a terminal illness, and 96% of hospice care is provided in the patient's home or place of residence.
2. The overwhelming majority of adults said they would be interested in the comprehensive program of care at home that hospice programs provide, yet most Americans know little or nothing about their eligibility for or availability of hospice.
3. When asked to name their greatest fear associated with death, respondents most cited "being a burden to family and friends," followed by "pain" and "lack of control." Addressing the whole range of physical and psychological needs of the patient and his or her family in an interdisciplinary way is what makes hospice care so special.
4. Ninety percent of adults believe it is the family's responsibility to care for the dying. Hospice provides families with the support needed to keep their loved one at home, and can provide the caretaker short "respite" periods.
5. Most adults believe that it would take a year or more to adjust to the death of a loved one. However, only 10% of adults have ever participated in a bereavement program or grief counseling following the death of a loved one. Hospice programs offer 1 year of grief counseling for the surviving family and friends.

From: National Hospice and Palliative Care Organization. What Americans Want. Caring Connections. Available at: www.caringinfo.org. Accessed February 2, 2006.

deal with the reality that children die too. The associated pain involved is overwhelming for the parents, patient, family, and caregivers including the health care workers. It goes against human nature of doing all that a parent can do to protect and prolong the life of the child. It is inconceivable to think that a parent would agree to withhold anything that would have a remote possibility of helping the child. These issues can be real barriers to the provision of hospice care as it is structured today.

POINTS TO REMEMBER

Barriers to Pediatric Hospice

Not all hospices or palliative care centers in the United States render care to the pediatric population. Some barriers to the cultural acceptance of pediatric hospices can include:

- the perception that the death of a patient is viewed as a failure in westernized healthcare,

- the expectation that children will outlive their parents,
- the acceptance that children die too, and
- the difficulty in withholding anything that may have a remote possibility of prolonging a child's life.

When Children Die

The causes of death in children are substantially different from the causes of death in adults. The leading cause of death in infants (<1 year old) is due to congenital anomalies, factors relating to prematurity and low birth weight, and Sudden Infant Death Syndrome. For a child between the ages of 1 and 21 years, the most common cause of death is an accident or unintentional injury. The leading cause of death in adults (age 45 years and older) is due to cancer or heart disease.[7]

Many hospice programs today were developed to address the needs of the adult who is dying, and their structure may not be appropriate for children.[6] The current requirement under Medicare that the patient has a life expectancy of 6 months or less is harder to predict in children.[6] Children with diseases that lead to a premature death may require services that improve their quality of life, but are not allowed or reimbursed under the current system. Many infants who die are born with rarely seen medical conditions, which make the prognosis uncertain.[7] In addition, the majority of children die in the hospital or on the way to the hospital.[8] Only a small percentage will die at home, which is the typical environment associated with the majority of adult hospice care.

POINTS TO REMEMBER

Leading Causes of Death

Infants (<1 year of age): congenital anomalies, factors relating to prematurity and low birth weight, and Sudden Infant Death Syndrome
Children (1 to 21 years of age): accident or unintentional injury
Adult (45 years or older): cancer or heart disease

There are also many issues related to medical ethics and decision making for and with children with a terminal illness. These issues are quite different from those for an adult, who has lived a long and productive life. Parents want to make the right choice but often struggle with the uncertainty of whether everything possible was done for their child. After all, this child's life is considered unnaturally shortened. In order for families to make such difficult decisions, a clear explanation relative to the outcome must be made and understood. Precise interventions or exclusions should be detailed and discussed. Continued clarification of the family's and child's priorities, throughout the provision of care, is essential for appropriate and sound decision making given the circumstances. Some of the more difficult and controversial issues that can arise include the decisions to withdraw or withhold life-sustaining medical treatment (LSMT), performing cardiopulmonary resuscitation (CPR) or carrying out do not resuscitate orders, and withholding or withdrawing artificial feeding.

When do health care providers cease to have a duty to attempt to prolong life? When does the potential for harm exceed the potential for benefit? Generally, a physician may recommend the *withholding or withdrawing LSMT* when:

There is brain death (this may be difficult to diagnose in the newborn and young infant);
There is a fatal condition, which is irreversible;
There is no effective treatment; or
There is a treatment that is effective but is unduly burdensome relative to the potential for benefits; or
There is a treatment but it is not proven to work.

Withholding or withdrawing LSMT is not viewed as an act of euthanasia.[9] If the treatment is withheld or withdrawn and the child dies, it is the underlying illness that causes the death.

CPR is indicated for the prevention of sudden, unexpected death. Therefore, a terminal illness where death is expected does not warrant CPR efforts. Interestingly age has not been shown to be a factor in the success of CPR. Some of the same conditions that make resuscitation attempts unsuccessful in the general population apply to children. What makes the decision to withhold resuscitation attempts on children so difficult is the overwhelming sense of loss for the parents and for the health care staff. For a parent to say "do not resuscitate" symbolizes the lost future of the child and lost hopes of the parents. The physician and other health care workers can help sort out the medical side of this decision. The more difficult part is letting go.[10] It might be helpful to reframe the question and discussion from "do not resuscitate" to "allow natural death."[11]

As difficult as it may be to *withhold or withdraw artificial feeding* from a failing 80-year-old patient, it is harder to make this decision for a child. With an elderly person who has always fed himself, it is usually accepted that the cessation of eating is a sign that the end of life is near. With a child, however, life is just beginning. The medical realities may be no different between the seriously ill child and the adult, but it feels different. Furthermore, it is not expected that an infant be able to feed himself even if he is healthy. Artificial hydration and nutrition might be seen as just another way of helping the child or infant to eat. From the first hours of a child's life, parents seek to feed their infant. These are difficult feelings to overcome as one considers refusing artificial feeding to a child.[10]

Physicians may also be reluctant to discontinue nutritional support. Many physicians have a difficult time with this issue as well. The ultimate concern is whether the obligation to act is in the patient's best interest by withholding or withdrawing a medical treatment or nutrition. These decisions are difficult. Time is needed for all persons involved to understand and emotionally accept such monumental decisions. For adults, there are ways to communicate wants and desires in the event of deterioration to the point of being unable to communicate. Adults have the advantage of making their wishes known through the execution of an advance directive. An *advance directive* is a legal document created by a competent adult communicating his desires about medical treatment if he cannot express his wishes. The advance directive provides the family, caregivers, and physicians specific information on how the adult wishes to be treated. Advance directives do not expire; they remain in effect until the adult changes it. There are two types of advance directives: a living will and the designation of a medical power of attorney. A *living will* allows the adult to convey instructions regarding interventions and treatment when those wishes can no longer be communicated. A living will lets the physician know what, if any, life-sustaining procedures the adult desires when death is imminent. A *medical power of attorney* allows the adult to designate one person (an agent) to make health care decisions when the adult is unable to do so. The agent follows the instructions about care, treatments, and extraordinary measures to be taken or withheld on behalf of the incapacitated adult. It is important to know that these legal documents are applicable to *adults only*; they do not apply to minors (children younger than 18 years). Although a child may execute such documents, legally those decisions are the responsibility of the parents.

POINT TO REMEMBER

Advance Directives

Advance directives, such as a living will or medical power of attorney, are all legal documents that express the wishes of an incompetent person and are commonly seen in health care environments. They do not legally apply to minors. The parents are the legal decision makers for children younger than 18 years.

PEDIATRIC HOSPICE

Children's Hospice International recently reported that >50,000 children die each year in the United States, and that <1% of children needing hospice care in the United States receive it. Box 9-2 lists some of the more common medical diagnoses of children with terminal illnesses who may benefit from hospice care. For children with complex chronic conditions (CCC), there are more adolescents and

BOX 9-2
Some Diagnoses That May Benefit from Palliative Care

- AIDS
- Cancer (Although rare, approximately 9000 children younger than 15 years are diagnosed annually)
- Chromosomal disorders (e.g., Trisomy 5,13,16,18)
- Congenital defects or anomalies (e.g., any cardiac defect for which transplantation is one therapeutic alternative)
- Hematologic abnormalities (e.g., aplastic anemia)
- Metabolic disorders (e.g., Menkes Kinky Hair Syndrome)
- Multiple major medical problems, which together are life threatening
- Muscular dystrophy (e.g., Duchenne muscular dystrophy, spinal muscular atrophy)
- Neurodegenerative disorders (e.g., adrenoleukodystrophy, mucopolysaccharidosis)
- Static encephalopathy (e.g., permanent vegetative state as a result of drowning, other ischemic or hypoxemic injuries, and congenital central nervous system defects, such as hydraencephaly)[9,12]

Premature death is likely or expected with many of these conditions.

young adults who might benefit from supportive care services than infants or children. The average number of living, hospice-eligible adolescents and young adults has, in relation to the other age groups, remained fairly steady over the last two decades, at approximately 1500 per year.[13]

Pediatric hospice programs have to be structured to provide appropriate services unique to the pediatric patient. A hospital-based hospice program that is structured to address the unique needs of the infant, or injured child, would have characteristics with a different emphasis as compared to the current adult hospice program that is prevalent today. The needs of the family to balance palliative care with life-prolonging interventions, decision-making strategies in a limited and uncertain time frame, and finding comfort and support in the medical environment are a few examples. Another aspect of pediatric hospice is the unique issue of the adolescent patient with a chronic life-shortening disease living at home. Adolescents who are ill may feel isolated from their peers. Their daily routines may be interrupted due to their illness, and they may not be able to participate in the routines and rituals of the family. In addition, the adolescent's health may keep him from attending school or other social functions that are important at this age. The pediatric hospice patient may be more mobile and active, requiring a broader view of the possible activities/services that would help improve his and his family's quality of life.

The American Academy of Pediatrics, Committee on Bioethics and Committee on Hospital Care, have identified the need for changes in the current regulations and reimbursement structure in order to improve access to hospice services for children and families.[6] They include:

1. A broader eligibility criteria concerning the length of expected survival
2. The allowance of concurrent provision of life-prolonging and palliative care
3. The provision of respite care and other therapies beyond those allowed by a narrow definition of "medically indicated."

Adequate reimbursement should also accompany these regulatory changes.

The NHPCO has identified that palliative care for children is not sufficient throughout the world. They are the sponsors of the Children's International Project on Hospice/Palliative Services (ChIPPS), which works to enhance the science and practice of pediatric hospice and palliative care, and to increase the availability of state-of-the-art services to families.[9]

The following Universal Principles of Pediatric Palliative Care have been defined by ChIPPS:

1. The sole admission criterion for palliative care programs is that the child is not predicted to survive to become an adult. Prognosis for short-term survival should not be required, as it interferes with the provision of critical support from the time of diagnosis.
2. The unit of care is the child and the family. Family is defined as the persons who provide physical, psychological, spiritual, and social comfort to the child, regardless of genetic relationships.
3. Palliative/hospice services should be accessible to children and their families in a setting that is desired and/or appropriate to their needs, whether home, inpatient hospice, hospital, or intensive care unit. Research indicates that the home is generally considered the preferred site of living until death, as bereavement outcomes are enhanced for family members who otherwise may have limited access to the child.
4. Palliative care is not viewed as shortening life. Symptom management is accomplished through means acceptable to the patient and the family.
5. Care provided focuses on the relief of physical, social, psychological, and existential or spiritual pain for the child and the family, whether or not they have chosen to continue with life-prolonging interventions.
6. Children and their families should have access to a team of caregivers, or at minimum, a "key worker" whose care is seamless, i.e., who cares for them where they prefer to be.

7. Care is designed to enhance the quality of life for the child and family. The child and family must be included in designing the priorities for care after being given as much information as is desired regarding the disease and treatment options.
8. The palliative care team recognizes the individuality of each child and his or her family, and upholds their values, wishes, and beliefs, unless unnecessary harm is at hand.
9. Pediatric palliative care is optimally delivered by an interdisciplinary team with pediatric knowledge, generally including trained volunteers, social workers, nurses, physicians, and spiritual counselors.
10. The palliative care team is available to the family 24 hours a day, 365 days a year.
11. The provision of respite, whether for a few hours or a few days at a time, is an essential service in palliative care.
12. Families should be able to refer themselves to a hospice and/or palliative care program.
13. Providing pediatric palliative care is difficult, although rewarding work. Direct caregivers must be provided formal or informal psychosocial support and supervision.
14. Regardless of cause of death, supportive and bereavement care should be provided to all those who are affected by the child's death, for as long as they need it.

After the decision is made to receive hospice services, an interdisciplinary hospice team will meet and schedule examinations and input in order to develop a *hospice plan of care* (see Appendix). The plan of care can include a variety of goals and objectives that are designed to provide palliative care and support to the patient and family during this period of the patient's illness. The interdisciplinary team of professionals and volunteers is central to making hospice care the highest standard of end-of-life care in the United States. Composed of a variety of professionals and specially trained hospice volunteers, the interdisciplinary team, the patient, and the family construct a plan of care.

PARENT PERSPECTIVE

THE STORY OF JUSTESS, AS TOLD BY HER HOSPICE NURSE

Justess is a 30-month-old girl who was diagnosed with leukemia. She underwent 10 months of medical treatment, which was not able to arrest the progression of the disease. Her physicians explained to her parents the current options at that time, which included a continued stay in the hospital with the provision of comfort care or caring for her at home with hospice support. Understanding that their child's kidneys and heart were beginning to fail, the parents chose to take her home. Her parents knew that Justess was always afraid of the hospital setting and wanted to bring her home where she could be more comfortable.

While at home, Justess appeared to be happy in her own room with her own things. The hospice team was able to provide palliative care until Justess died comfortably at home with her family by her side.

The parents felt that this choice of care was the best for their daughter. Even though this was their opinion and choice, controversy in the extended family existed. Justess' grandfather opposed the idea of hospice, at times becoming angry with the parents. He was not ready to "give up" and feared that she would die at home in pain.

The parents felt that Justess had a good death and were also pleased with the bereavement support that they received. Hospice reached out to Justess's 7-year-old sister with an invitation to attend a bereavement camp for children. It was very beneficial for her to know that what she was going through was something that other children also experienced. When speaking about Justess today, her sister will typically bring up pleasant memories about the time they shared.

When asked what convinced the parents to choose hospice, the mother responded that the nurse involved in the palliative care unit at the hospital clearly explained the concept of hospice and the services that were available. This explanation was very helpful to her and her husband when they had to make a decision during this very difficult period. When asked about advice they would give to other parents in similar situations, they noted "there needs to be more education and awareness about hospice for children to change the preconceived ideas about hospice. Hospice is wonderful!"

After Justess' death, her father enrolled in nursing school with the goal of working in pediatrics, specifically with children who have cancer.

The Hospice Plan of Care

The patient and the family unit are evaluated and re-evaluated continually in hospice by a variety of professionals. This is an important aspect of care because it can identify needs as they arise and provides the family or patient the opportunity to discuss emotional and difficult topics when they are ready.

It is important for the person involved in the examination process and collection of information to be sensitive to the family and patient's emotional state at this time. The grief cycle that is experienced can begin early on and can fluctuate dramatically. A parent's participation in an interview on the history of his child's illness and the current medical interventions may bring up feelings associated with grieving. Initially the patient or family may respond to the news of a terminal illness with calm and stability. The emotions that follow are characteristic of a roller coaster ride, fluctuating from anger to depression, from immobilization to acceptance. Elisabeth Kübler-Ross, in her book *On Death and Dying,* identified the stages of emotional response to life-altering information.[14] The health care provider should appreciate this sequence, which can provide some insight on how the family is dealing with the day-to-day issues of

caring for their child with a terminal illness. Listening and understanding can be the most important service that is provided on a particular day (see the Grief Cycle in Box 9-3). Acknowledging grief is often the first step toward facing the reality of the child's illness. Such acceptance may help parents focus on the quality of the child's remaining life.[15]

 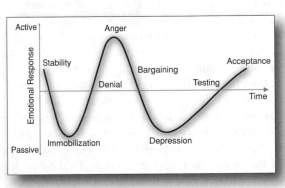

BOX 9-3
The Grief Cycle

Shock stage: initial paralysis at hearing the bad news
Denial stage: trying to avoid the inevitable
Anger stage: frustrated outpouring of bottled-up emotion
Bargaining stage: seeking in vain for a way out
Depression stage: final realization of the inevitable
Testing stage: seeking realistic solutions
Acceptance stage: finally finding the way forward

From: Kübler-Ross E. *On Death and Dying.* New York: Macmillan; 1969.

POINT TO REMEMBER

The Grief Cycle

Immobilization → Denial → Anger → Bargaining → Depression → Testing → Acceptance
Although discussed as a cycle of emotional responses, it should be remembered that the patient or family's emotions could vacillate.

A consistent component of hospice care is the examination and provision of psychosocial, emotional, and spiritual support. When a physician delivers a message to a patient and/or family that a terminal illness with a life-limiting prognosis is inevitable, imagine the response:

Why me?
Why, God?
What do I do now?
How can I go on?
Can I do this?

Actually, it's almost impossible to "go it alone." Psychosocial, emotional, and spiritual supports are imperative. A child with a terminal illness and prognosis is so inconceivable. People can rationalize that an elderly person with a terminal illness has had a quantity of life and now is entitled to a quality death, but a child is missing the quantity aspect. Although the child is entitled to a quality death as well, acceptance of that fact is difficult. Having a chaplain or spiritual counselor available allows some direction for the patient and family on this difficult spiritual journey. Some families may not have a religion or a higher power of reference. Care and support are directed at the individual needs. Occasionally, a patient or family member may have fallen away from his religious practice and now may have the need to be reconnected. An intervention to intercede may be necessary. Health care workers may find it difficult to discuss issues of spirituality or religion with the patient or the patient's family. This difficulty may be due to the fear of insulting the family's religious beliefs or a feeling of incompetence in discussing this topic. It is important to emphasize that *spirituality* is different from religion. It is a broader concept that includes religion as well as cognitive, experiential, and behavioral aspects of a person. It is important for the health care worker to understand this distinction, which can often be confusing and misinterpreted. In an attempt to clarify the attributes of spirituality, Martsolf and Mickley identified that spirituality can consist of the following attributes:[16]

- Meaning—significance of life; making sense of situations; deriving purpose in existance.
- Values—beliefs and standards of a person that are cherished.
- Transcendence—experience and appreciation of a dimension beyond self.
- Connecting—a relationship with self, others, God/a higher power, and the environment.
- Becoming—an unfolding of life that demands reflection and experience; includes a sense of who one is.

In addition, a health care worker should understand his or her own spiritual beliefs, values, and biases in order to remain patient centered and nonjudgmental.[17] Pastoral counselors, social workers, or nurses with education and training in this area typically do formal spiritual assessments, yet issues of spirituality can arise at any time with any provider during the provision of services to a patient in hospice. The HOPE Questions were developed to help medical students and physicians begin the process of incorporating a spiritual assessment into the medical interview.[17] These open ended questions will guide the interviewer in a discussion about spirituality, identifying concerns or needs of the patient or family which could lead to the services of a more trained professional in this area (Box 9-4).

The outcome of this assessment or screen may result in nothing but the patient's or family's comfort in discussing such issues, to a referral for a more formal evaluation or counseling by the appropriate professional. The goals often related to spirituality information can include:

Understanding and supporting individualized patient and family beliefs;

BOX 9-4
The HOPE Approach to Spiritual Assessment

H: Sources of hope, meaning, comfort, strength, peace, love, and connection

We have been discussing your support systems. I was wondering, what is there in your life that gives you internal support?

What are your sources of hope, strength, comfort, and peace?

What do you hold on to during difficult times?

What sustains you and keeps you going?

For some people, their religious or spiritual beliefs act as a source of comfort and strength in dealing with life's ups and downs; is this true for you?

If the answer is Yes, go on to O and P questions.

If the answer is No, consider asking: Was it ever?

If the answer is Yes, ask: What changed?

O: Organized religion

Do you consider yourself part of an organized religion? How important is this to you?

What aspects of your religion are helpful and not so helpful to you?

Are you part of a religious or spiritual community? Does it help you? How?

P: Personal spirituality/practices

Do you have personal spiritual beliefs that are independent of organized religion? What are they?

Do you believe in God? What kind of relationship do you have with God?

What aspects of your spirituality or spiritual practices do you find most helpful to you personally? (e.g., prayer, meditation, reading scripture, attending religious services, listening to music, hiking, communing with nature)

E: Effects on medical care and end-of-life issues

Has being sick (or your current situation) affected your ability to do the things that usually help you spiritually? (Or affected your relationship with God?)

Is there anything that I can do as a doctor to help you access the resources that usually help you?

Are you worried about any conflicts between your beliefs and your medical situation/care/decisions?

Would it be helpful for you to speak to a clinical chaplain/community spiritual leader?

Are there any specific practices or restrictions I should know about in providing your medical care? (e.g., dietary restrictions, use of blood products)

From: Anandarajah G, Hight E. Spirituality and medical practice: using the HOPE questions as a practical tool for spiritual assessment. *Am Fam Physician.* 2001;63:81–88.

Making community linkages with appropriate clergy;
Offering counseling to the patient and family members, and
Supporting the interdisciplinary team members;
Planning funerals or memorial services.

The health care provider should understand that spiritual pain is very real and can be overwhelming. Many times a family will focus on spiritual beliefs and behaviors to cope with the overwhelming emotions associated with a terminal illness.

Health care providers, including the physical therapist, have a role in providing spiritual support to persons who are dying, to persons who are caring for the dying, and to persons who grieve for their deceased loved ones. They can not change the outcome, but they can provide a presence, a listening ear, and a willingness to accompany and support the family through this experience. The health care provider might be able to facilitate forgiveness, to provide prayer support, and to arrange for deeply desired religious services that help the patient and family bear up under incredible sorrow.[18]

further developed with the individualized findings and concerns. If the child is alert and oriented, request his participation in this process. Keep in mind the need for the child to maintain some degree of control. As with many other types of evaluations, the physical therapist may begin with the question "What can I do for you?" This will allow the patient or family to identify and prioritize their needs and goals for the service. The outcome of the intervention ultimately is to optimize the quality of life for the child and the family. The physical therapist plays an important role on the team in the examination of pain, body mechanics, caregiver body mechanics, functional ability, burden of care, equipment, and environment accessibility.[19] Box 9-5 lists some examination information of the patient and caregiver that could be gathered at the initial evaluation as well as during each visit, if appropriate.

The examination of pain is a significant component of an evaluation. Examining the comfort level of a child differs from that of an adult, and the examination should be modified according to age of the patient. "Where is your pain?"

POINT TO REMEMBER

Spirituality

Spirituality is different from religion. It is a broader concept that includes religion as well as cognitive, experiential, and behavioral aspects of a person.

POINT TO REMEMBER

The Hospice Plan of Care

A patient who is receiving hospice services will have a hospice plan of care that will outline the parameters of service provision and the priorities of the patient and family.

Physical Therapy

Physical therapy services may be requested to help the patient accomplish a simple task, such as to be able to attend a particular function (family event, school, social, etc.), or to maintain his endurance. Physical therapy services, as one part of the interdisciplinary hospice team, should strive to maintain patient independence through the dying process and to provide the patient and family with a palatable support. Some of the common symptoms or impairments that may be experienced by a child with a life-threatening health condition that could be addressed include such things as pain, fatigue, dyspnea, dysphagia, skin breakdown, and limited mobility.

A clinical evaluation of the child should touch upon all the body systems. This evaluation will guide the physical therapist as a basic care plan is formulated and then

POINT TO REMEMBER

Physical Therapy and Hospice

Physical therapy services, as one part of the interdisciplinary hospice team, should strive to maintain patient independence through the dying process and to provide the patient and family with palatable support.

BOX 9-5
Examination Information

Patient
Vital signs: body temperature, blood pressure, pulse, and
   respirations
Level of consciousness
Pain level and response to medications for pain
Bed mobility
Skin integrity
Transfer skills
Balance
Functional mobility
Gait pattern
Safety
Use of assistive devices
Ability to participate in self-care
Ability to participate in age-appropriate activities

Parent or Caregiver
General emotional status at time of visit
Ability to cope with current situation or recommendations
Knowledge and understanding of instructions
Ability to participate in a home program

BOX 9-6
QUESTT

0	1	2	3	4	5
NO HURT	HURTS LITTLE BIT	HURTS LITTLE MORE	HURTS EVEN MORE	HURTS WHOLE LOT	HURTS WORST

Instructions: Explain to the person that each face is for a person who feels happy because he has no pain (hurt) or sad because he has some or a lot of pain. **Face 0** is very happy because he doesn't hurt at all. **Face 1** hurts just a little bit. **Face 2** hurts a little more. **Face 3** hurts even more. **Face 4** hurts a whole lot. **Face 5** hurts as much as you can imagine, although you don't have to be crying to fee' this bad. Ask the person to choose the face that best describes how he is feeling.

Rating scale is recommended for persons age 3 years and older.

Brief word instructions: Point to each face using the words to describe the pain intensity. Ask the child to choose face that best describes own pain and record the appropriate number.

From Hockenberry MJ, Wilson D, Winkelstein ML: *Wong's Essentials of Pediatric Nursing*, ed. 7, St. Louis, 2005, p. 1259. Used with permission. Copywrite, Mosby.

POINT TO REMEMBER

Being There

Throughout the practice of physical therapy with children, the concept of including the family's values, routine, and goals is often repeated and stressed. It is a common factor in the patient management process and delivery of services. Regardless of how much the physical therapist may disagree with a family's point of view, routines, parenting style, or family dynamics, it is never appropriate to give unsolicited advice. A family's behavior and dynamics are uniquely theirs, formed over years of association and rooted in family history, for which the physical therapist was not a part. The physical therapist is responsible for helping, as much as possible in the given situation, and should not try to change the larger family dynamics.

factors. It may be helpful to have the parents keep a record of the child's pain evaluations.

When evaluating pain in children, the physical therapist or any health care provider should take into consideration a broader view beyond the patient's response to questions or ratings of pain perception. An examination of a child's behavior, apparent physiologic changes, and the identified cause of the painful stimulus should be conducted. The acronym QUESTT summarizes the importance of evaluating the child's behavior and any physiologic changes, such as increase respiratory or heart rate, the parent's report, and the likelihood of pain from the source (e.g., a needle stick would likely result in some level of pain[21]) (Box 9-7). Facial grimacing and withdrawal from the painful stimuli are some of the key nonverbal responses associated with a painful stimulus.

is usually pertinent, but perhaps to a younger child it would be more beneficial to ask "Where does it hurt?" or "Where should I place a band-aid?" Referring to a doll or stuffed animal as the patient with a "boo-boo" may also provide assistance in asking the same questions.

Perhaps the most common pain assessment tool is the Wong and Baker cartoon faces ranging from a smiley face for "no pain" to a tearful face exhibiting the "worst pain"[20] (Box 9-6). This evaluation should be completed with each professional contact. Although the parents should be part of the process, questioning the child is the most important factor in the examination process. Understanding the child's previous pain history and the ability to recognize related concerns and behavioral changes are key

BOX 9-7
QUESTT

Q - Question the child
U - Use pain rating scales
E - Evaluate behavior and physiological changes
S - Secure parents involvement
T - Take the cause of pain into account
T - Take action and evaluate results

From: Meister L. The vitas innovative hospice care approach to pediatric palliative care at home. *Caring.* 2005;24:54–61.

When the evaluations are complete, a hospice care plan can be constructed with the core services (nurse, social worker, counselor or chaplain, and physician) developing basic goals such as:

1. Comfort related to pain and symptoms of disease;
2. Optimum nutrition; and
3. Adequate support for the patient and family during the end-stage periods of an illness.

The overriding goal of hospice intervention is to maintain comfort with pain and symptom management. The physical therapist could also provide interventions to promote patient independence, as long as possible, and to minimize complications such as contractures, falls, and skin breakdown, as the patient ultimately loses functional skills.

Physical Therapy Interventions

Although the physical therapist will often provide "hands on" interventions, a more important role is as an educator on movement and function.[22] Educating the caregivers on proper body mechanics for lifting, transferring, bathing, and use of special positioning equipment is important to assure that the primary caregivers to the child remain in optimal health as they care for their son or daughter. Education of the patient in mobility and energy conservation techniques can improve the efficiency of transfers and completion of activities of daily living. The physical therapist must demonstrate competence in clinical skills as well as the ability to communicate effectively, facilitate team interaction, and innovate extemporaneously.[22] Box 9-8 provides a list of some of the interventions that can be used by a physical therapist and their application in the hospice environment.

The pediatric patient should participate in the intervention to the fullest extent possible, given his illness experience, developmental capacities, and level of consciousness. Regardless of the prognosis, respect for the child requires that he be given a developmentally appropriate description of the condition along with the expected burdens and benefits of available management options, while soliciting and listening to the child's preferences.[1]

Although it may be difficult for the professional to have a child direct his care, always keep in mind the importance of keeping the patient in the decision-making process. Often the nurse or physical therapist wants to order standard DME and supplies assuming that this is what is best for the patient and family. This can quickly become a "cookie cutter" approach to care. Ordering equipment too soon, or having it available just in case, may be frightening as well as inconvenient for the patient and family. It is important that the child feel secure in his environment. Following repeated hospitalizations, home is a therapeutic and comforting environment. A hospital bed is usually not wanted. The professional must examine and intervene, incorporating creativity into the plan of care. A

BOX 9-8
Physical Therapy Interventions and Some Examples of Their Application in Hospice[23,24]

The physical therapist should be aware of the contraindications for the use of certain interventions and make an informed decision, along with the hospice team, including the patient and family, of the benefits versus the risk of an intervention application. In some cases, it may be determined that the contraindication does not outweigh the palliative benefit of the intervention, given the terminal diagnosis.

Coordination/Communication/Documentation: Coordination of information and interventions. Remember, in a hospice program time is of the essence.

Patient/Client Related Instruction: Body mechanics; transfers; positioning to optimize use of the upper extremities for eating or bathing; use of equipment. Reinforce pain management protocol. Instruct on nonpharmacologic pain control measures (e.g., heat, cold, Transcutaneous Electrical Nerve Stimulator Unit, massage, relaxation, deep breathing techniques). Instruct home program to maintain strength, range of motion, balance, positioning to promote comfort. Teach safety measures/injury prevention

Therapeutic Exercise: To maintain function; promote a feeling of self worth; pain management.

Functional Training: Self-Care/Home: Strategies to bathe, dress, eat, groom, use the toilet. Strategies to allow for participation in household chores or activities; being part of the family.

Manual Therapy (including mobilization/manipulation): For pain management.

Prescription, application, and fabrication of equipment and devices: Identification, prescription, acquisition, and utilization of assistive technology.

Airway Clearance Techniques: chest physical therapy, assisted cough techniques, proper positioning to promote optimal air exchange, suctioning.

Integumentary Repair and Protection: Education on risk reduction; skin inspection, or wound management.

Electrotherapeutic Modalities: For pain management.

Physical Agents/Mechanical Modalities: For pain management or to promote relaxation.

simple maneuver of furniture or borrowing a particular chair from another room may achieve the desired outcome.

Allowing the patient a choice provides a sense of control during these difficult times. Some examples include:

- Parents and caregivers are reminded to include the child when deciding what to wear (the red shirt or the blue shirt?) or what to eat (cereal or scrambled eggs?)
- The nurse can assist by directing questions to the child, such as "Do you want your medicine in a liquid or chewable tablet?"

TABLE 9-2 Children and Death

Age (yr)	Cognitive Development	How Death is Viewed	Behaviors	Interventions
3	Pre-operational	Temporary separation; abandonment; bad behaviors cause death	Nightmares; aggressive play; regression of behaviors; more infantile	Reassurance that they are loved, are not responsible for their illness, and they will not be abandoned.
6 to 11	Concrete operational	Death is a person, a skeleton, or a ghost. Death only happens to old people.	Nightmares about parents dying; active fantasy lives; changes in behavior both at home and at school	Talk about their fears and thoughts about death and dying.
12 to 15	Formal operational	Death happens to others but not them. Understand that death is inevitable and final. May challenge death by engaging in risky behaviors.	May become withdrawn, openly hostile; fantasize about their own death	Talk about their concerns regarding the loss of independence, being different, loss of bodily functions, being imperfect.

Adapted from: Russell PS, Alexander J. Bereavement management in pediatric intensive care units. *Indian Pediatr*. 2005;42:811–818.
and
Maish M. Developmental Stages and Grief. School Corner. Washington, DC: American Hospice Foundation. Available at: http://www.americanhospice.org/SchoolCorner/DevelopmentalStages.htm. Accessed May 1, 2006.

• The physical therapist can involve the child by asking, "Which exercise would you like to do first? Who do you want to assist you? Would you like to have a wheelchair?"

Although simple and basic, it is easy to forget to include the patient. However, when the patient is included in the development of the plan of care, cooperation and willingness to participate are often achieved.

In summary, the physical therapist should remember the following:

• Coordinate care plan with interdisciplinary group.
• Attend team meetings. You are the expert in your role.
• Set short-term goals.
• Transform rehabilitation goals to palliative goals.
• Provide instructions to both the child and caregiver.
• Allow autonomy when applicable.
• Include the child as much as possible in the decision-making process.
• Provide emotional support.
• Most therapeutic interventions will be nonaggressive.

Working collaboratively with other team members will facilitate the delivery of efficient and hopefully effective interventions, which should empower the family and patient, diminish anxiety, and most importantly provide dignity.[25]

TRANSITIONING

It is critical to include grief assessments at the time of admission to hospice. Bereavement services are available for the family after death has occurred. Actually bereavement concerns and support should be initiated at the time of establishing a diagnosis and formulating a plan of care. Medical staff should provide a realistic prognosis and an approximate time in which death is likely to occur. Some of the clinical signs associated with impending death include a noticeable increase in sleeping with difficulty in arousal, increased confusion, restless behavior, a decreased need or request for food or water, and a change in a child's breathing pattern. When death does occur, the child will be unresponsive and there will be no breathing, no heartbeat, and a loss of bowel and bladder control. The eyelids will be slightly opened, and the jaw slightly relaxed. For many physical therapists, being with a patient who is actively dying or dies is a rare occurrence.

Whether the child has a chronic illness or a life-shortening illness, parents may find it difficult to accept impending death. There is no routine for the grief and bereavement associated with this loss. In addition to that of the parents, the support of the siblings should not be excluded. The child should be reassured that he or she has done nothing wrong and is not responsible for this or his own illness or that of a sibling. Children should be encouraged to talk about their feelings of anger, sadness, fear, isolation, and guilt, or to express themselves through art or music therapy.[15] How children understand death depends on their level of development. There will be questions where there are no answers. Table 9-2 identifies the general relationship of a child's cognitive development and how he may view death, some typical behaviors that may be seen, and some suggestions for interventions.

Hospices are required to develop a bereavement plan of care, which includes a minimum time span of 1 year following the death of a loved one. Services may include:

1. An assessment of the family/caregiver needs, including coping abilities and support systems available;
2. Counseling for an individual or family;
3. Referral to resources within the community; and
4. Education related to the grief process.

The hospice team develops an individualized bereavement plan of care. Bereavement follow-up may include home visits, phone contacts, support groups, provision of written materials related to grief, and memorial services.

CASE STUDIES

David
A hospice patient presents with end-stage leukemia.

MEDICAL HISTORY

Ten-year-old David is referred to hospice with a primary diagnosis of end-stage lung cancer. At 10 years of age, he was diagnosed with squamous cell carcinoma of the lung following a long, complicated medical history beginning at the age of 10 months. At that time, laryngeal papillomatosis was diagnosed and treated with multiple laser oblation procedures. The disease progressed to a pulmonary papillomatosis within a 6-year time frame and then to squamous cell cancer 3 years later. A thoracotomy was performed at which time the tumor was found to be unresectable secondary to chest wall/mediastinal involvement. In the following months, a magnetic resonance imaging (MRI) revealed direct extension of the lung mass with involvement of C6-7 to T5. There was now compromise of nerve roots and the brachial plexus. Patient was treated with interferon and periodically with radiation until he could no longer tolerate procedures. David mainly received palliative care from the time of his diagnosis. Morphine sulfate was the mainstay, although many medicines were used to control his pain.

FAMILY CONSTELLATION

David lives with his mother and stepsister, age 5. Mother admits to alcohol abuse and domestic violence. Stepfather has been abusive to the child. Mother currently involved in Alcoholics Anonymous (AA) and receiving counseling, as she fears child's terminal illness. She verbalized guilt and wants to "do right" for her child now. This child spent 2 months in a hospital setting prior to admission to hospice due to multiple concerns.

AT ADMISSION

Height: 82". Weight: 19.2 kg. Patient presented with rapid heart rate, low-grade temperature, shortness of breath (SOB) with activity/transfers, very frail, gait unsteady, decreased breath sounds bilaterally with audible wheeze. Voice is hoarse and thrush noted to tongue and gums. He is very sensitive to touch. Mother requires a great deal of support and education. Groshong PICC infusing medications as ordered.

HOSPICE PLAN OF CARE

This complex treatment plan consisted of daily and prn nursing interventions with a focus on pain and symptom management and instructions and support for the caregiver. David participated in his care plan and was encouraged to direct care as much as he wanted to do so. Often, he refused to allow the nurse to take his vital signs. David requested the routes of administration with his medication regimen. Frequent contacts with the primary physician were necessary.

With team coordination, the interdisciplinary team determines that it is appropriate for the adolescent to be with his peers. The social worker counseled parents to allow this to happen, explaining the importance of quality of life and her son's decision-making efforts. The physician member of the team guided the nurse toward comfort concerns. The patient would be given medication prior to this event and would be allowed to participate in the dosing to achieve comfort but not extreme sedation. Physical therapy received a request to evaluate gait and balance and to provide appropriate exercises to optimize the patient's ambulation skills.

GOAL

To optimize ambulation skills that would allow David to go outdoors with friends in order to provide socialization.

SERVICES

Physical therapy provided visits at 2 times per week for 2 weeks duration then discharged. Patient refused any supportive device.

The following outline portrays the symptoms and associated treatments utilized.

Symptom	Treatment Protocol
Uncontrolled Pain	Morphine sulfate IV Hydromorphone (Dilaudid IV) Naproxen Gabapentin (Neurontin) (Note: the dose of morphine and hydromorphone escalated with increased pain.)
Nausea/Vomiting	Pepcid po Promethazine (Phenergan) po; Supp.
SOB	Morphine/dilaudid O2 @ 5 L/min
Fever	Acetaminophen (Tylenol) po; Supp.
Oral Thrush	Nystatin Oral Susp.
Productive Cough, Increased Secretions	Hyoscyamine (Levsin)
Constipation	PeriColace Sennosides (Senekot)

The social worker helped with financial assistance, acquired the necessary DME, and worked with the mother to make funeral arrangements. The patient deteriorated rapidly and the provision of ongoing support was necessary as the family attempted to cope with the inevitable. A great deal of grief counseling and support took place.

The spiritual counselor assessed religious and cultural variables. Although David and his family did not attend church, a pastor came to see him regularly. The mother carried a lot of guilt from the past. All communications with her related to a "higher power." She stated that she had David baptized in the hospital just "to make sure he was ok."

Concern also related to the 5-year-old stepsister. Counseling was provided. Mother was supportive to the child and provided excellent care. No other services were initiated. Hospice care was provided over the course of 12 days. He deteriorated rapidly and died comfortably at home with the nurse and his mother at his bedside. Bereavement services were initiated. The hospice staff made home visits and phone contacts, and attended the funeral service.

Reflective Questions

1. As the physical therapist assigned to David during the hospital stay, list possible physical therapy interventions.
2. Formulate two palliative goals versus rehabilitation goals.
3. What, if any, DME should be considered?

Oscar
Diagnosis: Nieman-Pick Disease, Type C

Part 1: See Case Study in Chapter 3
Part 2: Hospice Service: Physical Therapy
Oscar is presently enrolled in a hospice program through which he receives physical therapy services.

DIAGNOSTIC PATTERNS

Primary: Impaired Motor Function and Sensory Integrity Associated with a Progressive Disorder of the Central Nervous System.

Secondary: Impaired Ventilation and Respiration/Gas Exchange Associated with Ventilatory Pump Dysfunction.

Presently, Oscar demonstrates minimal voluntary movement of his trunk or extremities. Glasgow Coma Scale of 8. Ashworth Score of +3 in his lower extremities. He presents with flaccidity in his trunk, cervical region, and upper extremities. Oscar makes occasional eye contact and will visually track an object in his visual field (4 to 8 inches in front of his face), approximately 45 degrees to his left, and approximately 20 degrees from midline to his right, when supine. He has no head control when not supine. He will smile, occasionally. He cries when in pain or uncomfortable. He is on enteral feeding via a J-tube for 20 hours a day, PediaSure enteral formula. He receives oxygen via nasal cannula (1 liter). Oxygen saturation is monitored via a pulse oximeter and is typically at 95%.

Recently, Oscar was diagnosed with seizures (myoclonic) and a respiratory infection. Presently he is afebrile. Adventitious breath sounds are noted in the bilateral lower lobes of the lungs with auscultation. Tactile fremitus is noted bilaterally. He has a productive cough. He produces a moderate amount of sputum (which is thick and yellow) into his mouth. He has decreased cough strength. He is no longer verbal.

His present medications include Zyrtec syrup 5 mg/5 mL 1.5 teaspoon once a day. Topamax 25-mg tablets; 1½ tablet in AM and 2 tablets at night. Albuterol 0.083% in nebulizer four times per day or prn. Amoxil 250-mg 1½ tablets at hs. All medications are administered via his J-tube with the exception of the aerosol.

His physical therapy program includes passive range of motion to his extremities, rib cage, and cervical region. Sensory stimulation augments his educational program. (He continues to receive special education instruction from the local school district, home status.) Chest physical therapy (CPT) promotes adequate pulmonary hygiene. There is parental education on the use of the various positioning and medical devices, which include proper positioning when supine and side lying, supported sitting using Tumbleform chair with tray, and proper positioning in McClearan seating system and car seat. He has resting hand splints, an oral suction machine, a pulse oximeter, a nebulizer, and a pump for enteral feedings.

The use of Zyrtec aids in maintaining the patency of Oscar's airway while keeping him as responsive as possible. (This medication is nonsedating, although his Topamax is a sedative.) Timing the administration of Albuterol and physical therapy aids in the effectiveness of the CPT and Oscar's tolerance of the sensory experiences (rocking, swinging, massage, etc.). At times, when he is congested, his pulse oximeter reading can drop to 89%. Post treatment of medication, CPT, and suctioning can bring it up to 95%. Amoxil is used to address his respiratory infections, which are becoming increasingly more frequent. Use of the antihistamine, beta-adrenergic bronchodilator, and antibiotic are all aimed at maintaining Adam's airway and general health.

Reflective Questions

1. As a member of the hospice team, develop three goals for Oscar for which physical therapy services would be appropriate.
2. Identify and discuss the difference between interventions that are used to promote the acquisition of developmental skills (Part 1) versus interventions for palliative care (Part 2).
3. Identify three physical therapy interventions that could be used to improve Oscar's quality of life. How do the identified interventions improve his quality of life? How do they affect his mother's quality of life?

SUMMARY

Hospice is an option of care for a patient diagnosed with a life-limiting progressive illness. It focuses on promoting comfort and quality of life over a cure for the disease, and is an option for many adults made available by a benefit in the Medicare program. Hospice care for children may also be available, and reimbursed by Medicaid or private insurance, but is more difficult to accept or consider as an option, given the current societal views on death and children. Children are not adults. They do not die like adults do. The current system of hospice under Medicare, which is greatly influenced by the care and needs of adults with terminal illnesses, would require adjustments in the qualifications and services in order to address the unique needs of children with terminal illnesses and their families.

Hospice should be seen as a broader application of a combination of palliative care and interventions that promote functional skills delivered in a variety of settings from the hospital to the home. Being at home and participating in the family is a highly positive and much desired goal.[26] Children with terminal illnesses should be viewed as an inseparable part of the family unit with the goal of hospice care to promote an optimal quality of life for both the child and family.

REVIEW QUESTIONS

1. A family is unclear on the difference between hospice care and palliative care. Which of the following definitions best defines palliative care?
   a. Palliative care is synonymous with hospice care.
   b. Palliative care is the delivery of curative interventions with minimal amount of pain or discomfort.
   c. Palliative care is a package of health care services aimed at providing pain relief.
   d. Palliative care is interventions aimed at decreasing the many symptoms associated with a disease process without necessarily affecting the disease process itself.

2. Which of the following is the most common cause of death in a 2-year-old child?
   a. Sudden Infant Death Syndrome
   b. Cancer
   c. Death resulting from an unintentional injury
   d. Prematurity

3. Hospice programs for children are made more problematic due to the difference between a child's death and that of an adult. Which of the following is not a significant difference in between two age populations?
   a. Making a prognosis on life expectancy in a patient with a terminal illness
   b. Cultural beliefs regarding death
   c. Where death occurs
   d. The desire to die at home

4. Which of the following has the ultimate legal authority to direct the care of an adolescent who is in a hospice program and is unable to communicate or make decisions for himself?
   a. A living will which he signed before he was unable to make decisions for himself
   b. Power of attorney that he designated
   c. His parents
   d. The advance directive he had drawn up when he was admitted to the hospice program

5. A child should participate in the care planning process to the fullest extent possible

   a. given his illness experience, developmental capacities, and level of consciousness.
   b. at all times throughout the hospice care planning process.
   c. regardless of age or parental consent, when in a hospice program.

6. You are working with an 18-year-old man who has a diagnosis of Duchenne Muscular Dystrophy. He is presently using a power wheelchair as his primary means of mobility, and is having difficulty breathing. He asks you if you go to church on Sunday. This type of question could be an opening to a discussion on spirituality. Of the following, which would be the most appropriate course of action?
   a. Tell him that you do not discuss your personal life with patients and that you will refer him to a spiritual counselor if he wishes.
   b. Tell him that you do go to church on Sunday and ask if he would like to join you.
   c. Answer him honestly and ask if he is part of an organized religion.
   d. Tell him that it is out of your scope of practice to discuss spiritual issues with him.

7. Palliative care differs from conventional rehabilitative care primarily in its
   a. primary focus on patient comfort.
   b. ability to provide therapy in any manner that is comfortable to the physical therapist.
   c. focus on increased communication with the third party payers.
   d. none of the above. Palliative care does not differ from rehabilitative care.

8. Of the following, which would be considered, overall, the most important intervention a physical therapist could provide in a hospice setting?
   a. Airway clearance techniques
   b. Family and patient education
   c. Therapeutic exercise
   d. Integumentary protection or repair

9. Which of the following is not considered a sign of active dying?
   a. Restless behavior
   b. Incontinence
   c. Change in breathing pattern
   d. Crying

10. Which statement below best describes the provision of bereavement services in a hospice program?
    a. Hospices offer bereavement contacts for only the parents of the deceased child.
    b. Grief assessments begin at admission to hospice services, with bereavement services provided for up to 1 year following the child's death.
    c. Bereavement services are initiated after the child has died and the family portrays complicated grief.
    d. Bereavement care begins after the death of a child, with volunteer services.

Hospice Plan of Care

Albert Gallatin Hospice
Interdisciplinary POC

Patient Name:_____ Date: _____ M.R. #:_____ Office: _____

Pain	Inactive

GOAL: Pain control is adequate as measured by pt/family indicating a level of comfort on a standardized pain rating scale.

___Provide ongoing pain assessment
___Monitor current pain protocol/regime
___Instruct pt/family in medical pain management
___Instruct pt/family in non-invasive pain management (i.e. massage, distraction, relaxation, imaging, positioning, using heat/cold application, music therapy, art therapy)
___Monitor environmental facts, e.g. temperature, lighting, noise, etc.
___Instruct in safe narcotic use
___Explore spiritual/psychosocial barriers to pain management
___
___

Date Initiated:	Resolved:	Resumed:

Inadequate Nutrition/Hydration (Nausea/Vomiting)

GOAL: Pt's nutritional needs & hydration will be maintained for as long as possible. When nutritional status diminishes promote family acceptance.

___Nutritional assessment
___Develop nutritional plan in accordance with food/fluid preference
___Control symptoms that interfere with nutritional/hydration status.
___Consult nutritionist
___Pt./family teaching towards decreased nutritional intake to promote acceptance.
___Teach pt./family the effects of artificial nutrition in terminal illness.
___Support pt./family choices for nutritional support.
___Provide comfort measures
___
___

Date Initiated:	Resolved:	Resumed:

Sleep / Rest Disturbance

GOAL: Adequate rest will be maintained

___Assess sleep patterns.
___Control symptoms that interfere with sleep.
___Identify psychosocial factors that interfere with sleep.
___Instruct on medication regime.
___Instruct on measures to enhance sleep (relaxation, massage, environmental factors, positioning).
___Instruct pt./family in prayer/meditation techniques.
___
___

Date Initiated:	Resolved:	Resumed:

Bowel / Bladder Dysfunction	Inactive

GOAL: Elimination adequate for disease process & pt's comfort.
BOWEL:
___Assess bowel functioning
___Check for impaction & disimpact prn.
___Teach / perform care of ostomies including skin care around stoma.
___Instruct pt./caregiver on dietary factors.
___Increase fluid intake.
___Instruct on medication regime.
___

BLADDER:
___Monitor urinary output
___Teach incontinence measures & support pt/family preferences.
___Observe and report skin breakdown.
___Instruct on catheter care
___
___

Date Initiated:	Resolved:	Resumed:

Impairment of Skin Integrity

GOAL: Maintain skin integrity at optimal level & promote healing.
___Assess skin integrity.
___Provide pressure reducing devices.
___Reduce causative factors of skin breakdown.
___Reposition to reduce pressure.
___Provide personal care to improve skin integrity.
___Instruct caregiver on positioning and skin care to decrease potential pressure sores.
___Provide wound care as ordered.
___Assess for signs and symptoms of infection.
___Consult with RN ET for wound care.
___Instruct pt./caregiver on dietary factors.
___

Date Initiated:	Resolved:	Resumed:

Self Care Deficit

GOAL: Hygiene needs will be met with pt/family participation as appropriate.
___HHA to assist with hygiene/ADLs as directed by the RN.
___Caregiver instructions to maintain ADLs.
___Assist with homemaker needs as assigned.
___Meal preparation as requested.
___Comfort measures.

Date Initiated:	Resolved:	Resumed:

Patient Name:_____ Date: _____

Respiratory / Cardiac Impairment   Inactive

GOAL: Maintain adequate cardiopulmonary / respiratory status for current level of disease.

___Assess cardiac / respiratory status q visit.
___Assess need for O^2 therapy for comfort.
___Instruct caregiver / pt. on measures to conserve O^2 consumption & energy.
___Instruct on safe use of O^2 & O^2 precautions.
___Instruct on relaxation techniques to decrease dyspnea.
___Assess and instruct on medication regime.
___Assess for congestion, cough & sputum production.
___Instruct on deep breathing & coughing exercises.
___Initiate oro / nasal suctioning prn for excessive secretions & instruct caregiver on suctioning technique.

___

___

Date Initiated:	Resolved:	Resumed:

Knowledge Deficit

GOAL: Pt. / family will improve knowledge in identified teaching areas.

___Assess ability of family / caregiver to care for patient.
___Assess level of knowledge of caregiver.
___Review Hospice handbook with caregiver.
___Review medication teaching handouts.
___Staff to monitor caregiver.
___Review on-call access.

___

Date Initiated:	Resolved:	Resumed:

Declining Health Status

GOAL: Promote effective management of symptoms & acceptance of disease progression.

___Instruct regarding signs & symptoms of impending death.
___Assess patient's comfort.
___Provide feedback to family regarding proximity of death.
___Instruct caregiver in comfort measures / symptom control
___Assess for suicidal ideation
___Provide emotional support to pt./family
___Provide grief and loss counseling.
___Review Hospice Handbook with Caregiver.

___

___

Date Initiated:	Resolved:	Resumed:

Ineffective Functioning of Family System   Inactive

GOAL: Promote improvement of family system

___Explore pt./family concerns.
___Provide support/active listening/counseling.
___Clarify family role/support.
___Volunteer referral.
___Facilitate expression of fear/feelings.
___Assess caregiving ability/placement options.
___Evaluate support systems.
___Provide respite for caregiver.

___

Date Initiated:	Resolved:	Resumed:

Inadequate Finances/Support System

GOAL: Identify & promote effective use of available support systems & entitlements.

___Psychosocial assessment.
___Assess financial status.
___Refer to community resources.
___Educate pt./family on programs which can assist.
___Assist with long range plans.
___Refer to legal counsel.

___

Date Initiated:	Resolved:	Resumed:

Impaired Mobility

GOAL: Maintain optimal function, mobility & independence for as long as possible with attention to safety.

___Assess mobility limitations/impairments.
___Assess risk for injury.
___Evaluate need for DME.
___Consult physical therapy services.
___Instruct pt./caregiver on positioning/transfer techniques
___Instruct on ROM exercises.
___Provide active/passive ROM exercises.
___Assist with personal care as directed.
___Provide counseling to allow pt. to ventilate feelings with decreased activity.

___

Date Initiated:	Resolved:	Resumed:

GOAL:

Date Initiated:	Resolved:	Resumed:

Patient Name:_____ Date: _____

Seizures   Inactive

GOAL: Pt. will remain injury free with control of seizure activity.

___Seizure precautions and instruction to family.
___Drug levels as ordered.
___Monitor and instruct on medication regime.
___Provide calm environment.
___Promote family acceptance of declining health status.
___
___

Date Initiated:	Resolved:	Resumed:

Active Phase of Dying

GOAL: Promote a peaceful death with symptoms managed & provide support & comfort to family unit.

___Instruct caregiver/family on signs & symptoms of approaching death.
___Assess pt's comfort level.
___Provide comfort measures & symptom management.
___Assess coping ability of caregiver/family.
___Instruct caregiver on comfort measures.
___Inpatient care as needed for dying phase.
___Provide continuous care as needed.
___Provide emotional support.
___Provide counseling & spiritual support.
___
___

Date Initiated:	Resolved:	Resumed:

Spiritual Issues

GOAL: Pt. /family cope effectively, maximize spiritual support & integrate the dying process with spiritual value system

___Spiritual assessment
___Offer spiritual support to pt./family.
___Consult with pt's/family's church (religious leaders) for support.
___Allow pt./family to express spiritual concerns.
___Offer prayer/spiritual reading.
___Utilize music therapy.
___Facilitate reconciliation/forgiveness.
___Assist in practicing spiritual or religious rituals.
___Active listening regarding spirituality.
___
___

Date Initiated:	Resolved:	Resumed:

Diminished Care System   Inactive

GOAL: Augment effective provisions for pt/family care.

___Evaluate support system.
___Assess caregiving ability.
___Provide respite for caregiver.
___Volunteer referral.
___Refer to appropriate community organization.
___
___

Date Initiated:	Resolved:	Resumed:

Anticipatory Grief Issues

GOAL: Promote adaptation of the normal grief process.

___Provide for expression of grief.
___Assess for risk of pathological grieving.
___Assess support system of family.
___Initiate grief work.
___Promote use of support system.
___Provide counseling on grief process.
___Encourage life review with patient/family.
___Assess caregiver / family for bereavement plan.
___Foster communication / active listening.
___Consult support group therapy/community resources.
___
___

Date Initiated:	Resolved:	Resumed:

Coping Deficit

GOAL: Pt. / family will exhibit coping mechanisms that support a positive quality of life.

___Assess coping skills of caregiver/family.
___Identify contributing/causative factors.
___Instruct caregiver/family on coping strategies.
___Offer respite care.
___Offer volunteer support.
___Assess ability caregiver/family to provide adequate care of pt.
___Evaluate placement options/in home assist.
___
___

Date Initiated:	Resolved:	Resumed:

Admission & POC reviewed with input from:
___Attending MD (date:)_____
___Medical Director/Hospice MD (date:)_____
___Social Worker (date:)_____
___Spiritual Counselor (date:)_____

_____   _____
RN Signature   *date*

☒ Signatures on file

Albert gallatin Hospice. Albert gallatin Home Care and Hospice. Uniontown, PA. 2007, with permission.

REFERENCES

1. Nelson RM, Neff JM. Palliative care for children. *Pediatrics.* 2000;106:351–357.
2. National Hospice and Palliative Care Organization. What is Palliative Care? Caring Connections Web site. Available at: www.caringinfo.org. Last accessed February 2, 2006.
3. Kilburn LH. *Hospice Operations Manual: Hospice for the Next Century.* Dubuque: Kendall/Hunt Publishing Company; 1997.
4. Tax Equity and Fiscal Responsibility Act of 1982. PL 97-248.
5. National Hospice and Palliative Care Organization. Key Facts and Figures. Caring Connections Web site. Available at: www.caringinfo.org. Last accessed February 2, 2006.
6. American Academy of Pediatrics, Committee on Bioethics and Committee on Hospital Care. Palliative care for children. *Pediatrics.* 2000;106:351–357.
7. Fields M, Behram R, eds. When Children Die. Improving Palliative and End-of-Life Care for Children and Their Families. Committee on Palliative and End-of-Life Care for Children and Their Families Board on Health Science Policy. Institute of Medicine of the National Academies. Washington, DC: The National Academies Press; 2003:43–44.
8. Fields M, Behram R, eds. When Children Die. Improving Palliative and End-of-Life Care for Children and Their Families. Committee on Palliative and End-of-Life Care for Children and Their Families Board on Health Science Policy. Institute of Medicine of the National Academies. Washington, DC: The National Academies Press; 2003:66–70.
9. Levetown M, ed. Compendium of pediatric palliative care: children's international project on palliative/hospice services. Alexandria, VA: National Hospice and Palliative Care Organization; 2000.
10. Dunn H. *Hard Choices for Loving People.* Fourth ed. Herndon, VA: A & A Publishers, Inc.; 2001.
11. Carter BS, Levetown M. *Palliative Care for Infants, Children, and Adolescents. A Practical Handbook.* Baltimore, MD: The Johns Hopkins University Press; 2004.
12. Halamandaris VJ. Pediatric home care: continuing issues for the future. *Caring.* 2005;24:6–11.
13. Feudtner C, Hays R, Haynes G, et al. Deaths attributed to pediatric complex chronic conditions: national trends and implications for supportive care services. *Pediatrics.* 2001;107:e99.
14. Kübler-Ross E. *On Death and Dying.* New York: Macmillan; 1969.
15. Fitzgibbon EJ, Viola R. Parenteral ketamine as an analgesic adjuvant for severe pain: development and retrospective audit of a protocol for a palliative care unit. *J Palliat Care.* 2002;18:49–57.
16. Martsolf DS, Mickley JR. The concept of spirituality in nursing theories: differing world-views and extent of focus. *J Adv Nurs.* 1998;27:294–303.
17. Anandarajah G, Hight E. Spirituality and medical practice: using the HOPE questions as a practical tool for spiritual assessment. *Am Fam Phys.* 2001;63:81–88.
18. Benner Carson V, Koenig H. *Spiritual Caregiving: Healthcare as a Ministry.* Radnor, PA: Templeton Foundation Press; 2004.
19. Ebel S, Langer K. The role of the physical therapist in hospice care. *Am J Hosp Palliat Care.* 1993;10:32–35.
20. Wong D, Hockenberry-Eaton M. *Wong's Essentials of Pediatric Nursing, 6th ed.* St. Louis, MO: Mosby; 2001.
21. Meister L. The vitas innovative hospice care approach to pediatric palliative care at home. *Caring.* 2005;24:54–61.
22. Toot J. Physical therapy and hospice: concept and practice. *Phys Ther J.* 1984;64:665–671.
23. American Physical Therapy Association. *Guide to Physical Therapist Practice, 2nd ed.* Rev. Alexandria, VA: American Physical Therapy Association; 2003.
24. Himelstein BP, Hilden JM, Morstad Boldt A, Weissman D. Medical progress: pediatric palliative care. *N Engl J Med.* 2004;350:1752–1761.
25. Frost M. The role of physical, occupational, and speech therapy in hospice: patient empowerment. *Am J Hosp Palliat Care.* 2001;18:397–402.
26. Benini F, Ferrante M, Trapanotto M, Zacchello F. Palliative care in children: problems and considerations. *Riv Ital Pediatr.* 2004;30:205–209.

Additional Resources

The NHPCO is the largest nonprofit membership organization representing hospice and palliative care programs and professionals in the United States. The organization is committed to improving end-of-life care and expanding access to hospice care with the goal of profoundly enhancing quality of life for people dying in America and their loved ones. Web site: http://www.nhpco.org/

Carter BS, Levetown M. *Palliative Care for Infants, Children, and Adolescents. A Practical Handbook.* Baltimore, MD: The Johns Hopkins University Press; 2004.

Fields M, Behram R, eds. *When Children Die. Improving Palliative and End-of-Life Care for Children and Their Families.* Committee on Palliative and End-of-Life Care for Children and Their Families Board on Health Science Policy. Institute of Medicine of the National Academies. Washington, DC: The National Academies Press; 2003.

Hinds P, Schum L, Baker J, et al. Key factors affecting dying children and their families. *J Palliat Med.* 2005;8(suppl 1):S70–S78.

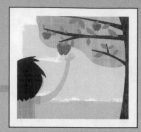

CHAPTER 10

After 21: Living and Working

Mark Drnach

LEARNING OBJECTIVES

1. Understand and evaluate the aspects of adulthood as they apply to a person with a disability.
2. Be familiar with key federal and state laws that address social issues of people with disabilities.
3. Understand and differentiate between state level programs of Medicaid, vocational rehabilitation, and worker's compensation.
4. Describe the options for living and employment available to people with disabilities.
5. Be able to perform a basic screen for physical accessibility in accordance with the Americans with Disabilities Act.
6. Be able to perform a basic evaluation for living and/or working for a person with a disability.
7. Understand Welfare and the general programs that may be available under this form of public assistance.

Congress periodically reauthorizes legislation, such as the Individuals with Disabilities Education Act (IDEA), which reflects the nation's commitment to children and adults with disabilities. In a reauthorization of IDEA Congress stated, "disability is a natural part of the human experience and in no way diminishes the right of individuals to participate in or contribute to society. Improving educational results for children with disabilities is an essential element of our national policy of ensuring equality of opportunity, full participation, independent living, and economic self-sufficiency for individuals with disabilities."[1]

The preceding chapters have provided a framework for the general provision of physical therapy services available to children from birth until the age of majority at which time the now young adult is expected to participate, as independently as possible, in society. With the passage of the Americans with Disabilities Act of 1990 (ADA) there has been a greater public awareness of the barriers to employment opportunities and public services for millions of people with a disability. Although public awareness has increased in these areas, "statistical evidence for real improvements in the lives of those with disabilities—more opportunities for employment and improved economic status, greater freedom of movement and ease of access, and increased levels of social integration—has been slow to materialize."[2] Low levels of participation in social, cultural, and commercial activities do not seem to have developed much since the passage of the ADA.[2]

This chapter will explore one framework in which physical therapy services could be provided to young adults after high school. Services are provided to promote full participation in society for adults who happen to have a disability.

DEFINING ADULTHOOD

The definition of adulthood is complex, as is the transition from childhood to adulthood. Traditionally, *adulthood* has been considered the age at which a person is a full member of society with responsibilities, not only for themselves but for the community as well.[3] These responsibilities include roles and rituals such as moving out of the family house, getting married, being employed, and voting. In addition to age, physical maturity, cultural and/or societal considerations, and mental capacity are common factors used to define the characteristics of an adult.[4] How a society defines adulthood has implications for the laws and rules that it adopts and follow.

Chronological age is used as to describe an adult from a physical perspective. The period after puberty is considered in many cultures to be the beginning of adulthood. Girls will reach their adult size around age 17 to 18 years. Boys will reach their adult size between ages 18 and 21 years.[5] Changes in muscle distribution, fat, and circulatory and respiratory systems lead to increased stamina and endurance in adolescents and bring them to the peak of their cognitive, visual, auditory, and strength levels.[6] At this level the person would be able to engage in social activities such as obtaining a driver's license, entering into marriage, voting, caring for children, choosing to live away from their parents, and working for financial gain, which are common characteristics of being an adult.

Cultural and/or societal definitions of adulthood include being *independent from parents* financially, structurally, and cognitively.[4] The ability of a person to be able to live on her own, pay bills, live in a place other than a parent's home, and be able to make decisions about her own life is a characteristic of an adult and a common goal that parents have for their child. Cognitive abilities are a major factor in the ability of a young adult to be able to make the decisions that would allow her to obtain employment and to make reasonably safe and rational choices. The potential for the person to live separately from her parents and to provide for herself is related to her cognitive ability and social support systems. Many adult children may choose to live with their parents and share financial responsibilities, but the potential to live without that structure and support is the key characteristic reflective of adulthood.

Historically *marriage* was a sign of being an adult and an expected part of adulthood. Cultural and societal influences can vary, making marriage either a necessity or nicety for being valued as an adult. Marriage is a reflection of the mental competence of the person who makes a decision to enter into a legally binding agreement. Although two people may love one another, their status as competent adults dictates the legal requirements to form this type of union. Although parents may disapprove of their adult child's choice of a spouse, a key difference for a person with a disability is that his or her parents may be able to legally stop the marriage by bringing into question the ability of the person with the disability to make such a decision.[4]

Consent is defined as the knowing, intelligent, and voluntary agreement to engage in a given activity.[7] Legal requirements that dictate the age of *sexual consent* are set up to protect children. In most states, the age of sexual consent is 16 years for a competent person. A person may be cognitively impaired, but it doesn't mean that he or she is sexually impaired. What are impaired are the social rituals that lead up to consensual sexual encounters. Developing social groups of same-age peers, which can lead to dating in groups, then to dating individuals, and finally, to dating exclusively, which is seen in the adolescent period, is often absent for individuals with developmental disabilities.

Being able to *vote* is a right and another indication of being an adult. This behavior reflects the society's opinion that the person voting is capable of making a decision about a potential law or another person who will represent her beliefs and opinions in the government. This is a right granted to any nonfelonious citizen of the United States who is 18 years old or older regardless of race, religion, gender, or intelligence quotient (IQ).[4] It is the *potential* to vote that is a characteristic of adulthood. Some adults may choose not to vote, but that choice doesn't make them any less of an adult.

Being an adult includes the characteristic of *self-determination*. Wehmeyer and Schalock[8] define *self-determination* as acting as the primary causal agent in one's life and making choices and decisions regarding one's quality of life free from undue external influence or interference. They describe four main characteristics of self-determination behavior: actions are autonomous; actions are self regulated; the person initiates and responds to events in a psychologically empowered manner; and the person acts in a self-realizing manner. If a person is declared incompetent, such as a person with a severe cognitive impairment, then he or she is considered unable to make reasonable choices regarding his or her life.[8]

Self-determination does not happen overnight. The characteristics of self-determination begin early in childhood and develop throughout a person's life. People who have a disability may be impaired in their ability to fulfill the rituals and roles that a society expects of an adult due to innate factors of the disability itself or to factors imposed upon them by societal attitudes or beliefs. Understanding and identifying the differences between an innate inability and an imposed external constraint is the first step in creating equal opportunity for all people.

 POINT TO REMEMBER

Adulthood

Traditionally, adulthood has been associated with physical maturity, chronological age, independence from parents, and the ability to vote, provide consent for sexual relations, marry, and display self-determination in actions and decisions.

THE PRACTICE ENVIRONMENT

According to the 2005 report from the United Nations Millennium Project, approximately one of 10 people in the world have a disability.[9] The U.S. Census Bureau in 2002 reported that 51.2 million Americans (18% of the population) have a disability, with 35.5 million (12% of the population) reporting that they have a severe disability.[10] Among the people with a disability, more than half of those aged 21 to 64 years (56%) were employed. People reporting having a severe disability have the lowest employment rate (43%) compared to those with a nonsevere disability (82%) and those with no reported disability (88%). Forty-four percent of individuals with nonsevere disability worked full time, year-round, compared to 13% of individuals with severe disabilities. The report also shows that the median annual income for people with nonsevere disability was $22,000.00, compared to that for people with a severe disability ($12,800.00), and for those with no reported disability ($25,000.00). The report defines a person as having a disability if he has difficulty performing a specific activity, such as seeing, hearing, bathing, or doing light housework, or has a specified condition, such as Alzheimer disease or autism.

POINT TO REMEMBER

Employment

People with a severe disability have the lowest employment rate, with 13% working year round for an annual income of approximately $12,800.00.

The Survey of Income and Program Participation (SIPP) provides an opportunity to examine disability and work using a definition of disability consistent with the ADA, with the inclusion of people who use wheelchairs, report functional limitations, or have other specified conditions but may be fully employed and report no limitation in the amount or kind of work.[11] This report shows that people who are disabled are less likely to be employed than are their nondisabled peers. The employment rate for people without a disability is 82.1%, but for those with a mental disability, employment drops to 41.3%. For individuals with any type of functional limitation, the percentage employed is 32.2%. For people who use a cane, walker, or crutch, 27.5% are employed; for those who use a wheelchair, 22.0% are employed.[11] Workers with functional limitations who are unable to walk three city blocks have an employment rate of 22.5%; unable to climb stairs, 25.5%; unable to lift and/or carry 10 lb, 27.0%; unable to see words and/or letters, 30.8%; and unable to hear conversation, 59.7%.[11] People who have a problem with mobility seem to have the lowest rate of employment. The survey also shows that the higher the educational level of the person, the more likely that person is to be working. This is true for people with or without a disability.

Both the federal and state governments have to be instrumental in facilitating the inclusion of people with disabilities in the workplace by the passage and implementation of various laws and programs.

POINT TO REMEMBER

Employment

People who have a problem with mobility have the least amount of job employment.

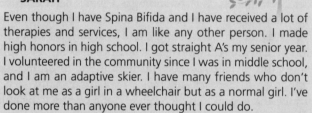

PERSONAL PERSPECTIVE

SARAH

Even though I have Spina Bifida and I have received a lot of therapies and services, I am like any other person. I made high honors in high school. I got straight A's my senior year. I volunteered in the community since I was in middle school, and I am an adaptive skier. I have many friends who don't look at me as a girl in a wheelchair but as a normal girl. I've done more than anyone ever thought I could do.

I started receiving many different therapies at the age of 6 months old up until I was 6 years old. I still benefit from services for people with disabilities. I was so little that it's hard to remember back when I had therapy, but I do remember that I always enjoyed it and I made many friends with the therapists. To me it was just something in life that I had to do. I met this girl in preschool and we are still best friends. I know the therapies have helped me with the way I move my body and the way I talk. In school, the services for people with disabilities were different and sometimes they weren't appropriate for me because I don't have any cognitive disability. I learned when to tell the teachers when I needed something and what I needed. Sometimes I had to push and prod to make them listen to me.

I feel a little nervous and scared about the future but I know that I am prepared and that I can tackle anything that comes my way. I've learned how to ask people for help, and if I face something in the future that I may need a little help with, I know that I can ask.

—Sarah

The Federal Government

The federal government has responded to the need for social reform through the enactment of a number of laws that address the needs of people with disabilities. In addition to the Rehabilitation Act of 1973 (PL 93-112) and the Education for All Handicapped Children Act of 1975 (PL 94-142), which are discussed in separate chapters of this book, the following laws have emphasized that the enablement of people with disabilities is a social responsibility.

The Social Security Act of 1935 (SSA; PL 74-271) was the most significant piece of social legislation passed by the U.S. government. This legislation established federal aid for public health and welfare assistance, maternal and child health, and children with disabilities services.[12] It also provided the first permanent authorization for the federal vocational rehabilitation program. The SSA would give rise in subsequent years to the programs of Medicare, Medicaid, and Supplemental Security Income (SSI).

The Social Security Amendments in 1956 (PL 84-880) established the Disability Insurance Trust Fund under Title II of the SSA and provided for payment of benefits to workers with disabilities under the *Social Security Disability Insurance* (SSDI) program.[13,14] Subsequent reauthorization extended the benefits to the dependents of the disabled worker.

Title XIX of the SSA (PL 89-97) is known as the *Medicaid* program, and was adopted in 1965. This federal–state medical assistance program is administered by the states with federal matching funds. The Medicaid program is available to all people receiving assistance under the public assistance titles (Title I, Title IV, Title X, and Title XIV) and to people whose income and resources are insufficient to meet their medical costs.[14] In 1971, Medicaid benefits were extended to cover services provided by intermediate care facilities (ICF). The purpose of this amendment was to provide a less costly alternative for the medically indigent, who do not need the institutional or intensive care provided in hospitals and skilled nursing facilities.

Title XVI of the SSA (PL 92-603), SSI, provides cash benefits to those persons older than 65 years, blind, disabled, or poor or to a child younger than 18 years with a disability or blindness. There are also benefits for persons who work despite a disabling impairment. It provides cash to meet basic needs for food, clothing, and shelter.[15] SSI is funded by general tax revenue, not Social Security taxes.

P O I N T   T O   R E M E M B E R

SSA

The federal government has responded to the need for social reform through the enactment of laws that address the needs of people with disabilities. One of the most significant pieces of federal legislation is the SSA, which gave rise to Disability Insurance, SSI, vocational rehabilitation, Medicare, and Medicaid Insurance.

The Architectural Barriers Act of 1968 (ABA) requires that buildings and facilities that are designed, constructed, or altered with federal funds, or leased by a federal agency, comply with federal standards for physical accessibility.[16] ABA requirements are limited to architectural standards in new and altered buildings and in newly leased facilities. This law marks one of the first efforts by the federal government to ensure access to the physical environment by people with disabilities.

The Civil Rights of Institutionalized Persons Act of 1980 (CRIPA) authorizes the U.S. Attorney General to investigate conditions of confinement at state and local government institutions, publicly operated nursing homes, and institutions for people with psychiatric or developmental disabilities. Its purpose is to allow the Attorney General to uncover and correct widespread deficiencies that seriously jeopardize the health and safety of residents of institutions.[16] The Special Litigation Section investigates covered facilities to determine whether there is a pattern or practice of violations of the residents' federal rights. The Special Litigation Section is not authorized to represent individuals or to address specific individual cases.

The Developmental Disabilities Assistance and Bill of Acts of 2000 (P.L. 106–402) allows for federal monies to be made available to the states to assist in providing comprehensive services and advocacy assistance to persons up to age 21 with developmental disabilities that promote self-determination, independence, productivity, and integration and inclusion in all facets of community life.[17]

Each state's Developmental Disability Council plans and implements projects to assist people with developmental disabilities to live in the least restrictive environment and to actively participate in their communities. State Councils pursue systems change (e.g., the way human service agencies do business so that individuals with developmental disabilities and their families have better or expanded services), advocacy (e.g., educating policy makers about unmet needs of individuals with developmental disabilities), and capacity building (e.g., working with state service agencies to provide training and benefits to direct care workers) to promote independence, self-determination, productivity, integration, and inclusion of people with developmental disabilities in all facets of community life.[18] State Council members are appointed by the governor and are individuals with developmental disabilities, parents and family members of people with developmental disabilities, representatives of state agencies that administer funds under federal laws related to individuals with disabilities, and representatives of local and nongovernmental agencies.

In addition, the Developmental Disabilities Act established Protection and Advocacy Organizations in each state charged with promoting and protecting the rights of individuals with developmental disabilities. These organizations provide legal assistance to individuals with developmental disabilities or to their families.[17]

The Voting Accessibility for the Elderly and Handicapped Act of 1984 generally requires polling places across the United States to be physically accessible to people with disabilities for federal elections. Where no accessible location is available to serve as a polling place, a political subdivision must provide an alternate means of casting a ballot on the day of the election. This law also requires states to make available registration and voting aids for voters who are elderly or disabled, including information by telecommunications devices for the deaf (TDDs), which are also known as teletypewriters (TTYs).[16]

The Fair Housing Act, as amended in 1988, prohibits housing discrimination on the basis of race, color, religion, sex, disability, familial status, and national origin. Its coverage includes private housing, housing that receives federal financial assistance, and state and local government housing. It makes it unlawful to discriminate in any aspect of selling or renting housing or to deny a dwelling to a buyer or renter because of the disability of that individual, an individual associated with the buyer or renter, or an individual who intends to live in the residence.[16]

The Fair Housing Act requires owners of housing facilities to make reasonable exceptions in their policies and operations to afford people with disabilities equal housing opportunities. For example, a landlord with a "no pets" policy may be required to grant an exception to this rule and allow an individual who is blind to keep a guide dog in the residence. The Fair Housing Act also requires landlords to allow tenants with disabilities to make reasonable access-related modifications to their private living space, as well as to common use spaces, although the landlord is not required to pay for the changes. The Act further requires that new multifamily housing with four or more units be designed and built to allow access for persons with disabilities. This includes accessible common use areas, doors that are wide enough for wheelchairs, kitchens and bathrooms that allow a person using a wheelchair to maneuver, and other adaptable features within the units.[16]

The ADA prohibits discrimination on the basis of disability in employment, state and local government, public accommodations, commercial facilities, transportation, and telecommunications.[16] To be protected by the ADA, a person must have a disability or have a relationship or association with an individual with a disability. An *individual with a disability* is defined by the ADA as a person who has a physical or mental impairment that substantially limits one or more major life activities, a person who has a history or record of such impairment, or a person who is perceived by others as having such impairment. The ADA does not specifically name all of the impairments that are covered.[16]

Title I of the ADA (Equal Opportunity Employment) requires employers with 15 or more employees to provide qualified individuals with disabilities an equal opportunity to benefit from the full range of employment-related opportunities available to others. It prohibits discrimination in recruitment, hiring, promotions, training, pay, social activities, and other privileges of employment. This Title restricts questions that can be asked about an applicant's disability before a job offer is made, and it requires that employers make reasonable

accommodation to the known physical or mental limitations of otherwise qualified individuals with disabilities, unless it results in undue hardship.[16]

Title II covers all activities of state and local government regardless of the government entity's size or receipt of federal funding. Title II requires that state and local governments give people with disabilities an equal opportunity to benefit from all of the state's programs, services, and activities (e.g., public education, employment, transportation, recreation, health care, social services, courts, and town meetings).[16]

State and local governments are required to follow specific architectural standards in the new construction and alteration of their buildings. They also must relocate programs or otherwise provide access in inaccessible older buildings, and communicate effectively with people who have hearing, vision, or speech impairments. Public entities are required to make reasonable modifications to policies, practices, and procedures where necessary to avoid discrimination, unless they can demonstrate that doing so would fundamentally alter the nature of the service, program, or activity being provided.[16]

The transportation provisions of Title II cover public transportation services, such as city buses and public rail transit (e.g., subways, commuter rails, Amtrak). Public transportation authorities may not discriminate against people with disabilities in the provision of their services. They must comply with requirements for accessibility in newly purchased vehicles, make a good faith effort to purchase or lease accessible buses, remanufacture buses in an accessible manner, and, unless it would result in an undue burden, provide paratransit where they operate fixed-route bus or rail systems. *Paratransit* is a service in which individuals who are unable to use the regular transit system independently (because of a physical or mental impairment) are picked up and dropped off at their destinations.[16]

Title III covers businesses and nonprofit service providers that are public accommodations, privately operated entities offering certain types of courses and examinations, privately operated transportation, and commercial facilities. *Public accommodations* are private entities that own, lease, or operate facilities such as restaurants, retail stores, hotels, movie theaters, private schools, convention centers, physicians' offices, homeless shelters, transportation depots, zoos, funeral homes, day care centers, and recreation facilities including sports stadiums and fitness clubs. Title III also covers transportation services provided by private entities.[16]

Public accommodations must comply with basic nondiscrimination requirements that prohibit exclusion, segregation, and unequal treatment. They also must comply with specific requirements related to architectural standards for new and altered buildings; reasonable modifications to policies, practices, and procedures; effective communication with people with hearing, vision, or speech impairments; and other access issues.

Additionally, public accommodations must remove barriers in existing buildings where it is easy to do so without much difficulty or expense, given the public accommodation's resources.[16]

Title IV addresses telephone and television access for people with hearing and speech impairments It requires common carriers (telephone companies) to establish interstate and intrastate telecommunications relay services (TRS) 24 hours a day, 7 days a week. TRS enables callers with hearing and speech impairments who use TDDs, and callers who use voice telephones to communicate with each other through a third party communications assistant. The Federal Communications Commission (FCC) has set minimum standards for TRS services. Title IV also requires closed captioning of federally funded public service announcements.[16]

POINTS TO REMEMBER

ADA

To be protected by the ADA, a person must have a disability or have a relationship or association with an individual with a disability. The various Titles of this law include:

Title I: Employment. Prohibits discrimination in recruitment, hiring, promotions, training, pay, social activities, and other privileges of employment

Title II: State and Local Governments. Requires that state and local governments give people with disabilities an equal opportunity to benefit from all of the state's programs, services, and activities, which include public transportation

Title III: Public Accommodations. Must comply with basic nondiscrimination requirements that prohibit exclusion, segregation, and unequal treatment; must comply with specific requirements related to architectural standards

Title IV: Telecommunications. Requires telephone companies to establish TRS 24 hours a day, 7 days a week (these include TDDs); also requires closed captioning of federally funded public service announcements

Section 255 and Section 251(a)(2) of the Communications Act of 1934, as amended by the *Telecommunications Act of 1996*, require manufacturers of telecommunications equipment and providers of telecommunications services to ensure that such equipment and services are accessible to and usable by persons with disabilities, if readily achievable. These amendments ensure that people with disabilities will have access to a broad range of products and services such as telephones, cell phones, pagers, call waiting, and operator services, which were often inaccessible to many users with disabilities.[16]

The Assistive Technology Act of 1998 was an amendment to Section 508 of the Rehabilitation Act of 1973. The Act covers access to federally funded programs and services. Its main purpose is to strengthen the already existing Section 508 of the Rehabilitation Act and access to technology provided by the federal government. Electronic and information technology are the focus. Federal agencies are required to make their buildings, web sites, and services accessible to people with disabilities.[19]

The Assistive Technology Act of 2004 is an amendment to the Assistive Technology Act of 1998. This amendment affects the states and their ability to provide assistance to millions of people with disabilities who depend on assistive technologies in their daily lives. This includes, but is not limited to early intervention, K–12, postsecondary, vocational rehabilitation, community living, and aging services programs. The purpose of this Act is to "provide states with financial assistance that supports programs designed to maximize the ability of individuals with disabilities and their family members, guardians, advocates, and authorized representatives to obtain assistive technology devices and assistive technology services."[20]

An advisory council carries out "consumer-responsive, consumer-driven advice" for planning, implementing, and evaluating programs. At least 60% of the funds available are used for state finance systems, device utilization, loans, and demonstration programs. A 40% maximum of funds is used on state leadership activities. These activities can include: training and technical assistance, public awareness, and coordination and collaboration.[20]

The device loan program involves loans to individuals or entities for devices. The device exchange program is for devices that are exchanged, repaired, recycled, or re-utilized. Demonstration of devices is a program that benefits individuals, communities, and entities.[20] Funds are not used for direct payment for an individual person's assistive device.

POINT TO REMEMBER

The Assistive Technology Act of 2004

Funds from the Assistive Technology Act are not used for direct payment for an individual person's assistive device.

According to a 1994 report from the Centers for Disease Control and Prevention (CDC) on the trends and usage of assistive technology devices, the number of people using assistive devices included 7.4 million with a mobility impairment, 4.6 million with an orthopedic impairment, 4.5 million with a hearing impairment (not including impairments fully compensated for by hearing aids), and 500,000 with a vision impairment.[21] Mobility impairment was the number one reason for the use of an assistive device, with a cane being most commonly used.[21] The age group with the most assistive devices used (hearing, mobility, and vision) was the >65 years age group. The majority of people who use any anatomic assistive device (a brace for any part of the body, such as a back, hand, or knee brace) were in the age group ≤44 years.[21]

The State Government

State governments have also passed laws and implemented programs that address the issue of employment or financial assistance for individuals with disabilities. The three most common of these state-run programs are workers' compensation, vocational rehabilitation, and the Medicaid program.

Workers' compensation was one of the first laws enacted that addressed work and disability. It is defined as the United States social insurance system for industrial and work-related injuries.[22] Workers' compensation is regulated at the state level. This statute requires the employer to pay benefits and to furnish care for job-related injuries sustained by employees, regardless of fault. It also requires payment of benefits to dependents of employees killed in the course of, and because of, their employment.

Each state has its own history on how its compensation laws were started. Workers' compensation laws were enacted to make litigation less costly and to eliminate the need for injured workers to prove their injuries were the employer's "fault." The first state workers' compensation law was passed in Maryland in 1902. By 1949, all states had enacted some kind of workers' compensation law.[23]

It is illegal in some states for an employer to terminate an employee for reporting a workplace injury or for filing a workers' compensation claim. Most states also prohibit refusing employment to a person who previously filed a workers' compensation claim. Those individuals who are disabled on the job and try to get another job somewhere else are protected from discrimination under the ADA.

Persons who are disabled on the job receive benefits depending on the resulting level of disability. The levels or categories of disability include permanent total disability, permanent partial disability, and temporary total disability. Each category has its own amount of compensation awarded and a specified length of benefit. Each state is different regarding the percentage of the workers' wage it will award and how long it will award the benefit. For example, for a permanent total disability the percentage of the workers' wage ranges from 60% to 80%. The length of the permanent total disability benefits can vary from 80 months to either the duration of disability or

until the age of 70. The average length of benefits corresponds to the duration of disability.[24]

Workers' compensation provides financial benefits for medical care related to the injury and lost wages, and pays for vocational rehabilitation if the worker cannot return to the job that he had prior to the injury. Putting people with disabilities to work, or enabling them to remain in their jobs with the onset of a disability, is one of the key elements of U.S. disability policy.[25]

Vocational rehabilitation refers to programs conducted by state vocational rehabilitation agencies operating under the Rehabilitation Act of 1973. Vocational rehabilitation programs provide or arrange for a wide array of training, educational, medical, and other services individualized to the needs of people with disabilities. The services are intended to help people with disabilities acquire, reacquire, and maintain gainful employment.[26] Services may include restoration of physical or mental functioning; academic, business, or vocational training; personal or vocational adjustment training; employment counseling; and job placement and referral. According to the Disability Statistics Abstract on Vocational Rehabilitation in the United States, among the most successfully rehabilitated people are those with an orthopedic impairment (20.8%), mental disorder (17.7%), or mental retardation (13.4%).[25] Successful participants spend approximately 2 years in the program, with 85.4% of the participants becoming competitively employed. Half of the participants find work in either industrial or service jobs.

Vocational rehabilitation programs are eligibility programs, not entitlements. The person must have a physical or mental disability, the disability must substantially impair the person's ability to work, and a reasonable expectation must exist that the provision of services will make the person employable.[27]

Probably the most well known of the state-run programs is the Medicaid program. Medicaid is a state-administered program with each state having its own guidelines regarding eligibility and services. People with a disability can qualify for Medicaid assistance (under the Optional Eligibility Groups) if they meet two criteria: one functional, the other financial. First, they have to be

BOX **10-1**
Social Security Administration's Definition of Disability

The SSA defines disability (for adults) as "inability to engage in any substantial gainful activity by reason of any medically determinable physical or mental impairment which can be expected to result in death or which has lasted or expected to last for a continuous period of not less than 12 months" [Section 223(d)(1)]. Amendments to the Act in 1967 further specified that an individual's physical and mental impairment(s) must be ". . . of such severity that he is not only unable to do his previous work but cannot, considering his age, education, and work experience, engage in any other kind of substantial gainful work which exists in the national economy, regardless of whether such work exists in the immediate area in which he lives, or whether a specific job vacancy exists for him, or whether he would be hired if he applied for work" (Sections 223 and 1614 of the Act).

BOX **10-2**
Medicaid Mandatory State Plan Services

Medicaid eligibility groups classified as categorically needy are entitled to the following services unless waived under section 1115 of the Medicaid law. These service entitlements do not apply to the SCHIP programs.

- Inpatient hospital (excluding inpatient services in institutions for mental disease)
- Outpatient hospital, including Federally Qualified Health Centers (FQHCs) and if permitted under state law, rural health clinic and other ambulatory services provided by a rural health clinic which are otherwise included under states' plans
- Other laboratory and x-ray
- Certified pediatric and family nurse practitioners (when licensed to practice under state law)
- Nursing facility services for beneficiaries 21 years old and older
- Early and periodic screening, diagnosis, and treatment (EPSDT) for children younger than 21 years*
- Family planning services and supplies
- Physician services
- Medical and surgical services of a dentist
- Home health services for beneficiaries who are entitled to nursing facility services under the state's Medicaid plan (intermittent or part-time nursing services, home health aides, medical supplies and appliances for use in the home)
- Nurse midwife services
- Pregnancy-related services
- 60 days postpartum pregnancy-related services

*Under the EPSDT program, states are required to provide all medically necessary services. This includes services that would otherwise be optional services. If an optional service is only available through the EPSDT program, it will not appear on this chart.

Centers for Medicare & Medicaid Services. Medicaid at a Glance 2005. A Medicaid Information Source. Washington DC: U.S. Department of Health and Human Services; 2005.

considered disabled as defined by the Social Security Administration's definition of disability (Box 10-1). To be financially eligible for disability benefits, a person must be unable to engage in substantial gainful activity (SGA). A person who is earning more than a certain monthly amount (net of impairment-related work expenses) is ordinarily considered to be engaging in SGA. The amount of monthly earnings considered as SGA depends on the nature of a person's disability.[28] In most states, an individual is automatically eligible for Medicaid if he or she is eligible for SSI.[29]

Services offered by Medicaid are extensive and usually free. States are allowed to provide a variety of services, but the federal government requires each state to make available certain basic services (Box 10-2).

POINT TO REMEMBER

Medicaid Eligibility

Medicaid is a state-administered program with each state having its own guidelines regarding eligibility and services. People with a disability can qualify for Medicaid assistance if they meet two criteria: one functional, the other financial. The Centers for Medicare & Medicaid Services provides information on the Medicaid programs in specific states.

Optional services that are important to people with disabilities may include prescription drug coverage; physical, occupational, and speech therapy services; prosthetic devices; eyeglasses; rehabilitation; ICFs; ICFs for mentally retarded persons (ICF-MR); and personal

care.[29] In 1971, Medicaid benefits were extended to cover services provided by ICFs. The purpose of this amendment was to provide a less costly alternative for medically indigent persons, who do not need the institutional or intensive care provided in hospitals and skilled nursing facilities.[30]

The Omnibus Reconciliation Act of 1981 (PL 97-35) further expanded the services provided by Medicaid, allowing states to apply for a waiver from the federal regulations in order to provide home- or community-based service packages to specific Medicaid populations.[29] These *waiver programs* [Section 1915(c) of the SSA] would allow an individual who meets the state requirements for the Medicaid nursing home benefit to receive services at home or in the community. The number of individuals served under a waiver program is limited by the state's ability to prove to the federal officials that the savings on nursing home care offsets waiver expenditures.[29] Most states share the cost of Medicaid services with the federal government at approximately a 50:50 ratio.[31]

POINT TO REMEMBER

Medicaid Waivers

A waiver allows the state to "give up the right" to comply with federal regulations for individuals who are eligible for nursing home services but demonstrate a cost savings by staying at home or in the community.

PARENT PERSPECTIVE

SALLY'S PERSPECTIVE (SARAH'S MOM)

When Sarah was a baby, during those impossibly difficult early years I would wish and dream for a time when my life would feel normal. Well, many years later, happily, life is normal. Spina Bifida is now just a part of life. Sarah's medical issues are always present, and the world always seems to present obstacles, but all of us now know how to meet these challenges with confidence. Sarah has received many different therapies over the years, all of which were helpful in their own ways. The common thread, the most important aspect, especially in those early years, was that we were all learning a new way of life. We took this new way of life very seriously, because we knew we were in this for the long haul, and, at the time, we didn't have the skills to get us through. We needed help, so we listened, we learned, we questioned, and we grew. When Sarah was young, we found ourselves in a very supportive environment, yet it was always made clear that we as a family would do the bulk of the work to help Sarah achieve all she could. The system seems more focused on young children. As Sarah has grown, we encounter many more people who seemed to have come up in the "dark ages" of disabilities. Sarah and I both find ourselves "training" principals, teachers, employers, and many people who should know better. Learning that new way of life in Sarah's early years has taught us how to politely demand, disagree, not give in, and advocate.

I am proud of Sarah. I am proud of the woman she has become. I am proud of how she has coped with all the challenges life has given her. I am proud of the excitement she feels about her future. I think she knows that she can accomplish anything. As parents, we plan for our children's independence from the moment they are born; if our child has a disability, we are even more aware of that goal. Each year, I have learned a little more about letting go. I will always have more to learn. I feel happy and secure knowing that Sarah can certainly take care of herself, thanks in part to her personality and the exceptional start she was given.

TRANSITIONING OUT OF HIGH SCHOOL

Transitioning out of high school is a critical time for all individuals. For young people with disabilities, the transition is an ending of entitlement programs and the related services they provided into the adult world of working, or postsecondary education, and possibly establishing living arrangements as a young adult. The student and family are leaving the relatively organized service delivery system of education, and entering one in which they are solely responsible for identifying, obtaining, and coordinating the services needed for employment and independent living.[27] All those years of educational instruction and planning have reached their zenith.

POINT TO REMEMBER

After High School

When the student leaves high school, he and his parents or guardian are responsible for identifying, obtaining, and coordinating the services needed for employment, independent living, or accommodations for college education.

Section 504 of the Rehabilitation Act states that "No otherwise qualified individual with a disability in the United States, as defined in section 706(8) of this title, shall, solely by reason of her or his disability, be excluded from the participation in, be denied the benefits of, or be subjected to discrimination under any program or activity receiving Federal financial assistance." [29 USC §794(a), 34CFR104.4(a)].[32] Nearly all postsecondary institutions receive federal financial assistance and would fall under this civil rights law. Many college campuses have an office for Disabled Student Services or Special Services.[27] But unlike education law (IDEA), colleges and universities are not mandated to provide services in accordance with an individualized education program. Accommodations, as identified under civil rights law, such as the Rehabilitation Act and the ADA, do come into play. Table 10-1 lists some of the general differences between secondary and postsecondary requirements for individuals with disabilities under Section 504 of the Rehabilitation Act.

Physical therapists can play an important role in preparing students for life after high school. Promoting functional skills that will carry over into the workplace or daily life of a student is an important aspect of a student's education. Such activities may include the strength and coordination to dress and perform daily hygiene tasks; the ability to manipulate not only the tools of education but the tools used in the workplace or at home; the ability to access communities, buildings, and classrooms; the ability to drive or access public transportation; or the endurance to attend to a job or academic program for several hours a day.

TABLE 10.1 A Comparison of Various Aspects of the Section 504 Regulations for School-Aged Children versus Postsecondary Education

	Preschool, Elementary, and Secondary	Postsecondary
Identification	Schools have an obligation to identify and locate children entitled to Section 504 protections.	No comparable obligation
Evaluation	Schools must undertake evaluation of children that they believe may be covered under Section 504.	Student is responsible for documentation concerning disability.
Entitlement to Education	Every child must be provided a free and appropriate public education. The educational program must be designed to meet an individual's needs.	Student has the right not to be excluded from educational programs or activities by reason of disability.
Planning Process	Schools must have in place policies and procedures that ensure the documentation and consideration of evaluative information.	No comparable provision for comprehensive planning for individuals.
Grievances	Schools must have in place grievance procedures and designate individuals responsible for 504 compliance.	Same
Due Process Rights	Schools need to provide notice to parents, an opportunity to examine records, an impartial hearing with opportunity for parental participation and representation by counsel, and a review procedure.	No comparable provision.

Adapted from: 504 Training. The Iowa Program for Assistive Technology. Training provided by John Allen (Clinical Professor of Law, University of Iowa), Mary Quigley (Co-Director, Iowa Program for Assistive Technology), and Lisa Heddens (Parent Training and Information Center of Iowa). Iowa City, Iowa. September 20, 2000. Available at: http://www.uiowa.edu/infotech/504Training.htm.

POINT TO REMEMBER

IDEA

IDEA does not apply to college level education. Because nearly all postsecondary institutions receive federal financial assistance, they have to comply with civil rights laws such as the ADA and the Rehabilitation Act.

LIVING OPTIONS

After high school, many children continue to live at home with their parents as they continue to mature socially, and then other living arrangements become desired or required. For a person with a severe disability, the options for living arrangements are dependent on caregiver availability and community resources. For many, the parent is the primary caregiver and the family home is the first choice for housing.

The cost of the services that family caregivers provide "free" is estimated to be approximately $257 billion a year. That is twice as much as is actually spent on home care and nursing home services.[33] The idea of a person with a disability living at home with his parents as the primary caregivers is socially acceptable and understandable, but several aspects of this arrangement should be clarified. First, does the person with a disability desire to live at home with his parents? Young adults, as they develop and mature, may desire their own living space

and environment in which they have more autonomy and privacy. The responsibility of maintaining one's own space also reflects independence and self-determination. Many children with disabilities may not see this as an option as they are growing up, because they are seldom exposed to the possibility. Also, do the parents of the adult child desire to have the child live with them? This is not the same as "will they," for the majority of parents will always welcome their children to live in the same house as they do. But do the parents of a child with a disability have the awareness and comfort of transitioning their child, who is more dependent on them than a child without a disability, into a new living arrangement? Are they knowledgeable of the services and support systems available that would allow their child to live in a type of arrangement other than the family home? Do the parents feel that this is important? Another obvious, but often not discussed issue is the fact that as parents age they may find it more difficult to care for their adult child at home. In the event that one or both parents die, the care for the adult child becomes an urgent issue, necessitating the need for community services or placement. Individuals and parents should be aware of their state programs and the various opportunities that may be available in their community. These can include such arrangements as independent living, the use of in-home services, and assisted or residential living.

Independent living is a philosophy for self-determination and equal opportunity. It does not mean that a person lives independently of everyone else. No one in society truly lives independently. Everyone has family, friends, and neighbors and lives in a community with grocery stores, parks, and shopping malls. Independent living for people with disabilities is the ability to live with the same opportunities and choices as your neighbor who does not have a disability. Many adults with disabilities choose to live in their own home and use a variety of community resources and supports. Adults who meet the criteria for Developmental Disabilities Waiver services are eligible for additional supports, like chore services, environmental modifications, and home-delivered meals. The National Council on Independent Living (NCIL) was founded in 1982 and represents more than 700 organizations and individuals including the Centers for Independent Living (CILs), Statewide Independent Living Councils (SILCs), individuals with disabilities, and other organizations that advocate for the human and civil rights of people with disabilities throughout the United States.[34]

POINT TO REMEMBER

Independent Living

Independent living is a philosophy of self-determination and equal opportunity. It does not mean that a person lives independently of everyone else.

Attendant services provide *in-home assistance* with activities of daily living (ADLs) and basic health maintenance activities. The goal is to provide support that enables a person with a disability to live in his or her own home. Some states offer Medicaid Waiver Assisted Living Services, which are provided in the home to Medicaid-eligible residents and can include such services as housekeeping, meal preparation, escort services, essential shopping, and medication assistance.

POINT TO REMEMBER

Waiver Programs

For more information on a specific state's home- and community-based waiver programs, contact the state's Medicaid office or access the Medicaid Web site.

Assisted living usually refers to a facility that is used by people who are not able to live on their own, but do not need the level of care that a skilled nursing facility offers. The term "assisted living" can have several different meanings, depending on the targeted population and services available. In 2001, the U.S. Senate created an Assisted Living Workgroup to develop recommendations

to assure consistent quality in assisted living services nationwide. One outcome was the following definition of assisted living:

> Assisted living is a state-regulated and monitored residential long-term care option. It provides or coordinates oversight and services to meet the residents' individualized scheduled needs, based on the residents' assessments, service plans, and unscheduled needs as they arise. Services that are required by state law and regulation to be provided or coordinated must include (but are not limited to):
>
> • 24-hour awake staff to provide oversight and meet scheduled and unscheduled needs
>
> • Provision and oversight of personal care and supportive services
>
> • Health-related services (e.g., medication management services)
>
> • Meals, housekeeping, and laundry
>
> • Recreational activities
>
> • Transportation and social services

These services are disclosed and agreed to in the contract between the provider and resident. Assisted living does not generally provide ongoing, 24-hour skilled nursing. It is distinguished from other residential long-term care options by the types of services that it is licensed to perform in accordance with a philosophy of service delivery that is designed to maximize individual choice, dignity, autonomy, independence, and quality of life.[35]

Residential care is an option for individuals who cannot live alone and require more supervision than is available through in-home community services. An ICF, as defined by the Centers for Medicare & Medicaid Services, is a facility that primarily provides health-related care and services above the level of custodial care to mentally retarded individuals, but does not provide the level of care available in a hospital or skilled nursing facility.[36] It is an optional Medicaid benefit. These residential facilities are licensed in accordance with state law and certified by the federal government as a provider of Medicaid services to persons with developmental disabilities (ICF-DD) or mental retardation (ICF-MR) in accordance with federal standards of operations. Hired staff provide, in a protected residential setting, ongoing evaluation, planning, 24-hour supervision, coordination, and integration of health or rehabilitative services to help each individual function at his greatest ability. Admission criteria will vary depending on the state program, but general criteria include the need for basic nursing care, assistance with ADLs, and care with physical and cognitive functioning or behavior problems. Most states do not allow admission of a person who needs 24-hour-a-day skilled nursing oversight. They are more appropriately referred to a skilled nursing facility.

EMPLOYMENT OPTIONS

Employment can be classified into three levels: competitive, supported, or sheltered. *Competitive employment* is defined as a full- or part-time job in the labor market with competitive wages and responsibilities in which the individual maintains the job with no more additional outside support than a coworker without a disability.[27] Many adolescents with disabilities leave high school with sufficient academic or vocational preparation to maintain competitive employment. These individuals only need assistance from an outside agency in order to locate an appropriate job.[27]

According to the Rehabilitation Act Amendments of 1986, *supported employment* is defined as competitive work in integrated work settings (with nondisabled peers) for individuals with the most significant disabilities. The provision of ongoing support distinguishes supported employment from competitive employment. Support is provided as long as the individual holds the job, allowing the person with a disability the opportunity to earn wages in job sites with their nondisabled peers.

Sheltered employment is the employment of individuals with disabilities in a self-contained work site, without integration with nondisabled coworkers. These employment sites can range from an adult day program, where the individual receives training in ADLs, social skills, and prevocational skills, to a sheltered workshop where the individual performs subcontracted tasks such as packaging, collating, or machine assembly.[27]

POINT TO REMEMBER

Employment Options

Competitive employment: Common type of employment for all people
Supported employment: Supports provided to enable a person to work in competitive employment
Sheltered employment: Employment in a self-contained work site

DRIVING

Access to public services and the community is a key aspect of independence and can be accomplished by accessing public transportation or private taxi services or by driving oneself. Obtaining a license to drive a car on public roads is a major activity in adolescence that adds to the teenager's independence and socialization. People who are disabled may require adaptive training or equipment to acquire this much sought-after skill. Learning to drive or relearning to drive after becoming disabled can aid in independence, return to work, and accessing public markets as well as providing an overall sense of autonomy and self-determination.

Learning to drive is not solely a physical skill. Driving is a multitask type of activity with a lot of visual processing and safety factors associated with it. No one test can determine the ability of a person to safely operate an automobile on public highways. This determination can only be made by taking a multidisciplinary examination and a "hands on" driving test. The ability to operate the car is only one aspect of driving. Appropriate mental actions and reactions and appropriate interactions with the highway environment while operating a car are crucial aspects of this highly skilled activity.[37] Awareness and observation of the activity in a person's immediate environment, visual scanning while moving, knowledge of the rules of driving, and eye–foot coordination are some of the key factors to consider when discussing the possible goal of driving.[38]

POINT TO REMEMBER

Driving

Driving is a multitask type of activity with a lot of physical skills, visual processing, and safety factors associated with it. A person with a disability can contact the state's Office of Vocational Rehabilitation to access programs on driver education.

AN EVALUATION FOR LIVING AND WORKING

Comprehensive evaluations are performed to identify the capabilities and impairments that may influence a person's ability to live as independently as possible as an adult member of society. The physical therapy evaluation can add to a comprehensive plan that should address not only the personal factors that affect disability but also the environmental and social factors as well. As with other formal plans, such as the Individualized Family Service Plan (IFSP) and Individualized Education Program (IEP), the outcome of the physical therapy evaluation is not to establish discipline- or impairment-specific goals, but rather to develop meaningful individualized goals and outcomes that will facilitate independence and autonomy for the person with a disability. These goals can include the identification and modification of environmental barriers, to independence with self-care and basic ADLs, to the identification of appropriate employment environments and activities.

The examination can include those common elements of any physical therapy evaluation, which are the demographic information, the medical diagnosis, current medications, current complaint or issue, and a systems review (see the Case Study). Examination of the person's ability to perform ADLs, instrumental ADLs (IADLs), and functional activities is vital to the evaluation of a person's capabilities and the development of strategies to promote independence (Box 10-3). The ability to perform

BOX 10-3
Definitions of ADLs, IADLs, and Function

ADLs: Everyday routines generally involving functional mobility and personal care and preparation[22,39]

Examples:

Personal Hygiene—Bathing, bowel and bladder management, brushing hair, brushing teeth, shaving

Dress—Getting dressed and undressed; donning shoes, socks, coat, gloves; manipulating fasteners (Velcro, hooks, buttons, zippers)

Feeding and Hydration—Eating, drinking, being able to cut meat, using utensils such as a spoon, fork, and knife

IADLs: Activities oriented to interactions with the environment, more complex than ADLs; optional (at times) or can be delegated[22,39]

Examples:

Financial Management—Going to the bank, keeping a checkbook, paying bills, managing spending

Meal Preparation—Preparing and cooking food, cutting, opening cans and jars, washing food, measuring items, keeping track of time

Shopping—For food, clothes, toiletries, household items

Medications—Preparing, organizing, buying, ordering, and managing medications, including safe and proper care, ability to dispense from container, and to take the proper dosage as prescribed

Telephone Use—Ability to operate a phone, call a person to talk, have appropriate conversations on the phone, call and talk in an emergency

Transportation—Ability to access public transportation, call taxi, or drive self

Housekeeping—Clean and maintain apartment, home, or living area

Function: Those activities identified by an individual as essential to support physical, social, and psychological well-being and to create a personal sense of meaningful living[39]

Functional activities can include ADLs and IADLs, in addition to activities such as standing, walking, carrying, squatting, and lifting or manipulating objects.

these activities can lead to the ability to hold a job and use public services, which in turn can lead to meeting people and developing relationships with others.

Part of the evaluation of a person's capability can include the use of *standardized tests*. By collecting objective information regarding functional skills, the physical therapist will have documentation that can be used to help evaluate a person's functional capabilities over time. Two commonly used standardized tests that can aid in this process are the Functional Independence Measure (FIM) and the Barthel Index.

The *FIM* is a criterion-referenced test that measures physical and cognitive disability in terms of burden of care.[40] Items are scored on a scale of 1 to 7, based on the amount of assistance a person needs to complete the item (1 = total assist to 7 = complete independence). The FIM includes 18 items categorized into areas of self-care, sphincter control, mobility, locomotion, communication, and social cognition. Ratings are based on observation or report. Total scores range from 18 to 126, with higher scores indicating more independent function in these areas. The psychometric properties of the FIM have been studied with several different populations, and the test has been shown to have good inter-rater reliability (0.86 to 0.96), content validity, and a strong correlation with the Barthel Index (0.84).[41–43]

The Barthel Index measures functional independence in personal care and mobility.[41] It can be done by a review of the person's medical record or from direct observation. Weighting of the items in the test reflects the aspect of disablement in impairment and disability as well as identifies the relative importance of that item in terms of care needed and social acceptability.[44] Total scores range from 0 to 100, with higher scores indicative of greater independence.

In the modified Barthel Index, eating and drinking are included as separate functions.[45] The modified version also has a range of total scores from 0 to 100. A total score of 60 is typically used as the threshold between marked dependence and independence. Shah et al.[46] suggest that scores of 0 to 20 (on either version) indicate total dependence, 21 to 60 severe dependence, 61 to 90 moderate dependence, and 91 to 99 slight dependence.

Reliability and validity have been established for both the 10- and 15-item tests with specific patient populations, namely inpatient rehabilitation for patients with traumatic brain injury or cerebral vascular accident and for adults with severe disabilities (inter-rater reliability = 0.89).[45,47] Two noted limitations of the Barthel Index are in the structure of the test, which may not detect low levels of disability, and that, unlike the FIM, the Barthel test has no specific cognitive test items.[48]

In addition to a person's functional capabilities, the type of *work* that the person is expected to perform can be evaluated with regard to the physical space and/or access as well as the specific tasks and body mechanics needed to perform the job. The physical space could be examined using the guidelines from the ADA regarding physical accessibility (a walk-through screen can be found in Box 10-4). An examination of the physical space begins with the approach to the work site and the ability to park a car or exit a transport vehicle and approach the building. Entrance into the building includes the ability to access the entrance doors and successfully open and pass through them into the building. Once inside, physical access to the primary work site as well as the ancillary sites, such as the lunchroom, rest rooms, emergency evacuation routes, and employee lounge, should be examined for accessibility. The actual task of work should also be

BOX 10-4
Quick Screen of Accessibility

BUILDING ACCESS
1. People with disabilities should be able to arrive and approach the building and enter as freely as anyone else.
2. Is there an adequate number of identified accessible parking spaces? (For every 25 under 100 spaces there should be one identified accessible space.)
3. Are the accessible parking spaces close to the accessible entrance?
4. Is there a route of entrance that does not require a step or stairs?
5. If there is a ramp for access, is the slope at least 1:12?
6. Is the entrance door at least 32 inches wide?
7. Is the door handle no higher than 48 inches? (Can you open the door with one hand?)
8. Is the threshold no more than 1/4 inch high?

BUILDING CORRIDORS
1. Ideally, the layout of the building should allow people with disabilities to access services without any more assistance than would be required by a person without a disability.
2. Is the path of travel at least 36 inches wide?
3. Are controls for public use accessible?
   a. Maximum height for side reach is 54 inches.
   b. Maximum height for forward reach is 48 inches.
4. Is the height of the elevator call button no more than 42 inches from the ground?
5. Do elevators provide an audible and visual signal?
6. At the cashier counter, is there a portion that is no more than 36 inches high?
7. Is there a water drinking fountain with a spout no higher than 36 inches from the ground?
8. If there are four or more public phones in the building, is one phone equipped with a text telephone (TT or TDD)?

PUBLIC REST ROOMS
Public rest rooms should be available to all members of the public, including people with disabilities.
1. If public rest rooms are available, is there at least one accessible rest room?
2. Can the door to the rest room be easily opened (5 lbf maximum force)?
3. Is there a 5-foot-diameter space/stall available in the rest room for a wheelchair to turn?
4. Is the toilet seat between 17 and 19 inches from the floor?
5. Is the sink 34 inches or lower above the floor?
6. Are the mirrors mounted with the bottom edge of the reflecting surface no higher than 40 inches from the floor?
7. Are soap and towel dispensers mounted no more than 48 inches from the floor?

Adapted from: ADA homepage. Available at: http://www.usdoj.gov/crt/ada/.

examined for the biomechanics needed to perform the task as well as the use of equipment or tools required for the job. The physical therapist can be instrumental in modifying the work space and tools in order to make the specific tasks of the job more ergonomically efficient and to decrease the risk of injury. Another aspect of work that should be examined is the work schedule. General questions that should be addressed include: Does the person have the endurance to sit or stand, or perform the movements, for the period of time needed to perform the job? Does the person have the ability to concentrate for an appropriate amount of time to perform tasks associated with the job? Does the person demonstrate appropriate behavior to perform the job safely? These questions will address the issue of endurance and concentration needed to perform the job well. Timing of medications, meals, rest periods, and the tasks associated with the job should be examined to make sure that the schedule fits the individual person and meets the needs of both the worker and the employer.

POINT TO REMEMBER

Work Evaluation

Work can be evaluated with regard to the physical space in which the job is performed as well as the specific tasks and body mechanics needed to perform the job. Complete information regarding accessibility guidelines under the ADA are available at www.ada.gov.

INDIVIDUAL HABILITATION PLAN

When the evaluation of the person, the physical environment of home or work, and the activities needed to participate in these environments is complete, the physical therapist can participate in the construction of an *Individual Habilitation Plan* (IHP), Individual Service Plan (ISP), or an Individual Program Plan (IPP). Much like the IFSP and IEP, the IHP is an individualized plan to address the needs and desires of a person who resides in an ICF. An interdisciplinary team, including the person with a disability (either in person or through his legal guardian), provides input into the development of the IHP which "must be directed toward the acquisition of the behaviors necessary for the individual to function with as much self-determination and independence as possible and the prevention or deceleration of regression or loss of current optimal functional status" [42CFR483.440(a)].[49] The physical therapist can provide key information on a variety of health-related issues, but most importantly on promoting functional skills in the areas of daily living and work ability. The Appendix shows one example of an IHP and the general type of information that is captured in this type of document. The structure of the IHP can vary from agency to agency.

When the team meets to construct an IHP, *goals* are identified and agreed upon. Goals on an IHP should be objective, measurable, and most importantly related to a functional activity in the person's life. According to Kettenbach,[50] appropriate goals in physical therapy should contain references to the audience, person, or caregiver (A), the identified behavior or what the person will do (B), the conditions in which the behavior will be observed (C), and the degree to which the behavior will be implemented (D). In addition, the physical therapist should keep in mind the education required of the caregiver or person in order to perform the behavior (E) and the functional relevance of the behavior in the person's everyday life (F).

POINTS TO REMEMBER

Goal Writing

When constructing goals, remember:
A: Audience
B: Behavior
C: Condition
D: Degree
E: Education needed
F: Functional relevance

When the IHP has been established, appropriate services are provided. The *interventions* used by the physical therapist when working with adults with disabilities is no different from any of the interventions used with adults without disabilities. The purpose when providing services is to maximize the person's ability to function within his daily life. In many instances, when working with a person who has a chronic condition, the goal is not to change the underlying condition but to make the person more able to function. This can be done by addressing those impairments to a specific ability that are inherent in the person, in the home or work environment, or in society (what other people believe he can do). As in other settings, coordination, communication, and documentation are vital components of intervention. Patient/client-related instruction, as well as caregiver instruction if appropriate, is necessary to assure implementation of the recommended interventions into the daily life of the individual. Specific procedural interventions may include functional training in self-care, home management, work, and leisure activities. As with all adults, physical activity and exercise can help promote a healthy lifestyle and maintenance of function for many years.

POINTS TO REMEMBER

Interventions

When choosing interventions, the physical therapist should keep in mind:

1. Coordination, communication, and documentation
2. Patient/client-related instruction, as well as caregiver instruction
3. Procedural interventions can include functional training.

FINANCIAL ASSISTANCE

In addition to the income generated through employment, common financial assistance programs available to adults include the federal government's welfare program, SSDI, and SSI.

The Merriam-Webster dictionary defines *welfare* as aid in the form of money or necessities for those in need and an agency or program through which aid is distributed.[51] Welfare has different meanings. What is generally considered welfare by politicians and the general public is the Aid for Families with Dependent Children (AFDC), which is today called *Temporary Assistance to Needy Families* (TANF).[52] The other meaning for welfare is the broad general term of all government programs providing benefits to needy Americans. These programs can include Medicaid, food stamps, SSI, and Housing and Urban Development (HUD) programs.[52]

TANF provides financial assistance and work opportunities to eligible families by granting states the federal funds to develop and implement welfare programs in the state. Citizens are able to apply at their local TANF agency. TANF is run through the U.S. Department of Health and Human Services, Office of Family Assistance.[53] It has four purposes: to assist families so that children can be cared for in their own homes; to reduce the dependence of parents by promoting job preparation, work, and marriage; to prevent out-of-wedlock pregnancies; and to encourage the formation and maintenance of two-parent families.[54]

The work requirements under TANF require recipients to work as soon as they are job ready or no later than 2 years after coming on assistance. Single parents are required to participate in work activities for at least 30 hours per week, and two-parent families must participate in work activities 35 to 55 hours per week. Failure to participate in work requirements can result in reduction or termination of benefits to the family. States cannot penalize a single parent with a child younger than 6 years for failing to meet work requirements if he or she cannot find adequate child care. States have to ensure that 50% of all enrolled families and 90% of two-parent families are participating in work activities.[54] These activities may include community service, on-the-job training, vocational training, and satisfactory secondary school attendance. There is a 5-year limit for families receiving TANF funding.[54]

Food stamps are another form of public assistance, which is based on household size and countable income after deductions are applied. Those households that have an elderly or disabled person are given special consideration. Food stamps are generally used to purchase food for human consumption and seeds and/or plants to grow food at home. There are limitations on the type of items that can be purchased with food stamps. These limitations may include certain household items, grooming products, tobacco, alcohol products, or pet food, to name a few.[55]

POINTS TO REMEMBER

Welfare

Welfare has several different meanings. It can be the aid provided by the TANF program or a multitude of other government programs ranging from food stamps to SSI. When taking a history, the interviewer should clarify what is meant by "welfare."

The Social Security Administration has two disability programs, SSDI and SSI. SSDI is funded through employees', employers', and self-employed persons' contributions and covers injured workers, their widows or widowers and dependents, and people with disabilities. In order to be eligible, a person must meet certain criteria. Income is one criterion and is based on the amount of benefit tied to a person's work history and earnings. Being disabled is another criterion.[56] A person has to meet the definition of disability according to the Social Security Administration, which is "being unable to perform the work that was done prior to becoming disabled or unable to adjust to other work because of a medical condition."[57] The disability must also last, or be expected to last, for at least 1 year or to result in death, and the person has to have a work history long enough and recent enough under Social Security to qualify.[58] In general, SSDI pays monthly cash benefits to people who are unable to work for 1 year or more because of a disability.[58] Other members of a family that may also qualify for SSDI may include a spouse, children, and children with a disability.[56]

SSI is a program administered by the Social Security Administration for eligible individuals (adults or children) who are disabled or blind, or who are 65 years old or older with limited income and resources (things they own). This program is funded by general tax revenue, not social security taxes. With SSI, a fixed monthly payment is provided, with some states supplementing this amount. The money from SSI is used to meet the basic needs of the individual for food, clothing, and shelter.[59]

POINTS TO REMEMBER

Disability Programs

The Social Security Administration has two disability programs, SSDI and SSI. Income level and disability are the criteria used for eligibility. To apply for SSI, you can do so on the Web at www.socialsecurity.gov. Parents or the guardian of a child who is disabled or blind can apply if the child is younger than 18 years.

■ CASE STUDY ■

Physical Therapy Evaluation: Resident in an ICF-MR

Name:	Margaret Alexander
Address:	1104 Kingstown Road
	Wheeling WV 39608
Date of birth:	05-20-57
Date of Evaluation:	05-30-05
Age:	48 years

Insurance: Medicaid

Guardian: Joe Weatherman		Phone: 304-589-6353
Physician: Tim Knierum, MD		Phone: 304-787-4598

Place of employment: County Workshop

Supervisor: Theresa Haddad	Phone: 695-243-4446

Medical Diagnosis: Mild Mental Retardation, Arteriosclerosis, Hyperlipidemia, Intermittent Explosive Disorder, Obesity, Gastroesophageal Reflux Disease, History of Seizure Disorder, Osteoarthritis

Medications: Lipitor 40 mg, Tegretol 200 mg, oyster shell 500 mg, Naproxen 500 mg, Zoloft 100 mg

Reason for referral: Annual review. Ms. Alexander, guardian (Joe Weatherman), and house staff report no concerns or needs at present.

Systems Review

Height	5'5"
Weight	197 lb
Vision	Wears glasses; nearsighted
Hearing	Intact
Behavior during examination	Cooperative; followed one-step request
Communication	Verbal; will communicate in complete sentences
Oral motor skills	Not impaired
Heart rate	71 bpm, regular
Shoe size	8½ wide
Edema	+1 in her lower extremities; capillary refill in feet <3 s
Sensation	Appears intact to light touch in lower extremities
Integumentary	No obvious surgical scars noted upon visual examination of her extremities and trunk
Assistive devices	Bilateral flexible orthotics with arch supports; adaptive equipment for eating, which includes a nonskid placemat, plate guard, and built-up handled spoon and fork

EXAMINATION FINDINGS

Musculoskeletal Status

The range of motion in the upper extremities is within functional limits. Her spine presents with a kyphoscoliosis, with a rib hump in the right thoracic region. Curve does not change with forward flexion. Range of motion in the lower extremities demonstrates asymmetrical symmetrical hip abduction RCL with 45 degrees of external rotation bilaterally, 45 degree of hip internal rotation on the left, and 30 degrees on the right. There is hip extension to neutral bilaterally, with a soft end feel noted. Hip flexion is 120 degree bilaterally. Popliteal angles were 55° measured bilaterally, ankle motions are within functional limits. She presents with pronated feet, for which she wears orthotics. The orthotics appear to fit well and were last replaced 4 months ago.

Calf girth measurements taken 10 cm distal to the tibial tubercle resulted in 39 cm on the right and 36 cm on the left. These measurements are unchanged from those taken 6 months ago. She has a long-standing history of edema in the lower extremities.

Neuromuscular Status

She is negative for clonus in the ankles. There is no report of falling in the last 6 months. Balance responses of ankle and stepping strategies were noted in stance. Ms. Alexander does not report pain in her hips. Her caregivers report that she appears to have hip pain occasionally as noted by an increase in limping, especially after she returns from work.

Cardiopulmonary Status

No adventitious sounds were heard with auscultation of the lungs. Ms. Alexander reports no episodes of shortness of breath. Her caregivers do not report her having any shortness of breath. Her present level of endurance is sufficient for her level of activity; it does not impair her ability to participate in daily activities, work, or social outings. She does not have a history of respiratory infection over the last year.

Functional Status

Bed mobility: Independent.

Transfers: Independent in transfers from sit to stand. She is able to transfer into and out of the bathtub. She is able to transfer onto and off of a standard toilet. Ms. Alexander will step onto and out of the van with handrail assistance.

Gait/Mobility: Ms. Alexander can ambulate 200' in 75 seconds. Gait pattern demonstrates a decreased stance phase on right and hip and knee flexion when walking. Trunk flexed at hips. She is able to ascend (step over step) and descend (step to step) five steps with the assist of a handrail. (There are five steps at her place of employment). She wears foot orthotics with a medial arch support.

Activities of Daily Living (by staff report): Ms. Alexander can dress herself, requiring minimal assistance for orientation and closure of fasteners. She requires assistance with bathing (preparing the washcloth and providing verbal cues) to complete the task sufficiently. She is able to eat her meals independently, using a plate guard and nonskid mat. She drinks from a regular cup. She will use the toilet when cued to do so. She requires only minimal assistance for hygiene. She does have episodes of bladder incontinence, approximately once a month by report. She is continent of bowel.

FIM Score: 63/126. Areas requiring the most assistance include sphincter control, self-care, and social cognition. Areas of most independence include locomotion, mobility, and communication.

Work

Ms. Alexander is employed by Belmont Workshop where she works as a laborer. Her main job is putting labels on boxes. Her job requires long periods of sitting, the ability to transition from sit to stand, and the use of bilateral upper extremities to manipulate labels and empty cardboard boxes, with dimensions typically 2' × 1' × 6". The job also requires the ability to rotate her trunk, to grasp and place boxes in front of her, and to stack boxes one on top of the other, three boxes high.

Leisure Activities

She enjoys rides in an automobile, watching movies at the local cinema, attending county fairs, going on brief walks of approximately 15 to 30 minutes, and picking wildflowers.

RECOMMENDATIONS

Consult with physician regarding gait deviation. Possible radiograph of right hip may be appropriate. Arch supports in shoes fit well, but may need to be replaced in 6 months due to general wear.

Reflection Questions

1. Identify the specific movements needed for Ms. Alexander to perform her job. What are the key muscles associated with the identified movements? Prescribe three exercises that Ms. Alexander could perform at home that would maintain her strength, flexibility, or endurance to perform her job.
2. Because she requires assistance with bathing, identify the features that would optimize safety for both Ms. Alexander and her caregiver during this task.
3. Identify appropriate assistive technology that would promote her independence in dressing.

SUMMARY

Throughout this book, transitioning has been presented as the movement from one program into another with their unique rules and regulations and expected role of the physical therapist. In this chapter on practice, transitioning is discussed in its broader application, from one phase of life into the next. Children with disabilities grow into adults with disabilities, who in turn age into seniors with disabilities. In the natural course of human events, as one ages there is a decline in physical activity and capability, accompanied by the loss of friends and family through death. The loss of a parent is an especially difficult transition, made even harder when that parent has been the primary caregiver for a person with a disability.

A key question arises at this time: Who will assume the role of caregiver? Death is not the only event that forces this question. Natural aging of both the parent and the dependent child will eventually lead to a decline in the physical capabilities of both. What happens when a 62-year-old mother can no longer lift her 37-year-old son? Who will assume this role?

A physical therapist, who is the family's practitioner of choice and has provided services to the family and child for several years, has a unique role in facilitating discussions on what can be a very emotional and oftentimes difficult topic about the future. Factors that affect an individual's ability to live on his own, to participate in some form of employment, or to acquire other characteristics commonly attributed to adulthood accumulate over years of growth and development on both the part of the individual and his or her parents. The physical therapist can educate the parents on the importance of fostering skills in their child that will develop into characteristics of self-determination and independence. Respecting a child's decisions, giving her true choices, letting her experience the effect of her choices and behaviors, and when appropriate, giving her freedom to be on her own (if only for one night at a sleepover or a few hours at home alone) can aid in the development of adult behaviors and characteristics.

Educating the family on the options and resources that are available in the community is an important aspect of the transitioning process that is continually occurring as the child ages. Each family is unique in their beliefs and in how they function as a family unit. Honest discussion on the role of the parents, siblings, and the child with a disability could facilitate a mutual understanding of each family member's needs. Periodic discussions on future plans and aspirations, caregiver support, and service options should be viewed as a natural part of life planning, just as many families discuss issues of the future for any child. What do you want to be when you grow up? Where do you think you would like to live? Where would you like to work? Who, or what supports, will be needed to achieve these goals? All children, regardless of their disability, should be presented with his or her options, including those that involve sheltered workshops and residential living arrangements.

By planning for these major life transitions, the physical therapist as well as other people involved in the life of a person with a disability can make one step forward to "ensuring equality of opportunity, full participation, independent living, and economic self-sufficiency for individuals with disabilities."[1]

REVIEW QUESTIONS

1. Self-determination is an important aspect of adulthood. When does an individual begin to learn the basic skills necessary to develop the adult attribute of self-determination?
   a. When he is a young child
   b. When he is an adolescent
   c. When he is a young adult
   d. When he begins to live on his own

2. Of the following, which group of people is most likely to have the highest unemployment rate?
   a. People who are unable to hear conversations
   b. People who are unable to clearly see words or letters
   c. People who are impaired in their mobility
   d. People who are unable to lift more than 10 pounds

3. You are performing an evaluation of a home to determine if the environment is suitable for wheelchair access. What is the recommended minimum width from left to right of a door opening that would allow a wheelchair user to pass through?
   a. 26 inches
   b. 28 inches
   c. 32 inches
   d. 36 inches

4. In the evaluation of a home for wheelchair access you note that there are five 6-inch steps that lead to the front door. What is the recommended minimum length of a ramp that is needed for a person using a manual wheelchair to access this height difference?
   a. 6 feet
   b. 11 feet
   c. 30 feet
   d. 70 feet

5. You are planning the annual budget for the physical therapy department. You want to make sure you have enough equipment to try on the patients to whom you will provide services in the coming year. Which of the assistive technology devices listed below is the most commonly used device?
   a. Computerized communication device
   b. Wheelchair
   c. TDD
   d. Cane

6. Medicaid is a state-administered program, and each state sets its own guidelines regarding eligibility and services. People with a disability can qualify for Medicaid assistance if they meet which of the criteria listed below?
   a. They have to demonstrate a financial need and be disabled as defined by the Social Security Administration's definition of disability.
   b. They have to demonstrate a financial need in accordance with the federal poverty guidelines.
   c. They have to be diagnosed by their physician as having a permanent disability.
   d. They must have a disability that is expected to last for at least 1 year or to result in death, and the person has to have a work history long enough and recent enough under Social Security to qualify.

7. As a physical therapist you are working with a family who is transitioning their 18-year-old son from high school to college. Of the following sentences, which would apply to their son who has been receiving special education instruction in accordance with his IEP while in high school?
   a. IDEA is applicable as long as the person is attending college.
   b. Universities are mandated to provide services in accordance with an individual education plan.
   c. Disabled Student Services is solely responsible for identifying, obtaining, and coordinating the services needed for employment and independent living after secondary school.
   d. Reasonable accommodations, as identified under civil rights law, such as the Rehabilitation Act and the ADA, apply to college programs and services.

8. This type of employment arrangement provides ongoing support and is integrated into a work setting with nondisabled peers for individuals with the most significant disabilities. Support is provided as long as the individual holds the job, allowing the person with a disability the opportunity to earn wages in job sites with their nondisabled peers.
   a. Competitive employment
   b. Supported employment
   c. Sheltered employment
   d. Attendant services

9. You have been asked to perform an evaluation on Harold Green, who is a resident of a local ICF-MR. The staff is concerned about Mr. Green's ability to transfer in and out of the van used to transport him to work. Until recently, he would transfer independently. Two weeks ago he began requiring some level of assistance to complete this task. Of the following, which would be the most appropriate goal for Harold Green?
   a. Mr. Green will increase the muscle strength of his quadriceps muscles from 4/5 to 5/5.
   b. Mr. Green will improve his gait pattern with noted dorsiflexion during the swing/through phase, perform consistently.
   c. Mr. Green will increase the active range of motion of his hip joint into extension.
   d. Mr. Green will improve his ability to step into and out of the van used for transportation.

10. Gregory is working at the local supermarket. His employer has requested help in making his place of employment more accessible and efficient for Gregory to complete his work during an 8-hour shift. After your examination, you do not note any physical barriers or biomechanical inefficiencies that would impair Gregory's ability to perform his job. Of the following, which one identifies another factor to consider for this request?
    a. Gregory's work schedule and his endurance to perform the specific job tasks
    b. Gregory's transportation to and from work
    c. Gregory's ability to manage his bank account and paycheck
    d. Gregory's eligibility for TANF assistance

A Habilitation Plan

DEPARTMENT OF HEALTH AND FAMILY SERVICES
Office of Quality Assurance
OQA-2371 (Rev. 10-06)

STATE OF WISCONSIN

INDIVIDUAL SERVICE PLAN (ISP)
(Model Form)

To be completed within 30 days of admission, updated every 6 months thereafter or more often when indicated by a change in the resident's condition

Name-Resident	Admission Date

Facility Name and Address

Date - Original ISP	Date - 6-Month Progress Review	Date - Annual Evaluation	Date - 6-Month Progress Review

SIGNATURE OF PARTICIPANTS

Resident or Guardian	Resident or Guardian	Resident or Guardian	Resident or Guardian
Agent or Designated Representative	Agent or Designated Representative	Agent or Designated Representative	Agent or Designated Representative
Licensee or Administrator	Licensee or Administrator	Licensee or Administrator	Licensee or Administrator
Others	Others	Others	Others

MEDICATIONS: (check one)
☐ Controls own medication (HFS 83.33(3)(b))
☐ Self administers own medication and staff supervises (HFS 83.33(3)(e))
☐ Medications administered by CBRF staff (HFS 83.33(3)(e)) (medical order from a practitioner is required)
☐ No medications

NURSING PROCEDURES:

☐ None   ☐ Yes (HFS 83.32(2)(a)3) If Yes, no. of hours per week

ALLERGIES: _____

_____

_____

_____

CAPACITY FOR SELF DIRECTION: (HFS 83.32(2)(a)7) **(check one)**

☐ Makes own decisions   ☐ Makes needs known
☐ Needs assistance   ☐ Cannot make needs known

RESIDENT HAS ADVANCE DIRECTIVES (HFS 83.33(2)(I))

☐ No   ☐ Yes   ☐ Activated   ☐ Not Activated

SUPERVISION: (HFS 83.33(2)(a) **(check one)**
☐ Capable of self supervision
☐ Needs some supervision; Describe: _____

_____

_____

☐ 24-hour supervision
☐ Other _____

CAPACITY FOR SELF CARE: (HFS 83.32(2)(a)6) **(check one)**

☐ Independent
☐ Needs some assistance
☐ Needs total assistance
☐ List any adaptive equipment _____

_____

_____

_____

MEDICATIONS

Current Medications	Reason	Physician	Side Effects	6-Month Progress Review	Annual Evaluation	6-Month Progress Review
				List any changes	List any changes	List any changes

PERSONAL CARE

	Current Status	Frequency of Service and Service Provided	Goal/Outcome	Service Provider Responsible	6-Month Progress Review List any changes	Annual Evaluation List any changes	6-Month Progress Review List any changes
Eating							
Special Diet							
Oral Care							
Dressing							
Grooming							
Bathing							
Toileting							
Other							

BEHAVIOR PATTERNS

	Current Status	Frequency of Service and Service Provided	Goal/Outcome	Service Provider Responsible	6-Month Progress Review List any changes	Annual Evaluation List any changes	6-Month Progress Review List any changes
Wandering							
Self-Abusive Behavior							
Propensity to Choke on Certain Foods							
Suicidal Tendencies							
Destruction of Property or Self, Physically or Mentally Abusive							
Evacuation Capability In Emergency							
Other							

PHYSICAL HEALTH HFS 83.32(2)(a)1

	Current Status	Frequency of Service and Service Provided	Goal/Outcome	Service Provider Responsible	6-Month Progress Review List any changes Date: Signature:	Annual Evaluation List any changes Date: Signature:	6-Month Progress Review List any changes Date: Signature:
General Health							
Chronic Illnesses							
Short-term illnesses							
Recurring Illnesses							
Physical Disabilities							
Hearing							
Eyesight							
Nursing Procedures							

MENTAL AND EMOTIONAL HEALTH

	Current Status	Frequency of Service and Service Provided	Goal/Outcome	Service Provider Responsible	6-Month Progress Review List any changes Date: Signature:	Annual Evaluation List any changes Date: Signature:	6-Month Progress Review List any changes Date: Signature:
Self Concepts							
Maturation							
Attitude							
Interaction with Others							
Aggressive/Combative							
Verbal							

SOCIAL PARTICIPATION

	Current Status	Frequency of Service and Service Provided	Goal/Outcome	Service Provider Responsible	6-Month Progress Review List any changes Date: Signature:	Annual Evaluation List any changes Date: Signature:	6-Month Progress Review List any changes Date: Signature:
Interpersonal Relationships							
Leisure Time Activities							
Family Contacts							
Community Contacts							
Religious Activities							
Other							

INDEPENDENT LIVING SKILLS Describe what skills are being taught to increase or maintain independence

	Current Status	Frequency of Service and Service Provided	Goal/Outcome	Service Provider Responsible	6-Month Progress Review List any changes Date: Signature:	Annual Evaluation List any changes Date: Signature:	6-Month Progress Review List any changes Date: Signature:
Educational Skills							
Vocational Skills							
Money Management							
Communication Skills							
Food Preparation							
Shopping							
Use of Public Transportation							
Seeking/Retaining Employment							
Housekeeping Skills							
Other							

REFERENCES

1. Individuals with Disabilities Education Improvement Act of 2004. 20 USC 1400. Title I. Sec. 601(c)(1).
2. Kaye S. Is the Status of People with Disabilities Improving? Disability Statistics Abstract. Disability Statistic Center. Washington, DC: U.S. Department of Education, National Institute on Disability and Rehabilitation Research; May 1998;21.
3. Arnett J. Emerging adulthood—a theory of development from the late teens through the twenties. *Am Psychol.* 2000;55:469–480.
4. Jordan B, Dunlap G. Construction of adulthood and disability. *Ment Retard.* 2001;39:286–296.
5. Porter RE. Normal development of movement and function: child and adolescent. In: Scully RM, Barnes MR, eds. *Physical Therapy.* Philadelphia, PA: JB Lippincott; 1989.
6. Culbertson JL, Newman JE, Willis DJ. Childhood and adolescent psychologic development. *Pediatr Clin North Am.* 2003;50:741–764.
7. Kaeser F. Can people with severe mental retardation consent to mutual sex? *Sex Disabil.* 1992;10:33–42.
8. Wehmeyer M, Schalock R. Self-determination and quality of life: implications for special education services and supports. *Focus Except Child.* 2001;33:1–16.
9. United Nations Millennium Project. Investing in Development: A Practical Plan to Achieve the Millennium Development Goals. Report to the U.N. Secretary-General. London: Earthscan; 2005;120.
10. Steinmetz E. Household Economic Studies. Current Population Reports. P70-107. Americans with Disabilities: 2002. U.S. Census Bureau. U.S. Department of Commerce. 2002. Available at: http://www.census.gov/hhes/www/disability/sipp/disab02/awd02.html. Accessed January 25, 2007.
11. U.S. Census Bureau. *Survey of Income and Program Participation.* In: Kraus LE, Stoddard S, Gilmartin D. Chartbook on Disability in the United States, 1996. An InfoUse report. Washington, DC. U.S. Department of Education, National Institute on Disability and Rehabilitation Research. Available at: http://www.infouse.com/disabilitydata/disability/index. php. Accessed May 17, 2006.
12. Sultz H, Young K. *Health Care USA. Understanding Its Organization and Delivery,* 4th ed. Boston: Jones and Bartlett; 2004.
13. University of Iowa. Major Disability-Related Legislation 1956-1999. Appendix 2. Available at: http://disability.law.uiowa.edu/csadp_docs/APPENDIX_2_APR.txt. Accessed April 2, 2006.
14. Kollmann G, Solomon-Fears C. Major decisions in the House and Senate on Social Security: 1935-2000. Social Security Administration. Legislative history: CRS legislative histories. Available at: http://www.ssa.gov/history/reports/crsleghist3.html. Accessed April 2, 2006.
15. Supplemental Security Income. Social Security Online. U.S. Social Security Administration. Available at: http://www.ssa.gov/notices/supplemental-security-income/. Accessed July 10, 2006.
16. U.S. Department of Justice, Civil Rights Division, Disability Rights Section. A Guide to Disability Rights Laws. Available at: http://www.usdoj.gov/crt/ada/cguide.htm. Accessed April 2, 2006.
17. The Developmental Disabilities Assistance and Bill of Rights Act 2000. (PL 106–402) Available at: http://www.acf.hhs.gov/programs/add/ddact/DDACT2.html. Accessed August 21,2007.
18. Developmental Disabilities Programs/Partners. Administration on Developmental Disabilities. Administration for Children and Families. U.S. Department of Health and Human Services. Available at: http://www.acf.hhs.gov/programs/add/addprogram.html. Accessed July 10, 2006.
19. Information Technology Accessibility & Workforce Division (ITAW), Office of Governmentwide Policy, U.S. General Services Administration. Assistive Technology Act of 1998. Available at: http://www.section508.gov/docs/AT1998.html. Accessed May 29, 2006.
20. Association of Assistive Technology Act Programs. Current Legislation. Available at: http://www.ataporg.org/publications.asp. Accessed May 29, 2006.
21. Russel JN, Hendershot GE, LeClere F, et al. Trends and differential use of assistive technology devices: United States, 1994. Advance data from Vital and Health Statistics; no. 292 of the National Center for Health Statistics, Centers for Disease Control and Prevention, 1997. Available at: http://www.cdc.gov/nchs/data/ad/ad292.pdf
22. *Stedman's Medical Dictionary for Health Professions and Nursing* Illustrated, 5th ed. Baltimore, MD: Lippincott, Williams & Wilkins; 2005.
23. Wikipedia Foundation, Inc. Wikipedia The Free Encyclopedia. Workers' compensation. Available at: http://en.wikipedia.org/wiki/Workers_compensation. Accessed May 17, 2006.
24. United States Department of Labor. Employment Standards Administration. Office of Workers' Compensation Programs. State Workers' Compensation Laws, List of Benefits Table. Available at: http://www.dol.gov/esa/regs/statutes/owcp/stwclaw/stwclaw.htm. Accessed May 17, 2006.
25. Kaye HS. Vocational Rehabilitation in the United States. Disabilities Statistics Abstract Number 20. Washington, DC: U.S. Department of Education, National Institute on Disability and Rehabilitation Research; 1998.
26. National Institute on Disability and Rehabilitation Research. Chartbook on Disability in the U.S. Appendices: glossary. Available at: http://www.infouse.com/disabilitydata/mentalhealth/appendices_glossary.php. Accessed May 17, 2006.
27. Valdivieso C. Transition Summary. Options After High School for Youth with Disabilities. National Information Center for Children and Youth with Disabilities (NICHCY) 1991;7:1–28.
28. U.S. Social Security Administration. Social Security Online. Substantial Gainful Activity. Available at: http://www.ssa.gov/OACT/COLA/SGA.html. Accessed June 3, 2006.
29. Tanenbaum S. Medicaid and Disability: The Unlikely Entitlement. *Milbank Q.* 1989;67(Suppl 2 Pt 2):288–310.
30. Social Security Online. Social Security History. Available at: http://www.ssa.gov/history/nixstmts.html#amend. Accessed May 17, 2006.
31. Clifton D. Disability management in long term care. In: Clifton D, ed. *Physical Rehabilitation's Role in Disability Management. Unique Perspectives for Success.* St. Louis, MO: Elsevier Saunders; 2005:57.
32. Section 504 of the Rehabilitation Act of 1973, 29 USC §794.
33. Arno P. Economic Value of Informal Caregiving. Presented at the American Association of Geriatric Psychiatry, Orlando, Fla; February 24, 2002.
34. History of the National Council on Independent Living. Washington, DC: National Council on Independent Living. Available at: http://www.ncil.org/about.html. Accessed July 12, 2006.
35. The Assisted Living Workgroup. Assuring Quality in Assisted Living: Guidelines for Federal and State Policy, State Regulation, and Operations. A report to the U.S. Senate Special Committee on Aging. 2003. Available at: http://www.aahsa.org/alw/intro.pdf. Accessed July 12, 2006.
36. The U.S. Department of Health & Human Services. Centers for Medicare & Medicaid Services. Available at: http://www.cms.hhs.gov. Accessed January 25, 2007.

37. Heikkila VM, Kallanranta R. Evaluation of the driving ability in disabled persons: a practitioners' view. *Disabil Rehabil.* 2005;17:1029–1036.

38. Marshall S, Man-Son-Hing M, Molnar R, et al. An exploratory study on the predictive elements of passing on-the-road tests for disabled persons. *Traffic Inj Prev.* 2005;3:235–239.

39. American Physical Therapy Association (APTA). *Guide to Physical Therapy Practice,* 2nd ed. Alexandria, VA: APTA; 2003.

40. Guide for the Uniform Data Set for Medical Rehabilitation (Adult FIM), version 4.0. Buffalo, NY. State University of New York at Buffalo; 1993.

41. Hamilton B, Laughlin J, Granger C, et al. Interrater agreement of the seven level Functional Independence Measure (FIM). *Arch Phys Med Rehabil.* 1991;72:790.

42. Keith R, Granger C, Hamilton B, et al. The Functional Independence Measure: a new tool for rehabilitation. In: Eisenberg M, Grzesiak R, eds. *Advances in Clinical Rehabilitation,* Vol 1. New York: Springer; 1987:6–18.

43. Rockwook K, Stolee P, Fox RA. Use of goal attainment scaling in measuring clinically important change in the frail elderly. *J Clin Epidemiol.* 1993;46:1113–1118.

44. Granger C. Outcome of comprehensive medical rehabilitation: an analysis based upon impairment, disability, and handicap model. *Int Rehabil Med.* 1985;7:45–50.

45. Granger C, Albrecht G, Hamilton B. Outcome of comprehensive medical rehabilitation: measurement of PULSES Profile and the Barthel index. *Arch Phys Med Rehabil.* 1979;60:145–154.

46. Shah S, Vanclay F, Cooper B. Improving the sensitivity of the Barthel index for stroke rehabilitation. *J Clin Epidemiol.* 1989;42:703–709.

47. Houlden H, Edwards M, McNeil J, et al. Use of the Barthel index and Functional Independence Measure during early inpatient rehabilitation after single incident brain injury. *Clin Rehabil.* 2006;20:153–159.

48. Mahoney F, Wood O, Barthel D. Rehabilitation of chronically ill patients: the influence of complications on the final goal. *South Med J.* 1958;51:605–609.

49. Centers for Medicare & Medicaid Services, Department of Health and Human Services. Requirements for States and Long Term Care Facilities. 42 CFR483.440

50. Kettenbach G. *Writing SOAP Notes with Patient/Client Management Formats.* 3rd ed. Philadelphia, PA: FA Davis Company; 2004.

51. Merriam-Webster Online Dictionary. Welfare. Available at: http://www.m-w.com/dictionary/welfare. Accessed June 15, 2006.

52. News Batch. Welfare Policy Issues. Available at: http://www.newsbatch.com/welfare.htm. Accessed June 15, 2006.

53. Administration for Children and Families. Office of Family Assistance (OFA). Available at: http://www.acf.hhs.gov/opa/fact_sheets/tanf_factsheet.html. Accessed June 15, 2006.

54. Administration for Children and Families. Welfare Reform/Social Services State Links. Available at: http://www.acf.dhhs.gov/programs/ofa/stlinks.htm. Accessed June 15, 2006.

55. West Virginia Department of Health & Human Resources, Bureau for Children and Families. Food Stamp Program. Available at: http://www.wvdhhr.org/bcf/family_assistance/fs.asp. Accessed June 15, 2006.

56. Social Security Administration. Disability Planner, How Much Work Do You Need? Available at: http://www.ssa.gov/dibplan/dqualify2.htm. Accessed June 15, 2006.

57. Social Security Administration. Disability Planner, What We Mean By Disability. Available at: http://www.ssa.gov/dibplan/dqualify4.htm. Accessed June 15, 2006.

58. Social Security Administration. Disability Planner, How You Qualify for Social Security Benefits. Available at: http:// www.ssa.gov/dibplan/dqualify.htm. Accessed June 15, 2006.

59. Social Security Administration. Supplemental Security Income (SSI). Available at: http://www.ssa.gov/pubs/11000.pdf. Accessed June 15, 2006.

Additional Online Resources

Centers for Disease Control and Prevention, National Center for Health Statistics. Classifications of Diseases and Functioning & Disability. Available at: http://www.cdc.gov/nchs/about/otheract/icd9/icfhome.htm. Accessed May 8, 2005.

The National Center on Secondary Education and Transition (NCSET). Established to create opportunities for youth with disabilities to achieve successful futures. NCSET provides technical assistance and disseminates information focused on four major areas of national significance for youth with disabilities and their families:
- Providing students with disabilities with improved access and success in the secondary education curriculum;
- Ensuring that students achieve positive postschool results in accessing postsecondary education, meaningful employment, independent living, and participation in all aspects of community life;
- Supporting student and family participation in educational and postschool decision making and planning; and
- Improving collaboration and system linkages at all levels through the development of broad-based partnerships and networks at the national, state, and local levels. Available at http://www.ncset.org/. Accessed July 11, 2006.

A comprehensive overview of information on a state's Medicaid programs for the aged, blind, and disabled is available at http://www.nasmd.org/eligibility/. Accessed June 3, 2006.

U.S. Department of Health and Human Services, State Residential Care and Assisted Living Policy: 2004. The purpose of this compendium is to inform residential care policy by providing detailed information about each state's approach to regulating residential care, as well as its funding for services in these settings. Available at http://aspe.hhs.gov/daltcp/reports/04alcom.htm. Accessed July 12, 2006.

For more information on Medicaid, visit http://www.cms.hhs.gov/MedicaidGenInfo/. Accessed August 21, 2007.

For more information on SSI, visit http://www.socialsecurity.gov/ssi/index.htm. Accessed August 21, 2007.

A listing of state councils can be accessed at: http://www.acf.hhs.gov/programs/add/states/ddcs.html. Accessed August 21, 2007.

More information on the ADA is available at http://www.usdoj.gov/crt/ada/adahom1.htm. Accessed August 21, 2007.

The Social Security Administration provides information on the vocational rehabilitation providers in specific states. Available at: http://www.ssa.gov/work/ServiceProviders/rehabproviders.html. Accessed August 21, 2007.

The Centers for Medicare & Medicaid Services provides information on the Medicaid programs in specific states. Available at: http://www.cms.hhs.gov/home/medicaid.asp. Accessed August 21, 2007.

Information on a state's center for independent living is available at: http://www.ncil.org/about.html. Accessed August 21, 2007.

State offices can be accessed through the U.S. Department of Education, Office of Special Education and Rehabilitation Services at: http://www.ed.gov/about/offices/list/osers/rsa/index.html. Accessed August 21, 2007.

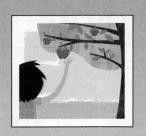

PART III

SELECTED TOPICS

Prenatal and Postnatal Exercises

Caterina Abraham

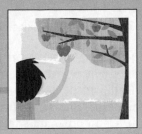

LEARNING OBJECTIVES

1. Comprehend the basic physical changes that occur during pregnancy.
2. Understand the benefits of pre- and postnatal exercises.
3. Understand the general indications, precautions, and contraindications of exercise for a woman who is pregnant or postpartum.
4. Be able to provide an outline of a basic exercise program with the appropriate prescription of exercises.
5. Be able to outline an exercise program for caregivers to promote strengthening of the back muscles and to understand the importance of back care.

Physical therapists who work with children and families are often working with women and men who are parents of a newborn child, whether that child is the patient/client or a new sibling of the patient/client. This situation provides an opportunity for the physical therapist to assist the parents, specifically the mother, with information on the importance of exercise and, if appropriate, exercises to aid in her recovery from pregnancy and childbirth.

All children need a healthy environment in which to grow, learn, and explore. This environment includes the environment of the fetus from the moment of conception and throughout the gestational period. It is important for the woman to prepare her body for the hard work of providing a healthy environment for the fetus in utero, as well as for the work that goes into the care of a newborn child. A woman can prepare for motherhood through proper diet and exercise prior to conception as well as during pregnancy.

Exercise and pregnancy have not always coexisted in a supportive way. It was once believed that a pregnant woman should limit all physical activity. The fear was that any overexertion could precipitate a miscarriage or injure the unborn child. However, many studies have since been published that not only disprove this philosophy, but support the opposite. Physical activity is healthy for the pregnant woman and is beneficial to the unborn child. This chapter will present some of the information currently available regarding the maternal effects of exercise during pregnancy, fetal effects of exercise during pregnancy, parameters for such exercise, and the overall benefit of an active lifestyle on the family. In addition, information will be provided on the topic of back care for the parents or primary caregivers of children. Due to the activities that are required of caregivers, such as picking a child up off of the floor and placing him in and removing him from a crib, to managing strollers and bags, a large amount of stress is placed on the musculoskeletal structures of the caregiver's body. For children with mobility impairments, parents are the primary providers of transfers and mobility beyond the infant and toddler stages of development. Back care is vital for the health and continued capability of the primary caregiver. Parents and caregivers should be educated about prevention of injury that includes core strengthening and stabilization, flexibility, and body mechanics training, in order to maintain their ability to perform their role in this vital aspect of the child's life.

HISTORY OF EXERCISE AND PREGNANCY

In the 1980s, James Clapp III, MD, began studying the maternal and fetal effects of increased physical activity levels in pregnant sheep.[1] Through various studies with this animal population it was found that, with prolonged periods of strenuous physical activity, the sheep were able to tolerate and compensate for an elevated body temperature and decreased blood flow and volume to the fetus. No detrimental effects were seen in either the sheep or their offspring. It was then decided that human trials were needed to determine if the same results could be expected from human mothers and their fetuses.

Human trials were begun in the 1980s and continue through today. Much of what is known about the maternal and fetal effects of exercise during pregnancy has been derived from this research. The human studies on hyperthermia and neural tube defects show a relationship between hyperthermia caused by exposure to high temperatures for prolonged periods of time in the first trimester (sauna, hot tub, fever) and the incidence of neural tube defects, when compared to neural tube defects in mothers who were not exposed to these hyperthermic conditions.[2] Human studies to date have not found that a rise in body temperature *from exercise* increases the risk of fetal anomaly.[3] Therefore, it is currently recommended that pregnant women exercise in a *thermoneutral* (not excessively hot or cold) environment and maintain appropriate hydration during the activity.

The exercise guidelines, published by the American College of Obstetrics and Gynecology (ACOG) and others, are based upon these research findings.[4] As studies continue to be conducted and published, the physical therapist is encouraged to continue to refer to the literature for updates and changes on this topic.

MATERNAL CHANGES DURING PREGNANCY

Before designing an exercise program for a pregnant woman, it is important for the physical therapist to be familiar with some of the maternal changes that occur during this period, specifically changes that occur in the musculoskeletal, cardiovascular/pulmonary, integumentary, and neuromuscular systems.

Changes in the *musculoskeletal system* are the most visually apparent in a pregnant woman. The woman's normal center of gravity (which generally sits anterior to S2) shifts superiorly and anteriorly due to the growing uterus, which influences balance reactions and joint forces throughout her body. The hormone relaxin, which continues to increase in amounts throughout pregnancy, contributes to an increase in ligamentous laxity in joints systemically. This puts a pregnant woman at a higher risk for ligamentous and joint injury due to the physiologic changes in the joint's support network. A pregnant woman is also at risk for nerve entrapment syndromes, such as

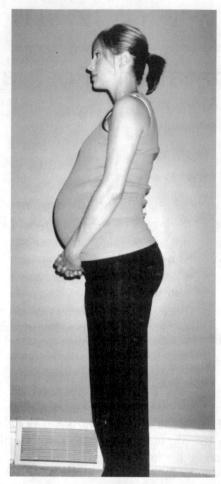

Figure 11-1 ■ Postural changes. Note the postural changes in this pregnant woman in her third trimester: increase in the lumbar lordosis, evidence of scapular protraction, and mild glenohumeral internal rotation.

carpal tunnel syndrome, due to the excessive fluid retention that occurs during this dynamic period.

Some of the major postural changes (Fig. 11-1) that may be seen during pregnancy include the following:[5,6]

- Forward head with increased upper cervical lordosis
- Scapular protraction and elevation
- Glenohumeral internal rotation
- Increased chest circumference[7]
- Increased lumbar lordosis
- Sacroiliac/iliosacral joint asymmetries
- Genu recurvatum
- Excessive foot pronation
- Increased base of support
- Systemic joint hypermobility

 POINT TO REMEMBER

The Center of Gravity

A woman's normal center of gravity is at the level of S2. During pregnancy, the growth of the fetus and uterus shifts the center of gravity up and out, changing a woman's postural alignment, joint forces, and balance.

The affects on the *cardiovascular/pulmonary system* are also evident, especially to the mother.[7,8] A woman can feel the changes in her cardiovascular system very early on in the pregnancy. When the fertilized egg fixes itself to the lining of the uterus, many processes begin that release hormones throughout the body in anticipation of fetal growth. These hormones will affect all maternal muscle tissue, which will decrease the resistance throughout the blood vessel walls as well. This phenomenon has a dilating effect on the vasculature structures, and the body will experience a drop in blood pressure. A drop in blood pressure can influence renal functioning, causing a decrease in excretion of water and salt, which leads to an increase in the blood plasma volume. The following changes are commonly seen in the cardiovascular/pulmonary system:

- Increase in blood volume
- Increase in blood plasma
- Increased cardiac output
- Increased stroke volume
- Increased heart rate
- Decrease in arterial blood pressure
- Increased oxygen consumption (by 15% to 20%)[5]
- Increased depth of respirations
- Increased tidal volume
- Dyspnea

Due to the expanding uterus, there are also mechanical changes that occur in this system. The ribs will flare up and out and the chest's dimension, both in the anterior/posterior and transverse direction, may increase up to two centimeters in each direction.[5] This, along with an elevation of the diaphragm, may produce an overall increase in chest circumference by 2 to 3 inches.

There are also conditions that affect the *integumentary system*, as seen in the various dermatologic conditions that may exist during pregnancy. The mother should notify her obstetrician of any new onset of a dermatologic condition during pregnancy, as the underlying condition could pose a risk to the developing fetus, although most of these conditions are benign. One common change that a pregnant woman may notice is a *linea nigra* (Latin for "black line"). This is an area of hyperpigmentation that runs from the pubis to the umbilicus along the same course as the linea alba. In most women, the linea nigra will fade to its prepregnancy state within a few months after delivery. *Pruritus gravidarum*, which causes severe itching in the third trimester, is another condition that may be experienced by up to 20% of pregnant women.[7] This condition is not associated with a rash, but is due to intrahepatic cholestasis (impaired bile flow) and bile salt retention.[7,9] *Herpes gestationis* is another skin condition that presents as a blister-like rash, primarily on the abdomen, during the second or third trimester. This condition typically resolves within 3 months of delivery.[7] Herpes gestationis is neither viral in nature nor associated with other herpes illnesses. The condition may reoccur in the mother with subsequent

pregnancies or with oral contraceptive use.[10] *Impetigo herpetiformis* results in a rash in the axillary and inguinal region, and occurs in the third trimester of pregnancy. Malaise, chills, vomiting, diarrhea, and at times tetany may accompany this rash. This condition achieves remission after delivery, but may recur with subsequent pregnancies. Impetigo herpetiformis has the possibility of resulting in fetal death or placental complications.[7,9] The reader is referred to other medical texts for complete lists and details on these and other dermatologic conditions.

The *neuromuscular system* can also be affected by pregnancy, specifically in the area of the mother's balance.[5] The altered center of gravity and impaired ligamentous support require static and dynamic compensations in order to maintain balance. Effects of these compensations may be seen in all functional activities. The physical therapist should educate the woman on these changes to increase her awareness of the risk of falling. It may become difficult for a pregnant woman to continue activities that require quick movements, movements with repeated changes in direction, or higher-level balance skills, such as seen in aerobic dancing. Attempts to squat, climb stairs, and reach outside her base of support, for example, may become difficult and could increase the risk for a loss of balance and falling.

EXERCISE DURING PREGNANCY

Exercise during pregnancy can be beneficial in addressing the systemic changes that occur such as controlling excessive weight gain, maintaining muscle strength and tone, elevating mood, maintaining necessary energy supplies, and decreasing the risk of gestational diabetes.[6,8] Exercise can also influence the delivery process by potentially decreasing the duration of labor, decreasing the musculoskeletal discomfort during labor, and increasing a woman's cardiovascular endurance so that she can better withstand the demands of labor.

Back pain can also be a common complaint during pregnancy due to the many musculoskeletal and neuromuscular changes that influence both the static and dynamic stabilizers of the trunk and the extremities. This discomfort can be quite debilitating, especially as the fetus and uterus continue to grow. Exercising to increase the strength of trunk muscles, as well as the muscles of the upper and lower body, can be used to address this common impairment.

Exercise can also affect a woman's mood by influencing the release of endorphins, which can occur during moderate-intensity exercise. This may assist in maintaining an emotional balance for the woman during a time of continued physiologic change and imbalance. Good exercise habits of both aerobic fitness and strength training can be the key to maintaining function, preventing disability, and sustaining a healthy emotional outlook throughout pregnancy, delivery, and the postpartum period.

The Benefits of Exercise During Pregnancy

Exercise during pregnancy can assist with preventing excessive weight gain, maintaining muscle strength, elevating mood, maintaining energy levels, and addressing the common complaint of low back pain.

The benefits of maternal exercise during pregnancy will also translate to the woman's growing and developing fetus. It is postulated that fetal size is affected by the frequency and intensity of maternal exercise; however, there are no current studies to date that confirm or refute this theory.[3] In studies where fetal size was observed to be less than normal, infants born to exercising women developed essential body parts and functions at the same rate as those born to nonexercising pregnant women, but did not gain as much fat weight.[8,11,12] It is also suggested that infants born with less fat mass are less likely to become obese adolescents and adults.[12]

A decrease in fetal blood flow was also once a concern regarding exercise during pregnancy; however, a >50% decrease in fetal blood flow is required to cause any change in fetal health.[5] There have been no human studies to date that demonstrate such a drastic decrease in fetal blood supply during a moderate intensity level of exercise. It is purported that the increased efficiency of the maternal cardiovascular system in the exercising mother prevents any change in fetal blood flow from becoming alarmingly low. Studies using ultrasonography of the human placenta during pregnancy found a greater placental growth and blood supply in women who exercise than in their nonexercising counterparts.[8,13]

Although exercise is appropriate for most women during pregnancy, the physical therapist should be aware of the precautions and contraindications to such intervention.

Contraindications and Precautions for Exercise

A woman who becomes pregnant should discuss the issue of exercise with her obstetrician. Generally, a woman who has been exercising prior to becoming pregnant should be able to continue her exercise routine throughout pregnancy as long as she is not experiencing any serious medical complications. A woman who has not previously been active on a regular basis should discuss beginning an exercise program with her obstetrician. She can begin exercising during pregnancy, but generally should start out slowly, at a low intensity level.

Discuss Exercise

A pregnant woman should discuss the issue of exercise with her obstetrician.

There are medical conditions that may limit a woman's ability to continue an exercise program throughout her pregnancy or will prevent her from starting a program at all. The following conditions are either absolute or relative contraindications to exercise and should be discussed with the obstetrician immediately.[4,5,7]

1. *Incompetent cervix.* This is a condition in which the cervix may dilate, efface, and shorten during pregnancy, which may precipitate labor. Treatments for this condition may include applying a suture at the cervix (*cerclage*), bed rest, and pharmacologic management to control premature contractions.[7] A woman with this condition may find herself on bed rest for an extended period of time in order to prolong the onset of labor.

2. *Pregnancy-induced hypertension.* Various forms of hypertension may be present during pregnancy. The categorization of the condition is based upon previous prepregnancy vital signs as well as other concurrent medical findings that may be present. One of the most significant concerns is when pregnancy-induced hypertension is associated with *proteinuria* (protein in the urine) and edema of the lower extremities. This can indicate the presence of *pre-eclampsia*; symptoms which can include persistent hypertension, swelling of the face, and proteinuria. This condition requires immediate medical attention.[7] If not controlled, this condition may lead to *eclampsia*, which is characterized by the progression of the symptoms of pre-eclampsia, and include the onset of generalized seizures.[7] This can be life threatening to the mother and indirectly to the fetus. Delivery of the fetus in these cases is usually recommended regardless of the gestational age.

3. *Premature rupture of membranes.* This condition exists in 10% to 12% of pregnancies and may lead to premature delivery of the fetus. This occurrence may be related to cervical complications such as cervical incompetence or an unripe cervix (one that is <80% effaced and <2 centimeters dilated).[7]

4. *Preterm labor.* Preterm labor is the onset of labor before full term or 40 weeks gestation. There are many factors, both intrinsic and extrinsic, that could initiate preterm labor. Hormones released during exercise have an effect on the uterus and could contribute to this process. During exercise, norepinephrine and epinephrine are released by the adrenal medulla. The increase in the levels of these hormones may have an effect on uterine activity. *Norepinephrine* primarily stimulates α-adrenergic receptors, which excite uterine contractile tissue. *Epinephrine* stimulates both α- and β-adrenergic receptors, but to varying degrees. Stimulation of β-receptors has a relaxation effect on the uterus. The combination and amount of these hormones can have a stimulating effect on the uterus, which may contribute to the increase in the intensity and/or frequency of uterine contractions. These contractions may cause the fetus to descend into the birth canal,

requiring birth. If the fetus does not descend into the canal with the contractions, he may be subject to stress due to uterine tightening, which decreases blood flow. A decrease in blood flow and lack of oxygen can subsequently lead to fetal distress.

5. *Persistent vaginal bleeding.* Persistent bleeding from the vagina may be an indication of a more serious complication and should be evaluated by the obstetrician.
6. *Intrauterine growth retardation.* Fetal growth retardation may be an indication of a more serious complication. There is evidence that pregnant women who have physically aggressive occupations or work long hours tend to deliver prematurely or deliver small for gestational age (SGA) infants.[14,15,16] These studies suggest that extremely aggressive exercise may affect fetal size. A woman who chooses to engage in these aggressive modes of exercise or training should be closely monitored to assure appropriate fetal growth throughout gestation. It must be said here, however, that SGA infants are not always problematic. For exercising pregnant women, some will deliver SGA infants, not because of retarded intrauterine growth, but due to a decrease in fetal fat tissue mass.
7. *Heart disease.* A pregnant woman with any history of cardiovascular pathology should be evaluated and cleared by her physician and/or obstetrician prior to beginning or continuing a current exercise program during pregnancy, due to the increased demand placed on that system throughout pregnancy.

Other relative or absolute contraindications of exercise in the pregnant woman include being extremely overweight or extremely underweight, having anemia or a previous sedentary lifestyle, and the presence of poor fetal growth.

POINTS TO REMEMBER

Contraindications for Exercise During Pregnancy[4,5,7,8]

Incompetent cervix
Pregnancy-induced hypertension
Premature rupture of membranes
Preterm labor
Persistent vaginal bleeding
Intrauterine growth retardation
Heart disease
Extreme under-/overweight
Anemia
Sedentary lifestyle
Poor fetal growth

During pregnancy, conditions may exist that may complicate the woman's ability to exercise, but not be an absolute contraindication. A woman should discuss the presence of these conditions with her obstetrician prior to

beginning or continuing an exercise program during pregnancy. A short list of some precautions to consider are outlined by Carolyn Kisner and Lynn Colby[5] and listed as follows:

- Multiple gestations (due to the risk of the premature onset of labor)
- Periodic uterine contractions persisting for several hours
- Presence of diastasis recti abdominis
- Anemia
- Systemic infection
- Extreme fatigue
- Musculoskeletal complaints and/or pain
- Phlebitis

There are positions and postures that should be avoided while exercising during pregnancy. A pregnant woman should not exercise on her back in excess of 5 minutes after the fourth month of pregnancy. In this position, the growing fetus and uterus compress the inferior vena cava and may alter venous circulation and decrease cardiac output. The woman should place a small wedge or towel roll under her right hip to encourage the left side-lying position. If a pregnant woman is experiencing vaginal bleeding or any type of placental detachment, she should avoid positions that place the hips and buttocks above the level of the chest, as this position places her at risk for an air embolism through the placental wound.[5]

An exercising pregnant woman should also bear weight through the lower extremities equally and avoid excessively long periods of single limb stance. Stretches should be done within the physiologic range of motion. Due to hormonal influences, overstretching can put the woman at risk for joint or soft tissue injury. While performing any exercise during pregnancy, the woman should be instructed in appropriate breathing techniques so as not to cause a *Valsalva maneuver* or become unnecessarily short of breath. The *Valsalva maneuver* occurs when an individual holds her breath and bears down as in having a bowel movement. This maneuver is sometimes used during exercise when the individual is straining to complete a task or difficult movement. This can place undue pressure through the uterus and down through the pelvic floor.

In general, as with any exercise regimen, a warm-up and cool-down period is important. It is recommended that a pregnant woman undergo a warm-up period of 8 to 12 minutes and a cool-down period of between 3 and 5 minutes.[17] Adequate hydration is also important during pregnancy, and women should be encouraged to drink water before, during, and after all physical activity. It is generally recommended that a pregnant woman drink 1 pint of water prior to the exercise session and 1 cup of water for every 25 minutes of exercise.[17] Fluid should also be replaced after exercise, as a woman could lose up to 1 to 2 quarts of fluid per hour through perspiration.

Pain is considered the fifth vital sign, and all pregnant women should be advised to discontinue exercising should they experience pain with the activity. Cessation of exercise should occur when any of the following signs are present:[4,5]

- Chest pain
- Calf pain or localized calf swelling
- Vaginal bleeding
- Shortness of breath prior to exertion
- Irregular heart beat
- Dizziness
- Faintness
- An increase in intensity or acute onset of back or pubic pain
- Headache
- Preterm labor
- Decreased fetal movement
- Amniotic fluid leakage

The ACOG guidelines for exercise during pregnancy state that most women who were previously active can safely continue their activity level during pregnancy as long as none of the complications listed above occur.[4] Any new or abnormal symptoms should be reported to the obstetrician. Contact sports and activities with risk of falling or abdominal trauma should also be limited due to the risk they place on the mother and fetus.

An exercising woman should also be instructed by her obstetrician or dietician in the necessary increase in caloric intake to meet the additional metabolic needs of pregnancy. Generally, a pregnant woman needs approximately 300 additional calories per day. This may increase to 500 calories if her activity or exercise level is high.

The physical therapist should be aware of the necessary precautions and contraindications to exercising while pregnant in order to provide an appropriate and effective program to the woman. After the woman has been cleared to participate in an exercise program, the physical therapist could prescribe the appropriate parameters to such an exercise program, and adjust them accordingly, as the woman progresses in her pregnancy.

POINTS TO REMEMBER

General Exercise Guidelines for the Pregnant Woman

Begin with an 8- to 12-minute warm-up period.
Do not exceed 5 minutes in supine for women after the fourth month of pregnancy (16 weeks).
Avoid postures that place the hips and buttocks above the level of the chest.
Weight bear through the lower extremities evenly.
Stretch within the physiologic range.
Breathe appropriately during movements. Avoid holding breath.
Cool down for 3 to 5 minutes.

BOX 11-1
Key Muscles and Muscle Groups Shortened Due to Postural Changes During Pregnancy

Suboccipitals	Low back extensors
Scalenes	Hip adductors
Levator scapulae	Piriformis
Scapular protractors	Hamstrings
Glenohumeral internal rotators	Gastrocnemius
Pectorals	Soleus

Exercise Prescription

The postural changes that occur during pregnancy cause some tissues to become tight and some to be weak due to overlengthening. (See Box 11-1 for a list of the muscles that tend to shorten due to the postural changes in pregnancy.) Postural changes during pregnancy will include an increase in the lumbar lordosis, scapular protraction with glenohumeral internal rotation, a forward head, and hyperextended upper cervical spine. The lower extremities are also affected by the postural and hormonal changes during pregnancy. Stretches should be held for a duration of 15 to 30 seconds and be repeated for three to four repetitions.[5] Stretching positions should not take the joint past its physiologic range of motion as this may increase the risk of joint or muscle injury. Education on proper technique and maintenance of proper posture will be important during the instruction of these exercises to assure that the woman is performing the techniques safely and effectively. No exercises, including stretching, should be performed for >5 minutes in the supine position after the fourth month of pregnancy.

A pregnant woman can choose a variety of modes to accomplish a stretching and flexibility routine during pregnancy. Traditional stretching techniques can be used as well as the more progressive forms of yoga, Pilates, and Tai Chi. Regardless of which mode is chosen, the previously mentioned safety considerations should remain in place. Especially with yoga, positions requiring the hips to be higher than the chest should be avoided during pregnancy and into the postpartum period until complete uterine healing takes place.

POINTS TO REMEMBER

Common Postural Changes Associated with Pregnancy

Increase in lumbar lordosis
Scapular protraction with shoulder joint internal rotation
Forward head
Hyperextended upper cervical spine

BOX 11-2
Key Muscle Groups To Be Strengthened During Pregnancy

Upper cervical spine flexors
Thoracic spine extensors
Scapular retractors
Scapular depressors
Abdominals
Pelvic floor
Hip extensors
Knee extensors
Ankle dorsiflexors

In addition to stretching the muscles that have shortened during this period, it is also important to strengthen those that have been elongated. Strength training during pregnancy is important not only for the musculoskeletal benefits, but also for the mental benefits as well. There are times during pregnancy in which the woman may feel out of control and fragile. By performing a strength-training routine throughout pregnancy, the woman can maintain muscle tone and strength throughout her body in preparation for the delivery process and the daily demands of the postpartum period. (See Box 11-2 for a list of muscles that may become weakened throughout pregnancy either due to being stretched or through general disuse.)

Strengthening exercises can take a variety of forms including: resisted exercise in the water; using isotonic exercise equipment, free weights, or resisted exercise tubing; or yoga, Pilates, or Tai Chi. Core stabilization is an important component to any strengthening exercise program during pregnancy. It helps to support the low back during pregnancy and prepares the body for the demands of childcare after delivery. Upper extremity strengthening should focus on the strength of the larger muscle groups and scapular stabilizers, which will take the brunt of carrying the newborn, as well as the rotator cuff muscles to assure normal glenohumeral arthrokinematics. Some key points to remember with instructing women in resisted exercise include the following:

Correct posture should be maintained throughout the performance of the entire exercise. As with instructing strengthening exercises to any population, if compensatory movements are noted, the resistance may be too much for the woman to handle. A good rule of thumb is that if the final two to three repetitions are a challenge to complete, but the woman is able to complete them without incorporating compensatory movements, the resistance level is appropriate. If the last two to three repetitions cannot be completed at all, or if they can be completed only with compensatory movements, the resis-

tance is too much. If the final two to three repetitions are as easy as the first, the resistance can be safely increased.

The pregnant woman should also be instructed in the *abdominal brace maneuver* for core stabilization in order to prevent excessive low back stress during strength training of the extremities. In this maneuver, the woman finds her neutral spine position and then contracts her abdominal muscles and maintains that position. Neutral spine position can be determined by having the woman assume the positions of hypolordosis (posterior pelvic tilt) and hyperlordosis (anterior pelvic tilt). She will then determine the midpoint between these two end-range positions. She is taught to maintain this position by performing abdominal isometric contractions without moving out of the neutral position. This will assist her with maintaining proximal stability while challenging the muscles of her extremities with resistance exercise. This isometric exercise can be done in multiple positions such as sitting, supine, standing, and quadruped, as dictated by her month of pregnancy.

> ### POINT TO REMEMBER
>
> **Core Stabilization**
> Core stabilization is an important component of any strengthening exercise program during pregnancy.

Aerobic and cardiovascular exercise should be included, if appropriate, in a prenatal or postpartum exercise program. In the prenatal period, this form of exercise can help to prepare the mother for the process of labor as well as for handling the increase in energy that it takes to care for a newborn child. In prescribing the parameters of a cardiovascular exercise program, it is important to consider the woman's general prepregnancy fitness level and any current complications that may be present.

The *rate of perceived exertion (RPE)* or *Borg scale* could be used to determine how hard, or intense, the exerciser is working[18]. This scale is a subjective scale in which the woman reports how hard she is working during an activity. The scale ranges from values of 6 to a maximal value of 20 and can be a valuable tool in determining exercise intensity. A moderate intensity level of exercise is described by the Centers for Disease Control and Prevention (CDC) as the level of exercise in which an individual can carry on a conversation, which corresponds to levels 12 to 14 on the Borg scale.[19] Levels 12 to 14 are considered to be safe levels of cardiovascular exercise for the healthy pregnant client. Cardiovascular exercise can include walking, running, participating in aerobic classes (including step aerobics), swimming, or participating in recreational sports. Depending on which type of cardiovascular exercise the woman chooses to perform, there are safety considerations with each.

A Moderate Level of Intensity

A moderate level of exercise intensity allows a woman to carry on a conversation while exercising.

WALKING AND RUNNING

It is important that the exercising pregnant woman uses appropriate footwear when walking or running. Due to the presence of ligamentous laxity and an increase in body weight that occurs during pregnancy, the joint alignment may begin to change at the midfoot, resulting in hyperpronation. It is important that the shoe be supportive and that the surface in which the walking or running is occurring be stable. As balance is affected by the change in the center of gravity, pregnancy may increase a woman's chance of losing her balance and falling. A woman who has not previously been a runner should begin the program very slowly with bouts of short duration and low-intensity walks, progressing to runs. Vital signs should be monitored to assure that she is physically adapting to added stress from the exercise.

AEROBICS AND STEP AEROBICS

Aerobics and step aerobics are very popular forms of exercise, and can be modified to accommodate the safety concerns that exist for the pregnant woman. As a general rule, if the woman can no longer see her feet, she should not be stepping on an aerobic step. This causes an increase risk of a misstep, or a loss of balance and fall, which may result in a musculoskeletal injury. A woman can continue to follow the class or step program on level ground without the step. Repeated movements should be kept to three or fewer, to avoid excessive stress on the low back and to the joints of the supporting leg.[17] When using the step, care should be taken when crossing over it, as the additional weight gained during pregnancy increases the load on the lower extremity joints. Asymmetrical forces through the lower extremities and pelvis could contribute to pelvic misalignment and low back pain.

Step Aerobics

Repeated movements should be kept to three or fewer.

AQUATIC EXERCISE AND SWIMMING

Swimming or exercising in the water is one of the safest forms of exercise to perform during pregnancy. When a woman is in waist- to chest-deep water, 50% to 80% of her body weight is counteracted by the buoyancy of the water.[17] The buoyancy and compressive forces of the water assist in allowing a pregnant woman to perform exercises that she may not have been able to perform on land. Aquatic exercise can be beneficial to the cardiovascular system as well as to the musculoskeletal system. Even though the woman may feel lighter in the pool, the resistance that the water provides is 12 times that of air.[17] Therefore, strengthening exercises can also be performed in the water with more control and comfort due to the physical properties of the water. It is generally recommended that a pregnant woman discontinue exercising in the water when the cervix begins dilating.[17] Cervical dilatation can begin weeks before the onset of true labor and may or may not be marked by the loss of the mucus plug, which tends to occur when the cervix begins to soften.

Exercising in Water

The use of water as an exercise medium is one of the safest forms of exercise for a pregnant woman.

RECREATIONAL SPORTS

There are many sports in which pregnant women can continue to participate during pregnancy. Each activity should be evaluated for safety, taking into consideration the type of movements and actions that are required in order to participate. Sports that have the potential for contact between participants should be avoided due to the potential risk to the uterus. (Generally, the uterus grows outside of the protection of the pelvic bones by the third month.) Examples of these types of sports are basketball, ice hockey, and soccer. Sports such as gymnastics, horseback riding, downhill skiing, and racquet sports have an increased risk of trauma due to falling and therefore should also be avoided due to the potential for injury to the pregnant woman and the fetus.[4]

POSTPARTUM

The physiologic and morphologic changes of pregnancy continue for up to 4 to 6 weeks into the postpartum period. Therefore, it is important for the woman to gradually return to her previous level of activity. The general guidelines for exercise during pregnancy can be applied to the woman postpartum as well. If a woman experienced an uncomplicated vaginal delivery, exercise may be appropriate soon after delivery. Bright red vaginal bleeding or an increase in the amount of postpartum bleeding is an indication to discontinue the activity. Care should continue with range-of-motion activities because decreased joint stability may persist, due to elevated hormonal levels.

During this time, the daily demands of caring for a newborn can cause new mechanical stresses to the mother's or caregiver's body. When feeding or nursing a newborn, for example, the mother or caregiver will assume a position of cervical flexion, side bending, and rotation. This position, if held for prolonged periods of time (as with nursing/feeding for 20 to 30 minutes every 2 to 3 hours), can cause mechanical stresses to the spine. This position will also encourage a forward head and rounded shoulder posture. It is important for the physical therapist to instruct the mother or caregiver on proper stretching and strengthening exercises in order to manage the long-term mechanical stresses to the body. Proper postural exercise may include scapular retraction, scapular depression, and lower cervical extension exercises.

POINT TO REMEMBER

Postpartum

Physiologic changes seen during pregnancy continue for 4 to 6 weeks postpartum. It is important for a woman to gradually return to her previous level of functioning and exercise.

SPECIAL CONSIDERATIONS

In addition, there are common conditions that occur in the postpartum period that can be addressed with physical therapy intervention. These can include impairments to the pelvic floor and rectus abdominis muscle, the impairments associated with prolonged bed rest, and back pain that may occur with lifting and caring for an infant or young child.

The Pelvic Floor

In normal anatomic alignment, the uterus sits posterior and superior to the bladder. As the fetus grows, so does the uterus. This places increased pressure on the bladder and pelvic floor musculature. These muscles, specifically the pelvic diaphragm or levatores ani, function to support the contents of the abdomen as well as the urethral and anal sphincters. Due to the increasing weight of the abdominal contents, the pelvic floor muscles may be stretched to the point that impairs their ability to function correctly. This can lead to problems of incontinence of bladder and bowel and to pain due to a pelvic misalignment. Strengthening the pelvic floor musculature is important in the prenatal period in order to prevent or minimize these occurrences. Prenatal pelvic floor activities will also increase a woman's awareness of her pelvic floor muscles, which will assist her with her ability to relax these muscles during the delivery of the infant. Especially after a vaginal delivery, the pelvic floor undergoes additional stretching that may lead to prolonged problems well into the postpartum period. Pregnant women should be instructed to begin exercises soon after giving birth and continue with their pelvic floor strengthening. The pelvic floor muscles respond quickly to training, and improvements in function should be evident within 2 weeks of consistently performing the exercises. As these muscles fatigue quickly, the woman should perform up to 80 repetitions per day of the pelvic floor exercises in multiple sets of 8 to 10 repetitions each. Variations in the exercises range from having the woman perform short quick contractions of the pelvic floor to the performance of graded exercises such as the "elevator" activity.

It is also important for the physical therapist to remember that asymmetry in the pelvic floor musculature can contribute to pelvic girdle misalignment and dysfunction resulting in pain with movement. The physical therapist should consider this area when pelvic girdle dysfunction is suspected. The examination of the pelvic floor is within the scope of practice for a physical therapist, but an internal examination of the pelvic floor during this time should be deferred to the woman's obstetrician.

Diastasis Recti

Diastasis recti is a condition in which the rectus abdominis muscle separates from the linea alba during pregnancy. This separation may occur in the second trimester, but is most common in the third trimester. This condition is generally not painful for the woman or the baby, and causes no serious complications. What it can do, however, is lead to back pain due to the inability of the rectus abdominis to sufficiently contribute to core stability. The pregnant woman will notice the impairment in the use of her rectus abdominis as she attempts to bring herself to an upright position. She will also notice that, as she contracts the abdominal muscles, a bulge will appear longitudinally on her abdomen. This separation can be measured by using calipers, or grossly by using finger widths. For the finger method, the fingertips are placed into the separation perpendicular to the line of the rectus abdominis. A separation of ≥2 finger widths, or ≥2 centimeters, is considered abnormal and is an indication for modifications in abdominal exercise.[5] Abdominal exercises are modified by having the woman in a hook-lying position, crossing her arms over her abdomen, and placing her hands at her side. She should then be instructed to pull her hands toward each other approximating the separation. From this starting position she can begin by lifting only her head off of the floor while exhaling. When she can perform this exercise successfully, she can progress by performing a posterior pelvic tilt and then lifting her head only off the floor.[5] These modified exercises should be continued after delivery until the separation returns to ≤2 finger widths or ≤2 centimeters.

Women may also experience a separation at the symphysis pubis called *diastasis symphysis pubis*. This condition can be severely debilitating to the woman's function and, if not treated or resolved, may limit her ability to walk or weight bear through the lower extremities. Physical therapists should consider this condition a possibility in a woman postpartum who complains of pain in the symphysis pubis region. The application of modalities, the use of crutches and a support belt or binder to immobilize the symphysis pubis may be appropriate.

Bed Rest

The obstetrician may order bed rest during a woman's pregnancy for reasons such as the presence of an incompetent cervix, placenta previa, premature rupture of membranes, pre-eclampsia, multiple gestation, or gestational diabetes. Bed rest is prescribed as an attempt to prolong the onset of labor until a safe gestational age is reached. These conditions alone can produce anxiety for the pregnant woman, which can be compounded by her inability to complete normal daily activities. The woman may be unable to work, unable to care for other children, or at times, be unable to rise from the bed or use the bathroom to perform general daily hygiene. Prolonged periods of bed rest can also lead to joint stiffness, intestinal motility problems, muscle aches, and depression. The initiation of gentle exercises during this time may assist in preventing or minimizing some of these consequences of bed rest as well as providing the woman with a sense of control over her present situation.

An exercise program for the pregnant woman on bed rest should always be discussed with the obstetrician to assure that the woman is cleared for the specific exercises suggested. The physical therapist will want to know if the woman is on *absolute bed rest*, during which she cannot leave the bed at all; or *modified bed rest*, where she is able to move about for certain activities, such as toileting, or for a specific amount of time. After her activity level has been clarified, the exercises can be performed in a variety of positions—supine, side-lying, quadruped, and/or sitting—depending on her medical clearance. Postural education and tips on total body positioning should be included to prevent the onset of muscle and joint soreness. The woman should be instructed to avoid the Valsalva maneuver to prevent any unnecessary increase in intra-abdominal pressure. Diaphragmatic breathing techniques could also be included. The woman should also be reminded to empty her bladder before beginning her exercise session, as a full bladder may stimulate uterine contractions.[5] All exercises should be performed in a smooth, controlled manner. The exercises should focus on mobility of all joints of the trunk and extremities, incorporating both stretching and active range-of-motion activities. Gentle, active range-of-motion exercises can be performed for the cervical, thoracic, and lumbar spines. Engaging the trunk will also assist the woman with transfers and bed mobility during her bed confinement. It will be important for the woman to demonstrate safe bed mobility and transfers without causing excessive increases in abdominal pressure. Performing trunk mobility exercises will also encourage intestinal movement. Upper extremity and lower extremity active range-of-motion exercises should address all joints through a full range of motion. Resisted exercise can also be performed during this time if cleared by the obstetrician. The woman can use homemade weights, dumbbells, or the weight of the extremity against gravity, to add some resistance to the muscle action. If abdominal exercises are prescribed, it is vital that the physical therapist ensure that the woman is correctly performing the exercises and that she is breathing through the activity. Abdominal exercise can be performed in the supine recumbent position, the side-lying position, and in the quadruped position. The physical therapist should evaluate the woman for the presence of a diastasis recti and modify the exercises as needed. It will be important to vary the exercise program in an attempt to stave off the boredom that can inevitably set in during long bouts of bed rest.

An outline of a possible exercise program for a pregnant woman on bed rest follows:[5,20]

Bed positioning and bed mobility (with breathing techniques):
  Left side-lying position to prevent vena cava compression;
  Scooting up, down, and side-to-side;
  Bridging (also assists with getting on and off the bedpan);
  Rolling (using log roll technique).
Stretching and active range-of-motion exercises to trunk and extremities.
Resisted exercise to the extremities and abdominals (if appropriate).
Pelvic floor activities.
Relaxation techniques.
Postpartum education.

Back Care

All people involved in the care of children should be educated on proper body mechanics for day-to-day activities. Putting a child in a car seat, placing the child in a bassinet for naps, and laying him on the floor for diaper changes or playtime can all take a toll on an unprepared body, especially the low back. Instructing caregivers on proper lifting techniques will assist them in maintaining their back health while caring for the child. The list below outlines some basic rules of safe lifting and body ergonomics.

1. Always keep the load close to the body and as close to the center of mass as possible.
2. Maintain a neutral (lordotic) position in the lumbar spine. Do not flatten the back.
3. Lift with the larger muscle groups of the lower extremities. Do not lift with the back.
4. Pushing is easier on the body than pulling is.
5. Avoid lifting heavy objects overhead as this may cause an increase in the lumbar lordosis.
6. When required to lift a load and move it away from the body, as when placing an infant in a bassinet or car seat, maintain the abdominal brace/contracted position to stabilize the trunk against the additional load.

General back care should also include stretching, strengthening, and cardiovascular endurance activities. Stretching should focus on the subcapital muscles, pectorals, erector spinae, hamstrings, and the gastrocnemius/soleus complex. Strengthening routines should focus on all major muscle groups of the body, particularly the larger muscle groups of the legs (in order to better assist in lifting and carrying), abdominal muscles, erector spinae, and scapular stabilizers (retractors and depressors). For the postpartum woman, it is also important to incorporate pelvic floor exercises as mentioned previously.

Cardiovascular endurance is important for the caregiver because the daily demands have increased, whereas time for rest may have decreased. Modes of cardiovascular exercise could include walking, swimming, cycling, rowing, aerobic dancing, Pilates, or any other activity that allows the caregiver to increase her heart rate for a prolonged period of time. The U.S. Surgeon General recommends that all adults exercise at a moderate intensity for at least 30 minutes most days of the week.[21]

At some point, all persons caring for a child will be required to place the child in a car seat to travel to doctor visits, etc. This task, although simple, can be stressful to the musculoskeletal system, especially if performed repeatedly on a regular basis. The caregiver would assume a trunk-flexed position, while loaded with the weight of the child, and potentially even the travel seat. To place the seat in the appropriate place in the automobile, the caregiver would have to extend the arms while still loaded with the child. This places a great amount of force on the spine. The caregiver should be instructed to keep a stable posture while performing all child care activities whenever possible, remembering that the abdominal brace is the starting point to stabilize the core in preparation for extremity loading.

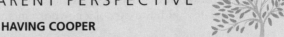

HAVING COOPER

When I found out that I was pregnant for the first time, I thought of how great it would be to be slim and trim with a basketball belly. Then reality set in. Morning sickness arrived causing the need to snack frequently throughout the day. I tried to exercise, but felt tired frequently, and exercised inconsistently throughout my first pregnancy. I gained 50 pounds and can honestly say that I did not feel all that great. My delivery and recovery were difficult, as I required a forceps delivery, and it took over a year to feel normal again.

When pregnancy number two came along, I was determined to feel better the second time. I had to accept the inevitable weight gain early on and realize that what was most important was my health and the health of my baby. I stayed focused on my nutritional needs early and maintained my exercise routine from the beginning of the pregnancy. I continued to perform step aerobics and progressed to aerobics without the step, treadmill running/walking, cycling, elliptical training, and weight training. This made a tremendous difference in my emotional and physical health during this pregnancy. I felt more in control, healthy, and proud of the abilities that I had maintained considering my ever-growing belly. The delivery was much simpler the second time, for many reasons. I was able to deliver the baby unassisted (except for the epidural), and my ability to immediately care for my newborn was amazing. I gained 38 pounds with the second pregnancy and getting it off was so much easier as my active lifestyle had been consistent throughout the entire 40 weeks.

An active lifestyle is now an important part of my family life as my husband and I try to instill these behaviors in our children. It is an activity that we can all engage in together, providing valuable family time, and we can all attest to how difficult that is to come by these days!

—C. Fox, wife and mother of two

SUMMARY

Physical therapists who work with children are working with mothers who were, or become pregnant. This situation provides an opportunity for the physical therapist to educate the pregnant woman on the benefits of safe exercise during and after her pregnancy. As the woman's pregnancy progresses, she may experience impairments in her movements and functional limitations secondary to the effects of pregnancy on her musculoskeletal, cardiovascular/pulmonary, and neuromuscular systems. Exercising during pregnancy can eliminate or lessen some of these impairments and provide the woman with a sense of control during this rapidly changing time. Exercise and the benefits gained from it may also help with the recovery process after birth and with some of the more common impairments associated with that process, such as impairment to the pelvic floor musculature.

Exercise is also important in promoting back health, which can be compromised by the new movements and activities associated with the care of a newborn infant.

REVIEW QUESTIONS

1. You are asked to develop an exercise program for a woman in her third trimester of pregnancy. During your examination, you would expect to find which of the following postural changes commonly associated with pregnancy?
   a. Decreased lumbar lordosis
   b. Excessive foot supination
   c. Forward head with increased upper cervical lordosis
   d. Scapular retraction and depression

2. You are treating a patient for a lateral ankle sprain she sustained while running. During her discharge, she informs you that she just found out that she is pregnant. She asks you if she could resume her exercise program, which consists of a 3-mile run and step aerobics. Which of the following would be the most appropriate course of action for the physical therapist?
   a. The physical therapist should educate the patient on the benefits of exercise while pregnant but refer her to her obstetrician for input on these activities, before she resumes her exercise program.
   b. The physical therapist should educate the patient on the benefits of exercise while pregnant and inform her that most women who exercise prior to becoming pregnant can continue exercising throughout pregnancy.
   c. The physical therapist should instruct the patient to resume her exercise program running fewer miles per day and at a decreased intensity, gradually increasing her intensity of exercise as tolerated.
   d. The physical therapist should instruct the patient to resume her exercise program educating her on the contraindications to exercise while she is pregnant. If she exhibits any of the contraindications she should not exercise.

3. Your patient has a diastasis recti which measures 3 centimeters in separation. You are initiating abdominal exercises to address this issue. This is the first session for these instructions. Which of the following exercise prescriptions is the most appropriate for the first session?
   a. Supine hook-lying with her hands over the midline of the diastasis; as she exhales, she lifts only her head off the floor.
   b. Supine hook-lying with her hands over the midline of the diastasis. She slowly lifts her head off the floor while simultaneously performing a posterior pelvic tilt.
   c. Supine hook-lying with her hands over the midline of the diastasis. She slowly lifts her head and scapula off the floor.
   d. Supine hook-lying with a posterior pelvic tilt. The client holds the pelvic tilt as she straightens one leg.

4. Prenatal exercise after the fourth month of pregnancy should
   a. decrease natural hyperthermia by increasing blood flow to the extremities.
   b. avoid the supine position for extended periods of time.
   c. not include performing abdominal exercises secondary to possibility of diastasis recti.
   d. only include low-intensity exercises.

5. As a general rule, a woman who is pregnant should exercise at an intensity (at) which
   a. her heart rate does not exceed 140 beats per minute.
   b. her body's core temperature does not rise 1°F.
   c. her exertion is such that she can still carry on a conversation.
   d. can be maintained for 15 minutes.

REFERENCES

1. Clapp JF. Acute exercise stress in the pregnant ewe. *Am J Obstet and Gynecol*. 1980;136:489–494.
2. Milunsky A, Ulcickas KJ, Rothman W, et al. Maternal heat exposure and neural tube defects [abstract]. *JAMA*. 1992;268:7.
3. Kelly A, Weiss K. Practical exercise advice during pregnancy. *Phys Sportsmed*. 2005;33:24–30.
4. American College of Obstetrics and Gynecology Committee on Obstetric Practice. Exercise during pregnancy and the postpartum period [Committee Opinion]. *Obstet Gynecol*. 2002;99:171–173.
5. Kisner C, Colby L. *Therapeutic Exercise: Foundations and Techniques*, 4th ed. Philadelphia: F.A. Davis Company; 2002.
6. Jeffreys R. The pregnant exerciser: an argument for exercise as a means to support pregnancy. *American College of Sports Medicine*. 2005;15:5–7.
7. Stevenson R, O'Conner L. *Obstetric and Gynecological Care in Physical Therapy*, 2nd ed. Thorofare, NJ: Slack Incorporated; 2000.
8. Clapp JF III. *Exercising Through Your Pregnancy*, Omaha, NE: Addicus Books; 2002.
9. *Stedman's Medical Dictionary for the Health Professions and Nursing*, 5th ed. Philadelphia: Lippincott, Williams & Wilkins; 2005.
10. Berkow R, ed. *The Merck Manual of Diagnosis and Therapy*, 16th ed. Rahway, NJ: Merck Research Laboratories; 1992.
11. Clapp JF III, Capeless EL. Neonatal morphometrics after endurance exercise during pregnancy. *Am J Obstet Gynecol*. 1990;163:1805–1811.
12. Synder S, Pendergraph B. Exercise during pregnancy: what do we really know? *Am Fam Phys*. 2004;69:1053–1054.
13. Clapp JF III. The effects of maternal exercise on fetal oxygenation and feto-placental growth [abstract]. *Eur J Obstet Gynecol Reprod Biol*. 2003;110:80–85.
14. Mozurkenich E, Luke B, Frni M, et al. Working conditions and adverse pregnancy outcome: a meta-analysis [abstract]. *Obstet Gynecol*. 2000;95:623–635.
15. Peoples-Sheps MD, Siegel E, Suchindran CM, et al. Characteristics of maternal employment during pregnancy: effects on low birth weight. *Am J Public Health*. 1991;81:1007–1012.

16. Savitz DA, Olshan AF, Gallagher K. Maternal occupation and pregnancy outcome. *Epidemiology.* 1996;7:269–274.

17. Kooperman S. *Moms in Motion: Pre/Post Natal Exercise.* Evanston: SCW Fitness Education; 2005.

18. Borg G. *Borg's Perceived Exertion and Pain Scales.* Champaign, IL: Human Kinetics. 1998.

19. Department of Health and Human Services, Centers for Disease Control and Prevention. Physical activity for everyone: measuring physical activity intensity. Perceived Exertion (Borg Rating of Perceived Exertion Scale) Last review date: 03/22/2006. Available at http://www.cdc.gov/nccdphp/dnpa/physical/measuring/perceived_exertion.htm. Accessed June 7, 2006.

20. Noble E. *Essential Exercises for the Childbearing Year,* 4th ed. Harwich, MA: New Life Images; 2003.

21. U.S. Department of Health and Human Services. The Surgeon General's Call to Action to Prevent and Decrease Overweight and Obesity. Available at: http://www.surgeon-general.gov/topics/obesity/calltoaction/fact_adolescents.htm. Last accessed June 7, 2006.

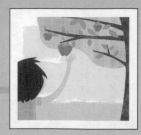

C H A P T E R **12**

Pediatric Pharmacology

Maureen McKenna

LEARNING OBJECTIVES

1. Understand the role of the physical therapist regarding medication management.
2. Have a basic understanding of the fundamentals of pharmacology and be familiar with the common methods of administration and action of medications taken.
3. Identify common over the counter (OTC) medications and how they are used in the health care of children.
4. Identify common prescribed medications and understand their general use in the health care of children.
5. Be familiar with the typical medications used in the treatment of common pediatric conditions.
6. Understand the role of the physical therapist in the primary prevention of drug and alcohol abuse.

The influence of chemicals on the health and recovery of a child or adult is becoming an increasingly important factor in patient/client management. Not only the medicines prescribed by the physician, but also the OTC medications and supplements, as well as the nutrients in foods are significant factors that influence the growth, development, healing, and general health and well-being of a child. A physical therapist should have a general knowledge of the basic issues of nutrition and pharmacology to aid in the patient/client management process and clinical decision-making regarding the effects of intervention. These factors can have a significant influence on the physical performance of the child in his care.

Physical therapists should address certain aspects of *medication management,* which should not be confused with prescribing medicines. Questions about basic nutrition, current medications, OTC medicines, and dietary supplements that the child is taking should be included as part of the history aspect of an evaluation. The parent's or, if appropriate, the child's knowledge of the purpose of the medication, both prescribed and OTC, and the ability of the parent to properly store (as prescribed), access (on a shelf or in the refrigerator), and handle the medicine (open the container and manipulate the pill or liquid) are aspects of management that could be addressed by the physical therapist. These aspects may be especially relevant to the adolescent or child with a chronic disability who learns to self-administer her medications. The parent or child should be able to articulate the schedule and dosage for taking the medication and the common side effects and adverse reactions that are listed in the materials provided with the medicine. Failure to demonstrate this aspect of health care should initiate a referral back to the prescribing physician or pharmacist. The scope of practice of physical therapy does not include the prescription of drugs actually, implicitly, or even by suggestion. By crossing this professional practice boundary, there could be serious legal consequences as well as the loss of the license to practice. However, there is a basic level of knowledge required in order to understand alterations in a child's abilities or behavior that may be the result of a medication or other substance. Physical therapists should be aware of the possible influences of diet and medication and be able to communicate any concerns to the appropriate professional.

The evaluation of the child's responses to a medication, particular diet, and her behavior is mainly the responsibility of the physician with the parent's input to monitor, to describe, and to evaluate, particularly when any recent changes have occurred in any of those areas. There is rarely an action, intended or otherwise, without a reaction of some kind. However, it may not always occur in an equal and opposite direction. A child's metabolism and the body's reactions to external factors often vary from those of an adult and may manifest in signs and symptoms that are very different from the way in which an adult would respond under similar conditions with the same medication.

In the pediatric population, serious illness and death can result from the inappropriate use of an OTC product, such as aspirin, that in the adult population could otherwise be considered harmless. Additionally, if dosage is exceeded or when used in combination with a prescribed or OTC medication, side effects that have serious consequences may occur. It is the physical therapist's professional duty to support the instructions given to the parent or child from the physician and the pharmacist on the importance of adherence to a medication regimen and to consider the possibility of a medication or dietary factor in the rehabilitation process. Any questions or concerns should be discussed with the appropriate professional.

The information in this chapter is intended to provide the reader with a basic understanding of pharmacology and to highlight a few of the common medicines, both prescribed and OTC, that are often seen in the pediatric population. The information is intended to provide the physical therapist with a working knowledge of basic pharmacology to allow him to participate in a discussion of the child's medications with the parent, physician, or pharmacist. It will begin with a general overview of the basics of pharmacology.

 POINTS TO REMEMBER

Medication Management

Aspects of medication management that can be addressed by the physical therapist include the patient's or parents':

understanding of the need and purpose of the medication, understanding of the correct dosage and side effects, ability to properly store and access the medication, and ability to effectively manipulate the container to access the individual tablets or liquid.

BASICS OF PHARMACOLOGY

There is some basic information to understand prior to reviewing specific drugs for the pediatric population. This introductory information will describe the ways in which drugs reach their desired target and how various impediments to that goal may be encountered along the way. This information emphasizes the importance of adherence to specific dosages depending on the individual child and some of the factors that go into the decision making regarding dosage and the route of administration.

There is a convention when documenting or describing a medication. The trade name of a drug is written with an initial capital letter (e.g., Valium), and the generic in lower case (diazepam). This should make it easier to discriminate between them and to reduce confusion, as there are numerous trade names for the same generic product.

Pharmacotherapeutics describes the function of drugs when they are interacting with the body. The two aspects of this function are pharmacodynamics and pharmacokinetics. *Pharmacodynamics* is the study of uptake, movement, binding, and interactions of pharmacologically active molecules at their tissue site(s) of action.[1] It is the analysis of what the drug does to the body, including the mechanism by which the drug exerts its effect.[2] These mechanisms are both physiological and mechanical. *Pharmacokinetics* is defined as the movement of drugs within biologic systems, as affected by uptake, distribution, binding, elimination, and biotransformation; particularly the rates of such movements.[1] It is the study of how the body deals with the drug in terms of the way the drug is absorbed, distributed, and eliminated.[2] Both pharmacodynamics and pharmacokinetics play a significant role in deciding how to administer the medication, how much to give, and the effects of the medicine on specific body systems.

Methods of Administration

There are several ways by which drugs can be introduced into the body. The most effective, convenient, and appropriate method for administering any given drug is largely determined by the type of drug, the dosage, the diagnosis, and the age and weight of the child or person taking it. The two main routes of administration are *enteral* (administered via the alimentary canal) and *parenteral* (administered via other routes besides the alimentary canal; examples are intramuscular or intravenous injections).

Enteral methods include oral intake, which is the most commonly used form of administration due to its ease and safety. When a drug is taken into the body by this route, absorption begins in the small intestine and then circulates to other parts of the body. This method has one caveat as it is subjected to the body's safe filtration process in the liver known as the *"first pass effect."*[1] After the drug has undergone the absorption process in the alimentary canal, it goes straight to the liver, which in turn determines the next action, which could be either metabolizing the drug or destroying a portion of it before it reaches the target organ or area. The dosage requires careful evaluation to ensure that a sufficient quantity is ingested, or injected, to manifest the desired result without being degraded by the liver and thus rendered relatively ineffective. This process makes for a somewhat unpredictable outcome as different individuals react differently to similar drugs and quantities, particularly when a drug requires a certain accumulation in the body to maintain a constant therapeutic effect. This accumulation is known as the *half-life* of the drug, described as the time that it takes for 50% of the drug that remains in the body to be eliminated. The other 50% is maintained, and additional doses are added on a regular basis to maintain a constant level, after the half-life time has been established.

There are both *lipid-soluble* and *non–lipid-soluble* drugs. Most of the drugs taken by mouth are the lipid-soluble type so that they can pass from the gastrointestinal tract's mucosal lining straight into the bloodstream. When a patient receives a general anesthetic, either by injection or inhalation, it is included in this category of lipid-soluble medications. There will be widespread distribution of the drug throughout the body, and it may be stored temporarily in the adipose tissue, gradually dispersing through the liver, the lungs, or a combination of both.[2] The more adipose tissue the patient has, the longer the recovery from those symptoms of disorientation and lethargy. Conversely, the non–lipid-soluble drug compounds (peptides and protein molecules, for example) are larger and poorly absorbed, which means that they often pass from the body in the feces without exerting their desired effect on the body. This type of drug was previously administered by a parenteral route and may now be administered orally when these agents are coated or encapsulated to enhance the effects of the absorption process, thereby avoiding most of it being excreted. However, many long-acting and coated medications have to be swallowed whole as chewing or cutting them will decrease the long-acting effect.

Another factor to be considered when taking an oral medication is whether it is to be taken with water, with food, before or after eating, and at what time of day. One of the main problems with oral administration is the likelihood of causing stomach discomfort, vomiting, or diarrhea.

The drugs administered by *buccal* and *sublingual* routes are not subject to the first-pass effect as they are absorbed directly through the mucosal lining of the mouth to the bloodstream. Nitroglycerin, which can be given to children intravenously and transmucosally, and to adults sublingually, is an example of this process.[3] Due to its rapid absorbance, the drug produces the desired response of chest pain relief much more quickly. The quantity of the drug administered in this way can be relatively small, and the form it takes must enable it to permeate through the mucosal lining.

Administering a medication *rectally* is another form of enteral administration, although the absorption rate is relatively poor. The drugs used are in the form of suppos-

itories that can create irritation to the mucosal lining. One of the main benefits is that it affords an opportunity to give medications to a patient who is vomiting, to an infant or a young child who is unable to take them orally, or to a patient who is comatose.[2]

POINT TO REMEMBER

Enteral Administration

The most common form of administration of medications is oral. Most drugs taken by mouth are lipid soluble.

Medication given by parenteral administration, on the whole, reaches the target area more quickly due to its bypass of the alimentary tract. By not passing through the alimentary canal, the drug is not subject to inactivation or degradation through the first-pass effect, and therefore has a more predictable outcome in reaching the target area.

Inhalation of drugs is one form of parenteral administration used commonly in the treatment of respiratory ailments. It is also the method by which a general anesthetic is administered and maintained. The effect of the drug takes place rapidly through the mucosal lining of the nose and pharynx initially as the small droplets in suspension can be administered through an aerosol device and can consequently permeate the entire respiratory tract with each inspiration.

Injections are another form of parenteral administration that is invasive as the skin and other tissues are punctured. These injections can be performed in many different ways depending on the type of condition being treated. The intravenous method delivers a drug directly into the venous system so that the drug can exert its effect on the target area. Sometimes this is a single event, and sometimes it is used over a prolonged period of time to maintain a consistent level of a medication or for hydration of the body using a saline solution. This intravenous method is especially common to see in the neonatal intensive care unit.

Intra-arterial administration of drugs is potentially more dangerous, because an error in the placement of the needle could cause significant damage by puncturing surrounding structures and by the seepage of blood or medication into the surrounding tissues. It is rarely used unless a patient is receiving chemotherapy or is having invasive diagnostic tests with the use of a contrast medium or a radio opaque substance.[2] The effect of the drug on a target organ administered this way will be even more rapid than that of one given intravenously.

Intramuscular injection is probably the most frequently used form of parenteral administration. Drugs can be injected into one or more specific skeletal muscles in the body for a local effect or for a longer lasting systemic effect when the drug is gradually absorbed into the circulatory system. The main drawback is the local discomfort and prolonged soreness at the injection site.[2] One of the main uses in the pediatric population is to administer the intermittent program of vaccinations for disease prevention.

Subcutaneous injections have a slower onset and dispersal rate throughout the circulatory system. They may be used to provide local anesthesia when a wound requires suturing, or patients with diabetes may use this method for self-administration of insulin.[2] Another function of this method of injection is the Mantoux tuberculin test done just under the skin on the ventral surface of the forearm.

Intrathecal injections are administered primarily to the spine in the subarachnoid or subdural spaces where the target is the central nervous system. The advantage of this method in some cases (particularly with antibiotics or with drugs used to treat cancer) is that the substance injected bypasses the blood–brain barrier.[2] The dosage is minimal compared to other forms of administration, thereby lessening the side effects. Intrathecal administration of baclofen is one form of medical management of muscle spasticity. The baclofen is continuously administered via a programmable pump placed superficially in the abdomen and a catheter that is inserted in the intrathecal space at L1-2 and threaded as high as T6.[4]

A medication is *topically* administered directly onto the surface either of the skin or the mucous membrane. The epidermis of the skin offers a greater impediment to absorption than the mucous membranes of the body and can be used to treat skin conditions at the site of the application. Examples of medications applied to the epidermis are antipruritic creams or lotions, counter-irritant products that contain properties feeling like heat or cold, and sunscreen protection against sunburn. Some other examples of the use of this method are the use of eye or nose drops as well as medications that are placed sublingually.

The *transdermal* method is not to be confused with the topical method of administration of a drug. The difference lies in the properties of the drugs that are designed for a slow and steady release of the active component into the peripheral circulation. These drugs would primarily include those used for the treatment of angina, smoking cessation, hormonal imbalance, pain, and motion sickness. In physical therapy, transdermal applications are used to drive the physician-prescribed anti-inflammatory and analgesic medications through the skin by either iontophoresis (which uses an electric current) or phonophoresis (which uses ultrasound).[2]

Absorption and Distribution

Bioavailability is the percentage of the drug that actually arrives at the desired destination. How the drug is administered initially, as well as the number of structures it has to pass through en route (including membranes and cells), will have a significant effect on its bioavailability. Ciccone[2] gives a simple example to illustrate this concept. If 100% of a drug is introduced into the body and only half of it actually gets to the target, then it is considered to be 50% bioavailable. When the drug leaves the systemic circulation, there are many obstacles in the form of membranes and cells through which it must pass to reach the target area. Different membranes provide differing barriers to absorption; some allow free passage, whereas others are more selective. This is another example of the body's safety mechanism that has the ability to monitor the distribution of substances introduced into it.[2]

If a child is actively receiving therapy in one of the rehabilitation disciplines, there may be optimal times for the patient to be seen based on the time for the therapeutic effect to be obtained from the medication. Each drug has its own period of efficacy with an initial administration and gradual onset lag time followed by the longer effective peak period, and finally the period when the drug is wearing off. The best time for the patient in therapy to be seen is during the peak period, so that the maximum benefit can be obtained from the therapy session. Some diagnoses and medications are affected by environmental factors or by the type of intervention used. For example, if a patient with diabetes participates in exercise, this can produce an insulin-like effect by lowering the blood glucose level.[5] The absorption and distribution of some medications are affected by heat, cold, exercise, and by massaging or manipulating the soft tissues of the body.

Most drugs eventually are eliminated from the body. However, in the interim, they may be stored in certain inert tissues and locations in the body, such as muscle, bone, or organs, which may not be the intended target site.

Storage and Elimination

The liver and kidneys are the primary organs where drugs are metabolized, eliminated, and may be stored. For this reason, their functioning is monitored when the child is taking a high dosage of medication or taking the medication for a prolonged period of time. This is commonly seen with antiseizure medications that may require periodic blood samples to analyze liver enzymes.

Adipose tissue is the primary site for the accommodation of lipid-soluble drugs as they are readily absorbed there. It is poorly vascularized, and its slow metabolic rate can provide a long-term storage site. A significant percentage of a child's body weight is composed of adipose tissue that provides a large repository for these drugs as well as for lipid-soluble vitamins (A, D, E, and K). Toxic agents, such as heavy metals like lead and mercury, as well as tetracycline (which is a common medication used in the treatment of acne) are stored in bone.[2]

Tetracycline may turn the teeth gray if used prior to the eruption of the child's permanent teeth.

Drugs entering the body are eventually expelled from either the target site or the storage areas in order to terminate their action. The main method of drug elimination is a combination of metabolism and excretion. The liver is primarily responsible for metabolism by altering the drug into a less active metabolite. The primary organ of excretion is the kidney. The drugs are not in their original active state by this time and have been altered or degraded by a process of *biotransformation* that can reduce the possibility of toxicity. Toxicity in the body can occur if the administration of the drug exceeds the ability to eliminate it. Conversely, if the drug is eliminated from the body faster than it is administered, it may not have attained the desired therapeutic effect.[2] One of the primary examples of this biotransformation process is that, after the administration of a general or a local anesthetic, it is necessary for it to be eliminated so that the child can return to the formerly alert and functional state.

There are alternative ways in which drugs may be excreted from the body other than by the kidneys; for example, the lungs can excrete inhaled substances, such as airway dilators or gaseous anesthetics. The gastrointestinal tract may receive bile from the liver, and if a drug has been in the tract for a period of time, it will be excreted eventually in the feces. Sweat, salivary, and mammary glands are also possible sites for the excretion of drugs, although they play a relatively minor role in this process.[2]

DIFFERENCES IN THE RESPONSE TO DRUGS

There are six main factors to consider in how the child's body will respond to a drug, particularly when a combination of more than one of these factors is included. These factors include age, size, weight, presence of disease, drug interactions, and diet.

Children present a special challenge with their varying size, weight, and age, particularly premature or newborn infants, some of whom may not have developed the enzymes needed for drug metabolism.[2] They are therefore at an increased risk for the prolongation of the effect of the drug in the system. At the other end of the age spectrum, elderly persons are more sensitive to most drugs because they are metabolized at a slower rate due to the changes that occur in organ function. This slow metabolism could result in a higher plasma concentration than that in a younger adult when given the same amount of the drug.[2]

If a child has an organ pathology, this may make a significant difference in the way in which the body responds to a drug, particularly the ability to excrete it. Problems can also arise if there is disease in some of the tissues where the drugs may be stored, or in the circulatory system transporting them.[2]

Drug interactions can be defined as "the pharmacological result, either desirable or undesirable, of drugs interacting with other drugs, with endogenous physiologic chemical agents (e.g., monoamine oxidase inhibitors [MAOI] with epinephrine), with components of the diet, and with chemicals used in diagnostic tests or the results of such tests."[1] The synchronous use of multiple medications may compound the effect the drug has on the body. This is why it is essential that the physician and the pharmacist obtain an accurate account of all the medications a child is taking, including OTC items, such as aspirin. These additional substances may have a significant effect when combined with another drug, could prolong the ability of the drug to be distributed, and could lead to potential toxicity. The family and the physical therapist have an important role in observing any changes in symptoms or behaviors the child may exhibit and should alert the physician to their findings.

The person's choice of diet (or, in the case of a child, what he is given to eat) may also have an effect on the response of the drug. Certain foods can interfere with the drug's absorption, making the prescribed medication less effective or quickening the body's elimination of the drug, which would also interfere with the intended effect. There are certain interactions of foods with drugs, some of which could be life threatening. One example is grapefruit juice, which can increase the absorption of some medicines used to treat high blood pressure, the "statin" family of drugs used to reduce blood cholesterol, and drugs used post-transplant and for the treatment of human immunodeficiency virus/Acquired Immunodeficiency Syndrome (HIV/AIDS).[6] Another example is MAOI used in the treatment of depression. Patients taking this medication must avoid ingesting any of the fermented foods such as aged cheese, some vinegars, and red wine. These foods contain a high proportion of tyramines, which are responsible for the release of epinephrine and norepinephrine in the body, whereas the MAOIs inhibit the release of catecholamines, resulting in a potential hypertensive crisis.[2] Also, if a child is taking Ritalin, medication should not be taken with food as it will be excreted from the body too rapidly before attaining the desired effect. The extended-release form can be taken with or without food. These examples show the importance of the interaction between specific foods and certain medications.

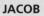
PARENT PERSPECTIVE

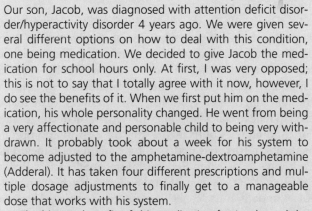

JACOB

Our son, Jacob, was diagnosed with attention deficit disorder/hyperactivity disorder 4 years ago. We were given several different options on how to deal with this condition, one being medication. We decided to give Jacob the medication for school hours only. At first, I was very opposed; this is not to say that I totally agree with it now, however, I do see the benefits of it. When we first put him on the medication, his whole personality changed. He went from being a very affectionate and personable child to being very withdrawn. It probably took about a week for his system to become adjusted to the amphetamine-dextroamphetamine (Adderal). It has taken four different prescriptions and multiple dosage adjustments to finally get to a manageable dose that works with his system.

The biggest benefit of this medication for Jacob, and the only reason he is on it, is that he can focus on the task at hand during the school day. Because of this medication, he has been able to maintain a B average. That is not to say that school is easy for him; he works and struggles like most children to get his grades. Homework has become a struggle lately. Because the drug is almost out of his system by the time he gets home, it becomes more difficult for Jacob to focus or remember how some of the work needs to be done.

If asked how I personally feel about having my son on *speed;* I hate it. This drug alters his personality and I lose my fun-loving child. With that being said, I do know that this drug does help him, and as his parent I must do what is best for him.

—*Laurie*

COMMON OVER-THE-COUNTER MEDICATIONS

OTC medications are popular in the health management of many Americans. Many commercially available drugs are purchased without a physician's prescription and are used for pain relief and/or fever reduction, as an anti-inflammatory, or for anticoagulation, respiratory congestion, and/or skin irritations.

Although a prescription is not needed to purchase these medications, specific directions regarding dosage, storage, and use should be strictly followed. Communication with the physician or pharmacist is important to minimize the adverse effects that can occur with drug interactions.

Nonsteriodal anti-inflammatory drugs (NSAIDs) are a large group of nonopioid and nonsteroidal drugs that are used for pain relief, inflammation, fever, and anticoagulation. They inhibit the synthesis of prostaglandin and thromboxane, both of which are implicated in the experience of pain, fever, inflammation, and blood clotting. *Aspirin* (acetylsalicylate, or abbreviated as asa) is one of the main generic drugs in this class. It is a systemic salicylate that primarily reduces fever and pain. It has many properties and uses in combination with other compounds. Some of the uses and applications are as an anti-inflammatory, antipyretic, antirheumatic, antithrombic, and as an inhibitor of platelet aggregation. Salicylates, including aspirin, should not be administered to a child or teenager if the child has a fever or has lost a large quantity of body fluid due to diarrhea or vomiting. In addition, salicylates should not be given to a child or teenager if there is any suggestion that the fever may be viral in origin, particularly if associated with symptoms of the flu or chicken pox.[7,8] This combination of conditions and the administration of aspirin or other salicylates to reduce the symptoms can result in the condition called *Reye Syndrome*, often misdiagnosed as encephalitis, meningitis, or a drug overdose. Reye Syndrome affects all organs of the body, but is most harmful to the brain and the liver, causing an acute increase of pressure within the brain and, often, massive accumulations of fat in the liver and other organs.[9] Symptoms include persistent or recurrent vomiting, listlessness, personality changes such as irritability or combativeness, disorientation or confusion, delirium, convulsions, and loss of consciousness.[9] Reye Syndrome has no cure and could lead to permanent brain damage or death if it is not diagnosed and treated promptly. Older children may inadvertently self-administer OTC preparations for minor symptoms, such as a headache or menstrual cramps, without the knowledge of their parents. Some of these products may contain salicylates. Additionally, there are topical products that older children may use for acne or dandruff, or as facial scrubs, moisturizers, and wart removers. Although they are not ingested, some of the ingredients may include salicylates that could be absorbed through the skin and therefore possibly be contributory to Reye Syndrome. If a product of this kind is not taken by mouth, there is no obligation by the manufacturer to list an aspirin warning on the package.[10]

Ibuprofen is sold under several trade names such as Advil, Excedrin, Nuprin, PediaCare Children's Fever, and Motrin. It has analgesic, anti-inflammatory, and antipyretic properties. Ibuprofen does not affect blood clotting which distinguishes it from aspirin. It does not incur the same consequences as a salicylate-based product. However, since April 2005, the U.S. Food and Drug Administration (FDA) has mandated that a warning be placed in or on the package regarding the potential for gastrointestinal bleeding, stroke, and heart attack. A specific instruction on the consumer-labeling leaflet states "Do not give this product to children under 12 except under the advice and supervision of a doctor."[11] Even though this source does not recommend the use of ibuprofen in children younger than 12 years without a physician's approval, it has been tested on children older than 6 months with no difference in side effects from those experienced by an adult.[7] Therefore, choosing one of these NSAIDs must be determined by the presenting problem and considered for the possible accompanying side effects that may occur in any of the body systems, but the most serious would be systemic anaphylaxis. Drug and herbal interactions may also produce unwanted side effects and even toxicity in some instances.[2,3]

Acetaminophen can be obtained in many different forms and compounds that determine the action they take in the body. These include acetaminophen alone (which has no anti-inflammatory properties), acetaminophen and salicylate combinations that include caffeine, and acetaminophen with narcotic analgesics.[7] The acetaminophen and salicylate combinations may reduce fever and relieve mild pain, although neither component is as effective as aspirin for relieving severe pain and inflammation associated with arthritis.[7] Some of these combination medicines may be too strong for use by children, so a careful check of the package is indicated in addition to making contact with the physician.[7] Acetaminophen has been tested in children, and side effects similar to those in the adult population have been found. These include nausea, vomiting, abdominal pain, stimulation or drowsiness, rash, and toxic reactions.[3] The signs of an overdose in children would include severe drowsiness, changes in behavior, and alterations in the depth and rate of breathing.[6] If acetaminophen with narcotic analgesics is given to a child younger than 2 years, breathing problems may occur. Children in this age group are much more sensitive to narcotics than adults are, and they may exhibit increased levels of restlessness and excitement.[7]

Children are prone to coughing, which is an important safety reflex to keep the airways clear of secretions. However, excessive coughing may be indicative of a more serious underlying condition. An acute cough comes on suddenly due to a cold, sinus infection, or the flu and usually resolves in less than 3 weeks, whereas a chronic cough lasts longer.[7] In many cases, the first approach is to use a remedy such as a humidifier or cool air vaporizer in the child's bedroom or a decongestant to relieve postnasal drip. Inhaling steam may also be beneficial for relieving a dry or nonproductive cough. For children older than 3 years, some kind of hard candy could be given, but be aware of the possibility of choking. If the cough secretions are thick, drinking extra amounts of fluid can help to thin the mucus.[3]

Guaifenesin is an example of an expectorant that works by stimulating a gastric mucosal reflex that, in turn, increases the production of lung mucus.[3] Guaifenesin is sold under several trade names, such as Robitussin. The commonly reported side effects are drowsiness, nausea, and vomiting.[3] *Pseudoephedrine* is an adrenergic drug that is used to relieve cold symptoms and as a nasal decongestant. For children with otitis media, this may be an appropriate medication. It is sold under many trade names, including Children's Congestion Relief, Children's Silfedrine, PediaCare Infant's Decongestant, and Sudafed. It acts on the vascular smooth muscle and causes constriction. The side effects of these remedies are the opposite of the expectorants as they produce anxiety, insomnia, and, in children, increased activity, and excessive agitation.[2,3]

Dextromethorphan is a nonopioid cough suppressant available under numerous trade names such as Benylin, Pertussin, St. Joseph Cough Suppressant, Children's Hold, Vicks 44, and Delsym, for example. This drug's mechanism of action is to depress the cough center of the brain. Common side effects are dizziness, sedation, and nausea. It is used primarily for nonproductive, persistent coughs.[3]

COMMON PRESCRIBED MEDICATIONS

Medications are an essential component of health care in the United States and have had a significant influence on the health and well-being of many individuals. Certain medications are available to the consumer only with a physician's prescription. The more commonly prescribed medications seen in pediatric patients include those that are used as an anti-inflammatory, for pain relief and/or sedation, and as a skeletal muscle relaxant.

Opioid analgesics are primarily used for moderate to severe pain relief and should only be used when necessary to treat the severity level of the child's pain. They inhibit synaptic transmission in the key pain pathways in the central nervous system to produce the analgesic effects. There are both central and peripheral side effects producing varying stages of mood alteration from sedation and drowsiness

POINT TO REMEMBER

Side Effects of Acetaminophen

Side effects of acetaminophen (which includes Tylenol) can include nausea, vomiting, abdominal pain, drowsiness or increased activity, and a rash.

to euphoria. One of the most serious side effects is respiratory depression, although this is not usually a major concern when the correct dose is given. These narcotic analgesics can lead to addiction, tolerance, or physical dependence if not used and monitored appropriately. They can also cause constipation as they slow down the peristaltic action and gastric motility of the gastrointestinal tract.[2] Additionally, opioids may be used in the short term to suppress coughs, control diarrhea, and reduce the experience of pain. Oral administration of these drugs is the most convenient method. Following surgery, and in children with cancer, they may be administered parenterally, in particular, by the use of a patient-controlled analgesia delivery system (PCA), which is the most commonly used method in children.

POINTS TO REMEMBER

Opioids

A common side effect of opioids is respiratory depression and constipation. Patients who are on opioids may not show an expected change in respiration with exercise or may need to be reminded to take deep breaths during movement activities. The decreased gastrointestinal motility can lead to discomfort.

Steroids, also called corticosteroids or glucocorticoids, are used primarily to reduce inflammation by inhibiting the inflammatory response. One of the most effective applications is in the treatment of respiratory conditions such as asthma and bronchospasm as well as in the relief of the effects of exposure to poison ivy and poison oak. They may be administered by inhalation, allowing the drug to reach the respiratory mucosa. This type of administration greatly reduces the adverse side effects that can occur with systemic application, which can produce some serious side effects, particularly with long-term use. Steroids can retard growth in children and cause osteoporosis, muscle wasting, breakdown of the skin and other tissues, and many other conditions.[2]

Drugs that induce sedation are prescribed for different conditions. The sedative effect may be either intentional or as an unintentional or unavoidable side effect. For example, children with epilepsy will probably have *barbiturates* or *benzodiazepines* prescribed for their condition, with sedation being the primary side effect.[2] Epilepsy is a chronic condition, and any of the drugs prescribed are intended to limit the damage to the central nervous system. Diazepam (trade name Valium) is a benzodiazepine used to treat muscle spasms, spasticity, as well as seizures and should not be administered to children younger than 6 months. Respiratory depression is a serious side effect with its use at any age.[3] Phenobarbital is a barbiturate that is used as an anticonvulsant for those children with all forms of epilepsy, for febrile seizures, for sedation, and for the treatment of *status epilepticus* (a prolonged seizure, at least 30 minutes in duration, which requires immediate medical attention). It can be administered via intravenous infusion, intramuscularly, rectally, or orally depending on the age of the child and the severity of the condition for which it is given.[3]

Skeletal muscle relaxants are used to decrease hyperexcitability of muscles without compromising muscle function. They are intended to normalize muscle excitability, decrease pain, and improve motor function. This type of drug is not to be confused with skeletal muscle paralytics, which are intended to prevent any muscle action, such as in a patient under general anesthesia.[3] Baclofen (Lioresal) is one of the most widely used drugs in this category, particularly for children with cerebral palsy. It acts on the spinal cord to reduce pain and spasticity. It is not a curative drug, but does permit interventions like physical therapy to take place with greater efficacy. Baclofen can be administered orally or intrathecally, by an implanted infusion pump.[3,7] Sometimes, if the orally administered dose is effective in controlling the spasticity, it is accompanied by sedation. Intrathecal administration is done by a physician and is an option for the control of severe and intractable spasticity. It is delivered very close to the spinal cord in the subarachnoid space that offers fewer side effects as it remains largely in the local area. There are a number of significant precautions with this method, and toxicity or withdrawal can be the result of pump malfunction.[2] The one side effect that has been documented with this method of administration is the temporary decrease in strength, or apparent strength, in those patients who had previously relied on the spasticity for attaining or maintaining a particular position. Any change in the child's symptoms could be due to the medication or pump operation, and the physician should be notified. There are numerous anecdotal reports of the benefits of intrathecal baclofen regarding improvement in activities of daily living, gait and wheelchair mobility, and improved efficiency in positioning, transfers, and dressing.[12] Some of the other commonly used drugs in this genre of antispasticity medications are dantrolene sodium (Dantrium) and diazepam (Valium).[3]

Botulinum toxin A (Botox) is a derivative of *Clostridium botulinum*, a bacterium that is often associated with food poisoning. It is administered by injection targeting the specific area of involvement. This neurotoxin prevents the release of acetylcholine at the neuromuscular junction creating a paralyzing effect on the muscle. It was initially used in the treatment of eye muscle imbalance problems such as strabismus and blepharospasm. It is now used to treat a wide variety of conditions in which unwanted muscle activity and spasticity is preventing movement or function such as in children with cerebral palsy or in those who have had traumatic brain injuries. Botox is often used in coordination with external support to maintain the length of the muscle and surrounding structures by the use of serial casting and supportive orthoses. Although anesthesia is not required, children may be anesthetized due to the pain associated with the procedure and to allow for a more accurate injection. The effects of Botox are temporary and may last for 3 to 4 months during which time the child participates in physical therapy to gain active range of motion, strength, and function.

MEDICATIONS FOR SELECTED PEDIATRIC CONDITIONS

Croup is a particular kind of cough and has been described as sounding like a seal barking. It tends to appear in children between 3 months and 5 years of age and commonly occurs between the months of October and March in the northern hemisphere. It has been reported as occurring a few days following a cold, as being much worse at night than in the day time, and as resolving usually within a week.[13] Remedies will depend on the severity of the condition which, at its worst, could cause death from respiratory distress. Conservative management and nondrug treatment for this condition can be implemented similar to that for coughs. Medications that may need to be used in severe cases typically contain steroids, such as oral dexamethasone, which has an almost immediate effect of relieving the symptoms of croup. Croup is still regarded as a potentially serious condition, and careful monitoring and contact with a physician or hospital is recommended.[13]

POINT TO REMEMBER

Croup

Croup has a distinct sound that has been described as a seal barking. Typically seen between the ages of 3 months and 5 years, it is considered a potentially serious condition and medical attention is recommended.

A common condition that can be alleviated by topical applications is that of *pruritis* or itching, in either localized areas or in a general area of the body. Itching may also be a side effect of medications. There are household remedies that can be implemented to reduce the discomfort: lukewarm baths, applying cold compresses to the affected area, and avoiding scratching and exposure to heat.[7] Itching can be caused by many different factors from parasites, insect bites, and reactions to external environmental factors. The pharmacologic remedies for each condition will be specific to the cause of the itching. Topical anesthetics such as benzocaine, lidocaine, or pramoxine can be used for minor itching due to insect bites. However, precaution must be exercised in administering these to children younger than 6 years and for longer

than 1 week. Hydrocortisone cream is included in the class of prescription topical glucocorticoids (also known as corticosteroids), which are also used as antipruritics and anti-inflammatories.[2,3] Exposing the area to the sun as well as prolonged use after 14 days are discouraged.[3] There are low strength (1%) hydrocortisone creams available OTC that do not have as potent an effect. Topical cortisone can have systemic effects due to absorption through the skin; therefore, it is advisable for a physician to determine the specific cause of the irritation and to prescribe the appropriate remedy. Oral antihistamines, diphenhydramine for example, may be taken, but there may be undesirable side effects such as drowsiness.

If an area of skin becomes infected, there are several OTC topical antiinfectives that may be used, such as bacitracin, gentamycin, and neosporin.[7]

Vitamins and mineral supplements are also available OTC. Children will generally receive adequate amounts of vitamins in their daily food intake even if they are finicky eaters. Infants who are either breastfed or fed infant formula will also acquire adequate amounts of vitamins if they have started on solid foods at approximately 6 months of age. The one vitamin that may need to be supplemented in breastfed infants is vitamin D, particularly if those infants do not get adequate sun exposure, live in a northern latitude, or during the wintertime. Vitamin D is naturally formed in the skin when exposed to sunlight, but deficiencies can cause alteration to the growth of bones and teeth. A deficiency of vitamin D can be easily remedied by administering daily drops.

Children are more vulnerable to *dehydration* than are adults. Caregivers need to watch for signs of this occurring, particularly if the child is taking a medication, because the concentration of the drug in the blood will be changed. Warning signs of dehydration can include a fever, the inability to produce tears, a low output of urine, light-headedness, fatigue, dry skin, and the inability to focus mentally. At a minimum young children require approximately 5 cups of liquid per day, older children more than that, and adults approximately 8 cups. It may be difficult to encourage a child to drink adequate amounts of plain water. However, there are several alternate sources that are acceptable to meet this minimal quantity and can be given in the form of flavored water, popsicle and juice sticks, and some fresh fruit and vegetables that provide a small fraction of this recommended intake. The use of beverages that are high in sugar is discouraged because they tend to increase dehydration. Beverages containing caffeine should also be discouraged as they contribute to dehydration.

If a child has had an illness during which there has been prolonged vomiting or diarrhea, taking fluids by mouth may be counterproductive. In this instance, the child may need to be admitted to the hospital for intravenous fluid replacement because not only has fluid been lost, but also essential electrolytes necessary for the body to function adequately. One product that is frequently used orally for children is Pedialyte, which contains those essential electrolytes.

There are many causes of diarrhea that can be due to any number of factors, such as bacterial and viral infections, parasites, and reactions to food and medications. In the newborn or young infant this can have serious consequences as these children do not have the reserves on which to draw to overcome the tendency for dehydration. Death can occur quite rapidly if not treated. However, before treating diarrhea, it is essential for the physician to identify the cause. Prescribing or suggesting an antidiarrheal medication may make the condition worse if it is caused by a bacterium. Preventing the purging of the organism can encourage it to proliferate in the intestines.[14]

POINTS TO REMEMBER

Dehydration

A child can become dehydrated quickly, especially if she is vomiting or has diarrhea. Signs of dehydration can include fever, inability to produce tears, a low level of urine output, feeling light headed, fatigue, and inability to mentally focus. Medical attention is required.

Children are prone to acquire various *infections*, particularly those of the ear, nose, and throat. The incidence tends to be more prevalent at the start of the school year or when children enter daycare due to the increased exposure to children who have an infection. Antibiotics are used to treat some of the secondary infections, although there has been some controversy over this practice due to the demands of the parents, the inaccurate diagnosis of the impression gained from the symptoms or assumptions made about the condition, resistance to the drugs, and the lack of effectiveness that has been occurring.[15] If a cough has been prolonged for more than 10 days, antimicrobial treatment may be indicated. It is recommended that an accurate culture be obtained prior to using any medication for an upper respiratory tract infection. Data from the National Center for Health Statistics indicate that, in recent years, approximately 75% of all outpatient antimicrobial prescriptions have been issued for five conditions: otitis media, sinusitis, bronchitis, pharyngitis, and nonspecific upper respiratory tract infection.[16] It is important to remember that antibiotics do not affect viral infections, but may be used to treat the complications.

Parents are often concerned about infants who tend to "spit up" a lot or who exhibit the projectile type of vomiting. These events are not uncommon, but would present a more serious concern if there is no weight gain, if these vomiting events occur more often than twice a day, or if it appears that the baby has an upper respiratory

infection, coughs a lot, or has sinus blockage or any other symptom that could be the result of aspiration. This condition is commonly known as reflux or *gastroesophageal reflux disease* (GERD). It is the result of the esophageal sphincter failing to constrict to prevent the stomach contents from backing up into the esophagus. If this persists, the stomach acid can eventually erode the walls of the esophagus and cause an inflammatory reaction. It is hoped that as the infant gets older, she will outgrow the tendency for this vomiting, which commonly occurs during or after feeding. It usually resolves when the infant is between 9 and 10 months of age. Some of the simple remedies to implement can be to have the infant in a more upright position during and after feeding, to increase the viscosity of the liquid, to slightly elevate the head of the crib, and to discourage a flat sleeping position. This condition is not unique to infants and can occur in people at any age. There should be an accurate diagnosis that can be obtained from the history, an active radiograph monitoring of a barium swallow, and by the use of various invasive procedures to view the upper gastrointestinal tract. Medication use or surgery in infants and very young children should be options to consider only when all other remedies have been attempted and have failed to reverse the severe symptoms. There are medications like cimetidine (Tagamet), ranitidine (Zantac), and antacids that are used in older children and adults.[17]

POINT TO REMEMBER

Gastroesophageal Reflux Disease

Some nonpharmacological interventions for GERD include remaining upright during and after eating for approximately 30 to 60 minutes, elevating the head of the bed 30 to 45 degrees, or increasing the viscosity of liquids consumed.

According to the U.S. Department of Health and Human Services, approximately 20% of American children have a mental disorder, with anxiety disorders, disruptive disorders (such as attention deficit and hyperactivity disorder) and mood disorders (depression) being the most common.[18] Antidepressants are sometimes prescribed for children and teenagers with mood disorders; however, there are many factors for the physician to consider in making this decision. The symptoms of *depression* need to be evaluated thoroughly, and the risks and benefits carefully weighed. The causes and the signs and symptoms are varied and are most often due to either biological or environmental issues. Causative factors may include the loss of a close relationship to a parent, the result of emotional or sexual abuse, or witnessing those events taking place. The warning signs that may manifest as depression are numerous and can include vague physical complaints, truancy from school, poor grades, intentions to run away from home, lack of interest in playing with friends, boredom, substance abuse, volatile emotions and outbursts, and alterations in sleep and food intake. Although parents may consider many of these to be normal occurrences in this age group, if they represent a marked change from prior instances, the behavior should be documented accurately as to date, time, behavior exhibited, and duration. This would provide the evaluating professional with tangible examples indicating a possible clinical depression. There are a number of clinical instruments to assess depression. Two tests that are appropriate for the pediatric population are the Beck Depression Inventory, which is used with adults and older children, and the Children's Depression Inventory, which measures the severity of symptoms of depression in children and adolescents ages 7 through 17 years. However, these and other similar assessment profiles are only available for use by a licensed mental health professional.[19]

Sometimes children feel out of control in their environment and may resort to the one behavior over which they feel that they can exert almost perfect control. Unless the child is being fed, he or she can choose what to eat, when, and how often. *Eating disorders* are basically divided into withholding food from the body or overindulging in it. Anorexia nervosa and bulimia nervosa are the two main categories. Children may develop these at an early age and become obsessed with the condition, attempting to control weight by many methods and completely denying that there is anything out of the ordinary in their behavior and choices, believing that they are grossly overweight. One of the most common methods of weight control is to purge by either vomiting or by the use of laxatives. There are life-threatening issues surrounding these conditions that can lead to suicide or severe metabolic disturbances due to the loss of fluid, muscle mass, and electrolytes, resulting in cardiac arrest.[19,20]

There are children and adolescents who have thoughts of taking their own life (*suicidal ideation*) or who have had incidents of self-inflicted injury for whom a prescription medication may be used to avert that tragedy. According to a statement by the FDA in 2005, the only drug approved to treat depression in pediatric patients is fluoxetine (Prozac). It is indicated for the treatment of major depression, but is not used to treat conditions like bipolar disorder or seasonal affective disorder (SAD). Prozac is one of the drugs in the class of *selective serotonin reuptake inhibitors* (SSRIs), which are thought to assist in increasing the brain's own supply of serotonin by preventing its uptake from the neurons of the central nervous system. There are many side effects of Prozac that may include headache, nausea, tremor, loss of appetite, dry mouth, drowsiness, insomnia, sweating, rash, fatigue, poor concentration, and abnormal dreams.[3]

There are some medications, however, that may actually induce suicidal ideation. Children at risk for suicide are those who have a family or personal history of

suicide or a diagnosis of bipolar disorder. The child's behavior when on antidepressant medication must be monitored closely for any alteration in mood or an increase in any of the following side effects: agitation, anxiety, sleep disturbance, indication of suicidality, or anything else that would be considered unusual for that particular child. It is essential that this behavioral or symptomatic information be communicated immediately to a licensed medical professional to avoid imminent danger. These drugs generally do not reach a therapeutic effect or steady state for approximately 3 to 6 weeks; they need to be taken on a regular basis in incremental doses, and must not be discontinued abruptly.

DRUG AND ALCOHOL ABUSE

According to the National Household Survey on Drug Abuse, in 2001 >6 million children lived with at least one parent who is dependent on or abuses alcohol or drugs.[21] This involved about 10% of children 5 years old or younger, 8% of children ages 6 to 11, and 9% of youths ages 12 to 17 years. It is not only adults who are using alcohol, tobacco, and illegal drugs, but also many adolescents and a growing number of preadolescents.[22] Approximately half (51%) of American youth have tried an illegal drug by the time they graduate from high school.[23] Also most adults who smoke began at an average of 12 years of age and were regular smokers by the age of 14 years.[23] Many times the use and possible subsequent abuse of legal (licit) or illegal (illicit) substances and drugs has it origins in childhood. According to the American Academy of Pediatrics, parents who abuse drugs and alcohol place their children at a high risk for substance abuse, especially if the exposure to such behavior occurs during adolescence.[24] Parents should be made aware that their dependence on or abuse of drugs and alcohol not only has negative effects on them, but also on their children. Even casual use of alcohol, tobacco, or other drugs by children and adolescents, regardless of the amount or frequency, is illegal and can have negative health consequences.[23]

The role of the physical therapist, as well as any other health care professional, is one of education and coordination between the family or patient and the physician. During history taking, the physical therapist should ask questions about medications. These questions could lead to questions or a discussion on the use of alcohol and tobacco around young children or the use of such substances by adolescent patients/clients. This may provide a nonthreatening opportunity to educate the parents on the risks of secondhand smoke, the casual use of alcohol and tobacco by underage persons, and the influence of dependence or abuse on the adolescent. It is a primary preventive measure taken to improve the health of children, which is as important as promoting the use of seat belts or appropriate car seats while riding in an automobile or the

BOX 12-1

CRAFFT Questionnaire. Questions to Identify Adolescents with Substance Abuse Problems

C	*car*	Have you ever ridden in a car driven by someone (including yourself) who was "high" or had been using alcohol or drugs?
R	*relax*	Do you ever use alcohol or drugs to relax, feel better about yourself, or fit in?
A	*alone*	Do you ever use drugs or alcohol while you are alone?
F	*forget*	Do you ever forget things you did while using alcohol or drugs?
F	*friends*	Do your family or friends ever tell you that you should cut down on your drinking or drug use?
T	*trouble*	Have you ever gotten in trouble while you were using alcohol or drugs?

From: Knight J, Sherritt L, Shrier L, et al. Validity of the CRAFFT substance abuse screening test among adolescent clinic patients. *Arch Pediatr Adolesc Med.* 2002;156:607–614.

BOX 12-2

Street Names

Street names of drugs can vary by time and region. Some of the more common street names are available through the Office of National Drug Control Policy available at: www.whitehousedrugpolicy.gov/streetterms/default.asp. Accessed August 6, 2006.
Additional lists and information are available at the National Institute on Drug Abuse at: www.drugabuse.gov. Accessed August 6, 2006.

use of protective equipment when riding a bike or skateboard. Early education, identification of children at risk, and early intervention must be promoted in the healthcare professions. Early intervention may be more effective in addressing the dependence or abuse than trying to address the issues after years of misuse.[24]

The *CRAFFT questionnaire* is a brief, valid screening tool that can be used to help identify adolescents who may need additional professional testing or evaluation regarding substance abuse or problems.[25] Box 12-1 lists the questions associated with the acronym. Two or more "yes" answers suggest further follow-up by a qualified professional. Also, because street names of drugs can change over time, and the nonuser may not be readily familiar with such terms as "beans" and "snappers," the White House Office of National Drug Control Policy and the National Institute on Drug Abuse are two organizations that have an internet site that provides a reference for street names of drugs, as well as other helpful information on this national health issue (Box 12-2).

The practice of physical therapy can take the professional into the homes of families or into other clinical settings that allow extended periods of time in which working relationships develop between the physical therapist, the child, and the family. This relationship can provide the opportunity to address the issue of substance dependence or abuse, in a nonthreatening and nonjudgmental manner, which can help the person obtain the necessary intervention by the appropriate professional. The physical therapist should feel comfortable discussing this primary preventive issue and make it a part of the examination process.

SUMMARY

Physical therapists play a role in the management of a patient's medications by supporting the prescribed regimen and evaluating the person's ability to physically access, manipulate, and administer the recommended dosage. A basic understanding of pharmacology and the usage of commonly prescribed and OTC medications allow the physical therapist to participate in a discussion regarding medications with the patient, family, physician, or pharmacist. Being aware of the possible influence of drug interactions between prescribed medications, OTC drugs, and diet opens the possibility for these factors to become potential causes for abnormal behaviors or adverse side effects seen in a child or patient. It is also important to realize that the factors that contribute to adult drug abuse or dependence can begin with a child's exposure to such behavior at a young age. Discussing the issue of drug or substance use in the home, in a nonthreatening manner, may possibly help address this social problem and is a primary preventive measure that can help to promote the health of all children.

REVIEW QUESTIONS

1. You are seeing a child through an outpatient clinic for rehabilitation following a hamstring tendon lengthening and a dorsal rhizotomy secondary to the movement impairments associated with muscle hypertonia. The mother reports that the child has been complaining of an upset stomach and that she has been giving him an OTC drug to combat the symptoms. As her physical therapist, you:
   a. instruct the mother that it is common to have an upset stomach after surgery.
   b. tell her to stop administering the OTC drugs to her child because of the possible side effects and drug interactions that may occur.
   c. ask her if she discussed this with her child's physician and instruct her on the importance of communicating

to the child's physician or pharmacist before providing her child with any OTC medications.

d. make a note in the medical record of the symptoms and instruct the mother to read the OTC drug label carefully.

2. Your patient is a 13-year-old boy who has cerebral palsy. You are working on his ability to don and doff his ankle–foot orthotics independently, stair negotiation, and functional activities that he will need for the next school year. During his visit today, you notice a significant decrease in his ability to walk, climb stairs, and perform the prescribed therapeutic exercise. He informs you that his physician recently increased his oral baclofen. Of the following options, which is the most appropriate physical therapist response?

a. Progress his therapeutic exercises to increase the strength of the key muscles for ambulation and stair climbing.

b. Discontinue the therapeutic exercises because of the sudden weakness and focus on donning and doffing the braces.

c. Consult with the physician and report the decrease in strength. This may be a factor in setting the correct dosage. Continue with the present physical therapy program as tolerated.

d. Discontinue physical therapy intervention until the appropriate baclofen dosage has been firmly established.

3. Your patient is a 17-year-old high school student who is being seen for rehabilitation of an ankle sprain that he sustained 2 days ago in a soccer game. His physician has ordered an air cast and ibuprofen for the pain and swelling. During your examination, the patient reports that his pain and swelling have not changed since taking the medication, which he began yesterday. Which of the following is the proper physical therapist response?

a. Instruct him to increase his dosage of medication.

b. Recommend a different type of anti-inflammatory that he can obtain OTC.

c. Instruct him to increase the frequency at which he takes the medication.

d. Instruct him that it may take a few days before he feels the effects of the anti-inflammatory medication. He should give the medication more time to take effect or consult his physician with his concerns.

4. Jenna is a 14-year-old girl who recently underwent a posterior spinal fusion secondary to adolescent idiopathic scoliosis. It is postoperative day one, and physical therapy has been ordered for gait and transfer training. She is presently receiving an opioid pain medication via PCA and is on 2 L of oxygen via nasal cannula. The percentage of oxygen in her blood (O_2 sats) is 96%. Upon standing, her O_2 sats drop to 92%, and she complains of stomach discomfort. Which of the following is the proper physical therapist response?

a. Instruct Jenna to sit down and rest. The change in her O_2 sats is indicative of exercise intolerance.

b. Instruct Jenna to take a deep breath in through her nose. Her drop in O_2 and her upset stomach could be side effects of the medication. Continue with the physical therapy intervention.

c. Discontinue physical therapy intervention at this time. According to the patient response to movement and her complaint of discomfort, she is not ready to get up and walk.

d. Instruct Jenna to lie down and perform therapeutic exercises in supine. She is unable to tolerate the upright position at this time.

5. You are providing services to a 13-month-old child through the local early intervention program in your state. The child has been diagnosed with a developmental delay. It is summer, very warm, and the apartment in which the family lives has no air conditioning. Her mother informs you that the child has a slight fever of 99°F and had an episode of diarrhea this morning. You are concerned about the risk of dehydration. Of the following statements reported by the mother, which one would least likely be associated with the signs of dehydration?

a. The child has not urinated today. Her diapers have been dry.

b. The child vomited once during the night.

c. The child does not appear to be sick. She is active.

d. The child does not appear to be interested in playing today.

ACKNOWLEDGMENT

I thank Ellen Kitts, MD, for her review and contributions to this chapter.

REFERENCES

1. *Stedman's Electronic Medical Dictionary* [book on CD-ROM], v6.0. Baltimore: Lippincott, Williams & Wilkins; 2004.

2. Ciccone CD. *Pharmacology in Rehabilitation,* 3rd ed. Philadelphia: FA Davis; 2002.

3. *Nursing Drug Reference*. St. Louis, MO: Elsevier Mosby; 2005.

4. Albright L, Barron W, Fasick M, Polinko P, Janosky J. Continuous intrathecal baclofen infusion for spasticity of cerebral origin. *JAMA*. 1993;270:2475–2477.

5. American Diabetes Association. Type I Diabetes. Available at: http://www.diabetes.org/type-1-diabetes.jsp. Accessed August 4, 2006.

6. Turner RE, Rampersaud GC. Using medications safely: interactions between grapefruit juice and prescription drugs. Institute of Food and Agricultural Sciences, University of Florida; 2002. Available at: http://edis.ifas.ufl.edu/FS088. Accessed August 1, 2006.

7. United States National Library of Medicine and the National Institutes of Health. Medline Plus. Drugs and supplements. Baclofen Oral. Available at: http://www.nlm.nih.gov/medlineplus/druginfo/medmaster/a682530.html. Accessed August 1, 2006.

8. Merck and Co: MerkSource. Physician's Desk Reference® Family Guide To Over-The-Counter Drugs. Available at: http://www.mercksource.com/pp/us/cns/cns_pdr_ frameset.jspzQzpgzEzzSzppzSzuszSzcnszSzcns_hl_pdrz-PzjspzQzpgzEzzSzppdocszSzuszSzcnszSzcontentzSzpdrotcz-Szotc_fullzSzalphaindexazPzhtm. Accessed August 1, 2006.

9. The National Institutes of Health, National Institute of Neurological Disorders and Stroke. Reye's Syndrome Information page. 2006. Available at: http://www.ninds.nih.gov/disorders/reyes_syndrome/reyes_syndrome.htm. Accessed August 1, 2006.

10. National Reye's Syndrome Foundation. What is the Role of Aspirin? 2005. Available at: http://www.reyessyndrome.org/aspirin.htm. Accessed August 1, 2006.

11. United States Food and Drug Administration: Center for Drug Evaluation and Research. Consumer Labeling Leaflet for Ibuprofen Tablets USP, 200 mg. 1997. Available at: http://www.fda.gov/cder/foi/anda/98/74931_Ibuprofen_Prntlbl.pdf. Accessed August 1, 2006.

12. Campbell SK, Almeida GL, Penn RD, Corcos DM. The effects of intrathecally administered baclofen on function in patients with spasticity. *Phys Ther*. 1995;75:352–362.

13. Van Voorhees B. United States National Library of Medicine and the National Institutes of Health. Medline Plus. Croup. 2006. Available at: http://www.nlm.nih.gov/medlineplus/ency/article/000959.htm. Accessed August 1, 2006.

14. United States National Institute of Diabetes and Digestive and Kidney Diseases: National Digestive Diseases Information Clearinghouse. Diarrhea. 2003. Available at: http://digestive.niddk.nih.gov/ddiseases/pubs/diarrhea/index.htm. Accessed August 8, 2006.

15. Dowell SF, Schwartz B, Phillips WR. Appropriate use of antibiotics for URIs in children: Part I. Otitis media and acute sinusitis. *Am Fam Physician* [serial online]. 1998;58:1113–1123. Available at: http://www.aafp.org/afp/981001ap/dowell.html. Accessed August 2, 2006.

16. Dowell SF, Schwartz B, Phillips WR, The Pediatric URI Consensus Team. Appropriate use of antibiotics for URIs in children: Part II. Cough, pharyngitis and the common cold. *Am Fam Physician* [serial online]. 1998;58:1335–1345. Available at: http://www.aafp.org/afp/981015ap/dowell.html. Accessed August 2, 2006.

17. National Institute of Diabetes and Digestive and Kidney Diseases, National Digestive Diseases Information Clearinghouse. Gastroesophageal Reflux in Children and Adolescents. 2006. Available at: http://digestive.niddk.nih.gov/ddiseases/pubs/gerinchildren/index.htm. Accessed August 7, 2006.

18. U.S. Department of Health and Human Services. U.S. Public Health Service. Mental Health: A Report of the Surgeon General. 1999. Washington, DC. Available at: http://www.surgeongeneral.gov/library/mentalhealth/chapter2/sec2_1.html. Accessed December 29, 2006.

19. U.S. Department of Health and Human Services, Substance Abuse and Mental Health Services Administration, National Mental Health Information Center. Child and Adolescent Mental Health. 2003. Available at: http://www.mentalhealth.samhsa.gov/publications/allpubs/CA-0004/default.asp. Accessed August 8, 2006.

20. Sullivan PF. Mortality in anorexia nervosa. *Am J Psychiatry*. 1995;152:1073–1074.

21. U.S. Department of Health and Human Services, Office of Applied Studies, Substance Abuse and Mental Health Services Administration, The National Household Survey on Drug Abuse. Children Living with Substance-Abusing or Substance-Dependent Parents. 2003. Available at: http://www.oas.samhsa.gov/2k3/children/children.cfm. Accessed December 14, 2006.

22. American Academy of Pediatrics Committee on Substance Abuse. *Substance Abuse: A Guide for Health Professionals.* Schydlower M, ed. 2nd ed. Elk Grove Village, IL: American Academy of Pediatrics; 2002.

23. Kulig JW; American Academy of Pediatrics Committee on Substance Abuse. Tobacco, alcohol, and other drugs: the role of the pediatrician in prevention, identification, and management of substance abuse. *Pediatrics*. 2005;115:816–821.

24. Biederman J, Faraone S, Monuteaux M, Feighner J. Patterns of alcohol and drug use in adolescents can be predicted by parental substance use disorders. *Pediatrics*. 2000;106:792–797.

25. Knight J, Sherritt L, Shrier L, Harris S, Chang G. Validity of the CRAFFT substance abuse screening test among adolescent clinic patients. *Arch Pediatr Adolesc Med*. 2002;156:607–614.

Additional Resource

Office of National Drug Control Policy. National Youth Antidrug Media Campaign. Keeping Your Kids Drug Free: A How-To Guide for Parents and Caregivers. A drug prevention brochure that provides parents and caregivers with real-life tips on how to keep kids drug free. Available at: http://www.theantidrug.com/pdfs/version3General.pdf. Accessed August 6, 2006.

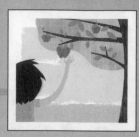

CHAPTER 13

Legal Issues

Bryan Warren

LEARNING OBJECTIVES

1. Understand the basic types of laws that influence the practice of physical therapy.
2. Understand the general concepts of child custody, confidentiality, and acting as a mandated reporter or an expert witness, as they apply to the practice of physical therapy with children.
3. Differentiate between a minor, a mature minor, and an emancipated minor and know how these affect clinical decision making.
4. Differentiate between an employee and an independent contractor.
5. Understand the basics of a business arrangement, including contracts.

Several federal and state laws impact the structure and delivery of health care in the United States. The practice of physical therapy is defined and influenced by a number of specific federal and state laws drafted and adopted by legislative bodies (*statutes*) and further defined and detailed in rules created by administrative agencies to help implement the statutes (*regulations*). Some examples can be found in the federal Medicare program that provides detailed regulations controlling the delivery of services and payment for treatment of Medicare patients; the concepts of informed consent and professional malpractice liability that arise from state-specific statutes and *common law* (the rule of law developed through court opinions); various employment laws that influence clinical practice and employment arrangements or business formation issues; and state-specific laws regarding family relationships, patient rights, and child custody.

Factors that influence the delivery of physical therapy services may involve several areas of law calling into play both federal and state statutes, regulations, and common law. The laws and regulations also can change very rapidly given the current climate of a particular legislative body. Accordingly, the reader cannot rely on the general nature of this chapter as guidance on his or her specific issue. Before taking up practice in a particular state, a physical therapist must become familiar with the relevant laws of physical therapy practice in that state and keep current on the changes that take place. Similarly, before treating patients under a federal program such as Medicare, Medicaid, or the Individuals with Disabilities Education Act, the physical therapist must understand the relevant laws and regulations that pertain to the delivery of services. Many resources are available to assist in this process, including the American Physical Therapy Association (APTA) and the agency in the state that oversees the practice of physical therapy. In most states, this is a physical therapy board. The Internet also provides a wealth of information, including state government web sites that contain statutes, regulations, and occasionally, summaries of relevant common law issues. A physical therapist should have a working knowledge of accessing and referencing the state and federal laws and regulations that apply to her specific area of practice.

Because of the serious nature of the physical therapist's legal obligations, she should access credible resources to understand the legal issues and influences involved in the delivery of health care services. This can be a daunting task, especially if the physical therapist is working in a variety of clinical settings, such as a hospital, an early intervention program, and hospice. Consultation with an experienced attorney is an efficient means of meeting this need. Although the cost of having a question answered by an attorney may seem prohibitive, it is often far less costly than the ramifications of acting without understanding the law. This chapter provides a brief overview of the general structure and principles of law that may be useful to the practicing physical therapist in pediatrics. Specific laws that pertain to certain settings are detailed in their respective chapters of this book.

POINT TO REMEMBER

Physical Therapy and the Law

Physical therapists are responsible for knowing the laws and regulations that affect the practice of physical therapy in their state. These laws may be found in statutes, common law, or regulations.

LAWS

The laws that impact a physical therapist come from many sources. The U.S. Constitution is at the heart of the American legal system. All laws and legal processes must be consistent with the Constitution. Although any court can determine whether a law is constitutional, the final say on the issue rests with the U.S. Supreme Court. For instance, cases before the Supreme Court have determined the constitutionality of laws related to abortion, patient autonomy, and informed consent. The U.S. Congress creates federal statutes such as the Social Security Act, which established the Medicare and Medicaid programs, and the Americans with Disabilities Act that protects the rights of Americans with disabilities. These statutes can be found in the *United States Code,* which is a collection of all federal statutes. Often these statutes require complex rules and regulations to clarify how they apply to various situations. For instance, the Center for Medicare & Medicaid Services (CMS) is a federal agency that drafts and enforces specific rules and regulations regarding Medicare and Medicaid programs.[1] The process of creating (or promulgating) and enforcing these rules and regulations makes up an area of law called administrative law.

Each state also has its own court system, including a state supreme court, which interprets state law. For instance, most medical malpractice (professional negligence) laws are state-specific laws, developed over time by state court decisions. This is the process of common law. Just like on the federal level, individual state legislatures are responsible for creating statutory law. Each state has some form of statute, sometimes referred to as an Act, which oversees the practice of physical therapy in the state, requires a license to practice, and defines what the practice of physical therapy is in that particular state. These statutes create and empower a state agency, commonly a state board of physical therapy, to create and enforce more specific rules and regulations such as the licensing process for applicants.

POINT TO REMEMBER

The Practice Act

Individual states control the practice of physical therapy in their state, which is outlined in some form of statute or Act, generally referred to as the Practice Act. The Practice Act is clarified through regulations created by a state agency such as the state board of physical therapy.

The board or agency controlling the practice of physical therapy in a state should not be confused with the state chapter of the APTA. The APTA is a national professional organization that promotes and protects the profession of physical therapy. Individual state chapters of the APTA serve that purpose on the state level. The APTA has a Code of Ethics and Guide for Professional Conduct that all APTA members are to follow. A violation of these professional guidelines is reported to, and handled by, that state's APTA chapter. The APTA may, in response, take action against the individual's APTA membership status. In contrast, a state physical therapy board exists to protect the public and to handle any violation of the state practice act and its regulations. The physical therapy board may, when appropriate, take action against the individual's license to practice physical therapy in that state.

POINT TO REMEMBER

APTA versus State Board

The APTA is a professional organization that promotes the profession of physical therapy. The State Board of Physical Therapy controls the practice of physical therapy in the state with the purpose of protecting the public.

FAMILY AND PATIENT ISSUES

A physical therapist working with children may frequently find herself in situations where several individuals are providing input with regard to a decision about a child or asking for information about the health or care of a child. Children generally cannot make decisions about their health care. They must rely on their parents. This can be a challenging aspect of the care of a child, especially if there is conflict between the parents. The physical therapist should be aware of the legal relationship between the parents and the child and understand her responsibility to ultimately advocate in the child's best interest. Unfortunately, the health care of a child may be an issue in a family lawsuit of some sort.

Lawsuits are usually the result of disagreements that cannot be settled through discussion or mutual agreement. Many times the person initiating the lawsuit feels that this is the only recourse available to address a perceived injustice. Although the legal system in the United States is arguably the best in the world, the lawsuit process, often referred to as *litigation*, can be time consuming and expensive, and may not reach a resolution with which either party is completely satisfied. Accordingly, it is almost always better to avoid litigation through prevention and pre-emptive intervention.

Often, the perceived need to initiate a lawsuit is a result of a series of misunderstandings, concealment of information, miscommunication, or a lack of honesty. This is particularly true in health care, where patients and their family members are vulnerable and situations involve intense emotions. Good health care provider businesses should have policies and procedures in place to ensure a clear understanding of the services to be rendered, the cost of such services, and the procedures to follow to assure family and patient safety and understanding. Following these policies and procedures will help minimize the risk of misunderstanding. They generally address requirements for documentation and communication with the patient and, when appropriate, the patient's family. Also, it is important that a physical therapist engage her superiors early when there is a situation that could give rise to a disgruntled patient or family member. It is better to address these situations early than to be surprised by a notification that a lawsuit has been filed.

During the first encounter with the child or family, it is important to clarify the rights of the adults who are with the child. The physical therapist should be aware of the parent who has authority to make decisions for the child, and the child's right to confidentiality.

PARENT PERSPECTIVE

LITIGATION

Getting a lawyer involved was the last thing I wanted to do. I just felt so overwhelmed, and was sure that my child was suffering due to the lack of care and compassion on the part of the health care provider. I honestly did not want another stress in my life, but I felt I had no other option. No one was listening to me. As soon as you mention a lawyer, then people seemed to take notice. It shouldn't be that way.
—*A parent.*

Custody

A central family law issue is child custody. Custody refers to either legal or physical custody. *Legal custody* means the right to make decisions affecting the child's life, including issues related to religion, medical care, and education. *Physical custody*, in contrast, means that the parent has a right to have the child reside with him or her, and that the obligation of that parent is to provide for routine daily care and control.[2] Either or both legal and physical custody may be granted to parents jointly or to an individual parent. State level courts, as opposed to federal level courts, make custody decisions. It is usually the state family or divorce court.

A child might not live in the state of the parents or other parties with custody interests. Accordingly, it might be difficult to determine which state's courts have *jurisdiction* (the authority) to make a custody decision. The majority of states resolve this issue by applying the Uniform Child Custody Jurisdiction Act (UCCJA) or the newer Uniform Child Custody Jurisdiction and Enforcement Act of 1997.[3] Under these Acts, jurisdiction will generally lie with the state with the closest connection to the child (other than the child's home state).

Generally, when determining who should have custody of a child, a court will apply the "best interests of the child" standard. In applying this standard, the court will consider multiple factors including parental wishes, wishes of the child, fitness of the parents, anticipated impact on the child's psychological development, interactions and relationships with parents and siblings, the child's adjustment to his or her home, school and community resources, and the mental and physical health of the parties.[2]

POINT TO REMEMBER

Policies and Procedures

Physical therapists should be familiar with, and adhere to, the facilities' policies and procedures, and take early steps to address any possible conflicts with the patient and/or family.

POINT TO REMEMBER

Custody

Legal custody is the right to make decisions affecting the child's life. Physical custody is the right to actually possess the child. Courts will generally look to the best interests of the child in making custody decisions.

In any situation in which a court must make a decision that will impact a child's life (including, particularly, custody disputes), the court may assert its authority to appoint counsel for the child. The attorney called upon to represent the child's interests is referred to as a guardian ad litem. The *guardian ad litem* has a duty to act on behalf of the child, even advocating for the child's custody preference if the child is too young or if the court for some other reason will not consider the child's expressed preference.[4]

In making custody decisions, courts will generally give deference to a natural parent's rights. The majority of states have statutes that encourage *joint custody* or custody that is shared between the parents, so that they both have an active role in the child's care and in important decisions about the child's welfare.[4] In instances where joint custody is not feasible or in the child's best interests, such as in the case of parents who have a hostile relationship, the court may recognize that, in the best interests of the child, a third party will be awarded custody. The third party may be a relative other than a parent, or a guardian appointed by the court.

The termination of any parent's rights regarding his or her child is a serious matter. Because of the fundamental nature of a parent's rights, any attempt to supersede them requires that the parents be accorded certain constitutionally protected procedural rights. These procedural rights are referred to as procedural due process. For instance, in any proceeding to terminate parental rights, a parent who cannot afford to hire an attorney will generally have an attorney appointed for him or her by the court.[5] Also, a state's allegations that are the basis for terminating parental rights must be proved by clear and convincing evidence.[6]

Legally created relationships can interfere with a parent's rights. *Adoption* is a proceeding whereby the legal relationship between the biological parent and child is terminated and a new legal relationship of parent and child is established with the adoptive parents.[2] In some cases, a court will see fit to establish a *guardianship,* forming a legal relationship between the individual (the guardian) and another person (in this case a minor or ward), giving the guardian the right, and the duty, to act on behalf of the child in all decisions affecting the child's life.

A parent's rights can also be subrogated with confirmation of child abuse or neglect. One area in which all adults should advocate for a child, regardless of their relationship, is in the area of abuse and neglect. Physical therapists and other health care professionals are required by statute in all 50 states to report incidents of suspected abuse or neglect.[7]

Abuse and Neglect

The U.S. Constitution provides parents with a fundamental right to raise their children as they see fit. State statutes covering child abuse and neglect, however, can take precedence over some parental rights. It may be in the child's best interests that one or both parents have all of their parental rights terminated. Termination of parental rights is generally based on parental misconduct involving serious physical harm to the child, including sexual abuse, abandonment, neglect and deprivation, and parental conduct that seriously harms the child physically or psychologically, including habitual drug and alcohol use and criminal conduct.[8] The Child Abuse Prevention and Treatment Act (CAPTA) is the federal statute that provides minimum standards for the definition of child abuse and neglect that states must incorporate into their statutory definitions.[9] Under CAPTA, child abuse and neglect means, at a minimum, any recent act or failure to act on the part of a parent or caretaker, which results in death, serious physical or emotional harm, sexual abuse, or exploitation, or an act or failure to act which presents an imminent risk of serious harm [42 USCA §5106g(2)].[9] A *mandatory reporter* is a person who is required by law to make a report of child maltreatment under specific circumstances.[10] Mandatory reporters are typically individuals who have frequent or routine contact with children, such as child care workers, school personnel, and health care workers, including physical therapists. Specific circumstances that would initiate a report of child maltreatment vary from state to state, but generally a report must be made when an individual working in his or her official capacity suspects or has reason to believe that a child has been abused or neglected.[10] State-specific information on child abuse definitions and reporting requirements can be accessed via the Internet from the Child Welfare Information Gateway (www.childwelfare.gov). Reports about abuse in any state can be made by calling Childhelp (800-4-A-Child) or the local child protective service agencies. All states have provisions in their statute to maintain the confidentiality of records regarding abuse or neglect. In most states, the identity of the reporter is specifically protected from disclosure.

POINT TO REMEMBER

Child Abuse or Neglect

A court may terminate parental rights due to abuse or neglect. Health care providers, generally, have a statutory obligation to report suspected abuse or neglect.

PHYSICAL THERAPIST AND PATIENT ISSUES

Health care providers work with information about patients that is highly sensitive and private in nature. Although health care providers including hospitals, physicians, and physical therapists own the medical record they create, under common law, state statutes, and federal law, including the Health Insurance Portability and Accountability Act (HIPAA), patients have the right to access the information contained in their medical records. Similarly, providers have certain obligations under these laws to protect the private nature of the information contained in these records. In the case of a child, the parents must also exercise these protections, because they are responsible for, and have control over the child.

In some situations, a minor who has reached the requisite age can petition a court to be *emancipated* from his parents. This status allows the minor to be treated as an adult (not subject to parental control). A minor who has been emancipated by court order has the right to access the information contained in his medical record and the right to make his own decisions as an autonomous individual. In this situation, the parents would have no right to invade the privacy of the child's medical information.[2]

Sometimes a parent who does not have custody of a child may want access to the child's medical records. As a general rule, parental physical custody does not impact a parent's access to a child's medical records. Accordingly, a parent who has legal custody cannot be denied access to the child's medical records even if the parent does not have physical custody unless, of course, a court has ordered otherwise.

POINT TO REMEMBER

Emancipated Minors

Minors, individuals under the defined age of the majority (usually 18 years), can petition the court to be emancipated from their parents. This emancipation allows them to be treated as an adult.

Informed consent is another legal principle by which a health care professional must abide in many situations. Informed consent means providing adequate disclosure of information to a patient in order to obtain that patient's consent to treatment. The basis of this principle lies in the ethical concept of autonomy—the right to determine what shall be done to a person's body.[2] Autonomy has been incorporated into American health care law, and all courts recognize some duty of health care providers to obtain informed consent. Below the age of majority (generally 18 years), parental consent is almost always required before medical treatment is administered. In certain situations, however, the state may override parental wishes in order to protect a child from irreparable harm. For instance, if a child is in extreme danger if he does not receive a blood transfusion, but the treatment is against the parents' religious beliefs, courts have stepped in to override the parental wishes.[7]

Although actual, explicit informed consent is always ideal, situations arise in which health care providers can rely on implied consent, such as in emergency situations in which it is impossible to obtain actual consent, but a life-threatening disease or injury requires immediate treatment. Under this principle, a minor can receive medical care in an emergency without the consent of a parent or guardian. All states allow the parental consent requirement to be waived in the event of a medical emergency, during which obtaining this consent is impossible or imprudent. Most states also allow minors to seek treatment for sexual abuse or assault without parental consent, but some states require that parents be notified of the abuse unless the provider has reason to believe that the parent was responsible for the abuse.[2] Similarly, some states have adopted a *mature minor* doctrine, whereby a minor of a certain age (generally 16 years) may consent to certain medical procedures if he can demonstrate sufficient maturity to make the decision on his own and if the medical procedure is not deemed serious.[2] For common medical procedures, the consent of one parent is generally sufficient for the health care provider to proceed with the treatment. However, if the procedure in question is more serious, or involves complex ethical issues, such as a treatment that may conflict with religious beliefs, the consent of both parents is advisable. A serious dispute between the parents may require court intervention.

With regard to divorced parents, if they have joint legal custody they share the right to make medical decisions. Therefore, either parent may consent to treatment unless the court order granting joint custody states otherwise. If one parent has sole legal custody, that parent has authority to make health care decisions for the child.

As a general rule, a legally appointed guardian has the same consent authority for a minor as a parent would have. Individual states may modify this rule and require biological consent for serious procedures. A stepparent, in contrast, will not generally have the authority to consent to care unless the stepparent has legally adopted the child or been appointed a legal guardian. The authority of foster parents to consent to treatment may also vary greatly between states. Some states will allow the foster parent to consent to ordinary medical care, but not to serious procedures such as surgery. As state law on these issues varies greatly and can be clarified only by looking at state-specific family law statutes, it is advised that the physical therapist clearly understand the relationship and responsibilities of the adult, as noted in the medical record, or seek the assistance of an attorney in order to understand the laws of a particular state.

Before a physical therapist evaluates or begins treatment of a pediatric patient, the following should be clarified: custody issues, who has the power to make health care decisions, and who is authorized to have access to information about the patient's care. This information may be available to the physical therapist in the patient's medical record. All programs that service children should have a policy of obtaining this information upon admission.

Joint Custody

If divorced parents have joint legal custody, they share the right to make medical decisions.

Informed Consent

Informed consent is the legal principle that health care professionals must make adequate disclosures of information to a patient or a parent of a minor in order to obtain the patient's consent to treatment. It is based on the ethical concept of autonomy. Parental consent for health care services is almost always required for a child younger than 18 years.

Custody

Either through chart review or during the history intake, the physical therapist should clarify custody issues and decision-making authority prior to proceeding.

AN EXPERT WITNESS

The physical therapist who treats children may be called upon at some point to serve as a witness in a legal proceeding. Complete guidance on serving as a witness is beyond the scope of this chapter, but some basic guidance is appropriate. In legal proceedings, a lay or *ordinary witness* may only provide testimony about facts: those things that the witness observed or heard. A physical therapist will generally be called, however, as an *expert witness*: someone who, because of professional training and expertise, can provide the court with opinion testimony. The physical therapist is called to give her professional opinion on issues such as a child's development or functional limitations. When called upon to serve in this capacity, the physical therapist should ask the attorney who is making the contact why she is being called and on what issues or topics will she be questioned. A thorough review of the patient's record is recommended in preparation for providing testimony. It should be remembered that the testimony provided should be honest, concise, and unbiased. The physical therapist should be prepared to provide the basis (such as research or references to appropriate resources) for her opinions and only provide answers to the questions

posed. Before anyone serves as an expert witness for the first time, it is advisable to speak with a respected colleague or mentor about how to prepare and what to expect. There are also numerous resources available, including the APTA, to assist the physical therapist in preparing for this important role.

BASIC EMPLOYMENT ARRANGEMENTS

In addition to laws that influence the practice of physical therapy, there are laws that influence the way in which physical therapists work. The majority of physical therapists practice as employees of hospitals, rehabilitation facilities, or home health agencies. This is the traditional work relationship in which the employee performs work, either full time or part time, under the direction and control of the employer in exchange for wages and benefits. Generally, this is in the form of an *"at will" employment* relationship where the parties have not agreed that the employment relationship will last for a defined period of time. In this situation, the employee or employer can terminate the relationship at any time, for any legitimate reason. The employer cannot, however, terminate the employee for an unlawful discriminatory reason such as gender, age, nationality, race, religion, or disability. Such prohibitions on discriminatory actions are based on the federal Civil Rights Act of 1964 and on individual state antidiscrimination laws.[11]

Employment at Will

In an employment at will situation, either party (the employee or employer) can terminate the relationship at any time, for any legitimate reason.

In contrast to the traditional employment relationship is the independent contractor relationship. This situation might exist when a physical therapist has her own company, providing physical therapy services to an early intervention program, home health agency, or other facility. In this case, the physical therapist is not an employee of the agency or facility, but enters into a contractual relationship whereby the physical therapist's company agrees to provide services to the agency or facility's patients.

The primary legal differences between an employee and an independent contractor are related to control and liability. An employer may be found to be legally liable for the negligence or misdeeds of an employee under the legal doctrine of *respondent superior*. Under this doctrine of "let the master answer," the employer is liable for the actions of the employee if the employee acted within the scope of employment. The negligence or misdeeds of an independent contractor, in contrast, are less likely to give rise to liability of the agency or facility. It is important to note, however, that how the parties define the relationship will not determine how a court defines the relationship. A physical therapist may enter into an independent contractor agreement with an agency, but upon the physical therapist's committing some negligent act, a court could find that the relationship was really more like an employment relationship, so the agency could face liability. Generally, if the agency has too much control over the work of the physical therapist, it will be seen as an employment relationship, no matter how the agreement characterizes it. It is important, therefore, to make sure that the contract between independent contractor and facility is properly drafted and that the commonly accepted characteristics of this relationship actually exist. For instance, the patient should understand who the physical therapist works for; that the independent contractor does not participate in the facility's employment benefit program and is not subject to its human resource policies; that the work is temporary (versus permanent); and that the physical therapist controls the hours of employment.

POINT TO REMEMBER

Employee versus Independent Contractor

The primary legal differences between an employee and independent contractor are related to control and liability.

In any business, including physical therapy, numerous contractual relationships arise, including contracts between physical therapists and agencies, physical therapists and employers, and physical therapists and equipment vendors. It is important to remember that a contract is not a document. The piece of paper often signed and referred to as a contract is merely the written evidence of mutual promises by two parties to do something; an agreement of sorts or, in legal terms, a contract. For instance, most physical therapists do not sign a written employment agreement with their employers. Rest assured, however, that they are working under a contract. The employer has agreed to employ the physical therapist and pay her, and the physical therapist has agreed to perform the agreed-upon work. If the employer fails to pay the agreed-upon wages, the employee could sue the employer for "breach of contract." Although there are requirements that certain types of contracts be in writing, as a general rule verbal contracts can be legally binding. The only difficulty arises when there is a dispute about the terms of the contract. In these situations, however, courts may turn to other evidence of the terms.

POINT TO REMEMBER

Contracts

It is important to remember that a contract is not a document. It is an agreement by two parties, to do something, and even without written evidence of the contract, it may be enforceable.

If a physical therapist decides that she wants to go into business for herself, the first thing she should do is contact a good business attorney and an accountant. There are many decisions to make and laws that need to be complied with when starting and running a business. One of the first decisions the physical therapist will need to make is what business form to choose. The laws of the state in which the business will be formed will define the options available. The simplest type of business form is the *sole proprietorship*. This form, as the name implies, involves a single person undertaking a business venture. Forming a sole proprietorship does not require the filing of any forms with state government, and the taxation of the entity is rather simple. The downside of a sole proprietorship, however, is that the physical therapist is individually responsible for the liabilities of the company. For instance, if "Jane's Therapy" fails to pay a vendor or a landlord, or is sued for professional negligence because of an injury sustained by a patient, Jane herself is liable to the vendor, landlord, or patient. This means that Jane's personal property (even if she kept separate accounting for the business) might be at risk.

If Jane chooses to take a partner, forming "Jane and John's Therapy," these two people have now formed a *partnership*. Like a sole proprietorship, the taxation of this business form is rather simple, and nothing is required to be filed with the state. It is strongly advisable though that all partnerships have a partnership agreement drafted and executed to define important terms such as what property or assets each partner brings to the business, how profits will be split, and how the partnership can be dissolved. Generally speaking, partners are seen as acting on behalf of the partnership and are jointly liable for their partners' actions. So, if John enters into a contract to purchase an expensive piece of equipment, the partnership is bound by that contract, even if Jane never consented to it. Similarly, if the contract is not honored, both John and Jane are subject to the likely breach of contract lawsuit filed by the seller.

POINT TO REMEMBER

First Thing

If a physical therapist decides that she wants to go into business for herself, the first thing she should do is contact a good business attorney and an accountant.

In order to limit the potential personal liability of a sole proprietorship or partnership, a business owner may choose to form a *corporation*. A single individual or a group may form a corporation. Because the corporation is a recognized distinct legal entity, each state requires that the corporation file certain forms with a state agency, usually the Secretary of State's office. These forms include Articles of Incorporation. Because the corporation is its own entity, it alone is liable for the obligations of the company. For instance, if the corporation defaults on bank loans, fails to pay vendors or is sued, the bank, vendors, or entity suing the corporation, in order to recover what they are owed, would only be able to go after the assets or property of the corporation, rather than those of the individuals. It is important to note, however, that merely filing Articles of Incorporation does not ensure this protection. If the company does not actually function as a corporation (for example, naming corporate officers, having annual meetings, and using "Inc." after its name), the owners may still face personal liability. This is another important reason to enlist the aid of a good business attorney familiar with the laws of the state.

 POINT TO REMEMBER

Inc.

Forming a corporation sets up your business as its own entity, making the corporation liable for the obligations of the business.

SUMMARY

The practice of physical therapy brings physical therapists in contact with diverse legal issues. Federal and state statutes, regulations, and common law control these issues. The practicing physical therapist should be familiar with the laws and regulations that influence the practice of physical therapy in a particular setting, as well as understand the rights of the custodial parent in the care of the child and in the decision-making process. Having a working knowledge of the rights and responsibilities of the physical therapist and parents may promote better communication and understanding, while protecting the rights of the child and family. Although these rights should always be at the forefront of care, the physical therapist, as a mandated reporter of child abuse and neglect, also has an obligation to the child that supersedes the rights of the parent(s) or guardian.

Physical therapists also interact with the legal profession through their role as expert witnesses and with the formation of business arrangements, either as sole proprietors or partners in a practice. Understanding these arrangements and seeking the assistance of a knowledgeable attorney with regard to business matters in the formation or running of a business is another step toward more autonomy in the practice and profession of physical therapy.

REVIEW QUESTIONS

1. Which of the following is responsible for enforcing a state's physical therapy Practice Act? Failure to practice in accordance with the Act gives this entity the power to revoke a physical therapist's license to practice in that state.
   a. APTA
   b. State Board of Physical Therapy
   c. State Supreme Court
   d. State Chapter of the APTA

2. Kate has been granted only physical custody of her 4-year-old daughter Emily, by the courts. This form of custody would allow Kate to do all of the following except:
   a. allow Emily to be released from the physical therapy session into Kate's custody.
   b. allow Kate to transport Emily to and from the therapy sessions.
   c. allow Kate to enroll Emily in a special education preschool program.
   d. allow Kate to be instructed in Emily's home exercise program.

3. Joey is a 5-year-old child who has been removed from his parents' home. The courts have considered it necessary to terminate the parental rights of both parents, making Joey a ward of the state. The courts also appointed another adult to act on Joey's behalf. This person has the authority to sign medical releases and consent forms. This person would most likely be which of the following?
   a. A guardian
   b. A foster parent
   c. A biological parent
   d. An emancipated minor

4. Alicia is a 15-year-old girl who has status post a posterior spinal fusion secondary to idiopathic adolescent scoliosis. She is 1 day postop., and you (the physical therapist) receive an order from the surgeon for an evaluation and treatment. Upon review of her medical records, you note documentation that identifies Alicia as an emancipated minor. What does this mean?
   a. Alicia is malnourished to that point at which it will negatively impair her recovery.
   b. Alicia used to be in foster care but is now eligible for adoption.
   c. Alicia is younger than the age of majority but has a designated guardian.
   d. Alicia, by court order, has been given adult status, eliminating the need for parental consent for treatment.

5. Of the following types of business arrangements, which ones would require notification or filing with the state government?
   a. Employment "at will" relationship
   b. Sole proprietorship
   c. Partnership
   d. Corporation
   e. All of the above

REFERENCES

1. U.S. Department of Health and Human Services. Centers for Medicare & Medicaid Services. Available at: http://www.cms.hhs.gov. Accessed January 9, 2007.
2. Oliphant R, Ver Steigh N. *Family Law, Examples and Explanations*. New York: Aspen Publishers; 2004.
3. Uniform Law Commissioners. The National Conference of Commissioners on Uniform State Laws. Uniform Child Custody Jurisdiction and Enforcement Act. 1997. Chicago, IL. Available at: www.nccusl.org. Accessed December 30, 2006.
4. DeWitt Gregory J, Swisher PN, Wolf SL, *Understanding Family Law*, 2nd ed. New York: LexisNexis; 2001.
5. M.L.B v S.L.J., 519 US 102 (1996).
6. *Sartosky v Kramer*, 455 US 745 (1982).
7. *Jehovah's Witnesses v King County Hospital*, 278 F Supp 488 (WD Wash 1967).
8. Atkinson J. *Modern Child Custody Practice*. New York: Kluwer Law Book Publishers; 1986.
9. The Child Abuse Prevention and Treatment Act of 1974 (PL 93-247). Amended and reauthorized by the Keeping Children and Families Safe Act (PL 108-36) 2003.
10. The Child Welfare Information Gateway. Mandatory Reporters of Child Abuse and Neglect: Summary of state laws. U.S. Department of Health and Human Services. Administration for Children and Families. Administration on Children, Youth and Families. Children's Bureau. 2005. Available at: www.childwelfare.gov/systemwide/laws_policies/statutes/manda.cfm. Accessed December 28, 2006.
11. Civil Rights Act of 1964 (PL 88-352). Title VII [42 USC §2000e(2)].

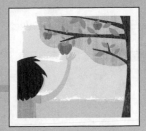

The Basics of Billing

Michael Drnach

LEARNING OBJECTIVES

1. Understand the basic concepts of health care finance.
2. Be able to develop a cost model for your practice.
3. Understand the basic role of government and private insurance in health care.

Health care has evolved over the past century into a multibillion-dollar business. The need to remain financially solvent has put pressure on both for-profit and not-for-profit organizations, whether it's a single provider or a group of providers working together as a single business unit. Constant pressure to achieve and maintain a positive bottom line (making a profit or surplus) has expanded the role and responsibilities of the physical therapist. No longer can he have a narrow focus on the treatment of the patients; he must also have an awareness of the revenues, expenses, and liabilities associated with the delivery of services to that patient. Even in the realm of not-for-profit or charitable health care organizations, pressure to manage or reduce expenses, and the focus on long-term financial viability is constant. Health care providers, including physical therapists, whether they are working in a for-profit or a not-for-profit organization have to report to many interested parties in order to justify and receive payment for the services rendered. These parties typically include educated patients who have access to more health care resources via the Internet, third party insurance companies that pay for the services rendered, outside accrediting agencies who advocate for the patient, as well as federal and state governmental agencies.

This chapter will cover the basic financial issues that can help a physical therapist understand the fundamentals of a business operation. In doing so, he will be better equipped to effectively participate in this aspect of health care.

THE BASICS

Whether it's a single practice or part of a larger group or organization, such as a hospital, the need to manage finances is an important and growing aspect of health care. Managing finances is a way to ensure that *expenses* (dollars spent) do not exceed *revenues* (dollars received). This can be thought of in terms of a personal checking account. Cash comes in from services provided, and cash flows out from checks written for items purchased. This is the same concept in health care but on a much larger scale. The services that a physical therapist provides generate revenue or cash-in. Revenue can include items such as cash paid by the patient for services rendered, third party billing fees generated through a practice or hospital setting, or consultant's fees for work done at a per diem (per day) rate. The items purchased to operate a practice are expenses or cash-outs, which include such items as salary and benefits, medical and office supplies, orthotic equipment, rent, and utility bills. Managing finances allows the physical therapist or owner of the business to better plan for the future and to assure the long-term success of his business by providing the necessary financial information to aid in the decision-making process. Having a basic understanding of

BOX 14-1
Common Financial Terms

Expense/Cost: any items for which you pay out funds. Cost is a cash term and Expense is an accrual term. The terms are used interchangeably throughout this chapter.

Revenue: income, funds generated through services rendered, investments, or sales of services or property

Fixed: any revenue or expense that does not change over time but remains constant from one period to the next (You tend to have little control over fixed items. Examples of fixed costs may include rent and malpractice insurance.)

Variable: any revenue or expense that changes over time and for which you have some control (Examples of variable costs include advertising expense, supplies, and equipment.)

Semivariable: costs that have both a fixed and variable component (An example of a semivariable cost is utilities. You have a fixed basic rate for your telephone as well as a per minute variable cost, which fluctuates based on usage.)

Fee Schedule: the list of services provided and the rate at which you charge for those services

Accrual Accounting: method of matching expenses with revenues, not based on cash flows.

Cash Accounting: method of accounting by which cash-in and cash-out are recorded at the time they are received or paid out

Profit: amount left over when you subtract your accrual expenses from your revenues

Gross Revenue: total amount charged for services prior to any reductions for contractual allowances or discounts

Net Revenue: gross revenue less contractual allowances or discounts

the terms used is one of the first steps in this process, and is necessary in order to participate in the conversation. Box 14-1 contains some common terms associated with finance. These terms will help the physical therapist better understand the structure and function of the fundamental financial documents of the budget, income statement, balance sheet, and cash flow statement.

The Budget

The first step in properly managing finances begins with preparing a budget. A *budget* is defined as a financial statement of estimated income and expenditures covering a specified future period of time.[1] The budgeting process involves completing a set of financial statements consisting of an income statement, balance sheet, and cash flow statement. Budgets can cover any specified period of time such as 6 months, 1 year, or 5 years, and

puts forth in financial terms what a business hopes to accomplish within a specified period of time. Most health care organizations budget annually but may make revisions to their budgets over the course of the year as the revenues and expenses fluctuate for any given month. Budgeting is an important process that establishes a business's financial or activity goals along with benchmarks to measure progress throughout the year. It also forces the examination of how revenues and expenses affect the overall financial performance of the business. It is important to remember that budgets are *pro forma* statements, meaning that they are a best guess of what is going to happen in the future. Therefore, changes in the budget are not necessarily bad. They could be reflective of significant changes in the business due to unforeseen factors or of changes brought about by external sources. The budget is also influenced by the information obtained through other financial statements, such as the income statement, balance sheet, or cash flow statement.

Financial Statements

Financial statements are a set of financial reports that include an income statement, a balance sheet, and a cash flow statement. All three of these statements are interrelated. Financial statements are used to view the financial health and stability, as well as growth potential, of an organization or business. Financial statements can be as simple or complex as the business and should always be prepared with the aid of a professional such as a Certified Public Accountant (CPA). For most independent providers of physical therapy, enlisting the help of a CPA is recommended. Check with friends, relatives, or professional associations for names and references of CPAs who have experience in health care. CPAs can be invaluable in establishing and maintaining the business, and aid in the management and review of the business's financial statements.

The *income statement* includes the revenues and expenses generated by the business in an organized report format. Revenues are listed first, followed by deductions to revenue, then expenses. Revenues are typically volume driven: An increase in the number of patients treated generates more revenue for the business. Revenues can also be contractually based, meaning that, for a stated service, a negotiated amount of revenue will be paid to the business. Offsets to revenue are typically third party *contractual allowances,* which are amounts agreed to between the business and the insurance company prior to billing for the service. These contractual allowances are accepted by the business in order to provide services to the people in the area who carry a specific health insurance. In this agreement, the business agrees to accept the payment of the insurance company as payment in full for the services rendered.

Expenses follow revenue on the income statement. Some expenses are volume driven, whereas others are fixed. The income statement is a summary of revenues generated minus the expenses incurred, which results in net income. Income statements are also known as *Profit and Loss Statements* because net income (revenues − expenses) shows how much of a profit or how big a loss is generated. Like budgets, income statements are prepared for a specific time period; however, this time period is in the past, not the future. The income statement will calculate the amount of profit or loss the business generated for the past month, year, or whatever time period is chosen. An income statement may also be called a *Statement of Operations* which lists the revenues and expenses of a business or department within a larger organization for a specified time period.

The second statement in the set of financial statements is the *balance sheet*. A balance sheet is a listing of the business's assets and liabilities. *Assets* are items that the business owns. They can include cash, *accounts receivable* (money due from patients treated who have not yet paid), and PPandE (Property, Plant and Equipment) such as offices and treatment equipment. *Liabilities* are items that the business has incurred or obligations that are owed to another party. They can include items such as *accounts payable*, which are expenses the business has incurred but not yet paid, such as dues and memberships, utilities bills, small equipment, or materials purchased on credit. Other types of liabilities include loans and notes payable, which include mortgages on the office or treatment space. The final section of the balance sheet is *owner's equity*. Owner's equity is the amount owed to the owners of the business or to the stockholders in the company. Equity is viewed as the value of the business to its owners whether the business is composed of one individual, a group, or an organization. At all times, Assets = Liabilities + Owner's Equity, which is called the balance sheet equation. Like the income statement, the balance sheet is for a past period of time and is prepared to reflect the business at a certain point in time.

POINT TO REMEMBER

Balance Sheet Equation
Assets = Liabilities + Owner's Equity

The final financial statement is the cash flow statement. A *cash flow statement* is a tool used to show inflows and outflows of cash and should be prepared by someone with knowledge of the business and is certified or a professional in the field of accountancy or financial statement preparation. Cash flow statements display when and how much cash flows in and out of a business over a given period of time. It is useful in financial planning and is usually required when seeking financial support from a bank or other financial institutions. The statement is prepared from the information on the balance sheet and income statement, and captures the changes in cash over a period of time. For example, if the cash balance on the balance sheet has increased over the year, the cash flow statement can answer the question of why it increased. It may show that the *accounts receivable* balance (what other people owe the practice) decreased or that payments due are being stretched out over a longer period of time. (A growth in the *accounts payable*; what the practice owes other people.)

POINT TO REMEMBER

Cash Flow
Cash flow statements are vital to a business's ability to pay its monthly bills; especially payroll.

PHYSICAL THERAPY PRACTICE

Whether working as an employee or as an independent physical therapist (whether as a new graduate or entering into a new venue of care provision such as hospice or pediatric care), it is important to understand how revenues and expenses are related to service provision. Most organizations have entire departments dedicated to monitoring, reporting, and controlling revenue and expenses. However, working as an independent practitioner, the physical therapist (or his designee) has control over revenues and expenses. Having a working knowledge of financial management will help to ensure that revenues exceed expenses and that the practice will survive. Identifying the expenses of the practice is one of the first steps in this process.

Identifying Expenses

Box 14-2 is an example of a cost worksheet. Using a cost worksheet is one method of calculating current costs or expenses. Identifying costs provides a baseline from which to work when calculating how much revenue is needed to reach a target profit level. Generating a profit is important for maintaining the practice, updating equipment, increasing salaries, or expanding a current practice into a new market. It is important to include all expenses when making expense projections. Many times independent practitioners may forget the obvious expenses such as home office space, office supplies, traveling expenses, and continuing education expenses. It is important, however, to be able to provide an explanation or support, in the form of receipts or purchase orders, to justify the expense to an outside agency.

After expenses have been identified, they can be classified as fixed, variable, or semivariable. Classification of expenses will help to identify how the expenses

BOX 14-2
Cost Worksheet

Cost Worksheet

DIRECT COST:

1.   Salary

        a.   base   _____
        b.   overtime   _____
        c.   **Total salary** =   _____

2.   Fringes (approx. 30% of 1c.)

        a.   FICA (7.65% of 1c.)   _____
        b.   Workman's comp. (4% of 1c.)   _____
        c.   State unemployment (av. $250/yr) _____
        d.   Fed. unemployment ($56/yr)   _____
        e.   Pension Plan (av. 3%–4% of 1c.) _____
        f.   Professional Liability (1% of 1c.) _____
        g.   Insurance (health, life, disability) (12% of 1c.) _____

        h.   **Total fringes** =   _____

3.   Other

        a.   mileage   _____
        b.   continuing education   _____
        c.   tuition reimbursement   _____
        d.   license/dues/subscriptions   _____

        e.   **Total other** =   _____

4.   **Direct Total** (1c + 2h + 3e) =   _____

5.   INDIRECT COST (allocation):
     Private Clinic or Home Health Agency
     (add 50 to 65% of direct total)   _____
     Hospital based (add 30 to 40% of direct total) _____

TOTAL COST (4 + 5) =   _____

TOTAL COST _____ **/ # HOURS PAID TO WORK PER YEAR =**
COST PER HOUR _____
Typically 2,080 hours per year for a 40-hour workweek; 1,950 for a 37.5-hour workweek
For a 10-month school year, 7 hours per day: 1,400 hours.

behave and how much control the physical therapist has over certain expenses.

Fixed expenses, such as salary and wages, rent, interest expenses on loans, and depreciation of equipment, are set (do not change) over an extended period of time. It is important to know, based on location, specialty, or the costs associated with an individual intervention, what is an appropriate level of fixed expense. To determine the level of fixed expenses, consider how many employees the practice may want or need to hire. Will the practice be a single provider practice with one employee, or will there be physical therapist assistants and support personnel to hire? What wages will be paid and how much? Will practice space be rented or purchased? What type of equipment will be needed, and how long will it last before needing replaced? These questions can be answered through careful planning and research or by consulting a financial professional such as an accountant. It is important to take the time to research and think about location and growth over a specific number of years so that an appropriate level of fixed expenses can be achieved.

Variable expenses are the expenses over which a physical therapist exerts the most control. These could include supplies such as office supplies, printing costs for brochures and pamphlets, and costs for small equipment and tools. It is important to document and track these costs and monitor the volume of activity in these areas. Variable expenses are costs that are the easiest to control and are generally the first to be affected in order to meet short-term financial goals.

Semivariable expenses are expenses over which the physical therapist has limited control. Unlike fixed expenses, which are static from one period to the next, semivariable expenses have a static or fixed component as well as a variable component. When purchasing phone or internet service, each package comes with a basic rate (no matter how many phone calls are made each month or how many times the internet is accessed). Coupled with the fixed rate is the variable rate, which is based on the number or length of calls or how many times the internet is accessed. Therefore, these costs have a fixed component and one that varies with the use of the item.

After the expected expenses are identified, the physical therapist can estimate the amount of revenue that would be expected from the practice, based on the knowledge of how much revenue is necessary to cover the basic expenses. Adding to that figure the amount of profit that would be needed to maintain and grow the practice, the physical therapist can then determine what fees to charge for the services provided.

POINT TO REMEMBER

Costs

Fixed costs are set for a period of time and do not vary depending on usage (e.g., payroll). Variable costs vary depending on usage (e.g., ultrasound gel). Semivariable costs have a combination of both fixed and variable costs (e.g., phone bill).

Estimating Revenues

Before the physical therapist can estimate revenues, a *fee schedule* needs to be created. The fee schedule is a listing of the services provided and the charge for each of those services. The fee can be based on a per hour or per minute rate of service, on the type of service or treatment, or on a per session rate for a set number of sessions. A *flat fee* is a fee that is charged to the patient no matter how long or complicated the treatment. Flat fees can be useful in school or hospice contracts whereby a physical therapist agrees to provide services for a specific number of hours per week for a flat fee, regardless of the number of students/patients seen. A per hour or per minute fee is the more common type of fee used by most professionals, especially in hospital outpatient settings, or private practice. Fees are charged to patients in time increments, usually minutes. Fees can also be based on the number of sessions or the number of patient consults. For example, in the case of a patient who needs 10 treatment sessions, the first evaluation session is charged at $150, but each subsequent treatment session is only $100. This is common in practices where multiple sessions over a short period of time are expected, such as with physical therapy.

The actual dollar amount of the fee can be calculated using several different methods: market or going rate, breakeven, or mark-up. The *market or going rate* is what others in the market are charging for the same or similar service. This method is easily established, but runs the risk of not covering all of the costs of the individual practice, as those costs may be significantly different from the costs of others in the market. The *breakeven method* requires the physical therapist to identify all of the expenses of his practice so the appropriate fee can be calculated to cover all of the costs. This method will cover costs, but may not provide the money to be able to update or expand the practice. The most common method is a mark-up method. The *mark-up method* is similar in most industries whereby a fee or price is estimated based on several factors such as cost, time, location, and type of service provided, and then a mark-up or additional percentage is added onto the fee to cover any unanticipated costs or to allow for additional revenue to fund updates or practice expansion.

Fee for service is the term used to describe the amounts charged by a physical therapist, or any health care provider, per the fee schedule. The revenues are service specific and generally reflect the market value of the service provided. Fee-for-service revenue can vary by the type of service (e.g., private or hospital-based) or the location of a service (e.g., rural or urban area). Typically, health care providers create a fee schedule, then set fees for certain services based on what the market will bear. For example, a physical therapist who practices in a city where the demand for physical therapy is high, might set a fee of $145.00 for 15 minutes of services, whereas another physical therapist practicing in a rural setting might set the same service at a fee of only $85.00 per 15 minutes of services. Every practice can have only one fee schedule and one fee for each type of service. It is illegal to charge different fees for the same services unless a true cost difference can be proven with the delivery of that service.

Identifying revenue and expenses and establishing a fee schedule are the starting points of an independent practice. Actually receiving cash for the services rendered is another important and vital aspect of any business.

POINT TO REMEMBER

Fee Schedule

A fee schedule is a detailed list of the services that are available and the charges associated with them.

Billing

Revenues can be very simple or extremely complex based on the type and length of service provided and how billing is done for those services. In a cash-based practice, services are delivered and the client or patient pays for those services directly, with cash. If the client or patient chooses to have a third party (i.e., an insurance company) pay for those services, additional steps have to be taken to secure payment. Most health care insurance companies incorporate their payment formula with *Current Procedural Terminology* (CPT) codes.[2] Established by the American Medical Association (AMA), CPT codes are five-digit codes used throughout the country by health care providers to designate the type of service or services provided. Physical therapists typically use codes in the Physical Medicine and Rehabilitation section, or 97000 codes. Examples of several common CPT codes used in physical therapy can be found in Table 14-1. CPT codes are reviewed and updated annually by the AMA. To ensure good coding and billing practices, it is recommended that all health care providers become familiar with all the codes associated with their specialty.

The Centers for Medicare & Medicaid Services (CMS) is a federal agency within the U.S. Department of Health and Human Services, which is responsible for setting the reimbursement rates at which the government pays health care providers. To assure that claims are processed efficiently, CMS uses the *Healthcare Common Procedure Coding System* (HCPCS), commonly referred to as "hicks picks" codes.[3] *Level I* HCPCS codes match the CPT codes, which are used primarily to identify medical services and procedures furnished by physicians and other health care professionals such as physical therapists. These health care professionals use the CPT code to identify services and procedures for which they bill public or private health insurance programs. To enhance a code or be more specific in coding, certain modifiers have been created to better define the code or the service provided. *Modifiers,* which are two digit numbers that help to more accurately define the CPT code used in billing, are more commonly used by specialists and can be found in any CPT book on the market. Modifiers are attached to CPT codes when the code alone is not adequate to explain exactly the service or treatment provided. The modifier does not change the definition of the code; it is used to denote that something has been altered due to certain circumstances. The two most frequently used modifiers used by physical therapists are the 22 and 59 modifiers. Modifier 59 is used when a physical therapist needs to indicate a distinct procedural service, meaning that two different procedures were performed on the same day on two different anatomic sites such as intervention for the shoulder as well as for the elbow. An example of the use of modifier 59 is as follows:

> Working one-on-one with a patient, the physical therapist performs therapeutic exercises. CPT code 97110 is billed for each 15-minute increment. Modifier 59 is only appropriate if the therapeutic exercises (97110) are performed on different regions of the body, such as the leg and shoulder.

Modifier 22 is used when additional work, above and beyond what is normally required, is needed. An example might be the provision of physical therapy to a patient who is noncommunicative, violent, severely disabled, or too heavy to transfer by one person (an additional person is needed to provide the intervention). Judgment must be used, and supporting documentation in the form of medical records and notes is required in order for modifier 22 to be paid.

Level II of the HCPCS is a standardized coding system that is used primarily to identify products, supplies, and services not included in the CPT codes, such as ambulance services and "durable medical equipment, prosthetics, orthotics, and supplies" (DMEPOS) when used outside a physician's office. Because Medicare and other insurers cover a variety of services, supplies, and equipment that are not identified by CPT codes, the level II HCPCS codes were established for submitting claims for these items. The development and use of level II of the HCPCS began in the 1980s. Level II codes are also

TABLE 14-1	Common Current Procedural Terminology (CPT) Codes Used in Physical Therapy
Code	**Definition**
97010	Application of a modality to one or more areas, hot or cold packs
97110	Therapeutic procedure, one or more areas, each 15 minutes, therapeutic exercises to develop strength and endurance, range of motion, and flexibility
97116	Gait-training therapy, includes stair climbing; therapist required to have direct (one-on-one) patient contact
97530	Therapeutic activities, direct (one-on-one) patient contact by the provider (use of dynamic activities to improve functional performance), each 15 minutes

referred to as alphanumeric codes because they consist of a single alphabetical letter followed by four numeric digits, whereas CPT codes are identified using five numeric digits.

When billing by CPT code, it is important that the ICD-9 code also be indicated, especially when billing Medicare/Medicaid and third party insurers. ICD-9 codes are taken from the *International Classification of Diseases*, Ninth Revision, developed by the World Health Organization.[4] These codes identify the patient's disease (or diagnosis) for which she is being treated. Since the passage of the Medicare Catastrophic Coverage Act of 1988, it is required by law that the ICD-9 code be submitted in order to receive reimbursement from Medicare. Since then, all insurers have required that an ICD-9 code be identified in order to be reimbursed for services provided. Books detailing the various ICD-9 codes can be found on the Internet or in most health care bookstores.

For several years, the National Center for Health Statistics and the Centers for Disease Control and Prevention have been working on an updated version of the ICD codes titled ICD-10. Although the final report has not been widely distributed, the ICD-10 incorporates changes in medical knowledge that have occurred over the years since the ICD-9 version was released. The ICD-10 update includes expanded detail for many conditions, and changes from using numeric codes to using alphanumeric codes.

Typically, revenues are shown at gross, meaning the amount listed on the fee schedule. However, what a physical therapist is actually paid is referred to as net revenue. The difference between gross and net is termed the "contractual allowance." Most organizations tend to confuse gross and net terminology; therefore, it is important

to be clear as to the actual payment received for services provided. Payments vary based on contractual agreements with various federal and state insurers or private and nonprofit insurers. For example:

A physical therapist charges $500 for orthotics fitting and training–extremities and/or trunk; CPT code 97660. The insurance company states that they will only pay $250 for the service. If the physical therapist performs five of these services in a given week, the total gross charges for the week would be $2,500 (5 × $500). The physical therapist's net revenue would be what he actually receives in payment for the services or $1,250 (5 × $250). The difference of $1,250 is termed the contractual write-off or allowance. In this example, the contractual write-off is 50% of the gross charge, leaving 50% as the payment rate or reimbursement rate.

Several payment factors have been developed over the years to assist health care providers in defining their revenues. Common payment factors are the *Resource-Based Relative Value Scale* (RBRVS) and *Diagnosis-Related Groups* (DRGs), which are ways of bundling like or related services or resources into one payment. These methodologies were viewed as ways to correct skewed financial incentives among various procedures and medical practices. For example, a physical therapist can not bill separately for services rendered to a patient who comes into the hospital for an orthopedic surgery and receives physical therapy while in the hospital. These services, the surgery, the physical therapy, and the nursing care would all be bundled under one DRG, and only one bill and payment would be issued. If follow-up physical therapy is ordered after the patient has left the hospital, then the physical therapist could bill for those services.

In the early 1990s, *Relative Value Units* (RVUs) were developed by Medicare to assign a value to a particular service or type of treatment. Although there are several types of RVUs, the *work RVU* (wRVU) is the one most commonly used to measure productivity. Other RVUs include *malpractice RVUs* and *practice expense RVUs*. A sample of several wRVUs related to physical therapy is shown in Table 14-2. In most cases, when a service or treatment becomes more complex or time-consuming, the wRVU increases. This provides one way to reduce geographic biases in payments by Medicare. No matter where in the country a practice is established, the wRVU

TABLE 14-2 Work Relative Value Units (wRVU)

Current Procedural Terminology Codes	wRVU
97010	0.06
97110	0.45
97116	0.40
97530	0.44

for a particular service remains the same. Analysis using wRVUs can be a useful tool, especially when working in a group practice, to increase overall productivity. Examining a health care provider's mix of wRVUs can assist the practice in determining the right mix of services or procedures needed to make a health care provider as productive as possible. To use the wRVUs to measure profitability, it is also important to know how the Medicare reimbursement is calculated. The Medicare provider fee schedule amounts are adjusted to reflect variations in practice expenses among various geographic regions. A geographic practice cost index (GPCI) has been established for every Medicare payment locality throughout the country. For each RVU (work, malpractice, and practice expense) there is a GPCI that is used to generate the applicable Medicare payment. To further add to the complexities of this calculation, Medicare has distinguished between a facility and nonfacility practice expense RVU, based on where a service is provided. Facility locations, under the resource-based system for calculating payments, include inpatient and outpatient hospital settings, emergency rooms, Skilled Nursing Facilities (SNFs), or Ambulatory Surgical Centers (ASCs). Outpatient rehabilitation services are usually reimbursed at the nonfacility practice expense RVUs. (See Box 14-3 for the formulas used in the Medicare calculations.) Using the Medicare formula, the higher the wRVU, the higher the pricing amount and payment. Although the formula is complex, it is a good way to estimate appropriate costs and proceeds for work performed.

BOX 14-3
Medicare Formulas

The 2006 formulas for calculating Medicare reimbursements are:

Nonfacility Pricing Amount = [(wRVU * wGPCI) + (Nonfacility peRVU * peGPCI) + (mpRVU * mpGPCI)] * Conversion Factor

Facility Pricing Amount = [(wRVU * wGPCI) + (Facility peRVU * peGPCI) + (mpRVU * mpGPCI)] * Conversion Factor

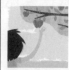

BOX 14-4
Example of Contractual Allowance

Your patient Timmy has Medicaid as his insurance. He receives two, 15-minute gait-training sessions (CPT code 97116). Your fee for this CPT code is $150.00 per every 15 minutes or $300.00 total for this session. The Medicaid reimbursement rate is $60.00 for a 15-minute session, or $120.00 for today's session. The difference of $180.00 is your contractual allowance.

RVUs are also linked to CPT codes. Without the proper CPT code, a bill will not be paid or not be paid correctly. It is important to correctly code for services, as wrongful coding is illegal and can lead to accusations of fraud. This is why many organizations and practices hire professional coders who have been trained and certified in proper coding. Ultimately, proper coding is based on the documentation provided by the physical therapist or other health care provider.

CMS generates Medicare and Medicaid rates, and through its programs of Medicaid and State Children's Health Insurance Program (SCHIP), it provides medical coverage for 1 in 4 Americans under the age of 18 years.[5] Most organizations and health care providers use these rates as a basis for calculating their own fees. For instance, a health care provider who sees both Medicaid and fee-for-service patients may create a fee schedule that is 250% above the Medicare/Medicaid fee schedule. As previously stated, it is illegal to charge two different fees for the same service; however, payers will only pay what has been negotiated. Thus, for a patient who has Medicaid health insurance, the Medicaid rate will be paid; however, for a patient with private insurance, the practice will receive 250% above the Medicaid rate. The same fee is being charged, but based on the individual contract the government will reimburse at a lower rate. By agreeing to treat a patient on Medicaid, the physical therapist is in fact agreeing to accept the lower reimbursement rates set by the government. In this case, the difference between the rate billed and the reimbursement actually received is considered a contractual allowance (Box 14-4).

POINT TO REMEMBER

Diagnosis-Related Groups

Using DRGs is a way to provide a specific payment for a type of patient group in the acute care setting. Using an RBRVS is a way to provide payment for a specific type of service or treatment.

Accepting a lower reimbursement than what is stated on a fee schedule is common practice in health care. There are many reasons for doing this including increasing volume, increasing market share, or establishing a new practice and recruiting patients. It is important when developing a fee schedule to consider things such as location, what the market will support, level of work experience, type of clientele targeted, and cost of living in a particular region. Every location and every market have certain limitations as to what the people in that area will be willing to spend for health care. It is important to know what these limitations are and how to work within them. A physical therapist should know the going rate for physical therapy services in the area. If prices for services are set too high, no patients will come, and if prices are set too low, the sustainability of a practice comes into question, as anticipated revenues may not match or exceed anticipated expenses. There are many ways to find out what the going market rate is, through either local government agencies or professional associations. Also, fees do not have to remain fixed, especially when first starting out in a new market. As skills improve and services expand, fees should be adjusted to reflect the change. It is important to review established fee schedules annually to ensure that fees are charged at a proper level. Most organizations and practices will review their fee schedule every time the CMS issues an update to the Medicare/Medicaid rates. It is also important to note that, by law, if a practitioner accepts Medicare patients and payment, he must also accept Medicaid patients. This does not have to have a negative effect on a practice, as these patients make up a considerable part of the economy and can help increase patient volume. However, because they are Medicare and Medicaid patients, reimbursement for services is typically lower than that from other insurers.

Billing third party payers for professional services is done by an independent physical therapist on a CMS 1500 (formally HCFA 1500) form, which was created by the Health Care Financing Administration (HCFA. Now CMS) and approved by the AMA Council on Medical Service. Basic information required on the CMS 1500 is patient name, address, insurance identification number, and insurance company's name and address. Treatment information in the form of CPT/HCPCS codes, dates of service, and ICD-9 codes are required as well. Finally, the health care provider's signature, credentials, address, and Unique Provider Identification Number (UPIN) or group insurance number are also required. A UB04 (formally UB90) form is used when the physical therapists are enrolled with the third party payer as a group, such as in a hospital setting. Which form is used for billing will depend on how the physical therapist is enrolled in the program.

In most instances, when working as an independent contractor a physical therapist provides a payment invoice that is broken down by time. Unlike the insurance companies or government agencies, which rely on CPT coding as a way of noting services, most independent contractors bill based on time. In order to correctly calculate an hourly rate, the physical therapist should have an estimate of the total annual cost of providing the services (Box 14-2). On average, a full-time employee works 2,080 hours per year, which breaks down to 40 hours per week for a 52-week year. Dividing the 2,080 hours by the total annual costs will produce the minimum hourly rate. A *mark-up*, as a percentage, is added to the actual cost of the service to come up with an hourly rate, which includes a profit. This can ensure that the financial targets for the year are met. A mark-up is arbitrary but should be reasonable based on the local market and skill level needed for the service provision, and should be an amount that can be easily calculated and explained (Box 14-5).

The physical therapist in private practice must have a basic understanding of these financial issues in order to make a profit from the services provided. Making a profit allows the practice to increase salaries, purchase new or updated equipment, and keep up with increases in the cost of living. *Profit* can be defined as revenue in excess of all expenses. It is the bottom line. On a cash basis, profit equals surplus, which is any excess cash left over after all costs have been subtracted from the cash-in. Having excess cash or a profit is beneficial to the livelihood of any practice. Understanding the payer source is helpful in generating a profit and is also necessary in order to comply with its billing rules and regulations regarding the provision of covered services.

BOX 14-5
Calculating an Hourly Rate Including a Mark-up

Tina is a physical therapist who has decided to become an independent contractor. She is considering an arrangement with a local school system to provide physical therapy services to students enrolled in the special education program. The school is in need of physical therapy services for three, 8-hour days a week, for 48 weeks of the year. (This includes the extended school year programs.) Tina has estimated her total costs to be $60,000 per year. Given the cost of living in her region and other market factors, Tina has estimated her mark-up to be 15%. Her hourly rate can be calculated as follows:

Total costs	$60,000
+ Mark-up (15%)	9,000
Annual target	$69,000
Annual hours	1,152 (24 hours per week for 48 weeks)
Hourly rate quoted	$59.89

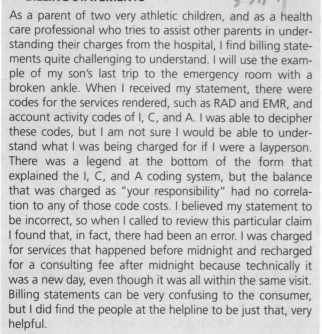

Understanding the Third Party

Understanding who is going to pay and how much they will pay is a very important aspect of managing a practice's finances. Depending on the situation, payers can be the government, third party insurance carriers, patients, families of patients, schools, or other organizations with whom a provider has a contract.

Each state has its own set of laws and regulations regarding health care insurance. Each insurance company also has its own rules and policies regarding covered services. It is best to check the local and state government's web page to get specific information for a particular state regarding insurance companies. The larger national insurance companies have their own web sites that provide useful information. A health care provider may find that, when dealing with patients who have regional or local insurance coverage, additional research may be required to ensure that payment is received. In most instances, the amount and type of insurance coverage is based on what the insurer (patient or patient's family) or the employer is willing to pay. Thus it is important to become familiar with the local insurance companies and governmental rules and regulations within a particular state. The rules and regulations can be very complex, and it is important to become familiar with them or to retain the assistance of someone who is familiar with them. In most cases, larger organizations have dedicated personnel whose only function is to keep abreast of governmental

and insurance company rules and regulations and to ensure that the practice is getting the appropriate level of reimbursement for their services.

Insurance companies and governmental agencies can also act as referral sources for a practice. By enrolling with an insurance carrier, a physical therapist becomes part of a larger network of health care providers who have access to a larger pool of potential patients. The enrollment process with an insurance company usually takes several weeks to months and requires that certain professional licenses be obtained and adequate paperwork be submitted. After the initial round of paperwork is completed, annual renewals are typically straightforward. The process of becoming credentialed or enrolled begins with obtaining a state license to practice. After receiving a state license, the health care provider can then apply for a Medicare UPIN. To enroll with Medicare, the physical therapist must contact the CMS regional office in the state where he plans to practice. Typically, the application process takes 30 to 60 days. An advantage to participation in the Medicare program is that Medicare fees are 5% higher for participants than for nonparticipants. After the health care provider has a Medicare UPIN, he can enroll in other insurance programs, both public and private. Although the process can be arduous due to the excess amount of paperwork, it is well worth it financially. On average, it can take from 3 to 9 months to become credentialed with all the various insurance agencies in an area.

When working with schools, community organizations, home health agencies, or other groups for which services are provided, an annual contract may be all that is needed. In this capacity, the physical therapist can work as an independent contractor. It is important when negotiating such contracts that all expenses related to the terms of the contract are considered in order to remain financially healthy.

SUMMARY

The physical therapist is faced with a myriad of hurdles to navigate in order to develop a successful practice in the health care industry today. No more can he be concerned only with patient management; he must also be able to manage finances, or at least participate in the discussion of finances, to help make well-planned business decisions. Consideration must be given to the market, the location, external factors that may inhibit or promote growth in the area, as well as the local and state government laws and regulations pertaining to the delivery of health care services. Preparation and analysis of potential revenues and expenses must be examined along with the anticipated cash flow, to ensure that the business is profitable. The physical therapist should seek the advice of a qualified accountant to assist with preparing financial documents (balance sheet, income statement, cash flow statement, and budget) as well as with understanding and preparing an appropriate fee schedule and billing systems.

REVIEW QUESTIONS

1. As the manager of a physical therapy department, you want to get better control over the expenses of the department. Of the following, which group reflects the three common classifications of expenses?
   a. Fixed, variable, and semivariable
   b. Static, dynamic, and volatile
   c. Fixed, dynamic, and automatic
   d. Static, variable, and semivariable
2. In your practice, you use CPT codes when billing for services rendered. Of the following, which best defines CPT and its purpose?
   a. Calculated Payment Threshold: the highest amount that can be charged for a health care service in a particular geographical region
   b. Current Procedural Terminology: a five-digit code used nationwide to designate the type of health care service provided
   c. Correlated Payment Term: the fee that is the payment basis for a health care service or services provided, which is related to Physical Medicine and Rehabilitation
   d. Current Procedural Task: a numeric descriptor for a particular health care service, defined by the AMA
3. It is the beginning of the financial year for your practice, and you are thinking of increasing your fees in order to keep up with inflation and the cost of living adjustments to your business's payroll. You access the practice's fee schedule in this process. What is a fee schedule?
   a. A CMS 1500
   b. A listing of services provided and the associated charge
   c. A schedule of charges and expected payments based on insurance type
   d. A statement of operations
4. As an independent contractor, you would like to make a profit during your first year on the job. Which of the following best defines the concept of profit?

   a. Owner's equity
   b. Expenses in excess of revenue
   c. Revenue in excess of expenses
   d. Assets greater than liabilities
5. As a physical therapist in private practice, you submit a bill or invoice to third party payers every week. Of the following, which is the official form used for billing for professional services to a third party payer?
   a. A fee schedule
   b. An ICD-9 cost form
   c. A UB04 form
   d. A CMS 1500 form

REFERENCES

1. The Living Webster Encyclopedic Dictionary of the English Lanuage. Kellerman E, ed. The English Language Institute of America Inc. Melrose Park, IL.1975:128.
2. *Current Procedural Terminology. CPT 2004 Professional Edition.* Chicago: American Medical Association Press of the American Medical Association; 2003.
3. U.S. Department of Health and Human Services, Centers for Medicare & Medicaid Services. HCPCS Background Information. Available at: http://www.cms.hhs.gov/Med-HCPCSGenInfo/. Accessed January 5, 2007.
4. *2006 Professional International Classification of Disease, Ninth Revision (ICD-9), Clinical Modifications,* 6th ed. Salt Lake City, Utah: Ingenix; 2005.
5. National Center for Health Statistics. Health, United States, 2006. With Chartbook on Trends in the Health of Americans. Hyattsville, MD: 2006:30.

Additional References

1. Finkler SA. *Finance and Accounting for Nonfinancial Managers,* 3rd ed. Paramus, NJ: Prentice Hall Press; 2002.
2. Turner ML. *The Unofficial Guide to Starting a Small Business,* 2nd ed. Hoboken, NJ: Wiley Publishing; 2004.
3. Shim JK, Siegel JG. *Complete Budgeting Workbook and Guide.* New York, NY: Simon and Schuster; 1994.

Additional Online Resources

A complete listing of codes can be obtained from the AMA online at: http://www.ama-assn.org/ama/pub/category/3113.html.
A listing of HCPCS codes can be found on the CMS web site, at: http://www.cms.hhs.gov. ICD-9 codes can also be found at: http://www.cms.hhs.gov/icd9ProviderDiagnosticcodes.
More information about the ICD-10 can be found at: http://www.cdc.gov/nchs/about/otheract/icd9/abticd10.htm.
A local CMS office can be found at: http://www.cms.hhs.gov/medicareprovidersupenroll/01_overview.asp?.

APPENDIX

Chapter Questions Answer Key and Rationales

CHAPTER 1

1. **B.** Physical therapists commonly work with a variety of specialists, including doctors of osteopathic medicine and physiatrists. In many rehabilitation settings, a physiatrist works closely with the therapy department in the rehabilitation of patients. Physiatrists are physicians who specialize in physical medicine and rehabilitation.

2. **A.** The Individualized Education Program (IEP) is the contractual agreement made between the school district and the parents of a student enrolled in special education. Although a physician may indicate the frequency and duration of therapy services in a prescription, the IEP takes precedence in establishing the parameters of service delivery. As a member of the IEP team, a physician may recommend services but the IEP team decides which services and frequency are necessary and appropriate.

3. **A.** The need for a physician's referral for physical therapy services is dictated by state law and is found in the physical therapy practice act for that state. The state's Medicaid program may also require a physician's prescription for physical therapy services as a requirement of payment of health-related services in special education, which is allowed under the 1988 Medicare Catastrophic Coverage Act (PL 100–360).

4. **C.** The behavior of this team, performing discipline-specific evaluations and providing discipline-specific interventions is reflective of a multidisciplinary team. There would be more emphasis on role release and the identification of a primary provider in a transdisciplinary model. The fact that the physical therapist is working with other disciplines would not make it unidisciplinary.

5. **A.** The Nagi model of disablement shows the relationship between a pathology (cell death), an impairment (impaired movement), a functional limitation (inability to roll), and a disability (unable to participate in day care or preschool). The sequence moves from a cellular or systems level to a disability level.

6. **C.** The physical therapist groups the collection of examination findings into a defined category or practice pattern that best describes the presentation of the patient. Medical tests such as arthroscopic examinations, MRIs, or genetic testing diagnose meniscus tears, osteogenesis imperfecta, and demyelinization in the CNS. The diagnosis of impaired mobility associated with local inflammation can be appropriately diagnosed by the knowledge and tests that a physical therapist can apply.

7. **D.** A physical therapist may utilize information from a variety of sources even if she cannot order the tests. Radiology reports and laboratory values are very instrumental in aiding in the selection of the interventions used and the intensity of treatment that can be tolerated by a patient.

8. **A.** Intra-rater reliability relates to the ability of a test to produce consistent results if the same person does the testing (when one person takes repeated measurements). This is different than inter-rater reliability (between two people).

9. **B.** Sally began treatment with 50 degrees of ROM in her right shoulder. With each visit, she demonstrated 10 degrees more range than she demonstrated the previous visit. It could be expected that, in order to obtain 20 degrees more range in her right shoulder, she would need two additional visits. This forecast is based on her rate of attainment of her range of motion.

10. **B.** Moderate assistance is defined as two points of contact required to complete the task safely. One hand on each shoulder would give two points of contact.

CHAPTER 2

1. **A.** Today a family can consist of one or more parents, same-sex parents, a blended family, foster care family, adoptive family, an aunt, uncle, grandparent, or other related or nonrelated people. Understanding this concept will aid the physical therapist in understanding each child's unique family structure.

2. **A.** Rubella is a mild, febrile, highly infectious viral disease most commonly seen in childhood. A mother who acquires the infection while pregnant could pass it to the fetus. Understanding this relationship can aid the physical therapist in parental education or help her to understand the examination findings of a child.

3. **A.** Family routines are defined as those interactions within the family that occur frequently, are episodic, have a clear beginning and end, and reflect the broader concept of family organization. Identifying them may help the physical therapist integrate certain interventions into a family's daily activities.

4. **D.** Rituals are defined as family routines that convey a message about who we are as a group and are defined by each family. The physical therapist, when providing suggestions for modifications to home activities, should appreciate a family's association or level of importance for certain activities.

5. **D.** Implantation outside the uterus is termed ectopic pregnancy and ultimately ends in death of the fetus.

6. **A.** As a newborn, an infant will show complete head lag during PTS, and progressively develop better head control until approximately 5 months of age, when there will be no head lag noted when he is pulled to sit. All of the other skills listed should not appear until later in the year.

7. **B.** Spontaneous stepping is a reflex that is seen from 27 weeks' gestation until approximately 2 months of age. The parents often interpret the stepping movements as the child's desire to walk. The apparent walking is a reflexive movement.

8. **B.** Physical growth in middle adolescence is the most remarkable period of growth with an average growth in height of 3 inches per year. This may be relevant to a physical therapist who is ordering equipment for an adolescent during this time. Rapid changes in growth should be anticipated.

9. **C.** It is recommended that children participate in at least 60 minutes of age-appropriate physical activity on all, or most, days of the week. The duration should be in smaller increments of 15 minutes at a time. Providing the child a variety of activities, as well as spreading them over the course of a day, may encourage the child to participate.

10. **C.** In late adolescence, girls will reach their adult size around 17 to 18 years. Boys will reach their adult size between 18 and 21 years. Cathy still has the potential to grow.

CHAPTER 3

1. **A.** The classic symptom of autism is the inability of the child to relate to others, even his parents. The inability to pay attention, or impairments in language or coordination, may be associated with other disorders.

2. **C.** Osteosarcoma is the most common primary malignant bone tumor in children. The tumor occurs most commonly in the femur followed by the tibia and then the humerus, but any bone can be involved.

3. **D.** Type III deformities cannot be realigned with passive movement because of the rigidity of the forefoot. This foot is treated with serial casts.

4. **B.** Immobilizing the hip in 100 degrees flexion and approximately 30 degrees abduction will properly position the head of the femur in the acetabulum.

5. **A.** This is called a Gower maneuver or Gower sign. The other tests listed are used in the examination of the hip joint.

6. **C.** Although passive stretching is important in the management of torticollis, active movement is necessary to strengthen the cervical muscles. With the head rotated to the right, it is the left SCM that is shortened. (The SCM rotates the head to the opposite side.) Active rotation to the left would strengthen the right SCM.

7. **A.** Involvement of a hemibody, with lower extremities involved more than the upper extremities, is the definition of CP, spastic diplegia.

8. **A.** Pressure ulcers are placed into four categories, depending on their stage of development. Stage I ulcers are characterized by a nonblanchable erythema on intact skin. Stage II ulcers include the epidermis, dermis, or both. Stage III ulcers extend to the subcutaneous tissue. Stage IV ulcers involve muscle, bone, and/or supporting tissues. This patient would present with a Stage I ulcer on the posterior aspect of his left calcaneus.

9. **C.** Signs and symptoms of increased intracranial pressure may include the presence of a headache, double vision, projectile vomiting, and lethargy. It requires immediate medical attention. You should notify the nurse or primary physician immediately.

10. **C.** Arnold Chiari malformation is defined as a prolapse or displacement of the medulla and cerebellum into the foramen magnum. This impairs CSF flow and leads to the development of hydrocephalus.

CHAPTER 4

1. **C.** The average gestational period is 40 weeks and has a range of 37 to 42 weeks. Generally, an infant born before 37 weeks is considered to be premature.

2. **B.** Low birth weight is defined as a weight <5.5 lb (2,500 g) but >3.3 lb (1,500 g). Maria would be considered low birth weight.

3. **A.** Tolerance to handling can be monitored through the infant's vital signs. Each examination should be unique to the patient and circumstances. Performing an examination based on the physical therapist's amount of time or until the infant cries would be inappropriate.

4. **C.** This is the quiet alert state, which is the optimal state for learning in the infant.

5. **C.** In this position, the upper extremities and hands naturally come together allowing the infant to explore and manipulate objects placed in her hands. This gravity-eliminated position for elbow and shoulder flexion would also make hand-to-mouth movements potentially easier.

6. **A.** Providing care to an infant in the NICU is a coordinated process. The infant's nurse would be able to provide the physical therapist with the current status of the infant and be able to provide information on additional tests or procedures that were recently performed or are scheduled for that day.

7. **B.** It takes approximately 10 minutes for most patients to feel the effect of intravenous pain medications. Oral medications take longer. Planning physical therapy interventions when the pain medication is taking an effect may be appropriate, depending on the role of pain in the rehabilitation process.

8. **C.** Typically, a child who is 6 years old would be old enough to understand the concept and importance of nonweight bearing and have the sufficient coordination skills to use axillary crutches. A child younger than this may need the support of a walker.

9. **C.** The most common mode of transmission of VRE is by physical contact; therefore, contact precautions should be used.

10. **B.** All information disclosed to another party must have the authorization of the legal guardian or parent. Even if the physical therapist feels that it is in the best interest of the patient, the physical therapist must obtain the consent of the parent or legal guardian prior to disclosing information in this case.

CHAPTER 5

1. **A.** Working in an outpatient setting and coordinating services can be very different from an inpatient setting, where all the services are provided by one agency. HIPAA requires that parental authorization be obtained prior to any discussion or coordination of services with other agencies.

2. **B.** This is the definition of an Ashworth grade 2.

3. **B.** Typically, in outpatient facilities physical therapy services are billed according to the service provided, such as an evaluation, gait training, or therapeutic exercise. Individual contracts with third party payers may vary this arrangement.

4. **B.** Children younger than 8 years may require a less abstract method of objectively rating their pain. Having a very young child evaluate his pain using a visual analog scale may not be the most appropriate method due to the level of his cognitive development.

5. **C.** Although obtaining a history from the parent may be perceived as being more time efficient from the physical therapist's point of view, a review of the medical record prior to beginning the interview may provide the physical therapist with valuable information to make the interview with the family more efficient. It can also provide information that the family may unintentionally leave out.

6. **A.** A CARF accreditation signifies that the facility has demonstrated a commitment to continually enhance the quality of their services and to focus on the satisfaction of the patients served. Part of this process is to gather information to use as part of an outcomes management system to measure the performance of a program, to make improvements, and to benchmark the program with similar programs across the country.

7. **C.** Pediatric inpatient rehabilitation hospitals generally follow the CMS criteria for number of hours of therapy as part of their admission criteria, as well as a patient who is medically stable and has the potential to benefit from interdisciplinary rehabilitation services.

8. **A.** Functional training begins from the time of admission to decrease the activity limitations that may be present at the time of discharge. Early functional training includes bed mobility and transfers and should be carried out by all team members. For functional training to be effective for the patient, communication among staff and with the family is important as well as daily practice.

9. **B.** According to the information given, Kevin continues to show impairments in his stair negotiation and balance skills. Physical therapy would still be warranted, but on an outpatient basis as his parents appear competent to manage him at home at this stage.

10. **A.** Functional assessments are not meant to replace other assessment tools, so other measures such as developmental assessments, balance tests, and timed tests may also be used to complete the examination and develop a plan for intervention.

CHAPTER 6

1. **A.** There are many federal laws that affect children and their families. The IDEA established certain early intervention services for eligible children and their families under Part C of the law.

2. **C.** Child find is the title and process by which an early intervention program attempts to identify children in the state who are eligible for Part C services.

3. **B.** The IDEA defines this process as an evaluation. It is a picture of a child at a moment in time that is used to determine if the child or family is eligible for early intervention services as defined by the federal law and state definitions.

4. **B.** The 45-day timeline is a federal government requirement. Failure to meet this deadline could affect a state's federal funding.

5. **D.** Natural environments for children in an early intervention program are defined as those settings in which children learn to develop everyday abilities

and skills. This environment is not limited to one place. Answer D best reflects this concept.

6. **B.** The family is the greatest resource for a child. It should be the first place a physical therapist should explore for resources to aid in the development of a child.

7. **A.** The federal government requires that the services provided to children and their families be based on current research to the extent that that information is available in the literature.

8. **C.** Strategies in early intervention should be integrated into the daily routines of the family as much as is appropriate and necessary for each individual child and family. Answer C reflects that integration the most, incorporating encouragement, strengthening, and daily practice of the desired goal.

9. **D.** If the state allows, Jack can continue receiving early intervention services until he is 5 years old. States have a right to stop early intervention services when the child turns 3 years old, but the federal law does allow for early intervention services to continue until the age of 5 years, if the state is willing to provide these services.

10. **A.** No more than 9 months before she is eligible for preschool services but no less than 90 days before she is eligible for preschool.

CHAPTER 7

1. **C.** The Rehabilitation Act's definition of a person with a disability includes an impairment that substantially limits one or more major life activities. A major life activity would include walking, speaking, and breathing, as defined in the law. The teacher should talk to the student's other teachers to determine if in fact the asthma is associated with the tardiness.

2. **D.** As defined in the law, an individual with a disability means any person who has a mental or physical impairment that substantially limits one or more major life activities. Given the limited information, having a history of multiple fractures would not be readily associated with any current impairment that would limit a major life activity.

3. **C.** No formalized test is required under Section 504 to determine the student's eligibility, but the Section 504 Committee should consider a variety of information from more than one source. This could include health records, information from the parents, and physical therapy evaluations.

4. **A.** The Section 504 Plan is less structured than either the IEP or IFSP, and is not required by federal law to contain any of the items listed in the answers provided.

5. **D.** The Rehabilitation Act requires periodic re-evaluation of the education program (34CFR104.35). Periodic as defined under IDEA is at least every 3 years.

6. **C.** The Office of Civil Rights has the authority to enforce Section 504. Remember that The Rehabilitation Act is a civil rights law, not an educational law.

7. **B.** Screening for scoliosis is a common practice in many of our public schools for grades five through eight.

8. **A.** Fitness is a measurement of physical condition or being in shape. Answer **A** incorporates aspects of strength, agility, and flexibility and therefore reflects attributes of fitness more than the other choices do.

9. **C.** Although all the choices listed are important, in order for the athlete to be able to perform at a competitive level both effectively and safely, the athlete must have strong core musculature (strength).

10. **C.** Grade 3 is the only grade associated with a loss of consciousness.

CHAPTER 8

1. **B.** Students who have multiple disabilities statistically spend the least amount of time with their nondisabled peers. Physical therapists are in a unique position to help facilitate this process through consultation and education with the teachers and staff on selected interventions and techniques or use of assistive technology to aid in the integration of students with disabilities.

2. **C.** As a member of the IEP team, the physical therapist works collaboratively with other personnel and parents to optimize the student's ability to learn as outlined in his individualized education program. It is the main focus on the use of physical therapy as a related service in special education.

3. **A.** FAPE was introduced in 1975 with the passage of PL 94-142, the Education for All Handicapped Children Act. It clearly states that children with disabilities are entitled to a free appropriate public education. It also identified physical therapy as a related service in special education.

4. **B.** A physical therapist must provide services in a state in accordance with that state's Practice Act.

5. **D.** It depends if the student was placed in a private school in order to obtain a free and appropriate public education.

6. **A.** The physical therapist would evaluate the student to gain information to aid in the discussion and development of an individualized education program.

7. **C.** The evaluation does not establish discipline-specific goals to be added to the IEP. The evaluation pro-

vides information that aids in the development of the IEP goals during the IEP meeting.

8. **C.** The goals in the IEP should clearly relate to the student's education. For each goal listed in the IEP, the answer to "How would this optimize the student's ability to learn?" should be obvious.

9. **D.** It is not inappropriate to pull a student from a classroom and provide an intervention that ultimately would aid in that student's ability to learn in the classroom. At certain points in learning a motor skill, it may be necessary to control the environmental conditions to allow for learning, before generalizing that skill into the classroom.

10. **B.** A physical therapist should be aware of a student's transition program and assist the student and parents in that process. Planning for life after high school does not occur at graduation, but rather years before the transition actually takes place. The IDEA requires that a transition plan be identified on a student's IEP by the time he is 16 years old. This would allow 2 to 5 years for additional planning and implementation.

CHAPTER 9

1. **D.** Palliative care is comfort care and can be provided to any person, not just those in a hospice program, to relieve pain and other symptoms, such as nausea or fatigue, which may be associated with a disease.

2. **C.** Death resulting from an unintentional injury is the most common cause of death in children 2 years of age, so safety should be emphasized as an important primary prevention measure.

3. **D.** All of the answers listed differ significantly between an adult and child with regard to death or dying with the exception of the desire to die at home.

4. **C.** Until a competent child reaches the age of majority (18 years), the ultimate authority to direct care rests with his parents. The execution of advance directives by a minor can be a way of allowing the child to make known his wishes, but his parents are legally responsible.

5. **A.** It is appropriate, and encouraged, to allow a child to participate in his care planning to the best of his abilities. At times, there may be a need to make decisions or implement interventions without his participation, such as when there is an immediate need to start a new intervention, or if his cognitive or current health status does not make his participation possible.

6. **C.** Spirituality is more than a religion. It includes factors such as a person's experiences, behaviors, and

beliefs, which can provide meaning and acceptance of the present situation. It is an important aspect of hospice, as well as health care in general. A physical therapist should be honest with the patient and feel comfortable discussing this aspect of a person. The pain felt with spiritual issues is very real and at times can be overwhelming. It should not be ignored.

7. **A.** Palliative care focuses on the comfort of the patient, whereas rehabilitative care focuses on the patient's recovery.

8. **B.** All of the interventions listed could be important given the individual circumstance, but family and patient education would apply in all circumstances and be especially important during this emotionally charged time.

9. **C.** Of the behaviors listed, crying would be least likely associated with active dying, which is generally not associated with this process.

10. **B.** Bereavement services are a vital part of a hospice program and begin at the time of admission. Services are provided to family members, or other appropriate individuals associated with the family or child, for up to 1 year following the death of the child.

CHAPTER 10

1. **A.** Self-determination is not learned overnight. The characteristics develop over time, beginning with the experiences of childhood. Physical therapists should encourage their young patients to make choices, experience the consequences of their behaviors, and act autonomously (when appropriate), realizing that what children experience can influence their behavior as adults.

2. **C.** Physical therapists can play a vital role in promoting mobility and environmental access for individuals with disabilities. This may help to address the higher unemployment rate seen in people who are impaired in their mobility.

3. **C.** According to the ADA guidelines, the recommended minimum width is 32 inches.

4. **C.** According to ADA guidelines, the slope of a ramp should be 1:12. If there are five 6-inch steps, the height between the two surfaces would be 30 inches (5 × 6 = 30). 30 inches × 12 = 360 inches or 30 feet. The minimum length of the ramp would have to be 30 feet.

5. **D.** According to the CDC, the most used assistive technology device is the cane.

6. **A.** There are two criteria, one functional and the other financial.

7. **D.** The IDEA does not apply to higher education programs, but because most colleges and universities

receive federal funds, they must comply with civil rights legislation.

8. **B.** The integration of people with and without disabilities is a key factor in supported employment.

9. **D.** Goals for individuals who reside in ICF should focus on function. The most appropriate goal, of those listed, would be to improve his ability to step into and out of a van. Addressing his impairment to this activity would be part of the interventions.

10. **A.** The ability to perform a task does not automatically translate into a person's ability to perform that task over a period of time. An examination of his endurance and work schedule would be appropriate.

CHAPTER 11

1. **C.** Changes in the woman's musculoskeletal system are the most visually apparent during pregnancy. Expected changes, such as a forward head and increased cervical as well as lumbar lordosis, should be expected and noted during the examination. Identification of these postural changes throughout her pregnancy will aid in the design of an appropriate and safe exercise program.

2. **A.** To assure that the interventions are safe and appropriate, a multidisciplinary approach to client management should be followed when providing services to women who are pregnant. A woman's obstetrician should be consulted.

3. **A.** This is the first level of this exercise that focuses on contracting the rectus abdominis muscle.

4. **B.** After the fourth month of gestation, the size of the uterus and fetus can compress the inferior vena cava and affect a woman's circulation.

5. **C.** As a general rule, a pregnant woman who performs cardiovascular or aerobic exercises should be able to carry on a conversation while performing the exercise. According to the CDC, this corresponds to a level 12 to 14 on the Borg scale.

CHAPTER 12

1. **C.** The use of OTC products can have a significant influence on the prescribed medication taken by a patient. In the pediatric population, serious illness and death can result from the inappropriate use of an OTC product that alone could be considered harmless. Communication with the physician and pharmacist is important.

2. **C.** Significant changes in a child's functioning should be reported and discussed with the physician. Some medications require adjustments in their dosage in order to produce the desired effect in a specific and unique patient. Communication with the physician prescribing the medication is important.

3. **D.** Physical therapists do not prescribe medications or make recommendations on dosage outside of the prescribed orders or the information provided in OTC products. They can educate the patient on the pharmacodynamics of a medication and support the adherence to the physician's prescription.

4. **B.** A common side effect of opioids is respiratory and gastrointestinal motility depression. Instructing the patient to take a deep breath will allow her to breath in more oxygen. Her physical therapy interventions should continue. Appropriate breathing and mobility exercises may help to eliminate the medication used in surgery from her system.

5. **C.** Warning signs of dehydration can include fever, low output of urine, light-headedness, fatigue, and the inability to focus mentally. Of the list provided, being active would least likely be associated with dehydration. The physical therapist should be aware that dehydration could occur quickly in infants, especially in the presence of diarrhea and vomiting.

CHAPTER 13

1. **B.** The state board of physical therapy is responsible for protecting the public. It does this by issuing a license to practice in a state, and it has the power to revoke that privilege if the physical therapist fails to adhere to the state regulations on the delivery of physical therapy services.

2. **C.** Kate has been awarded physical custody, which would not allow her to enroll her daughter into a program that would require parental consent, including the authorization to evaluate, provide services, and release information.

3. **A.** A guardian is appointed by the courts and would have the authority to consent to medical interventions and to act on behalf of the child's best interest.

4. **D.** This is the definition of an emancipated minor.

5. **D.** Forming a corporation limits the potential personal liability of a sole proprietorship or partnership. Because the corporation is a recognized distinct legal entity, each state requires that the corporation file Articles of Incorporation with the Secretary of State's office.

CHAPTER 14

1. **A.** Understanding how to classify expenses, based on their behavior, is an important step in the process of financial management. This will allow the physical therapist to attempt to control those costs,

variable and semivariable, that are influenced by their utilization.

2. **B.** This is the correct expansion of CPT.

3. **B.** The fee schedule is a list of the services provided and the charge for each of those services. Typically, fees are charged to patients in time increments, usually minutes.

4. **C.** Revenues in excess of expenses best defines profit. All businesses, whether they are for-profit or not-for-profit, must make a profit in order to update equip-

ment, give pay raises, and make other financial investments for the practice.

5. **D.** Billing third party payers for professional services is done on a CMS 1500 form. The CMS 1500 is a form created by the Health Care Financing Administration and approved by the AMA Council on Medical Service. The UB 90 is used when physical therapists are enrolled with the third party payer as a group, such as in a hospital setting.

A

abdominal brace maneuver – a maneuver in which the woman finds her neutral spine position and then contracts her abdominal muscles and maintains that position during an exercise

acanthosis nigricans – excessive axillary pigmentation

accounts payable – expenses that a business has incurred but not yet paid, such as dues and memberships, utility bills, or small equipment or materials purchased on credit

accounts receivable – money due to a business which has not yet been paid

activity-based instruction – a type of intervention that observes what the child's interests are and works on functional skills that are applicable to the child versus what a developmental book states that the child should be doing at a certain age

adaptability – how well a family responds to change

adoption – a proceeding whereby the legal relationship between the biological parents and child is terminated and a new legal relationship is established with the adoptive parents

adult patient – a patient who is older than 18 years

adulthood – the age at which a person is a full member of society with responsibilities, not only for himself, but for the community as well

advance directive – a legal document created by a competent adult communicating his desires about medical treatment if he cannot express his wishes in the future

Americans with Disabilities Act – U.S. civil rights legislation that prohibits discrimination and ensures equal opportunity for individuals with disabilities in employment, public transportation, public accommodations, and telecommunications

anhedonia – loss of enjoyment in activities that would normally be enjoyable

Apgar score – a common test done on newborn infants immediately after birth. A total score takes into consideration the newborn's heart rate, respiratory effort, muscle tone, reflex irritability, and color at 1 and 5 minutes after birth.

apnea – the cessation of spontaneous respirations lasting 20 seconds or more

arachnodactyly – long and slender feet and hands

Arnold Chiari malformation – a prolapse or displacement of the medulla and cerebellum into the foramen magnum

assessment – the ongoing procedures to identify (i) the child's unique strengths and needs; (ii) the services appropriate to meet those needs; (iii) the resources, priorities, and concerns of the family; and (iv) the support services needed to enhance the family's capacity to meet their child's developmental needs

assets – items that the business owns

assisted living – a facility or style of living that is used by people who are not able to live on their own, but do not need the level of care that a skilled nursing home offers

assistive technology – any item, piece of equipment, or product system whether acquired commercially off the shelf, modified, or customized that is used to increase, maintain, or improve functional capabilities of individuals with disabilities

"at will" employment – an employment relationship in which the parties have not agreed that the employment relationship will last for a defined period of time. Either party may terminate the relationship at any time.

aura – subjective symptoms that precede a seizure

autonomy – the right of an individual to determine what shall be done to his or her body

B

balance sheet – a financial statement that lists a business's assets and liabilities

bioavailability – the percentage of a drug that actually arrives at the target organ or tissue in the body

biotransformation – the process of a drug conversion from its original state to one that is altered or degraded after administration into the organism

Blount disease – idiopathic growth disorder of the tibia that results in tibia vara; bowlegs

Borg scale – a subjective scale used to determine how hard, or intense, the exerciser is working

brachycephaly – a malformation of the head noted by a decreased anterior/posterior diameter

Braxton Hicks – false contractions that may be felt after the third month of pregnancy

breakeven method – a method of estimating revenues in which the business identifies all of the expenses of the practice so that the appropriate fees can be calculated to cover all of the costs

breech – the presentation of the fetus when the head has not descended into the birth canal first

budget – a financial statement of the estimated income and expenditures covering a specific period of time in the future

C

capitated reimbursement – a payment system that pays the service provider in advance a fixed dollar amount for each child enrolled in the program

care coordination conference – a formal or informal meeting of the health care professionals involved in the care of a patient in order to communicate, develop, or modify the plan of care

CARF (Commission on Accreditation of Rehabilitation Facilities) – an independent, nonprofit accreditor of human service providers in the areas of rehabilitation, employment, child and family, community, and aging services. Accreditation is voluntary.

cash flow statement – a financial statement that shows the inflows and outflows of cash for a specific period of time

central line – an intravenous catheter that is inserted into a large vein, typically located on the chest, neck, arm, or groin. It is used to deliver medicine or parenteral nutrition.

cerclage – the suturing of the cervix using nonabsorbable sutures. Cerclage may be done for an incompetent cervix during pregnancy.

Cesarean section – the delivery of a fetus by abdominal surgery requiring an incision through the uterine wall

child find – a federally required state system to identify, locate, and evaluate all children with disabilities who reside in the state and are in need of early intervention, special education, and related services

Civil Rights Act of 1964 – the major piece of federal civil rights legislation that prohibits discrimination based on race, color, religion, sex, or national origin

clostridium difficile (C Diff) – a bacterium that causes abdominal pain and diarrhea. C Diff can lead to more serious intestinal disorders, but rarely results in death.

common law – the rule of law developed through court opinions

competitive employment – full- or part-time employment in the labor market with competitive wages and responsibilities in which the individual maintains the job with no additional outside support

computed tomography – commonly known as a CT scan or CAT scan. It is a diagnostic imaging technique that uses x-rays, detectors, and computers to create images of anatomy in slices, allowing for a more refined examination.

concussion – a mild traumatic brain injury noted by a brief period of unconsciousness that occurs immediately following a head trauma

consent – the knowing, intelligent, and voluntary agreement to engage in a given activity

contractual allowances – the amount agreed upon between the business and the insurance company prior to billing for the service. This allowance may differ from the business's typical fee.

contusion – a mechanical injury that results in hemorrhaging and swelling

corporation – the legal entity of the business itself, which exists separately from the people who own the business

corrected chronological age – the difference between the infant's gestational age at birth and 40 weeks (typical gestational period), subtracted from the infant's current chronological age

corticotrophin-releasing hormone – a substance released from the hypothalamus believed to cause a release of oxytocin from the posterior pituitary

cost-based reimbursement – a form of reimbursement that looks at the number of children cared for per year and then bases future annual payments on the historical numbers of children served

croup – a particular kind of cough in children that has been described as sounding like a seal barking

Current Procedural Terminology (CPT) – five-digit codes used throughout the country by health care providers to designate the type of service or services provided

cytomegalovirus – a group of herpes viruses that are the most common cause of congenital infection; asymptomatic in the majority of cases

D

Department of Health and Human Services – the U.S. government's principal agency for protecting the health of all Americans and providing essential human services, especially for persons who are least able to help themselves

diabetic ketoacidosis – a condition in which the arterial blood pH is < 7.25, serum bicarbonate level is < 15 meq/L, and ketones are present in the serum or urine

diagnosis – evaluation of the results of the examination, which includes a history, a systems review, and the results of tests and measurements, which allows the physical therapist to categorize a child into a specific group, aiding in the selection of interventions and possible outcomes

Diagnostic-Related Group (DRG) – a common payment arrangement in which there is bundling of like or related services or resources into one payment

diastasis recti – a condition in which the rectus abdominis muscle separates from the linea alba during pregnancy

diastasis symphysis pubis – a separation at the symphysis pubis

direct access – the ability to access physical therapy services without a physician's referral

direct service – the provision of an intervention by a physical therapist directly to a student in the classroom or in the community

dolichocephaly – a disproportionately long narrow head, elongated from front to back, as a result of prolonged positioning

domains of development – categorization of developmental skills into five areas or domains: motor, language, cognitive, social–emotional, and self-help skills

due process – the right to be heard

Durable Medical Equipment (DME) – adapted or assistive devices that are used in the course of an illness or disability to provide assistance or promote function. These items can be used for a period of time. Examples include canes, walkers, wheelchairs, and hospital beds.

Dynamic Systems Theory – a theory of movement acquisition that identifies the interdependence of multiple systems, including the external environment as well as the internal biological environment of the child, in the acquisition of movement skills

E

echolalia – nonsense rhyming, repetition of a spoken word or sentence

eclampsia – a condition seen in pregnancy resulting from pregnancy-induced hypertension; it includes the onset of generalized seizures

ectoderm – an outer layer of cells of an embryo that gives rise to the skin and nervous system

ectopic pregnancy – implantation of the zygote outside the uterus

Education for All Handicapped Children Act – a federal law that provided for a "free and appropriate public education" (FAPE) for all children with disabilities, beginning whenever the individual state provides public education to children who are not disabled

Educational Amendments to the Civil Rights Act – Under Title IX of this law, boys and girls are expected to receive fair and equal treatment in all areas of public schooling: recruitment, admissions, educational programs and activities, course offerings, financial aid, scholarships, and athletics

effacement – thinning of the cervix

Elementary and Secondary Education Act – federal legislation that provided a plan for addressing the inequality of educational opportunity for economically underprivileged children and became the statutory basis upon which early special education legislation was later drafted

eligibility meetings – a meeting held prior to the implementation of services in order to determine if the child qualifies for services based on federal and state guidelines for eligibility

emancipated minor – a court-ordered status that allows a minor to be treated as an adult and therefore not subject to parental control

embryo – the developing human for the first 8 weeks of gestation

embryonic period – the period 6 weeks in duration beginning after the first 2 weeks of conception as the zygote is implanted into the uterine wall

endoderm – an inner layer of cells of an embryo that gives rise to the digestive and respiratory systems

engagement – a process in birthing when the baby's head passes through the pelvic outlet and descends into the birth canal

enteral – administration of nutrition via the alimentary canal

enthesopathy – a disease process that occurs at the site of the tendon insertion

episiotomy – a surgical opening of the area from the vagina to the rectum done to minimize the damage to the mother during delivery of the infant

episode of care – an unbroken sequence of care provided to address a given condition

equilibrium reactions – sequential movements of the body to maintain the center of mass over the base of support. Rotational movements are incorporated into this higher level of balance.

erythematous – marked by redness

evaluation – clinical judgments made from the information gained from the examination data

evidence-based medicine – a combination of the utilization of published research, clinical expertise, the patient's values, and the patient's unique circumstances in the provision of medicine or health care

expenses – dollars spent

expert witness – someone who, because of professional training and expertise, can provide the court with opinion testimony on a specific topic

extended school year (ESY) – special education and related services that are provided beyond the normal school year to a child with a disability

F

family activities of daily living – activities that are the work of the family unit

Family-centered approach – the provision of services and interventions based on the concerns and priorities of the family and not primarily on the diagnosis or level of developmental delay of the child

Family Systems Theory – a theory that assumes that all members of the family are involved in each other's lives, so what happens to one member will affect the entire family

fee-for-service – the term used to describe the amount charged by a health care provider for a service rendered, based on the business's fee for that service

fee schedule – a business's listing of the services provided and the charge for each of those services

fetal alcohol effects – physical or mental birth defects associated with Fetal Alcohol Syndrome, but to a lesser degree

Fetal Alcohol Syndrome (FAS) – a combination of physical and mental birth defects resulting from the mother consuming alcohol during pregnancy

fetus – the developing human after 8 weeks of gestation

financial statements – a set of fundamental financial reports that typically include an income statement, a balance sheet, and a cash flow statement

first pass effect – the body's filtration process. It occurs in the liver.

first trimester – weeks 1 through 12 of a pregnancy

fixed expenses – expenses of a business that are generally constant for the fiscal year. Examples include salary and wages, rent, interest expenses on loans, and depreciation of equipment.

flat fee – a set fee that is charged to the patient no matter how long or complicated the intervention

frog-legged position – a position of the lower extremities that consists of hip abduction and flexion, excessive hip external rotation, and knee flexion

G

gastroesophageal reflux disease (GERD) – reflux which is the result of the esophageal sphincter failing to constrict to prevent the stomach contents from backing up into the esophagus

germinal period – begins at conception when a mature ovum (egg) is fertilized by the sperm. It lasts for 2 weeks, until implantation in the uterus.

gestation – period of time in which an embryo develops within the mother's womb. It typically averages 40 weeks in humans.

glycosuria – urinary excretion of carbohydrates

gravidity – the number of pregnancies

guardian ad litem – the attorney called upon to represent the child's interests in court

guardianship – a legal relationship between the individual (the guardian) and another person (in this case, a minor or ward), giving the guardian the right, and the duty, to act on behalf of the child in all decisions affecting the child's life

Guide to Physical Therapist Practice (The Guide) – a fundamental document of the profession of physical therapy that provides an outline of the profession's body of knowledge and describes the boundaries within which physical therapists design and implement appropriate plans of care for specific patient/client diagnostic groups

gynecomastia – excessive development of a man's breasts due to increased estrogen levels. Mild gynecomastia may occur in normal adolescents.

H

half-life – the time that it takes for 50% of the drug that remains in the body to be eliminated

Health Insurance Portability and Accountability Act (HIPAA) – a federal law that establishes patients with privacy standards to protect their medical records and other health information provided to insurances, hospitals, physicians, and other health care providers. The Act also gives patients access to their medical records and increased control over how their health information is disclosed and used.

Healthcare Common Procedure Coding System (HCPCS) – codes used to identify medical services and procedures furnished by physicians and other health care professionals and products, supplies, and services not included in the CPT codes

herpes gestationis – a skin condition that presents as a blister-like rash, primarily on the abdomen, that may be seen during the second or third trimester of pregnancy

herpes simplex virus – a viral infection that causes lesions in the genital areas and can be passed to the fetus in utero, but infections are more common during the birthing process

Hill–Burton Hospital Construction Act – federal legislation that came about in 1946 that had a major influence on the expansion of the hospital industry and the physical therapy departments that they housed

hospice – a philosophy of care that is available to anyone with a terminal prognosis, providing palliative and supportive services to patients and their families. Intervention is provided by an interdisciplinary team of professionals and volunteers who are available to provide assistance at home and in specialized settings.

hospice plan of care – the plan of care developed by a hospice team designed to provide palliative care and support to the patient and family during the patient's illness

human immunodeficiency virus (HIV) – a virus that suppresses the function of the human immune system that progresses to the development of acquired immunodeficiency syndrome, AIDS

hypercapnia – increased arterial CO_2 tension

hyperuricemia – increased concentration of uric acid in the blood

I

impact seizure – a generalized seizure occurring within seconds of an injury to the head

impetigo herpetiformis – a rash in the axillary and inguinal region sometimes occurring in the third trimester of pregnancy

income statement – a financial statement that includes the revenues and expenses generated by the business for a specific period of time. This is also referred to as a statement of operations.

incubator – an enclosed bed that is used to regulate the external environment of a neonate, in order to minimize the child's energy expenditure in maintaining body temperature

independent living – a philosophy of living that promotes self-determination and equal opportunity

indirect service – the provision of an intervention by a physical therapist for a student in the classroom where the recipient of the intervention shifts more towards the teacher, classroom staff, school environment, or parent, rather than directly to the student

Individual Habilitation Plan (IHP) – a formal individualized plan to address the needs and desires of a person who resides in a group home or Intermediate Care Facility (ICF)

individual with a disability – defined by the Americans with Disabilities Act as a person who has a physical or mental impairment that substantially limits one or more major life activities, a person who has a history or record of such impairment, or a person who is perceived by others as having such impairment

Individualized Education Program (IEP) – a legal document that describes the educational program for an individual student enrolled in special education. The IEP is mandated under the Individuals with Disabilities Education Act (IDEA).

Individualized Family Service Plan (IFSP) – a legal document in early intervention programs that is written in family-friendly language and addresses the family's primary concerns, priorities, and resources (CPR). It also identifies how the team can work together to improve the family's situation. The IFSP is mandated under the Individuals with Disabilities Education Act, Part C.

Individuals with Disabilities Education Act (IDEA) – federal law that provides federal funds to states to assist them in structuring and providing a public education to children with disabilities

infantile paralysis – another name used for poliomyelitis

informed consent – a legal principle that requires adequate disclosure of specific information to a patient in order for the patient to make a knowledgeable decision regarding the intervention or treatment

inotropic – influencing the contraction of muscle tissue

inpatient rehabilitation – a program of coordinated and integrated medical and rehabilitation services that is provided 24 hours per day. It is an intensive comprehensive interdisciplinary approach to the restoration of function for children and adolescents who have sustained injuries or have undergone surgical procedures that have impacted their activity and participation levels

integrated approach – a collaborative effort by all persons involved in the care or education of a child that attempts to assure that the most appropriate level and type of intervention is being incorporated into the child's daily routines and activities. This approach is used in the educational setting to optimize a student's ability to benefit from the individualized educational program.

Intermediate Care Facility (ICF) – a facility that provides health-related care and services above the level of custodial care to individuals with mental retardation but does not provide the level of care available in a hospital or skilled nursing facility

International Classification of Diseases (ICD) – the World Health Organization's codes to classify diseases. The codes are updated periodically, and are commonly known as ICD-9 codes or the more current updates (ICD-10).

interventions – interactions of a physical therapist using various techniques or procedures to produce a change in a patient or client

intrathecal injections – injections administered primarily to the spine in the subarachnoid or subdural spaces, where the target is the central nervous system.

J

Joint Commission on Accreditation of Healthcare Organizations (JCAHO) – A nonprofit, nongovernmental accrediting agency that develops professional standards and evaluates and accredits health care organizations in the United States regarding compliance with these standards. Accreditation is voluntary.

joint custody – custody of a child that is shared between divorced parents or both parties involved in the dispute. Forms of joint custody are further defined as physical or legal custody.

jurisdiction – the authority to grant or make a legal decision

K

kangaroo care – a type of care for a newborn that involves holding the child upright against the mother's chest, providing skin-to-skin contact. The infant wears nothing but a diaper.

ketoacidosis – acidosis attributed to an enhanced production of ketone bodies

L

Landau posture – a posture in prone, with the head, shoulders and hips extended above the horizontal

lead agency – an identified group or agency within a state, responsible for the supervision of services and coordination of resources in early intervention or special education programs

least restrictive environment (LRE) – a term used in federal law that refers to the education of students with disabilities. To the extent appropriate, students with disabilities should be educated in a regular classroom with students who are not disabled.

legal custody – a form of custody that gives the parent or guardian the right to make decisions affecting the child's life, including issues related to religion, medical care, and education

liabilities – items that the business has incurred or obligations that are owed to another party; a business's bills

linea nigra – an area of hyperpigmentation that runs from the pubis to the umbilicus along the same course as the linea alba. The linea nigra is seen sometimes in women who are pregnant.

litigation – the lawsuit process

living will – an advance directive that allows a competent adult to convey instructions regarding interventions and treatment when those wishes can no longer be communicated

M

magnetic resonance image (MRI) – a diagnostic image produced through the use of magnetic fields, radio frequency waves, and computers to create an image of anatomy. The MRI is used to visualize soft tissues.

mandatory reporter – a person who is required by law to make a report of a child's maltreatment or neglect

market or going rate – the price of an item or service that is based on what others in the marketplace are charging for the same or similar item or service

markup – the business process of adding to the actual cost of a service to come up with an hourly rate or fee that includes a level of profit

mature minor – a court-appointed status of a minor (person younger than 18 years) that allows the minor to consent to certain nonserious medical procedures

Medicaid – a joint federal and state program under the Social Security Act (Title XIX) that provides financial assistance and health programs to eligible populations, namely the poor

medical power of attorney – a legal arrangement created by a competent adult that designates one person (an agent) to make health care decisions when the adult is unable to do so

medication management – the ability to understand the purpose of medications as well as the physical ability to store, retrieve, open, and manipulate the medication for proper administration

mesoderm – the middle layer of cells of an embryo that gives rise to the skeletal, muscular, and circulatory systems

Methicillin-Resistant Staphylococcus Aureus (MRSA) – a strain of *Staphylococcus aureus* that developed a resistance to all forms of penicillin. It is seen in hospital patients or people residing in nursing homes who have an impaired immune system.

modifiers – used with CPT codes. These are two-digit numbers that help to more accurately define the code.

multidisciplinary – working with more than one discipline, especially in the examination and ongoing assessment processes, but generally providing interventions solely within one's professional boundaries

muscular endurance – the ability of a muscle to perform repeated movements without premature fatigue

myelinization – the process by which some of the nerve fibers throughout the body are coated with a layer of protein and lipids that acts to increase the rate of signal transmission along the nerve fiber

N

natural environments – the home, community, or other early childhood settings in which all children learn to develop everyday abilities and skills

neuromaturation theories of motor development – theories that correlate changes in motor development with observable changes in the central nervous system

No Child Left Behind Act – a federal law that addresses accountability in education by requiring a statewide system of accountability for all public school students, including students with disabilities

O

obesity – having an excess of body fat >35%, a body weight >20% of the ideal body weight, adjusted for age and height, or a body mass index (BMI) ≥30

Olympic lifts – a method of strength training that promotes total body strengthening within the context of explosive multiplanar movements, which simulate sport-specific movement patterns

ordinary witness – a lay witness who may only provide testimony about facts; those things that the witness observed or heard

outcome – the result of the provision of a service

outpatient rehabilitation – a type of rehabilitation, less intense than inpatient, conducted in a hospital department or a freestanding clinic. Services are provided for an identified activity limitation for a defined episode of care.

owner's equity – the portion of a business's assets that belongs to the owner

oxytocin – a hormone released from the posterior pituitary gland that facilitates contractions of the uterus to help with the expulsion of the fetus and subsequently the placenta. It also promotes milk release during lactation.

P

palliative care – comfort care; a component of hospice care directed toward physical comfort, emotional support, and quality of life

paratransit – a service in which individuals who are unable to use the regular transit system independently (because of a physical or mental impairment) are picked up and dropped off at their destinations

parenteral – administered via other routes besides the alimentary canal

parenting – the act of teaching and raising a child

parity – the number of births

partially capitated reimbursement – method of repayment that looks to combine the fee-for-service and capitated systems, in which the payer will reimburse the service provider on a fee-for-service basis up to a certain number of visits and no more

pathologic reflex – name given to a primitive reflex when the reflex is present after the time when it is expected to be integrated

Patient-controlled analgesia (PCA) – personally administered dosage of pain medication via an IV line; time limited

Patient Self-Determination Act – a federal law that requires health care facilities that participate in Medicare and Medicaid to give adults information regarding the facility's policies regarding advance directives

pharmacodynamics – the uptake, movement, binding, and interactions of pharmacologically active molecules at their tissue site of action or receptor level

pharmacokinetics – the movement of drugs within biologic systems; how the body deals with the drug in terms of the way the drug is absorbed, distributed, and eliminated

pharmacotherapeutics – the function of drugs when they are interacting with the body. It includes pharmacodynamics and pharmacokinetics.

physical custody – a form of custody of a child in which the parent or guardian has a right to have the child reside with him or her and the obligation to provide for routine daily care and control

Physical Therapist Assistant (PTA) – a professional who assists the physical therapist in the provision of physical therapy interventions and services

Physical Therapy Practice Act – a state law intended to protect the public from imposters or fraudulent billing practices in which the services are not rendered by a physical therapist or physical therapist assistant

physiologic flexion – the presence of a somewhat flexed body posture seen in full-term infants; a by-product of intrauterine positioning

physis – growth plates in bones

plagiocephaly – flattening of the skull noted in infancy, often resulting from external forces applied to the relatively soft skull

plyometric exercises – exercise that utilizes the stretch-shortening cycle of a muscle. Plyometric exercises incorporate an eccentric muscle contraction immediately followed by a concentric contraction of the same muscle.

Poland syndrome – an idiopathic congenital birth defect that includes the unilateral absence or underdevelopment of the pectoralis major muscle, associated ribs, and webbing of the fingers on the same side

poliomyelitis – a viral infection that causes an inflammatory process involving the gray matter of the spinal cord. Replication of the virus in motor neurons of the anterior horn cell and brain stem result in cell destruction and the general manifestation of paralysis.

polycythemia – an increase in the number of red blood cells

polydipsia – excessive thirst

polyuria – excessive urination

postictal – the period following a seizure

power – in regard to muscles, the product of strength (force) × speed (velocity)

Power of Attorney (POA) – a legal arrangement created by a competent adult that designates one person (an agent) to act on his or her behalf. A POA may be limited to certain actions.

precipitous labor – a rapid cervical dilation accompanied by severe, violent contractions that results in the birth of the infant usually within 1 hour

pre-eclampsia – a condition seen in pregnancy with symptoms that include persistent hypertension, swelling of the face, and proteinuria

preterm infant – an infant born at <37 weeks' gestation

primary family – one definition of a family in which members are living in the same house, have a biological relationship to the patient or child, or are involved in the care of that person

pro forma – when used with financial statements, it designates a document that is provided in advance of the information. Budgets are examples of pro forma statements.

profit – revenues in excess of expenses

protective reactions – a balance reaction; generally single-plane movements incorporating little or no rotation, elicited when a child is suddenly and quickly pushed off of her base of support

proteinuria – the presence of protein in the urine

pruritis – itching

pruritus gravidarum – a condition that may be experienced by up to 20% of pregnant women in the third trimester that causes severe itching due to intrahepatic cholestasis (impaired bile flow) and bile salt retention

psychometric properties – quantifiable attributes, such as validity and reliability, that relate to the item's statistical strength or weakness

ptosis – drooping eyelid or any body part

public accommodations – under Title III of the Americans with Disabilities Act, refers to private entities that own, lease, or operate facilities such as restaurants, that must comply with basic nondiscrimination requirements that prohibit exclusion, segregation, and unequal treatment

pulse oximeter – a device that records the oxygen saturation of arterial blood. This is typically found attached to a finger, toe, or ear lobe.

R

radiograph – commonly known as an x-ray; a diagnostic imaging technique that uses x-rays to produce images of body structures, namely bone, on film

Rate of Perceived Exertion (RPE) – a subjective scale used to determine how hard, or intense, the exerciser is working; also known as the Borg Scale

rebound test – a quick screen to ascertain whether an athlete is physically able to complete a plyometric exercise. The athlete is placed on a box (typically 12 inches in height) and asked to step off and immediately jump as high as he can after contacting the ground. The height jumped after rebounding is recorded. If the athlete is able to rebound to the height of the box jumped from, then he can be cleared for plyometric training.

reconstruction aide – early designation of a person who was trained and worked to rehabilitate military personnel in the early 1900s; a precursor to the physical therapist in the United States

regulation – a legal rule created by a governmental administrative agency to help implement statutes

Rehabilitation Act – a federal law that prohibits the discrimination against an individual based on his or her disability in any program that receives federal funds

related services – those services necessary in special education for a student to benefit from special education; defined in the Individuals with Disabilities Education Act

Relative Value Units (RVU) – units developed by Medicare to assign a value to a particular service or type of treatment for billing purposes. The fee schedule amounts then reflect variations in practice expenses among various geographic regions.

relaxin – a hormone produced by the corpus luteum that plays a role in the relaxation of connective tissue throughout pregnancy; results in the ability of the pelvic outlet to expand to allow for the passage of the fetus during birth

Resource-Based Relative Value Scale (RBRVS) – scale in which a relative value is assigned to certain procedures, adjusted for the geographic region, and multiplied by a fixed conversion factor. It determines how much a health care provider will be paid by the third party payer. It is used by Medicare and other insurance companies.

respondent superior – a legal term that means that the employer is liable for the actions of the employee if the employee acted within her scope of employment

revenues – income received

Reye syndrome – an acquired encephalopathy, causing an acute increase of pressure within the brain and often massive accumulations of fat in the liver and other organs; associated with aspirin use in children

righting reactions – midbrain reactions that develop during the first 6 months of life that generally orient the head to the horizontal, or a body part that is rotated or displaced from the symmetrical posture back into proper alignment

rituals – family routines that convey a message about family identity (who the family is as a group)

rounds – a formal meeting at which multiple health care disciplines discuss the clinical case of one or more patients

routines – those interactions within the family that occur frequently, are episodic, have a clear beginning and end, and reflect the broader concept of family organization

rubella – a mildly febrile, highly infectious disease caused by the rubella virus commonly seen in childhood; associated with a high incidence of birth defects in children from maternal infection during the first several months of pregnancy

S

saddle anesthesia – loss of sensation around the anus, perineum, and inner thighs

scarf sign – a test to examine muscle tone in a newborn. The newborn's arm is horizontally adducted with his hand placed on the opposite shoulder (like a scarf). In a term newborn, the hand does not pass the opposite shoulder and the elbow does not pass the midline of the body.

school readiness – a concept that a child should demonstrate certain developmental skills determined to be necessary in order to succeed in the school environment

second trimester – weeks 13 through 26 of a pregnancy

secondary family – another definition of a family that may emerge when major health issues arise. Other members besides those of the primary family may be involved or become important. These individuals are more evident in situations of illness, death, when difficult decisions regarding health care need to be made, or when violence or abuse is suspected.

Section 504 Committee – a group of people who are knowledgeable about a specific student, the meaning of any evaluation data, placement options, least restrictive environment requirements, and comparable facilities who meet to discuss a student who is eligible for services in the public school under Section 504 of the Rehabilitation Act

Section 504 Coordinator – a person responsible for assisting the school in meeting the requirements of Section 504 of the Rehabilitation Act by providing resources and helping the school make the necessary accommodations for the qualified students

Section 504 Plan – an accommodation plan for a student who qualifies for services under Section 504 of the Rehabilitation Act

selective serotonin reuptake inhibitor – a drug that assists in increasing the brain's own supply of serotonin by preventing its uptake from the neurons of the central nervous system

self-determination – acting as the primary causal agent in one's life and making choices and decisions regarding one's quality of life, free from undue external influence or interference

semivariable expenses – expense items that have a fixed component and a variable component. Phone service is one example.

service coordinator – a person who is responsible for identifying, contacting, facilitating, and coordinating health care or developmental services provided to a patient or family

sheltered employment – employment of individuals with disabilities in a self-contained work site, without integration with workers without disabilities

sliding scale fee schedule – an adjustable fee schedule that is based on a family's income level

Social Security Act – one of the most significant pieces of social legislation in the United States. It established federal aid for public health and welfare assistance, maternal and child health programs, and services for individuals with disabilities.

Social Security Disability Insurance (SSDI) – a program of financial assistance administered by the Social Security Administration for eligible individuals. The program covers injured workers and their widows or widowers, dependents, and people with disabilities.

sole proprietorship – a single person undertaking a business venture who is solely liable for the actions of the business

spasticity – resistance of a muscle in joint motion determined by the angle and velocity of motion

spica cast – a cast that immobilizes the hip or shoulder joint in an abducted position

spirituality – a broad concept that includes religion as well as cognitive, experiential, and behavioral aspects of a person

Sprengel deformity – congenital in nature, resulting in one or both scapulae being underdeveloped and relatively high on the thorax; more common in women

Standard Precautions – Guidelines published by the CDC to reduce the risk of the transmission of microorganisms from infectious materials. Standard precautions apply to all health care providers and patients regardless of diagnosis or possible infectious status.

status epilepticus – a prolonged seizure, at least 30 minutes in duration, that requires immediate medical attention

statutes – federal and state laws drafted and adopted by legislative bodies

Sudden Infant Death Syndrome (SIDS) – sudden and unexplained death of an infant, typically younger than 1 year

suicidal ideation – thoughts of taking one's own life

Supplemental Security Income (SSI) – a federal program administered by the Social Security Administration for eligible individuals (adults or children) who are disabled or blind or are aged 65 or older, with limited income and resources

supported employment – competitive work in an integrated work setting (with nondisabled peers) for individuals with disabilities

swaddling – wrapping an infant snugly in a blanket so that limb movement is restricted

syphilis – an acute and chronic infectious disease caused by the bacterium *Treponema pallidum* and transmitted by direct contact, usually through sexual intercourse

T

teratogen – a drug or environmental factor that may hinder fetal growth and lead to malformations or neurologic problems

thermogenesis – production of body heat by the body's break-down of fat.

thermoneutral – not excessively hot or cold

third trimester – weeks 27 through 40 of a pregnancy

TORCHHS – an acronym for a common group of teratogens that can affect a developing fetus. The acronym stands for **T**oxoplasmosis, **O**ther Infections, **R**ubella, **C**ytomegalovirus Infection, **H**uman Immunodeficiency Virus, **H**erpes Simplex Virus, and **S**yphilis.

total parenteral nutrition (TPN) – the delivery of nutrition other than through the gastrointestinal tract; via IV line

toxoplasmosis – an infection caused by the *Toxoplasma gondii* organism; most commonly transmitted by inadequate hand washing after handling cat feces or by eating undercooked pork, lamb, or eggs

transdisciplinary – working and collaborating with team members from more than one discipline, which may include cross-training and the sharing of traditional intervention roles among members of the team

transition plan – a formal plan that moves an individual from one program to another. A transition plan is mandated for early intervention and special education programs under the Individuals with Disabilities Education Act to assure a seamless transition into the school system or another appropriate setting.

transition services – a coordinated set of activities for a student, designed within an outcome-oriented process, that promotes movement from school to postschool activities, including postsecondary education, vocational training, integrated employment (including supported employment), continuing and adult education, adult services, independent living, or community participation

transitioning – the process that prepares a family or child to move from an early intervention program into the school system or from school to postschool activities

Trendelenburg sign – associated with various hip pathologies or impairments. This sign results in the pelvis dropping on the opposite side of the involvement when the person is in single leg stance on the involved leg. It is associated with weakness of the hip abductor muscles.

triennial – at least every 3 years; applied to a student's periodic re-evaluation for special education services

trisomy 21 – the most common autosomal chromosomal abnormality that exists in the human species with an extra chromosome (chromosome 21) present in the cells of the body

U

Unidisciplinary – a team of one professional discipline

United States Code – the codification of the federal laws of the United States

uveitis – inflammation of the iris, ciliary body, and choroids

V

Valsalva maneuver – any forced expiratory effort against a closed airway, as when an individual holds a breath and bears down. This maneuver can increase intrathoracic pressure.

Vancomycin-resistant enterococcus (VRE) – *Enterococcus* is a bacterium that colonizes the gastrointestinal tract and can become resistant to vancomycin therapy. Patients with prolonged hospital stays or who received antimicrobial therapy are at risk of developing this infection. VRE can be life threatening in people with compromised immune systems.

variable expenses – expenses of a business that vary with use. Office supplies are one example.

varicella – a contagious disease often seen in childhood caused by the *varicella zoster virus*. Sparse eruptions and itching are the classic signs. Varicella is also referred to as chicken pox.

vocational rehabilitation – programs conducted by state Vocational Rehabilitation agencies operating under the Rehabilitation Act of 1973. Vocational rehabilitation programs provide or arrange for a wide array of training, educational, medical, and other services individualized to the needs of people with disabilities. The services are intended to help people with disabilities acquire, reacquire, and maintain gainful employment.

W

waiver programs – States may apply for a waiver from federal regulations, in order to provide home- or community-based service packages to specific Medicaid populations. These programs would allow an individual who meets the state requirements for the Medicaid nursing home benefit to receive services at home or in the community. The number of individuals served under a waiver program is limited.

welfare – federal and state financial aid in the form of money or necessities provided to those in need

Workers' compensation – the United States social insurance system for industrial and work-related injuries

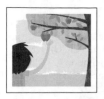

INDEX